Introductory Management
and Leadership
for Clinical Nurses

The Jones and Bartlett Series in Nursing

Introductory Management and Leadership for Clinical Nurses
A Text-Workbook

Russell C. Swansburg, RN, PhD, CNAA

Consultant in Nursing and Hospital Administration
San Antonio, Texas

Jones and Bartlett Publishers

Boston   *London*

To my wife—
Laurel C. Swansburg, RN

Editorial, Sales, and Customer Service Offices

Jones and Bartlett Publishers
One Exeter Plaza
Boston, MA 02116

Jones and Bartlett Publishers International
P O Box 1498
London W6 7RS
England

Library of Congress Cataloging-in-Publication Data

Swansburg, Russell C.
    Introductory management and leadership for clinical nurses :
a text-workbook / Russell C. Swansburg.
        p.   cm.
    Includes bibliographical references and index.
    ISBN 0-86720-338-2
    1. Nursing services—Administration.   I.   Title.
    [DNLM: 1.   Administrative Personnel.   2.   Nurse Administrators.
3. Nursing, Supervisory.   WY 105 S972i 1993]
RT89.S885 1993
362.1'73068—dc20
DNLM/DLC
for Library of Congress   93-7042
                                                              CIP

Production service: TKM Productions
Design: Helane M. Prottas
Cover design: Bruce Kennett
Printing and binding: Courier Companies, Inc.

Printed in the United States of America
97 96 95 94 93   10 9 8 7 6 5 4 3 2 1

Contents

Preface

This book is organized around the four major management functions of planning, organizing, directing (leading), and controlling (evaluating). It is specifically designed for beginning management development of professional nurses. It can be used in all nursing programs as a first course in nursing management as well as staff development programs in health care agencies. Each chapter contains specific experiential exercises.

Among the goals are to provide theoretical and practical knowledge that will aid each clinical nurse manager in meeting the demands of constantly changing patient care services. The extreme nurse shortages are closely related to the management process. Financial considerations have dominated the health care industry in recent years, making the job of managing scarce and costly human and material resources even more important. As health care has moved out of hospitals, more nurse management positions have evolved in skilled nursing facilities, ambulatory care centers, hospices, home health care agencies, and staffing agencies. New nurse management positions are developing.

This book focuses on management competencies needed by clinical nurse managers, including knowing how to manage nursing activities so that a professional nurse will be able to practice the primary functions of clinical nursing: assessment, diagnosis, prescription, and evaluation. It provides essential theoretical and practical knowledge in several areas including learning about leadership skills and employee motivation, and learning to make sound decisions that contribute to progress.

Clinical nurses oversee many tasks involving many people with specialized knowledge and skills. The management role may be played by clinical nurse managers of shifts, and head nurses or supervisors of units, departments, clinics, and agencies. This book is intended as an aid to improving communication, enhancing assignment planning and priority setting, and developing training and education programs that lead to staff satisfaction. Through the evaluation process, nurse managers determine whether they are satisfied with the results, from both their viewpoints and that of their constituents.

I wish to thank my wife, Laurel C. Swansburg, RN, who has put this manuscript on a word processor. Her encouragement and knowledgeable input have supported my writing throughout the past 30 years. Also, Mr. Steve Simmons, administrator of the University of South Alabama Medical Center, Mobile, Alabama, has unhesitatingly permitted me to use illustrations for my book.

Russell C. Swansburg

•1•

Theory of Nursing Management

WHAT IS MANAGEMENT?

Modern management theory evolved from the work of Henri Fayol, who identified the administrator's activities or functions as planning, organizing, coordinating, and controlling.[1] Fayol defined management thus:

> To manage is to forecast and plan, to organize, to command, to coordinate, and to control. To foresee and provide means examining the future and drawing up the plan of action. To organize means building up the dual structure, material and human, of the undertaking. To command means binding together, unifying and harmonizing all activity and effort. To control means seeing that everything occurs in conformity with established rule and expressed demand.[2]

Although some persons believed these were technical functions to be learned only on the job, Fayol believed that they could be taught in an educational setting if a theory of administration could be formulated.[3] He also stated that the need for managerial ability increased in relative importance as an individual advanced in the chain of command.[4]

Fayol listed the principles of management as follows:[5]

1. Division of work
2. Authority
3. Discipline
4. Unity of command
5. Unity of direction
6. Subordination of individual interests to the general interest
7. Remuneration
8. Centralization
9. Scalar chain (line of authority)
10. Order
11. Equity
12. Stability or tenure of personnel
13. Initiative
14. Esprit de corps

Another theorist in the development of the science and art of management was L. Urwick. He indicated that administrative skill is a practical art that improves with practice and requires hard study and thinking. The administrator has to master intellectual principles, the process being reinforced by general reflection about actual problems. From his work Urwick concluded that there are three principles of administration. He described the first principle as that of *investigation* and stated that all scientific procedure is based on investigation of the facts. Investigation takes effect in *planning*. The second principle is *appropriateness*, which underlines *forecasting*, entering into process with *organization* and taking effect in *coordination*. Exercising the third principle, the administrator looks ahead and organizes *resources* to meet future needs. Planning enters into process with *command* and is effected in *control*.[6]

Throughout management literature, the original functions of planning, organizing, directing (command and coordination), and controlling as defined by Fayol, Urwick, and others have been accepted as the principal functions of managers. Managing means accomplishing the goals of the group through effective and efficient use of resources. The *manager* creates and maintains an internal environment in an enterprise in which individuals work together as a group. *Managing* is the art of doing, and *management* is the body of organized knowledge underlying the art. In modern management, staffing is frequently separated from the planning function, directing has been labeled "leading" or "supervising," and "controlling" is used interchangeably with "evaluating."

Theories, Concepts, and Principles

The knowledge base of management science includes theories, which in turn include concepts, methods, and principles. The principles are related and can be observed and verified to some degree when they are translated into the art or practice of management. *Concepts* are thoughts, ideas, and general notions about a class of objects that form a basis for action or discussion. *Principles* are fundamental truths, laws, or doctrine on which other notions are based. Principles provide guidance to concepts and to thought or action in a situation.[7] In nursing management, research—Urwick's "investigation of facts"—becomes part of the theory of the field.

If nursing is going to base its theories on laws, nurses will need to validate principles through research. This is a difficult task, as theorists in the social sciences have discovered. It is difficult to reduce human behavior to laws. Nurses deal with human behavior in all roles, but particularly so in nursing management.

Nurse managers learn to merge the disciplines of human relations, labor relations, personnel management, and industrial engineering into a unifying force for effective management. Many nurse managers would add the theory of nursing to this list. A successful synthesis of these disciplines would promote employee commitment, increased productivity, good labor relations, and competitiveness in health care. If these goals are not achieved, the work force is poorly managed. However, there are contradictions in management theory because of a lack of agreement about sets of ideas and concepts among and within disciplines.[8]

General Systems Theory

General systems theory is an organismic approach to the study of the general relationships of the empirical universe of an organization and human thought. It grew out of biology as an analogy between an organism and a social organization. Boulding describes nine levels of general systems theory.[9] One approach to a framework in nursing is that nursing persons apply the nursing process in giving care to patients. There are many similarities between nursing process and nursing management. See Figure 1–1.

Another version of the key concepts of general systems theory is summarized in Figure 1–2.

NURSING MANAGEMENT

In nursing, management relates to planning, organizing, staffing, directing (leading) and controlling (evaluating) the activities of a nursing enterprise or division of nursing departments and of the subunits of the departments. A nurse manager performs these management functions to deliver health care to patients. Nurse managers or administrators work at all levels to put into practice the concepts, principles, and theories of nursing management. They manage the organizational environment to provide a climate optimal to provision of nursing care by the clinical nurses. In turn, clinical

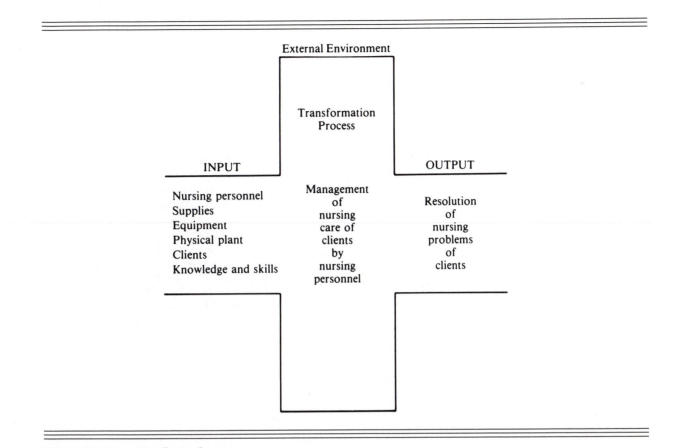

External Environment

Transformation Process

INPUT

Nursing personnel
Supplies
Equipment
Physical plant
Clients
Knowledge and skills

Management
of
nursing
care of
clients
by
nursing
personnel

OUTPUT

Resolution
of
nursing
problems
of
clients

Figure 1–1 • An Open System

nurses manage selective personnel and material resources and give additional input into the management process.

Management knowledge is universal; so is nursing management knowledge. It uses a systematic body of knowledge that includes concepts, principles, and theories applicable to all nursing management situations. A nurse manager who has applied this knowledge successfully in one situation can be expected to do so in new situations. Nursing management occurs at the clinical nurse, head nurse, supervisor, and director or executive levels. At the director or executive level, it is frequently termed "administration." The theories, principles, and concepts remain the same. They can all be classified under the major functions of nursing management or nursing administration.

Nursing administration is the application of the art and science of management to the discipline of nursing. Nursing management is also the group of nurse managers who manage the nursing organization or enterprise. Finally, nursing management is the process by which nurse managers

practice their profession. Although many nursing management jobs do not require specialty certification, such certification is available. The American Nurses' Association awards management certification in nursing administration and in advanced nursing administration. The American Organization of Nurse Executives has in the past certified nurse managers at the nominee, candidate, and fellow levels. Both programs require education, experience, and examination.

Who Needs Nursing Management?

All types of health care organizations, including nursing homes, hospitals, home health care agencies, ambulatory care centers, student infirmaries, and many others, need nursing management. Even the nurse working with one client and family needs management knowledge and skills to help people work together to accomplish a common goal. A primary nurse working with several clients prioritizes their care to assist them to improved health or, sometimes, peaceful death.[10]

Subsystems or Components. A system by definition is composed of interrelated parts or elements. This is true for all systems—mechanical, biological, and social. Every system has at least two elements, and these elements are interconnected.

Holism, Synergism, Organicism, and Gestalt. The whole is not just the sum of the parts; the system itself can be explained only as a totality. Holism is the opposite of elementarism, which views the total as the sum of its individual parts.

Open-Systems View. Systems can be considered in two ways: (1) closed or (2) open. Open systems exchange information, energy, or material with their environments. Biological and social systems are inherently open systems; mechanical systems may be open or closed. The concepts of open and closed systems are difficult to defend in the absolute. We prefer to think of open–closed as a continuum; that is, systems are relatively open or relatively closed.

Input-Transformation-Output Model. The open system can be viewed as a transformation model. In a dynamic relationship with its environment, it receives various inputs, transforms these inputs in some way, and exports outputs.

System Boundaries. It follows that systems have boundaries that separate them from their environments. The concept of boundaries helps us understand the distinction between open and closed systems. The relatively closed system has rigid, impenetrable boundaries; whereas the open system has permeable boundaries between itself and a broader suprasystem. Boundaries are relatively easily defined in physical and biological systems, but are very difficult to delineate in social systems such as organizations.

Negative Entropy. Closed physical systems are subject to the force of entropy, which increases until eventually the entire system fails. The tendency toward maximum entropy is a movement to disorder, complete lack of resource transformation, and death. In a closed system, the change in entropy must always be positive; however, in open biological or social systems, entropy can be arrested and may even be transformed into negative entropy—a process of more complete organization and ability to transform resources—because the system imports resources from its environment.

Steady State, Dynamic Equilibrium, and Homeostasis. The concept of steady state is closely related to that of negative entropy. A closed system eventually must attain an equilibrium state with maximum entropy—death or disorganization. However, an open system may attain a state where the system remains in dynamic equilibrium through the continuous inflow of materials, energy, and information.

Feedback. The concept of feedback is important in understanding how a system maintains a steady state. Information concerning the outputs or the process of the system is fed back as an input into the system, perhaps leading to changes in the transformation process and/or future outputs. Feedback can be both positive and negative, although the field of cybernetics is based on negative feedback. Negative feedback is informational input which indicates that the system is deviating from a prescribed course and should readjust to a new steady state.

Hierarchy. A basic concept in systems thinking is that of hierarchical relationships among systems. A system is composed of subsystems of a lower order and is also part of a suprasystem. Thus, there is a hierarchy of the components of the system.

Internal Elaboration. Closed systems move toward entropy and disorganization. In contrast, open systems appear to move in the direction of greater differentiation, elaboration, and a higher level of organization.

Multiple Goal-Seeking. Biological and social systems appear to have multiple goals or purposes. Social organizations seek multiple goals, if for no other reason than that they are composed of individuals and subunits with different values and objectives.

Equifinality of Open Systems. In mechanistic systems there is a direct cause-and-effect relationship between the initial condition and the final state. Biological and social systems operate differently. Equifinality suggests that certain results may be achieved with different initial conditions and in different ways. This view suggests that social organizations can accomplish their objectives with diverse inputs and with varying internal activities (conversion processes).

SOURCE: F. E. Kast and J. E. Rosenzweig, "General Systems Theory: Applications for Organization and Management," *Academy of Management Journal,* December 1972, 447–464. Reprinted with permission.

Figure 1–2 • *Key Concepts of General Systems Theory*

General Principles of Nursing Management

Nursing Management Is Planning. Planning is primary to all other activities or functions of management. Planning is a thinking or conceptual act that is frequently committed to writing. Although many people in nursing make plans informally, the commitment of plans to paper is essential to their accomplishment. If plans are not written down, they probably will not be implemented.

Planning is the forecasting of events—the building of an operational plan. Planning is also a management function of every nursing leader—from *professional clinical nurses* to nurse managers, supervisors, directors, and administrators.

Planning is an important management function that helps reduce the risks of decision making, problem solving, and effecting planned change. The clinical nurse manager who learns to plan will aim to use all resources—money, supplies, equipment, and, of course, personnel—to the maximum.

Planning will help workers achieve job satisfaction. All people plan their activities to some extent. Individual plans may include a weekly schedule of personal events, a sequential list of daily activities, or an appointment calendar. A predetermined fire evacuation route is a special kind of plan—a disaster plan.

Planning requires a knowledge of the characteristics of the planning processes and the relationships within a system; planning elements; planning standards; knowledge of and skill in implementing the planning process, including applying standards to the work situation; and acquisition of the skills necessary to bring the planning process up to the set standards. Planning makes possible effective use of time. During planning, nurse managers analyze and assess the system, set organizational and personal long-range (strategic) and short-range (tactical or operational) objectives, assess present organizational resources and capabilities, and specify and prioritize the activities, including alternatives.

Management plans are business plans. They specify goals, strategies, responsibilities, policies, and budgets. They use directions, progress, adjustments, and measurement. Management planning forces clinical nurse managers to analyze unit activities and structure. It is a process of human action and interaction, the work environment being a microcosm of society.

Health care organizations are social entities in which cooperation and competition conflict. They have life and character as well as patterns of behavior that become entrenched. Personal success is tied to organizational success in the form of pay-checks, promotions, careers, and job security. Peer pressure among nurses may create conflict with the goals of the organization.

Ratcliffe and Logsdon specify six stages in the planning process:

1. Design stage
2. Delegation stage
3. Education stage
4. Development stage
5. Implementation stage
6. Follow-up stage (performance evaluation and feedback)

Personnel are involved in goal setting, performance evaluation, and feedback on a continual basis. Business planning takes into account the behavioral process.[11]

Nursing Management Is the Effective Use of Time. Because management is the effective use of time, successful clinical nurse managers plan in order to use their time effectively. In nursing, management is affected by the abilities and limitations of the clinical nurse manager, who has a theory or systematic set of management principles and methods that relate to the larger institution and the nursing organization within it, including each unit. Such a theory will include knowledge of the mission or purpose of the institution but may require development or revision of the mission or purpose of the nursing division. From a clearly defined mission statement, the nurse manager develops clear and realistic objectives for nursing services. This theory will also provide the foundation on which the nurse manager makes operational or management plans, sets priorities, formulates strategies, and assigns work. Managerial jobs and structures are designed from this theory. Decisions of top managers—at least those of the chair of the nursing division—will be affected by input from lower levels of highly knowledgeable and skilled clinical nursing personnel. It is good management practice to seek this input rather than block or discount it, because it is often a source of imaginative proposals that can be incorporated into improvements in personnel management and, ultimately in nursing practices and patient care services. Application of knowledge of a theory or systematic set of principles and methods of nursing management is necessary for the effective use of time. See Figure 1–3.

Clinical nurse manager's decisions will be influenced by time elements, because all management decisions are so influenced. Management decisions take into account the future, particularly with regard to human resources. Nursing manage-

1. The chief nurse executive keeps an appointment schedule that relates to management plans. This schedule is followed for all activities—organizational meetings, divisional meetings, professional meetings, travel, rounds, individual appointments, and so on.

2. The head nurse of a home health care agency has planned staff meetings at the beginning and end of each week. Schedules of individual nurses are reviewed at each meeting and are compared with productivity goals that balance the budget.

3. A home health care nurse reviews the schedule each day. It must be tightened so that five more patient visits can be added during the 40-hour workweek. Otherwise, a merit pay increase will not materialize.

Figure 1–3 • *Examples of Effective Use of Time*

1. A staff nurse decides whether to apply for a clinical promotion. If the application is accepted, a performance results contract will require additional productivity, including continuing education and increased participation on committees and in special nursing activities such as discharge planning and quality assurance studies. It will also result in higher pay.

2. The chief nurse executive makes a decision about whether to increase the number of clinical nurse III positions in the budget or allocate more funds to nurse manager development. Both are needed, and the pros and cons of splitting limited resources have to be weighed.

Figure 1–4 • *Examples of Managerial Decision Making*

ment performs in the present while planning for future performance, growth, and change.

All resources are finite, including nursing personnel and the supplies and equipment used. Resources are managed for efficiency and effectiveness to achieve productivity—output of a given amount during a specified time that generates enough income to exceed expenses and realize a profit. Effective use of time requires the implementation of plans by an organization directed toward productivity.

Nursing Management Is Decision Making. Nursing management requires decisions to be made by nurse managers at every level, from division to department to ward or unit. This is especially true where a service is provided 24 hours a day. The process of decision making will vary depending on whether traditional patterns of communication are followed or decision making is decentralized to the level of its implementation. See Figure 1–4.

Meeting Patients' Nursing Care Needs Is the Business of the Nurse Manager. The patient is the starting point at which the business of nursing is defined, and it is the patient who is to be satisfied. Nursing management performs the activities needed to determine what patients see, think, believe, and want. Part of the performance is to be sure patients are asked, because they buy their care, and therefore buy satisfaction of wants. Anticipatory management means building into objectives a determination of what the business of

nursing is, will be, and should be, discarding the obsolete through systematic abandonment.

To achieve these objectives, clinical nurse managers perform three major tasks in which they manage human and material resources. These are:

1. Perform to achieve a specific purpose or mission for the division, department, and ward or unit.
2. Make work productive.
3. Manage social impacts and social responsibilities.

Management and practice are involved in all three tasks of clinical nurse managers. The end product, the work of the personnel other than managers, is the practice of nursing. The social impact and social responsibilities of nursing have been highly visible when nurses have gone on strike or serious shortages of nurses have occurred.

Professional nurses are primarily knowledge workers, applying their knowledge to the gathering of data, the making of nursing diagnoses and nursing prescriptions, the supervision of the implementation of the nursing care plan by skilled workers, and the evaluation and adjustment of the plan. They are clinical decision makers. Their work involves skills and the training of skilled workers; however, nurse managers recognize that the primary functions of professional nurses are based on expert, in-depth knowledge. Nurses earn their livelihood and probably gain their greatest job satisfaction with knowledge gained in an educational institution and put to work in a service institution.

That same knowledge is used to build the society within which those institutions exist and to achieve institutional goals. According to Drucker, "To make our institutions perform responsibly, autonomously, and on a high level of achievement is thus the only safeguard of freedom and dignity in the pluralistic society of institutions.[12]

Nursing as an institution does not make decisions; nurse managers do. Management is essential to the institution of nursing. It is independent of ownership, rank, or power, being an objective function that ought to be grounded in the responsibility for performance. Nurse managers are the professionals who practice the discipline of nursing management, carry out its functions, and discharge its tasks.

Nursing performance results in care that will meet patients' needs, the care being a product potentially desired by all people at a cost they can afford. Care given is the end product of management of a division of nursing. Nurse managers design a model organization that will provide this product. Nursing workers see themselves as resources who have the opportunity of producing nursing care services. Nurse managers will build and manage new nursing organizations and at the same time manage the old or existing ones.

People are the true resources of the division of nursing, and people are made productive by effective nursing management. Through the nursing function they earn their livelihood and find access to their needs for social status, community and individual achievement, and satisfaction. Nurse managers make the work environment suitable for practicing nurses to meet needs related to their personalities, to controls over quantity and quality of work, and to citizenship. The satisfaction of these needs requires opportunity for the individual to assume responsibility, to be an active participant in planning work, to gain satisfaction, to receive incentives and awards, to give leadership to others, to achieve status, to be motivated, and to fulfill a function. See Figure 1–5.

Nursing Management Is the Formulation and Achievement of Social Goals. Social innovation is essential in dealing with the health needs of poor people, people who live in large cities, and people confronted by environmental pollution. The goal of meeting such needs is also partly dependent on the nurse manager. The nurse manager manages the institution's social impacts and discharges its social responsibilities relative to nursing. Formulating these goals and supporting clinical nurses in

1. Nursing personnel—Human resources with expert knowledge and skills, they practice nursing to produce patient care.

2. Nursing functions—Ms. Williams practices clinical nursing to earn a living. Other functions of nursing are management, teaching, and research.

Ms. Allen proudly tells people that she works as a registered nurse at the general hospital. Through her work she is satisfying social needs, community needs, and personal needs. She is also a nurse person.

3. Nurse managers—Ms. George tries to place personnel where they desire to work. This is a function of management, and Ms. George is working to satisfy needs related to employee personalities and controls over quantity and quality of work.

Mr. St. Clair makes full use of the recognition program. He sees all performance appraisals and has supervisors make recommendations for recognition of all personnel who are outstanding or who perform unique humanitarian acts. Through his leadership workers will receive incentives and awards, achieve status, and be motivated to provide health care to patients.

Figure 1–5 • *Examples of Nursing Personnel, Nursing Functions, and Nurse Managers*

achieving them are managerial tasks. See Figure 1–6.

Nursing Management Is Organizing. Organizing is identifying the organizational needs from mission statements and objectives and from observations of work performed, and adapting the organizational design and structure to meet these needs. Like planning, organizing is primarily a thinking act.

There are four building blocks for organizational structures:

1. Unit
2. Department
3. The top; the division or executive level of organizational management
4. The operational level, including all phases of work within the organizational structure

During the organizing process, activities are grouped, responsibility and authority are determined, and working relationships are established

1. *Health needs of poor people.* A director of nursing in a rural area has sponsored a meeting with other nurse managers from institutions in the area. Their agenda will include discussion of "people who have no health insurance and cannot afford it: identification of their health needs and of ways to meet them." Invited guests include the state Medicaid director and other public health officials.

2. *Health needs of people in large cities.* A nurse manager of an institution in a large city has asked the local nurses' association to assist with a project to identify elderly people with fixed incomes who are in need of health care. Their goal will be to find ways of providing needed health care that is affordable through negotiating with HMOs, PPOs, physicians, hospitals, and other agencies.

3. *Health needs of people confronted with environmental pollution.* After much publicity about lead poisoning of children from local industrial pollutants, the chair of the division of nursing consults with the hospital administrator on determining the health care needs of children involved. As a consequence nurses are being educated to assist with providing this needed health service to these children.

Figure 1–6 • Examples of Areas of Goals of Nurse Managers

to enable both the organization and the employees to realize their mutual objectives. The organizational structure relates to the effectiveness of communication. Organizing is a continual process that may take from 1 week to 5 or 10 years. Organizing for decentralization and the participatory management process could fall in the strategic planning category of 3 to 10 years.

Nursing Management Denotes a Function, a Social Position or Rank, a Discipline, and a Field of Study.   A division of nursing has a management function of fulfilling purposes and objectives, management tasks, and management work. These activities are performed by nurse managers with titles denoting increasing responsibilities using nursing management theory. As in leadership, a title does not make a nurse a manager. A title indicates the position is one of management. See Figure 1–7.

As a discipline, management is a branch of knowledge or learning. The discipline of nursing

1. *Nursing management function.* Several of the positions within the organization do not fulfill the purpose for which they exist. The nurse administrator will review the organization and functions of the entire division.

2. *A social position or rank.* Ms. Joliet is assistant chair of a division of nursing.

3. *A discipline.* Ms. Fisk has learned management theory and has been trained to be proficient in all the management skills that make her a strong clinical nurse manager. She is strong in the discipline or nursing management.

4. *A field of study.* Mr. Wilbur is majoring in the management of nursing services in his university program.

5. *Nursing management task.* One of the pieces of work to be done by the clinical nurse manager was to plan a holiday schedule based on the expected workload.

6. *Nursing management work.* Ms. Zeller's primary nursing team gives good nursing care to their patients. They produce under Ms. Zeller's management.

Figure 1–7 • Examples of Nursing Management as Function, Social Position or Rank, Discipline, Field of Study, Task, and Work

management draws from the generic discipline of management. Through adoption and application of the methods of the discipline of management, clinical nurse managers are able to extend their knowledge or learning in the discipline of nursing management. Thus they develop a field of study.

Nursing Management Is the Active Organ of the Division of Nursing, of the Organization, and of the Society in Which It Functions.   Every health care institution is an organ of society and exists for society. The division of nursing exists for the good of people—clients or patients. The organization, through the division head, has power and authority over its employees. It has an effect on the community as a source of services, jobs, and waste products and pollutants. It has a concern for the quality of life and may be seen by consumers as ethically above that of economic institutions of the business world. It must have the support of society, which needs its services.

In business and industry it takes a profitable organization to make a social contribution, as a bankrupt one can neither employ personnel nor provide services to patients. Patients or consumers keep the health care institution and the division of nursing in existence and people employed. Their use of nursing services makes it a success and keeps it operational. Nurse managers work to have the organization through its personnel produce what these patients need and want. Nursing management functions to manage the nursing business or industry and make nursing profitable in fulfilling its social contribution.

The chair of the division of nursing manages the total nursing operation, and each nurse manager manages the nursing activities of a department or unit. Although it is often carried on the overhead rather than the profit side of the ledger, the division of nursing performs for society and as a business. Nursing care provides for some of human beings' needs and wants. Nursing management recognizes that nursing as an institution exists for its contribution and performance rather than for the convenience of employees. To accomplish this nurse managers show a contribution by nursing personnel, whom they manage for performance.

Clinical nurse managers satisfy clients, physicians, other nurses, technicians, clients' families, employers, labor unions, and numerous professional entities.

Clinical nurse managers look to managers in business and industry for the exemplars who have built sound institutions. Following their example means learning to provide needed primary nursing care services to clients on an economically feasible basis.

Nursing practice is the means by which nurses use their knowledge to practice their skills and use supplies, equipment, and other resources effectively to give satisfactory health care to people. As an organ of the nursing organization, nursing management acts to accomplish the nursing work and ultimately clients' health goals.

Organizational Cultures Reflect Values and Beliefs. The institutional culture within which nursing management is performed is built up over a number of years in all organizations. Managers in nursing have a common purpose of making productive the values, aspirations, and traditions of employees who are individuals, as well as members of communities and of society. Social and economic development of nursing will thus take place, resulting in satisfactory services to clients. See Figure 1–8.

Responses to change reflect the values inherent

---

1. Clients place high value on nursing care they recognize as good.
2. Nursing management is well developed in an organization where professional nurses have equal status with physicians, dentists, pharmacists, and members of other disciplines.
3. All nursing workers have values and beliefs, which an effective nurse manager will learn to use.
4. It is important for a clinical nurse manager to know and support the needs of all nursing workers, including their desire to have time to participate as citizens, how they see their jobs, and what they hope to become.

Figure 1–8 • *Examples of Nursing Management as a Culture and a System of Values and Beliefs*

in an organization's culture and behavior of its members. Clinical nurse managers are assessed against values and responses to change. Values include autonomy for nursing's practitioners, prestige, and a regard for advanced preparation.[13]

Shared values create bonds among clinical nurse managers and nurse workers. Clinical nurse managers articulate moral values and beliefs, basic attitudes and loyalties, concepts and policies as shared entities, value being placed on both process and results. Maidique indicates that strategy and strategic planning are overintellectualized, indicating they are overvalued. Workers who attend to product, customer, and marketplace produce better results than does a grand strategy. To achieve success one coordinates and integrates workers and specialized talents.[14]

Nursing Management Is Directing or Leading. Directing is an action element of nursing management—the interpersonal process by which nursing personnel accomplish the objectives of nursing. It is the process of applying the management plans to accomplish the objectives of nursing.

Directing is often called the leading function of nursing management. It includes the processes of delegating, supervising, coordination, and controlling the implementation of the organized plan. The nurse administrator's philosophy will determine whether directing is authoritarian or democratic.

A Well-Managed Division of Nursing Motivates Employees to Perform Satisfactorily. Nurse employees provide health-care services for an institution within an institutionalized society dependent on its members' performances. Health care institutions are among the most complex social institutions. Their members or employees will give satisfactory performances in return for their livelihood, opportunities for advancement, opportunities for status within society, self-esteem, and self-actualization. Satisfactory performance results from job satisfaction, a condition requiring that clinical nurse managers stimulate motivation of nurse employees. See Figure 1–9.

Nursing Management Is Effective Communication. Effective communication assures that all levels of personnel know the mission or purpose, the philosophy or beliefs, and the specific objectives of the institution and the division of nursing. Effective communication will result in fewer misunderstandings and will give employees a common vision, common understanding, and unity of direction and effort. Compatible decisions can then be made. Poor communication results in failures and frustrations due to lack of clear purpose, philosophy, and objectives. See Figure 1–10.

Nursing Management Is Controlling or Evaluating. Controlling is an action element of nursing management. It includes the process of evaluating

---

1. Employees are rewarded for satisfactory performance by a system of merit pay increases and chances for promotion.

2. Personnel policies provide for time off with pay for continuing education related to the job.

3. Salary compensation provides for annual or biannual longevity pay increases, *during an entire span of employment.*

4. A public relations program provides for publicity that tells the story of nursing and of contributions made by people in different nursing jobs.

5. The chief nurse executive hires a consultant to assist nurses interested in writing for publication.

Figure 1–9 • *Examples of Directing or Leading*

---

1. As an exercise, the clinical nurse manager had clinical nurse staff read the written statements of mission, of philosophy, and of specific objectives for their units and for the division and departments of nursing. They then discussed how their work related to each objective at each level. They wrote a summary of their discussion, including some recommended revisions of the specific unit objectives for the clinical nurse manager to implement and to forward to senior nursing management as applicable. People working here achieved a common vision, a common understanding, and unity of direction and effort as a result of the exercise.

2. The nursing practice committee prepared an article to tell why the division of nursing existed, what its personnel believed in, and what their goals were. They took it to the local paper where it was printed in the Sunday edition.

3. All new employees joining the division of nursing receive orientation that teaches them the mission, the philosophy, and the objectives of the division of nursing and of the department or unit to which they are assigned. When they transfer to another department or unit, they are taught its mission, philosophy, and objectives.

Figure 1–10 • *Examples of Nursing Management as Effective Communication*

the implementation of the adopted plan, the given orders, and the established principles through establishing standards, comparing performance with standards, and correcting deficiencies. The controlling function of nursing management is frequently called evaluating.

All of these major functions of nursing management operate independently and interdependently. They will be examined in detail in succeeding chapters.

SUMMARY

A theory of nursing management evolves from a generic theory of management governing effective use of human and material resources. Four major elements of a theory of management are planning, organizing, directing or leading, and controlling or evaluating. All management activities, cognitive, affective, and psychomotor, fall within one or more of these major functions that operate simultaneously.

A main thrust of nursing management is that the focus is on human behavior. Nurse managers educated in the knowledge and skills of human behavior manage professional nurses, as well as nonprofessional nursing workers, to achieve the highest level of productivity in patient care services. To do this they acquire the management competencies of leadership to stimulate motivation through communication with the work force.

General principles of nursing management include the following:

1. Nursing management is planning.
2. Nursing management is the effective use of time.
3. Nursing management is decision making.
4. Meeting patients' nursing care needs is the business of the nurse manager.
5. Nursing management is the formulation and achievement of social goals.
6. Nursing management is organizing.
7. Nursing management denotes a function, social position or rank, a discipline, and a field of study.
8. Nursing management is the active organ of the division of nursing, of the organization, and of the society in which it functions.
9. Organizational cultures reflect values and beliefs.
10. Nursing management is directing or leading.
11. A well-managed division of nursing motivates employees to perform satisfactorily.
12. Nursing management is efficient communication.
13. Nursing management is controlling or evaluating.

A theory of nursing management evolves from the theory of nursing and the nursing process. Just as data are collected and analyzed by the clinical nurse to make the nursing care plan, so does the clinical nurse manager collect and analyze data to do planning. The clinical nurse organizes the care of individual patients as well as the care of a group of patients (a total practice). Likewise, the nurse manager organizes work at division, department, or unit level. Although the clinical nurse performs the directing or leading function with other nursing personnel, patients, and families (applies nurs-

ing orders), the nurse manager performs the directing or leading function of larger groups of personnel and the use of more material resources. Controlling or evaluating is performed by the clinical nurse in assessing the results of nursing advice in terms of patients' outcomes. Clinical nurses also evaluate those personnel who assist or work for them. Nurse managers perform the controlling or evaluating function at division, department, and unit levels. They evaluate programs, personnel performance, and outcome (qualitatively and quantitatively). Development of nursing management theory will transform theory of nursing and theory of management. Research in nursing management will validate the theory of nursing management.

The primary role of the nurse manager is to manage a clinical practice discipline. This requires numerous competencies that support a theory of nursing management.

EXPERIENTIAL EXERCISES

1. In your own words, define nursing management as it relates to your job. Observe the work of a nurse manager and define nursing management in terms of your observations.

2. List a belief you have about nursing management in the organization in which you are doing clinical practice. Discuss your belief with your clinical group of practicing peers or students and nurse manager or instructor.

Summarize the conclusions. Is your belief valid? Totally? Partly? Not at all? Validity can be established by comparing your conclusions with viewpoints found in publications or by obtaining agreement from practicing nurse managers. You will be codifying selected theory of nursing management.

3. Translate the management of time as nursing management theory into an example such as "A nurse who practices good management will know how to use time effectively." The example may apply to you as clinical nurse manager/student or to observed behavior of a nurse manager. To do this you can keep a log for a day. Make entries at 15-minute intervals using the following format:

TIME	ACTIVITY	DELAYS, BOTTLENECKS

Analyze your log. How much of your day was productive? How much was unproductive? What can be done to increase productive time? Make a management plan to use your time better. Use the following format:

MANAGEMENT PLAN

OBJECTIVE: To manage my time better.

ACTIONS	TARGET DATES	ASSIGNED TO	ACCOMPLISHMENTS

Based on your observations from this exercise, write a theory statement that describes management as the effective use of time.

4. The following functions originate from a theory of the institution or organization and the division of nursing:

- Make plans for accomplishing objectives
- Formulate strategies for accomplishing plans
- Organize activities by priority
- Assign work
- Design managerial jobs
- Evolve an organizational structure

Describe how each of these activities is evident in your place of practice.

5. *Scenario:* Ms. Apple is chair of the division of nursing in a medical center. She is concerned that even though they have ward clerks and unit managers, professional nurses are performing too many clerical duties. Also, an RN is on night duty on every ward or unit. In counseling with nurses, Ms. Apple has discovered they are bored, because many patients require minimal care on these shifts. She has met with a representative group of clinical nurse managers and asked for suggestions and changes to consider. The clinical nurse managers have asked for 4 weeks' time to identify specific areas where changes are needed and to formulate recommendations for change. They are keeping a log of their activities on all shifts to decide which tasks can be performed by other workers.

Answer the following questions:

5.1 What evidence is there that Ms. Apple is influenced by time elements in making her decisions?
5.2 What evidence is there that Ms. Apple is considering the future and human resources in making her decisions?
5.3 What evidence is there that Ms. Apple is taking care of the present while planning for the future?

6. *Scenario:* When Ms. Apple met with her group of clinical nurse managers, the recommendations were as follows:

• Make optimal use of intensive care units: surgical, coronary, and newborn and pediatric. Keep them optimally staffed with RNs around the clock.

• Have an RN for clinical nurse manager of each ward each shift. Other RNs would carry case loads and would assess patients' needs through history taking, making nursing diagnoses and prescriptions, write the nursing care plans, teach LPNs and nursing assistants to carry them out, and be on call 24 hours a day for their patients. They would cover each other as needed. A minimal number of RNs would be available for immediate need including at least one physically present in intensive care units at all times.

• Eliminate evening and night supervisors by giving key personnel responsibilities for on-call management advice.

• In cooperation with hospital administration, develop new programs for patient care. Give different rates: highest for total care; medium for care in which patient participates to limit of ability; and lowest for care in which family assists in every possible way with specific duties.

• Restructure clinic jobs, making them focus on primary care.

Answer the following questions:

6.1 What evidence is there that Mrs. Apple is an entrepreneur?
6.2 What evidence is there that the cost of health care is a consideration?
6.3 What evidence is there that health care services will be better?
6.4 At least two areas for development of nursing goals can be identified in the nurses' recommendation to Ms. Apple. List them.

7. How is the definition of planning, as it relates to a theory of nursing management, evident in a nursing unit, department, service, or division with which you are or have been associated?

8. How is the definition of organizing, as it relates to a theory of nursing, evident in a nursing unit, department, service, or division with which you are or have been associated?

9. How is the definition of directing or leading, as it relates to a theory of nursing, evident in a nursing unit, department, service, or division with which you are or have been associated?

10. How is the definition of controlling or evaluating, as it relates to a theory of nursing, evident in a nursing unit, department, service, or division with which you are or have been associated?

11. Write a short theory of nursing management based on information presented in Chapter 1. Remember that a theory of nursing management is an accumulation of concepts, methods, and principles that can be or have been observed and verified to some degree when translated into the art or practice of nursing management.

NOTES

1. H. Fayol, *General and Industrial Management*, trans. by C. Storrs (London: Pitman & Sons, 1949), 3.
2. Ibid., 5–6.
3. R. M. Hodgetts, *Management: Theory, Process, and Practice* (Orlando, FL: Academic Press, 1986), 40.
4. Fayol, op. cit., 8–9.
5. Ibid., 19–20.
6. L. Urwick, *The Elements of Administration* (New York: Harper & Row, 1944), 14–15.
7. L. C. Megginson, D. C. Mosley, and P. H. Pietri, Jr., *Management: Concepts and Applications*, 2d ed. (New York: Harper & Row, 1986), 15. They define theories as part of knowledge and as statements of cause-effect relationships involved in a set of phenomena. They include principles, rules, methods, and procedures that form the knowledge base of science. According to them a principle is a general belief or proposition sufficiently applicable to a situation to provide a guide to thought or action in that situation. A concept is "an abstract or generic idea generalized from particular instances that serves as the basis for an action or discussion. . . . A law is a statement of an order or relation of phenomena, that, so far as is known, is invariably true under the given conditions."
8. W. Skinner, "Big Hat, No Cattle: Managing Human Resources, Part 1," *Journal of Nursing Administration*, July-Aug. 1982, 27–29.
9. K. E. Boulding, "General Systems Theory: The Skeleton of Science," *Management Science*, Apr. 1956, 197–208.
10. V. Henderson, *The Nature of Nursing* (New York: Macmillan, 1966), 15.
11. T. A. Ratcliffe and D. J. Logsdon, "The Business Planning Process—A Behavioral Perspective," *Managerial Planning*, Mar.-Apr. 1980, 32–38.
12. P. F. Drucker, *Management: Tasks, Responsibilities, Practices* (New York: Harper & Row, 1973, 1974), x.
13. M. A. Poulin, "Future Directions for Nursing Administration," *Journal of Nursing Administration*, Mar. 1984, 37–41.
14. M. A. Maidique, "Point of View: The New Management Thinkers," *California Management Review*, Fall 1983, 151–160.

FOR FURTHER REFERENCE

Arndt, C., and Huckabay, L. M. D., *Nursing Administration: Theory for Practice with a Systems Approach*, 2d ed. (St. Louis: Mosby, 1980).

Clark, M. D., "Loss and Grief Behavior: Application to Nursing Managerial Practice," *Nursing Administration Quarterly*, Spring 1984, 53–60.

DeWeese, S., and Satecki, D., "Combining Management Education with an Assessment Center," *Nursing Management*, Aug. 1986, 80–81.

Drucker, P. F., *The Frontiers of Management* (New York: Truman Talley Books, 1986).

Fralic, M. F., and O'Connor, A., "A Management Progression System for Nurse Administrators, Part 1," *Journal of Nursing Administration*, Apr. 1983, 9–13; "A Management Progression System for Nurse Administrators, Part 2," *Journal of Nursing Administration*, May 1983, 32–33; "A Management Progression System for Nurse Administrators, Part 3," *Journal of Nursing Administration*, June 1983, 7–12.

Freund, C. M., "Director of Nursing Effectiveness: DON and CEO Perspectives and Implications for Education," *Journal of Nursing Administration*, June 1985, 25–30.

Gentleman, G., "Power at the Unit Level," *Nursing Administration Quarterly*, Winter 1983, 27–31.

Gleeson, S., Nestor, D. W., and Riddell, A. J., "Helping Nurses through the Management Threshold," *Nursing Administration Quarterly*, Winter 1983, 11–16.

Hillestad, E. A., "Is It Lonely at the Top?," *Nursing Administration Quarterly*, Spring 1984, 1–13.

Koontz, H., and Weihrich, H., *Management*, 9th ed. (New York: McGraw-Hill, 1988).

Kroner, K., "If You're Moving Into Management . . .," *Nursing 80*, Nov. 1980, 105–114.

Marriner, A., "Development of Management Thought," *Journal of Nursing Administration*, Sept. 1979, 21–31.

McClure, M. L., "Managing the Professional Nurse: Part 1. The Organizational Theories," *Journal of Nursing Administration*, Feb. 1984, 15–21; "Managing the Professional Nurse: Part 2. Applying Management Theory to the Challenges," *Journal of Nursing Administration*, Mar. 1984, 11–17.

Nugent, P. S., "Management and Modes of Thought," *Journal of Nursing Administration*, Feb. 1982, 19–25.

O'Leary, J., "Do Nurse Administrators' Values Conflict with the Economic Trend?," *Nursing Administration Quarterly*, Summer 1984, 1–9.

Poulin, M. A., "The Nurse Executive Role: A Structural and Functional Analysis," *Journal of Nursing Administration*, Feb. 1984, 9–14.

Reeves, D. M., and Underly, N., "Nurse Managers and Mickey Mouse Marketing," *Nursing Administration Quarterly*, Winter 1983, 22–27.

Spicer, J. G., "Dispelling Illusions with Management Development," *Nursing Administration Quarterly*, Winter 1983, 46–49.

Swansburg, R. C., *Management of Patient Care Services* (St. Louis: Mosby, 1976).

———, *Nurses and Patients: An Introduction to Nursing Management* (Hattiesburg, MS: Impact III, 1978).

Taylor, B. A., and deSimone, A., "Taking the First Steps to Become a Nurse Manager," *Nursing Administration Quarterly*, Winter 1983, 17–22.

Wagner, L., Henry, B., Giovinco, G., and Blanks, C., "Suggestions for Graduate Education in Nursing Administration," *Journal of Nursing Education*, May 1988, 210–218.

White, V., "Nursing Theory: A Viewpoint," *Journal of Nursing Administration*, July-Aug. 1984, 6, 15.

• 2 •

The Planning Process

INTRODUCTION

Definition

Planning, a basic function of management, is a principal duty of all managers within the division of nursing. It is a systematic process and requires knowledgeable activity based on sound managerial theory. The first element of management defined by Fayol was planning. He defined it as making a plan of action to provide for the foreseeable future. This plan of action must have unity, continuity, flexibility, and precision. Fayol outlined the contents of a plan of action for his business, a large mining and metallurgical firm. This plan included annual and 10-year forecasts. Forecasting takes advantage of input from others. It improves with yearly experience, gives sequence in activity, and protects a business against undesirable changes. Fayol's concept was that planning facilitates wise use of resources and selection of the best approaches to achieving objectives. Planning facilitates the art of handling people; it requires moral courage, because it can fail. Effective planning requires continuity of tenure. Good planning is a sign of competence.[1]

Urwick wrote that research in admininstration provides needed information for forecasting. According to Urwick, investigations should be carried out and their results expressed in concrete terms. Planning should be based on objectives, which should be framed in terms of making a product or providing a service that the community needs. Simplification and standardization are basic to sound planning procedures. The product or service should be of the right pattern. Planning provides information to coordinate work effectively and accurately. A good plan should be based on an objective, be simple, have standards, be flexible, be balanced, and use available resources first.[2]

Douglass stated that "planning is having a specific aim or purpose and mapping out a program or method beforehand for accomplishment of the goal."[3] She further defined planning as being "a continuous process of assessing, establishing goals and objectives, and implementing and evaluating or controlling them, which is subject to change as new facts are known."[4]

Alexander stated that planning *"is deciding in advance what to do, how to do it, when to do it, and who to do it."* [5] She dealt with long- and short-term planning, decision making, strategies, policies, programs, rules, and procedures as elements of planning. [6]

Steiner defined planning as a process beginning with objectives; defining strategies, policies, and detailed plans to achieve them; achieving an organization to implement decisions; and including a review of performance and feedback to introduce a new planning cycle. [7]

Planning is an administrative function that takes some of the risk out of decision making and problem solving. It ensures that the probable outcome will be desirable and effective in terms of use of human and material resources and production of the product or service. In nursing, planning helps to ensure that clients or patients will receive the nursing services they want and need and that these services are delivered by satisfied nursing workers. [8]

Purposes of Planning

Douglass listed the following as reasons for planning:

1. It leads to success in achieving goals and objectives.
2. It gives meaning to work.
3. It provides for effective use of available personnel and facilities.
4. It helps in coping with crisis situations.
5. It is cost-effective.
6. It is based on past and future, thus helping reduce the element of change.
7. It can be used to discover the need for change.
8. It is needed for effective control. [9]

Among the activities of planning that Douglass addresses are assessment by collection, classification, analysis, interpretation, and translation of data; strategic planning; development of standards; identification of needs and priority setting; management by objectives; and formulation of policies, rules, regulations, methods, and procedures. [10]

Donovan wrote that planning has several benefits, among which are satisfactory outcomes of decisions; improved functions in emergencies; assurance of economy of time, space, and materials; and the highest use of personnel. She included decision making, philosophies, and objectives as key elements in planning. [11]

Several factors relative to successful planning should be known and put into action by successful managers. These are:

1. A knowledge of the characteristics of planning.
2. A knowledge of the elements of the planning process.
3. A knowledge of the strategic or long-range planning process.
4. A knowledge of the tactical or short-range planning process—functional versus operational.
5. A knowledge of planning standards.
6. A knowledge of and skill in applying the planning processes, including standards, to the work situation.
7. Skill in bringing the planning process up to the standard set, *when there are deficiencies.* [12]

Characteristics of Planning

What is the nature of planning? What is so distinctive about it that requires a nurse manager to have the knowledge and skills requisite to engage in planning? In an environment of changing technology, mounting costs, and multiple activities, there is a need for the chief nurse administrator and subordinate managers to plan. The forecasting of events and the laying out of a system of activities or actions for accomplishing the work of nursing and of the organization are prerequisites to success. Koontz and Weihrich defined planning as "selecting missions and objectives and the actions to achieve them; it requires decision making, that is, choosing future courses of action from among alternatives." [13] They view planning as an elementary function of management. In planning, the nurse manager would avoid leaving events to chance; the nurse manager would apply an intellectual process to consciously determining the course of action to accomplish the work of the total nursing organization. Donovan stated that the planning process must be deliberate and analytic to produce carefully detailed programs of action that will achieve objectives. [14]

The clinical nurse manager plans effectively to create environments in which nursing personnel will provide the nursing care desired and needed by clients. In this environment clinical nurses will make decisions about the form or modality of practice, and nurse managers will work with nursing personnel to establish and meet their personal objectives while meeting the objectives of the organization. According to Hodgetts, planning establishes a path to where managers and subordinates want to go. [15] It should be comprehensive, with nurse managers carefully determining objectives and making detailed plans to accomplish them. It has generally been implied that top administrators in nursing focus on long-range or strategic planning while operational nurse managers focus on short-range or tactical planning. This process is outmoded. All managers and representative clinical nurses should have input into strategic planning.

Rowland and Rowland state that planning begins with a philosophy about nursing. They list these phases of planning: determining objectives, collecting data, developing a plan of action, setting goals, and evaluating.[16]

Planning involves the collection, analysis, and organization of many kinds of data (the *how*) that will be used to determine both the nursing care needs of patients and the management plans that will provide the resources and processes to meet those needs. Accepting the fact that nursing is a clinical practice discipline providing a human service, nurse managers plan in order to nurture the practitioners who provide the service.

Some of the kinds of data that must be collected and analyzed for planning purposes include:

1. Daily average patient census
2. Bed capacity and percent of occupancy
3. Average length of stay
4. Number of births
5. Number of operations
6. Trends in patient populations
   a. Diagnoses
   b. Age groups
   c. Acuity of illness
   d. Physical dependency
7. Trends in technology
   a. Diagnostic procedures
   b. Therapeutic procedures
8. Environmental analysis
   a. Forces impacting on nursing from within: availability of nurses, turnover, other departments
   b. Forces impacting on nursing from outside: government, education, accreditation bodies, and others
   c. Trends in health care and in nursing, including changes in characteristics
   d. Threats to the nursing profession
   e. Opportunities for the nursing profession

Figure 2–1 demonstrates examples of data that would be collected and analyzed for planning purposes by nursing managers.

- Live births have decreased 30 percent in the 3 years since the institution of a family planning program.
- Sixty-three percent of live births are discharged within a 24-hour period.
- The number of deliveries with complications has increased from 210 to 257 in one year.
- A new cardiac catheterization laboratory has been completed.
- The hospital planning board has decided to coordinate with other hospitals in the area to consolidate specialty services for newborn care, cardiovascular surgery, and neuroscience services.
- Enrollment of students for clinical nursing affiliation has decreased from 450 to 392 in one year.
- Enrollment of students in the nursing cooperative education program has decreased from 102 to 87 students.
- Medicare reimbursement pays $____ per patient for ____ days of home care.

Figure 2–1 • *Planning Data for Nurse Managers*

Data on diagnostic and therapeutic procedures will be used to plan for new procedures, to revise old procedures, and to make new procedures known to nursing personnel. This is certainly not an exhaustive list of sources of data that will be used for planning purposes. Other sources will be listed in this chapter.

Planning has the characteristics of an open system, being a dynamic organizational process. It leads to success rather than failure. It prevents crisis and panic planning that is costly, unrealistic, chaotic, distorting of achievement, and dominated by a single person. Planning thus improves nursing unit performance. Planning identifies future opportunities and expectations based on conditions, through forecasting techniques that range from simple to complex. Simple forecasting techniques follow the process of gathering data and analyzing them to determine alternative decisions and what effects each will produce. Strengths, weaknesses, opportunities, and threats are part of this analysis, which leads to decision, choice, and implementation. In complex forecasting, computer-based mathematical models are available. They are high in cost, require a lot of time and specialized skills, and extend from 3 to 15 years.

Planning is viewed as resting on logical, reflective thinking that is neither cast in concrete nor all encompassing. If needed, leadership or top management will effect change to do effective planning. They will obtain input from all levels to ensure success through format, procedures, time frames, maintenance, and input review.

Planning is the key element of nursing that gives it direction, cohesion, and thrust. It causes all nursing personnel to focus on goals and objectives and stimulates their motivation. Through the planning process nurse managers select and retain the elements of past and present plans that work. They focus on the future and they implement. Thus they successfully manage nursing personnel and material resources to achieve the objectives of the nursing enterprise.

Elements of Planning

Although planning is characterized as being a conceptual or thinking process, it produces specific elements or constituent parts that are readily identifiable. These include written statements of mission or purpose, philosophy, objectives, and detailed management or operational plans—the blueprints by which the purpose, philosophy, and objectives are put into measurable actions. Management or operational plans include decision-making and problem-solving processes. They include strategies, policies, and procedures.

The nursing division's strategic and operational plans are road maps that describe the business by name and location. Nurse managers will make them informative by including a description that summarizes the work of the division.

The summary describing the nursing division will include enough information to give outsiders a bird's-eye view of its totality. This will include the nursing products and services provided by quantity, which can be admissions, discharges, patient days, number of patients by acuity categories, research projects, education programs, students, outpatient visits, and other products and services. The description will summarize marketing activities of the nursing division, including total revenues and expenses. It will describe the managerial style of the division and its impact on employees. This will be related to the organizational plan of the division of nursing.

Planning is the assessment of nursing division's strengths and weaknesses, covering factors that affect performance and facilitate or inhibit the achievement of objectives. This assessment process will have both long-range and short-range objectives of its own. As an example, if the clinical promotion ladder is a strength in nurse retention but is weakly applied by selective nurse managers, the problem will be addressed by written objectives.

Planning entails formulation of planning premises by extrapolating assumptions from the information analyzed.[17] If data indicate nurses will be in shorter supply because of decreased enrollments in schools of nursing and increased opportunities for women to enter other fields, this finding should be translated into a premise. Other premises evolve related to increased salaries and fringe benefits and improved conditions of work. These will lead to further premises for marketing a career in nursing to high school students.

Planning implies writing specific, useful, realistic objectives (the *why*) that will reflect both strategic and operational goals for the division of nursing and its personnel. Objectives become the reasons for an operational nursing management plan (the *what*) that will detail activities to be performed, the target dates or time frames for their accomplishment (the *when*), the persons responsible for accomplishing them (the *who*), and strategies for dealing with technical, economic, social, and political aspects. These operational plans will have control systems for monitoring performance and providing feedback. Objectives and operational plans are discussed in detail in Chapter 3.

Good management according to Meier,

starts with a coordinated purposeful organization of people who collectively on a functional responsibility basis are responsible for:

1. *Setting objectives*
2. *Planning strategy*
3. *Setting goals—short-term objectives*
4. *Developing company philosophy*
5. *Setting policies—the plan*
6. *Planning the organization*
7. *Providing personnel*
8. *Establishing procedures*
9. *Providing facilities*
10. *Providing capital*
11. *Setting performance standards*
12. *Initiating management programs*
13. *Developing management information systems*
14. *Activating people*[18]

Good management keeps the nursing division successful, ensuring its growth, success, and direction and a return on investment in the future.

STRATEGIC PLANNING

Nurse managers can increase effectiveness through strategic planning, which can promote professional nursing practice and the long-range goals of the organization and the division of nursing. Strategic planning is defined as "a continuous, systematic process of making risk-taking decisions today with the greatest possible knowledge of their effects on the future; organizing efforts necessary to carry out these decisions and evaluating results of these decisions against expected outcome through reliable feedback mechanisms."[19]

Strategic planning in nursing is concerned with what the division of nursing should be doing. Its purpose is to improve allocation of scarce resources, including time and money, and to manage the division of nursing for performance. Strategic planning provides strategic forecasting from 3 years up to more than 20 years. It should involve top nurse managers and can effectively involve representatives of all levels of nursing management and practice. It will include analysis of projected technological advances, the internal and external environments, the nursing and health care market and industry, the economics of nursing and health care, availability of human and material resources, judgments of top management, and other factors.[20]

In today's world the strategic planning process is used to acquire and develop new health care services and product lines. These include new nursing services and products. Strategic planning is also used to divest outdated services and products. Both activities present moral and ethical dilemmas for the managers and practitioners of nursing. Strategic planning can foster better goals, better corporate values, and better communication about corporate direction. It can lead to changes in operating management and organization. Strategic planning can produce better management strategy and analysis and can forecast and mute external threats.

Figure 2–2 lists ways in which strategic planning can be used to improve management.

Participants in the strategic planning process will range from top nursing management to a cross-section of all levels of management. Including input from clinical nursing personnel promotes professsional satisfaction throughout the nursing division.

Among the benefits of strategic planning is the giving of a sense of direction to all managers and practitioners of nursing within the organization. The strategic plan becomes a flexible control mech-

To provide accountability and monitoring of performance, tie merit to performance.

To set up more formal planning programs and require divisional and unit planning.

To integrate strategic plans with operational and financial plans.

To think more and concentrate on strategic issues.

To improve knowledge of, and training in, strategic planning.

To increase top management involvement and commitment.

To improve focus on competition, market segments, and external factors.

To improve communication from top administration and nursing management.

To allow better execution of plans.

To use more realism and less rationalizing and vacillating.

To improve the development of nursing management strategies.

To improve the development and communication of nursing management goals.

To put less emphasis on *raw* numbers.

Figure 2–2 • How Strategic Planning Can Be Used to Improve Nursing Management

anism that can be modified to deal with variables, conservation of resources, and professional satisfaction. The strategic plan deals concretely with complex projects or programs in multistage time sequences.[21]

Human Resources Planning

Human resources strategic planning is undertaken as part of the strategic planning process. This is essential to retention of outstanding professional talent. It is not enough to address only the business activities of nursing such as management processes and functions, budgets, objectives, staffing, and the like. The goals of the division are accomplished through its people. Nurse managers serve in dual roles, as managers of human resources and managers of nursing operations. Nurse managers need to enlist the good offices of the human resource department and use it. They also need to develop understanding between other operational departments and nursing.[22]

Strategic human resources planning decides how the full spectrum of human resources will affect the strategic and operational plans. If the human resources do not fit the strategic plan the nurse manager decides what action to take. This can include locating new people with special skills or upgrading the skills of senior people. There will be a statement of objectives for the human resource program in the strategic plan. It can be developed with input from clinical nurses.[23]

Conclusions about the Strategic Planning Process

Strategic planning is a goal-setting process largely carried out by top management. However, although long-range plans are often made, many times they are not put to use. In truth, many operating nurse managers need to be trained in the strategic planning process. This training would include techniques to involve operational managers and thereby to commit them to decisions. Development of global goals and strategies broadens the identification and solution of problems, thereby reducing threats to and unveiling opportunities for the organization.

The demonstrated usefulness of scientific planning will influence the behavior of operating managers. Rewards, in the form of both pay and praise, will motivate these operating managers.

PRACTICAL PLANNING ACTIONS

Practical day-to-day planning actions of value to the nurse manager include the following:

1. At the beginning of each day, make a list of actions to be accomplished for the day. Cross off the actions as they are accomplished or at the end of the day. At the beginning of the next workday, carry over actions not accomplished; either do them first or decide whether they really need to be done. Do not hold tasks over from one day to the next indefinitely.

2. Plan ahead for meetings. If the meeting is a nursing responsibility, prepare and distribute the agenda in advance. Have a secretary call members for their items to be listed on the agenda. Forward nursing items for the agenda of organizational meetings to the appropriate chair in advance. Prepare for the presentation.

3. Identify developing problems and put them in the appropriate portion of the division's operational or management plans.

4. Review the operational or management plan on a scheduled basis. Do this with key managers so that each knows personal responsibilities for accomplishment of activities.

5. Review the appropriate portions of the department operational or management plan with subordinate nurse managers when they are being counseled. Department, unit, or clinic plans will be reviewed at the same time.

6. Plan for discussion of ideas gleaned from professional publications. This can be part of a job standard, with different managers assigned specific topics or journals. This may help to integrate research results into practice.

7. Suggest similar practical planning actions to nursing department heads and other nurse managers.

Planning will also be necessary to provide programs for orientation and continued learning of nursing personnel, so that all will have current knowledge and be current in practice. Improvement of patient care and of other administrative and hospital services necessitates initiation of, use of, and participation in studies or research projects in the health care field.

Two additional large and important areas for planning are, first, educational programs that include student educational experience in the division of nursing and, second, evaluation of clinical and administrative practices to determine if the objectives of the division are being achieved.

UNIT PLANNING

Planning should extend to the operational units. The processes involved are the same. It is here that the work for which the division of nursing exists takes place. Planning should be done on a daily, weekly, and long-range basis. Daily planning is related to patient care and includes history taking, assessment, and nursing diagnosis and prescription. It involves matching people to jobs, developing policies and procedures specific to the types of clients cared for, identifying training needs, preparing and conducting training programs, coordinating all patient care activities, supervising personnel, and evaluating.

Unit objectives should be clearly defined, and a sound management or operational plan should be made to achieve them. An operating instruction from one division of nursing states, "The division of nursing has a stated philosophy and objectives.

Personnel of each unit within the division willl have their own philosophy and will set up their own objectives. The objectives will be continuously evaluated, and a written statement as to progress will be sent to the chair's office each August and February." Figure 2–3 is a plan for accomplishing objectives related to management improvement and resource management for an intensive care unit.

1. Management improvement: Unit Objectives February 1, 1993

    1.1 Precipitate imaginative thinking to improve existing procedures, capitalize on time expenditure, and introduce modern concepts and materials that directly enhance unit accomplishment.

1.2 Promote creativity in improving the existing patient environment.

1.3 Provide more modern concepts of total patient care by constant review and revision of unit administrative/managerial policies.

Plans for Achievement of Objectives	Actions	Target Dates	Accomplishments
1.1–1.2 Plan and implement a continuing unit improvement program.	1. Conduct a continuous review and analysis of unit improvement efforts through:	February	Reviewed and found current for following reasons: Turnover in personnel is fast. All objectives were not adequately met. We need to establish a better way of accomplishing them.
	1.1 Monthly unit conferences to review and update philosophy and objectives. Strive to accomplish more in each objective area.	February–July	
	1.2 Patient suggestions.	Review each month.	
	1.3 Suggestions of superiors.	Daily	
	1.4 Revise unit procedures.	April	Done.
	1.5 Brief all personnel. Discuss philosophy, objectives, job descriptions, performance standards, hospital and nursing service policies and procedures, and unit procedures.	February	Done. In addition all nurses were counseled by the clinical nurse manager. Nursing technicians are presently receiving counseling and all is being documented. Counseling had not been documented in 6 years except for remarks such as, "Things went well

Figure 2–3 • *Unit Operational Plan—Intensive Care Unit*

(Continued)

Plans for Achievement of Objectives	Actions	Target Dates	Accomplishments
			and we did our job, so no counseling was needed."
	2. Review equipment and supplies for improvement by addition or deletion.		
	2.1 Submit work order to alter a locker as a drying cabinet for respirator parts, because moisture provides a growth medium for *Pseudomonas* bacteria.		Disapproved. Disposable tubing was approved, ordered, and in use by June.
	2.2 Check on status of new floor, piped-in compressed air system, and cardiac monitors.	February–April	New floor to be done by August 1. Compressed air started by March 15. Cardiac monitors arrived April 3. Patient units 1, 3, and 4 were equipped. Unit 4 was designated the maximum monitoring site and is to be used to monitor patients with Swan-Ganz arterial lines and questionable cardiac conditions.
1.3 Review standardized policies and procedures to find ways to implement more current concepts of improved care.	3. Evaluate all areas of management for current standardized efficiency. 3.1 Check all areas of infection sources.		
	3.1.1 Culture floors and equipment to check cleaning procedures.	February	This was done, and cleaning procedures were looked at and improved when they appeared poor. Adhesive floor mats were placed at entrance and exit areas to control dust carried in by personnel and visitors. Air conditioning filters were replaced in February. Wall suction valves were replaced. Pipelines were found to be clogged with secretions, and system had to be purged. Shelves were mounted on wall by four units to replace bedside stands. Respirators,

Figure 2–3 •   *(Continued)*

(Continued)

Plans for Achievement of Objectives	Actions	Target Dates	Accomplishments
			nebulizers, and blenders were mounted on wall above each patient unit. Suction bottles were relocated and outlets changed to isolate them from the oxygen nebulization units. Swan-Ganz catheters were standardized, and requisitioning was transferred from the unit to central supply. Ambu bags were equipped with corrugated tubing to serve as an oxygen reservoir and deliver a maximum concentration of 99% to 100%. The disposable Aqua-pack nebulizer was deleted, resulting in a $40-per-case saving.
	3.1.2 Clean air conditioning filters.	February	
	3.1.3 Check wall suction, which is not working adequately.	February	
	3.1.4 Eliminate messy bedside stands.	February	
	3.2 Improve safety.		
	3.2.1 Secure equipment.	April	
	3.2.2 Isolate oxygen nebulation units from suction.	April	
	3.2.3 Send all equipment to central supply for processing.	April	
	3.2.4 Improve efficiency of Ambu resuscitators.	April	
	Projected: An anesthesiologist will be assigned to the intensive care unit. All bronchoscopies will be done here. Open heart surgery is still an open and current topic.		

Myra C. Breck, RN, Clinical Nurse Manager, ICU

Figure 2–3 • *(Continued)*

(Continued)

2. Resources management

   2.1 Provide, secure, and maintain the appropriate and economical use of supplies and equipment that will permit unit personnel to devote maximum time and care to patient activities.

   2.2 Provide the unit with adequate tools for safe and effective patient care.

   2.3 Provide the unit with conservative utilization and centralization of unit supplies and equipment, thus promoting peak efficiency in meeting patients' needs.

Plans for Achievement of Objectives	Actions	Target Dates	Accomplishments
2.1 Plan, evaluate, and project needed supplies and equipment that will enhance effective and safe nursing care.	Identify projected needs with unit manager through review of: 1. Unit inventories of equipment and budgetary estimate. 2. Standards for supplies. 3. Availability of supplies and equipment. 4. Economical use of supplies and equipment.	February	Items ordered (projected replacements for 1993–1994): 1 Thermometer—electronic, $300. 1 IV pump, $700. 5 transducers, $385. 1 Mark 8 Bird respirator, $275. 1 sphygmomanometer, $655. 1 Wright respirometer, $275. 4 metal storage cabinets. 4 Ambu bags. Vertical venetian blinds. 1 blood gas analyzer, $7455. New cubicle curtains.
2.2–2.3 Plan and execute appropriate use of materials	1. Economical use of expendable supplies and adequate safeguards to prevent misuse and loss. 2. Knowledge of principles of operation of appropriate mechanical equipment and procedures for effecting prompt servicing and repairs.		Items replaced: ECG and defibrillator. Portable ECG machine. MA1 filters. Spirometers. Suction regulators. Items deleted: 1 electric thermometer. 1 internal/external defibrillator (to dog lab). 2 compressor units. Miscellaneous: File card supply system revamped. Shelving obtained for lower doors. Personnel turnover—projected losses: Ms. Speich, RN, June. Ms. Ullman, RN, Aug. Ms. Urbom, RN, May. Ms. Malloy, RN, June. Mr. Falco, ward clerk, April. Projected gains:

Figure 2–3 • *(Continued)*

(Continued)

Plans for Achievement of Objectives	Actions	Target Dates	Accomplishments
			Ms. Tishoff, RN, May.
			Mr. Robertshaw, RN, May.
			Mr. Angelus, RN, April.
			Mrs. Figuera, unit secretary, April.

Myra C. Breck, RN, Clinical Nurse Manager, ICU

SOURCE: R. C. Swansburg, *Management of Patient Care Services.* St. Louis: Mosby, 1978, 49–53.

Figure 2–3 • *(Continued)*

RELATIONSHIPS TO ORGANIZATION

Planning within the division of nursing is intended to assist in fulfilling the mission of the health care facility. It supports the organization's objectives and meshes with the plans of all other departments contributing to provision of total health care needs, whether direct or indirect (such as planning for the environment). Planning includes delineation of the responsibilities of nurse managers in relation to activities in other departments in which nursing participates. The organizational chart will show the relationship of the division of nursing to the board of control, the administrator, and other departments.

Plans will provide for optimum support of the nursing division by other departments providing services, supplies, and equipment used by nursing service. There will be plans for regular meetings with the hospital administrator for participation on all hospital committees concerned with general administrative policies and activities and the total program of the organization. There will also be plans for periodic reports to the board of control, through administrators, concerning the programs, major plans, and problems of the division of nursing.

SUMMARY

Planning is a mental process by which all nurse managers use valid and reliable data to develop objectives and determine the resources needed and a blueprint for their use in achieving the objectives. The major purpose of planning is to make the best possible use of personnel, supplies, and equipment.

Strategic planning sets objectives for long-range nursing activities of 3 to 5 years. Although traditionally done by top managers, it is an important skill to be developed by all nurse managers. It ensures survival. Human resource planning will assure effective use of a scarce commodity, the professional nurse. Strategic planning has a mission; collects and analyzes data; assesses strengths and weaknesses; sets goals and objectives; uses strategies; operates on a timetable; gives operational and functional guidance to nurse managers; and includes evaluation.

EXPERIENTIAL EXERCISES

1. Determine the length of the planning process for a nursing unit. Use the checklist from Figure 2-4. From your survey, summarize the effectiveness of the planning process. How can it be improved? Can you initiate this improvement? If not, who can?

2. Interview a chief executive officer and a chief nurse executive officer of an organization. Determine their orientation to strategic planning. Compare the results. Possible questions to ask are stated in Figure 2-5.

Standards	Yes	No
1. The plan is written.		
2. It defines the nursing business.		
3. It contains objectives (general and specific goals).		
4. It defines strategies.		
5. It supports the mission.		
6. It details forecasted activities for 1 year.		
7. It details forecasted activities for longer than 1 year.		
8. It has been developed with input from clinical nurses and line managers.		
9. It addresses resources (personnel and facilities).		
10. Changes are evident.		
11. Financial plans are included.		
12. Needs are identified and supported.		
13. Priorities are listed.		
14. Timetables are listed.		
15. It is based on current data analysis.		
16. It assesses both strengths and weaknesses.		
17. It derives from a good nursing management information plan.		
18. It is used and modified consistently.		

Figure 2–4 • *Standards for Planning Process*

1. Do you have a strategic plan?
2. What length of time does it cover?
3. Who develops it?
4. Who uses it?
5. What products and services will be affected by it?
6. How will it impact professional nurses and nursing?
7. How will they impact it?
8. Can professional nurses initiate new products and services?
9. How will managers be updated?
10. Will products and services be divested?
11. What moral and ethical dilemmas could evolve?
12. What new nursing skills and roles will be needed?
13. How will they be obtained?
14. How does the strategic plan position nursing technically?
15. How does it position nursing as a profitable enterprise?
16. What have been the results of employee attitude surveys?
17. How are accomplishments celebrated?
18. How are employees made successful, supportive of one another, more communicative, and more trusting?

Figure 2–5 • *Planning Interview Questions*

3. Make a management plan for your work for a
day.

MANAGEMENT PLAN

OBJECTIVE:

ACTIONS	TARGET DATES	ASSIGNED TO	ACCOMPLISHMENTS

4. Make a management plan for a meeting.

MANAGEMENT PLAN

OBJECTIVE:

ACTIONS	TARGET DATES	ASSIGNED TO	ACCOMPLISHMENTS

NOTES

1. H. Fayol, *General and Industrial Management*, trans. by C. Storrs (London: Isaac Pitman & Sons, 1949), 43–50.
2. L. Urwick, *The Elements of Administration* (New York: Harper & Row, 1944), 26–34.
3. L. M. Douglass, *The Effective Nurse: Leader and Manager*, 3d ed. (St. Louis: C. V. Mosby, 1988), 92–93.
4. Ibid., 94.
5. E. L. Alexander, *Nursing Administration in the Hospital Health Care System*, 2d. ed. (St. Louis: C. V. Mosby, 1978), 132.
6. Ibid., 134–150.
7. G. A. Steiner, *Top Management Planning* (New York: Macmillan, 1969), 1.
8. M. Beyers and C. Phillips, *Nursing Management for Patient Care*, 2d ed. (Boston: Little, Brown, 1979), 41–48.
9. Douglass, op. cit., 95–96.
10. Ibid., 96–106.
11. H. M. Donovan, *Nursing Service Administration: Managing the Enterprise* (St. Louis: C. V. Mosby, 1975), 50–64.
12. P. F. Drucker, *Management: Tasks, Responsibilities, Practices* (New York: Harper & Row, 1973), 121–129.
13. H. Koontz and H. Weihrich, *Management* (New York: McGraw-Hill, 1988), 16.
14. Donovan, op. cit., 63–64.
15. R. M. Hodgetts, *Management: Theory, Process, and Practice*, 4th ed. (Orlando, FL: Academic Press, 1986), 97.
16. H. S. Rowland and B. L. Rowland, *Nursing Administration Handbook*, 2d ed. (Rockville, MD: Aspen, 1985), 24–27; *Nursing Administration Handbook*, 3d ed. (Rockville, MD: Aspen, 1992), 29–32.
17. W. E. Reif and J. L. Webster, "The Strategic Planning Process," *Arizona Business*, Apr. 1976, 14–20.
18. A. P. Meier, "The Planning Process," *Managerial Planning*, July/Aug. 1974, 1–5, 9.
19. Drucker, op. cit., 125.
20. D. H. Fox and R. T. Fox, "Strategic Planning for Nursing," *Journal of Nursing Administration*, May 1983, 11–16; R. N. Paul and J. W. Taylor, "The State of Strategic Planning," *Business*, Jan.-Mar. 1986, 37–43.
21. Fox and Fox, op. cit.
22. E. J. Metz, "The Missing 'H' in Strategic Planning," *Managerial Planning*, May/June 1984, 19–23, 29.
23. E. C. Smith, "How to Tie Human Resource Planning to Strategic Business Planning," *Managerial Planning*, Sept./Oct. 1983, 29–34.

FOR FURTHER REFERENCE

Ackoff, R. L., "Our Changing Concept of Planning," *Journal of Nursing Administration*, Oct. 1986, 35–40.

Bryan, E. L., and Welton, R. E., "Let Your Business Plan Be a Road Map to Credit," *Business*, July-Sept. 1986, 44–47.

Cushman, R., "Norton's Top-Down, Bottom-Up Planning Process," *Planning Review*, Nov. 1979, 3–8, 48.

Forman, L., "Which Comes First, the Planning Process or the Planning Model?," *Business Economics*, Sept. 1979, 42–47.

Gray, D. H., "Uses and Misuses of Strategic Planning," *Harvard Business Review*, Jan.-Feb. 1986, 89–97.

Joint Commission on Accreditation of Healthcare Organizations, *Accreditation Manual for Hospitals* (Chicago, IL: American Hospital Association, 1989), 133–139.

Mercer, Z. C., "Personal Planning: An Overlooked Application of the Corporate Planning Process," *Managerial Planning*, Jan./Feb. 1980, 32–35.

Nylen, D. W., "Making Your Business Plan an Action Plan," *Business*, Oct.-Dec. 1985, 12–16.

Palesy, S. R., "Motivating Line Management Using the Planning Process," *Planning Review*, Mar. 1980, 3–8, 44–48.

Paul, R. N., and Taylor, J. W., "The State of Strategic Planning," *Business*, Jan.-Mar. 1986, 37–43.

Pearce, W. H., "I Thought I Knew What Good Management Was," *Harvard Business Review*, Mar.-Apr. 1986, 59–65.

Redman, L. N., "The Planning Process," *Managerial Planning*, May/June 1983, 24–30, 40.

Singleton, E. K., and Nail, F. C., "Guidelines for Establishing a New Service," *Journal of Nursing Administration*, Oct. 1985, 22–26.

Mission, Philosophy, Objectives, and Management Plans

INTRODUCTION

Statements of mission or purpose, of philosophy or beliefs, of objectives, and of an operational or management plan have already been referred to; in this chapter, these basic tools of management are discussed in greater detail. Knowledge of their use is part of the theory of nursing management. They are part of the planning function of nursing management, and skill in using them successfully is part of the strategy of nursing management planning.

Written statements of purpose, philosophy, and objectives, and written operational plans are the blueprints for effective management of any enterprise, including a health care institution. They are a component of planning at each management level. Statements at the corporate level serve the top managers of the organization. Those at the division level serve the managers of major divisions such as nursing, operations, and finance. These statements evolve from and support those of the institution. Services, departments, and units each have written statements of purpose, philosophy, objectives, and written operational plans that are developed from and support the documents at division and corporate levels.[1] See Figure 3–1.

Operational plans
Mission (purpose) statements
Philosophy (beliefs) statements
Objectives statements
Operational (management) plans

Corporate→
Division→
Department→
Unit→

Figure 3–1 • *Evolution of Mission, Philosophy, and Objectives Statements and Operational Plans*

MISSION OR PURPOSE

Each organization exists for specific purposes or missions and to fulfill specific social functions. For health care organizations this means providing health care services to maintain health, cure illness, and allay pain and suffering. Business enterprises and government provide most of the economic resources to pay for these services. Although nursing has not been considered a profit-making enterprise, this condition is changing as third-party payers require better cost-accounting procedures.

Defining a mission or purpose allows nursing to be managed for performance. It describes what it will be and what it should be. It describes the constituencies to be satisfied. It is the professional nurse manager's commitment to a specific definition of purpose or mission.

One purpose of a nursing entity is to provide nursing care to clients. This can include promotion of self-care concepts. Thus the statement should include definitions of nursing and self-care as defined by professional nurses.

Virginia Henderson has defined nursing as follows:

The unique function of the nurse is to assist the individual, sick or well, in the performance of those activities contributing to health or its recovery (or to peaceful death) that he would perform unaided if he had the necessary strength, will or knowledge. And to do this in such a way as to help him gain independence as rapidly as possible.[2]

Yura and Walsh describe the nursing process as

an orderly, systematic manner of determining the client's health status, specifying problems defined as alterations in human need fulfillment, making plans to solve them, initiating and implementing the plan, and evaluating the extent to which the plan was effective in promoting the optimum wellness and resolving the problems identified.[3]

King defined nursing as

a process of action, reaction, interaction, and transaction whereby nurses assist individuals of any age group to meet their basic human needs in coping with their health status at some particular point in their life cycle. Nurses perform their functions within social institutions and they interact with individuals and groups.

Therefore, three distinct levels of operation exist: (1) the individual; (2) the group; and (3) society.[4]

Orem defined nursing as follows:

Nursing is an art through which the nurse, the practitioner of nursing, gives specialized assistance to persons with disabilities of such a character that more than ordinary assistance is necessary to meet daily needs for self-care and to intelligently participate in the medical care they are receiving from the physician. The art of nursing is practiced by "doing for" the patient with the disability, by "helping him do for himself," and/or by "helping him learn how to do for himself." Nursing is also practiced by helping a capable person from the patient's family or a friend of the patient learn how "to do for" the patient. Nursing is thus a practical and didactic art.[5]

Kinlein suggested that "nursing is assisting the person in his self-care practices in regard to his state of health."[6] Emerging from these and other theories of nursing is a commonality of terms central to the definition of nursing: nurse, patient or client, individual, group, society, nursing process, self-care, and health.

A further mission of nursing is to provide a public good, which should be indicated in the statement of mission or purpose. The statement of mission or purpose tells why the nursing entity exists. It is written so that it can be known by all people working within the organizational entity, because it states the reason for their employment. An ultimate strategy is to have nursing personnel participate in developing mission statements and in keeping them updated, so that they will know, understand, and support them.

The mission should also be known and understood by other health care practitioners, by clients and their families, and by the community. A statement of purpose must be dynamic, giving action and strength to evolving statements of philosophy, objectives, and management plans. Statements of purpose can be made dynamic by indicating the relationship between the nursing unit and patients, personnel, community, health, illness, and self-care. Figures 3–2, 3–3, and 3–4 represent examples of mission statements from three different levels: the organization, the division, and the unit, respectively.

Mission statements are used in successful business and industrial organizations to provide a clearly defined reason for being. They are simple statements to move the organization forward and

1. It is the mission of the University of South Alabama Medical Center to provide the best possible health care services and resources for the people of the community and the state and to provide a high-quality setting conducive to the medical education and research activities of the College of Medicine.

2. To provide good quality and cost-effective acute care services to patients to get them discharged to self-care as safely and quickly as possible.

3. To provide a dynamic innovative setting for clinical experiences for postgraduate education, medical students, nursing students, and allied health students.

4. To provide a setting for the conduct of funded medical, nursing, and allied health research.

5. To establish and maintain sound financial practices and procedures, recognizing the patient care and education missions will only be achieved through the protection and growth of hospital assets.

6. To provide a safe and comfortable environment that is conducive to learning and which provides an environment that allows the patient and family to feel their emotional and medical needs are being satisifed.

SOURCE: Courtesy of the University of South Alabama Medical Center, Mobile, Alabama.

Figure 3–2 • *Mission and Purpose of the University of South Alabama Medical Center*

are formulated for performance, products, and services. They contain statements of ethics, principles, and standards that are understood by workers. Workers who clearly perceive that they are pursuing meaningful and worthwhile goals through their individual efforts are more committed and dedicated than those who do not.[7]

Proprietary changes have brought change and competition to the hospital industry. They have also brought business techniques, moving the hospital industry from being facilities-dominated to being market-driven. The corporate structures of for-profit hospitals consider product line and function. They focus on mission. This focus has been adopted by not-for-profit hospitals that now look at mission statements relative to new markets, market share, and diversification. These new not-for-profit corporate structures are organized like chains and

The purposes of this organization shall be:

1. To assess, plan, implement, and evaluate nursing care in keeping with the standards for professional nursing practice, as defined by professional nurses of the staff and the ANA Standards of Nursing Practice. Believing that health is not merely the absence of disease or infirmity but a state of optimum physical, mental, and social well-being, nursing care promotes self-care concepts and enables clients to meet their basic human needs in coping with their health status throughout their life cycles.

2. To develop and continuously evaluate systems and methods of nursing management with open channels of communication between all levels of practitioners and other disciplines. This system holds final authority and accountability for the quality of nursing care delivered by each professional practitioner at every level.

3. To strive to constantly improve the quality of nursing care delivered by providing and promoting staff development programs, ongoing nursing research programs, and formal mechanisms for evaluating the level of care provided, including quality assurance, patient classification systems, and a quality monitoring system. In addition, to develop and implement formal client education programs fostering self-care abilities.

4. To be accountable for providing quality nursing care at the lowest cost to our clients utilizing the nursing process to set attainable self-care goals for them.

5. To evaluate, make changes and additions as needed.

SOURCE: Courtesy of the University of South Alabama Medical Center, Mobile, Alabama.

Figure 3–3 • *Purposes—Division of Nursing*

look at regionalization and integration as linkages. Their leadership is dynamic and future-oriented rather than being focused on maintenance.[8]

PHILOSOPHY

A written statement of philosophy sets out values and beliefs that pertain to nursing administration and nursing practice within the institution or organization. It verbalizes the nurse manager's and nurse practitioner's visions of what they believe

The purposes of the sixth floor are consistent with the purposes of the Division of Nursing.

1. To assess the physical, emotional, and spiritual needs of patients, their families and/or significant others so as to provide optimal care.

2. To provide each patient with an individualized plan of care, in regard to their needs, in a cost-effective manner to the patient and the hospital.

3. To serve as the patient's, family's, and/or significant other's advocate to assure complete care with regard to the patient's, family's, and/or significant other's needs.

4. To provide and promote continuing education through in-services, research projects, and patient care conferences to improve the quality of our health care.

5. To incorporate all disciplines related to patient's care, in evaluating the needs of the patient, family, and/or significant others.

6. To assess and evaluate our quality of nursing care on an ongoing basis through quality assurance and monthly audits.

SOURCE: Courtesy of the University of South Alabama Medical Center, Mobile, Alabama.

Figure 3–4 • *Purposes—Sixth Floor*

nursing management and practice are. It states their beliefs as to how the mission or purpose will be achieved, giving direction toward this end. Statements of philosophy are abstract and contain value statements about human beings as clients or patients and as workers, about work that will be performed by nursing workers for clients or patients, about self-care, about nursing as a profession, about education as it obtains to competence of nursing workers, and about the setting or community in which nursing services are provided. The character and tone of service are set by planning that evolves purpose and philosophy statements, one from the other, for the organization, division, department or service, and ward or unit.

Hodgetts indicates that all managers in any organization have a set of values, each generation being different from the preceding one.[9] Predictions of future values for the 1990s will reflect the future values of society. Nurse managers will be involved and will reflect the values of the times in their statements of philosophy. The philosophy of an or-

ganization is very often implicit and is not written down.

As with mission statements, philosophy statements evolve from higher levels of management and practice.

Figures 3–5, 3–6 and 3–7 are examples of philosophy statements for the organization, division, and unit levels, respectively.

OBJECTIVES

Objectives are concrete and specific statements of the goals that nurse managers seek to accomplish. They are action commitments through which the mission will be achieved and the philosophy or beliefs sustained. They are used to establish priorities. They are stated in terms of results to be achieved and focus on the production of health care services to clients. Like the statements of mission and philosophy, they must be functional and useful. They must be alive. Moore has stated, "If objectives are presented in terms of what can be observed, they can serve as useful tools for evaluation of nursing care and personnel performance, and as a basis for planning educational programs, staffing, requisition of supplies and equipment, and other functions associated with the nursing department."[10]

According to Moore, there should be objectives for evaluation of patient care, evaluation of personnel performance, planning educational programs, staffing, and requisition of supplies and equipment.

Drucker indicates that mission and purpose, as well as the basic definition of a business, have to be translated into objectives if they are to become more than insight, good intentions, and brilliant epigrams never to be achieved. Objectives are the concrete statements that become the standards against which performance can be measured. Objectives are the basic tactics of any business, including the business of nursing management. Objectives must be selective rather than global and they must be multiple rather than single, so as to balance a wide range of needs and goals related to nursing services to clients or patients; productive use of people, money, and material resources; updating through innovation; and the discharge of a social responsibility to the community. Objectives must be used, and one way to use them is to develop them into specific management and operational plans.[11]

The nursing staff—specifically, the nurse manager—must decide where efforts will be concen-

Policy. We believe that:

- The University of South Alabama Medical Center is dedicated to excellence in the fields of patient care, teaching, and research.
- We are dedicated to providing the most effective and efficient patient care.
- We are committed to provide services for patients requiring highly specialized and unique medical treatment.
- We are committed to providing a safe environment for patients, staff, and guests. We assure the rights of patients to confidentiality, full disclosure of risks involved in care, and involvement in decision making.
- Continuing education is essential to competence of staff. Professional growth and development is both a personal and organizational responsibility.
- Research should be fostered to the extent possible and should follow acceptable guidelines for protection of human subjects.
- We have an obligation to monitor all activities through quality assurance and to initiate corrective measures when indicated.
- Everyone should be treated with dignity.

- There are fiscal limits to what we can do, therefore every employee must market the hospital to obtain revenues to maintain financial stability.
- Health care for the medically indigent is the responsibility of society and the community from which they come. Our capacity and obligation for providing indigent care is limited to what the community supports.
- We have an obligation to use our finances and limited resources responsibly and maintain and improve the fiscal integrity of our institution.
- Health care should focus on wellness as well as illness. We promote and plan for patients to care for themselves from time of admission.
- We are the leaders in health care in this community. We believe in supporting laws and regulations and in working to make changes that benefit our mission.
- Our staff are our best asset and they will be treated with respect.
- Our staff have a responsibility to provide learning experiences for all students in the health care field, including providing appropriate clinical settings and role models.

SOURCE: Courtesy of the University of South Alabama Medical Center, Mobile, Alabama.

Figure 3–5 • *Philosophy of the University of South Alabama Medical Center*

trated to achieve results. Some areas of concentration have already been mentioned. Others may be similar to those related to business and industry. They include marketing and the development of health care services in areas of need. As an example, there has recently been increased activity in the area of physical and mental wellness or fitness. There is potential for much more in the area of prevention of disease and injury.

Another area for objectives is innovation. This would include the introduction of new methods and particularly the application of new knowledge.

Organization and use of all resources—human, financial, and physical—are areas for objectives. They address the need to develop managers, the needs of major groups within the division including nonmanagerial workers, labor relations, the development of positive employee attitudes, and maintenance and upgrading of employee skills. Objectives provide for attractive job and career op-

portunities. They provide activities to control worker assignment and productivity. Objectives are the means by which productivity in nursing is measured.

Objectives are also needed in the area of social responsibility. Society must believe that nursing is useful and productive and that it does a desired job; see Figure 3–8.

Management balances objectives. Some will be short range with their accomplishment in easy view or reach. Others will be long range, and some may even be in the "hope to accomplish" category. The budget is the mechanical expression of setting and balancing objectives. The nurse manager plans two budgets, one for operations and one for future capital expenditures.

Objectives are the fundamental strategy of nursing, because they specify the end product of all nursing activities. They must be capable of being converted into specific targets and specific assign-

We believe that:

- The philosophy of the Division of Nursing is consistent with the philosophy of the University of South Alabama Medical Center.
- We are dedicated to excellence in patient care, teaching, and research and to providing the most effective and efficient care.
- Everyone should be treated with dignity.
- Health is not merely the absence of disease or infirmity but a state of optimum physical, mental, and social well-being.
- Nursing care promotes self-care concepts, enabling patients to meet their basic human needs in coping with their health status throughout their life cycles. Nursing involves a broad approach of health care aimed at a healthy society through education of the public.
- Professional nursing care at University of South Alabama Medical Center is provided equally to all patients accepted for treatment.
- Patients and their families have a right to be kept informed about all aspects of their health status and to participate in decisions affecting their care to the fullest extent possible.

- The physical, mental, spiritual, and social needs of our patients can be achieved by striving to maintain goal-directed multidisciplinary plans of care.
- The highly specialized care offered at the Medical Center requires qualified staff for all positions. The most important assets of the institution are the staff and they will be treated with respect.
- We have an obligation to manage personnel and finances to achieve maximum productivity.
- Improvement of the quality of nursing is assured by the continuous evaluation of nursing care and positive modifications to nursing techniques and activities.
- Continuing education is essential to the delivery of quality professional nursing and is both a personal and organizational responsibility.
- We have a responsibility to provide appropriate learning experiences and role models for all students in the health care field.
- We accept the responsibility of being involved in nursing research.

SOURCE: Courtesy of the University of South Alabama Medical Center, Mobile, Alabama.

Figure 3–6 • *Philosophy of the Division of Nursing*

- We believe that all patients should be given equal, individualized care by all nursing staff incorporating physical, emotional, and spiritual needs.
- We believe the goal of health care should be assisting the patient to progress toward a level of optimal health.
- We believe that the patient should be encouraged by all nursing staff to progress toward self-care and independence.
- We believe that it is the responsibility of all nursing staff to act as a patient advocate to

provide quality care according to the wishes of the patient, family, and/or significant others.
- We believe that continuing education is a necessary component of continuing improvement in health care.
- We believe that nursing is an integral part of health care, and the nurse is an important member of the health care team.
- We believe that patients, their families, and/or significant others have the right to be well informed about the patient's state of health, prognosis, and care.

SOURCE: Courtesy of the University of South Alabama Medical Center, Mobile, Alabama.

Figure 3–7 • *Philosophy of Sixth Floor*

- *Evaluation of patient care*. To develop methods of measuring the quality of patient care.

  Evaluation of personnel performance. The patient benefits from close nursing supervision of all nonprofessional personnel who give patient care and from continuous appraisal of the nursing care given and the performance of all nursing personnel based on professional standards.

- *Planning educational programs*. The patient benefits from a continuous, flexible program of in-service education for all division of nursing personnel, adapted to orientation, skill training, continuous education, and leadership development.

- *Staffing*. To establish a systematic staffing pattern for patient care so that all members of each department can function in accordance with their skill levels for the maintenance of continuity of nursing care and management of nursing service.

- *Requisition of supplies and equipment*. To supply nursing personnel with adequate resources to facilitate patient care; to anticipate future nursing needs and plan for the acquisition of needed resources.

- *Marketing*. To collaborate and consult with intradepartmental health team members for maximal effectiveness in promoting health care and disease prevention. New programs will be developed to meet identified needs.

- *Innovation*. To influence progressive nursing practices and research training programs in supporting changing trends that improve the quality of patient care.

- *Organization and use of all resources (human, financial, and physical)*. To apply standards for decentralization of decision making and increase efficiency and effectiveness of staffing and budgeting.

- *Social responsibility*. To support, publicize, and sustain service to the community in health endeavors.

Some of these objectives are not as clearly stated as they could be; however, each was fully developed in the operational plan for its accomplishment.

Figure 3–8 • *Examples of Categorical Areas for Writing Objectives*

ments so that nurses will know what they have to do to accomplish them. Objectives become the basis and motivation for the nursing work necessary to accomplish them and for measuring nursing achievement. They make possible the concentration of human and material resources and of human efforts. Objectives are needed in all areas on which the survival of nursing and health care services depend. In nursing all objectives should be performance objectives that provide for existing nursing services for existing patient groups. They provide for abandonment of unneeded and outmoded nursing services and health care products. They provide for new nursing services and health care products for existing patients. They provide for new groups of patients, for the distributive organization, and for standards for nursing service and performance.

Objectives are the basis for work and assignments. They determine the organizational structure, the key activities, and the allocation of people to tasks. Objectives make the work of nursing clear and unambiguous, with measurable results, deadlines, and specific assignments of accountability. They give direction and make commitments that mobilize the resources and energies of nursing for the making of the future. Objectives are needed for the organization, division, and all wards or units. They should be changed as necessary particularly when there is a change of mission or when current objectives are no longer functional.[12] Refer to Figure 3–9 for examples of these categories of objectives. Figures 3–10, 3–11, and 3–12 are examples of objectives for an organization, a nursing division, and a nursing unit, respectively.

THE OPERATIONAL PLAN

Objectives must be converted into actions: activities, assignments, and deadlines, all with clear accountability. The action level is where nurse managers eliminate the old and plan for the new. It is where time dimensions are put into perspective and new and different methods can be tried. It is where nurse managers answer these questions over and over again: What is it? What will it be? What should it be?

An operational plan is the written blueprint for achieving objectives. It specifies the activities and procedures that will be used to achieve them and sets timetables for their achievement. It tells who the responsible persons are for each and every ac-

- *A performance objective.* The patient receives individualized care in a safe environment to meet the total therapeutic nursing needs—physical, emotional, spiritual, environmental, social, economic, and rehabilitative.
- *Existing nursing services for existing patients.* Nurse consultants have been made available from medical nursing, surgical nursing, mental health nursing, and maternal and child health nursing. Their services can be requested by any professional nurse or physician.
- *Abandonment of outmoded nursing services and products.* New isolation procedures have been implemented and the old handwashing basins have been discarded.
- *New nursing services for new groups of patients.* Plans are being made to offer consultative nursing services from the general hospital to nursing homes in the area. In the future this will be extended to retirement homes. Both actions are the result of market surveys.
- *Distributive organization for new nursing services.* The nurse manager has evaluated the necessity for restructuring the organization of the division of nursing to provide the new nursing services.
- *Standards of nursing service and performance.* The nurse manager has decided to use the Standards of Nursing Practice developed by the ANA Congress for Nursing Practice for all nurses within the division.

Figure 3–9 • *Examples of Categories of Objectives*

tivity and procedure. It describes ways of preparing people for jobs and procedures for evaluating care of patients. It specifies the records that will be kept and the policies needed. It gives individual managers freedom to accomplish their own objectives as well as those of the institution, division, department, ward, or unit. The operational plan is sometimes called a management plan. Refer to Figures 3–13 and 3–14.

STRATEGY

Planning is the strategy of an organization. It is essential to any and all businesses including those providing health care. Top management has to answer planning questions like these:

1. Where do we go and what do we want to become? Such questions seek to define the organization's mission and objectives.
2. What and where are we now? The purpose here is to examine and define the organization's philosophy and objectives.
3. How can we best get there? The answer to this question will take the form of ongoing plans that include organizing, directing, and controlling concepts.

Such activities constitute the strategy of top management. They are developed into the strategy of the nursing division's top management and subsequently into the strategy of nursing and other business units of the organization. Planning is neither a top-down or a bottom-up proposition. Each level must harmonize their strategies with those below and above.[13]

Focusing on development and use of planning strategies is a key element that gives direction, cohesion, and thrust to the nursing division. Nurse employees involved in achieving objectives and goals are motivated. These goals and objectives should be clearly defined and focus on the future without losing sight of the present. Successful implementation of management plans to achieve mission, objectives, and goals while sustaining philosophy results in productivity, profitability, and achievement. This process is managing and it is performed by managers.[14]

SUMMARY

The basic tools of management planning are statements of mission or purpose, philosophy or beliefs, and objectives, and an active operational or management plan. All managers use such documents to accomplish the work of nursing.

The statement of mission or purpose tells the reason an entity exists, be it the organization, division, department, or unit. The nursing mission statement pertains to the clinical practice of nursing supported by research, education, and management.

The statement of philosophy reflects the values and beliefs of the organizational entity. It is translated into action by nursing personnel.

Objectives are concrete statements describing the major accomplishments nurses desire to

Global Goals

Increase paying patients.

Increase awareness of resources among public.

Short-term plan of what we sell.

Long-term plan of what we sell.

Increase in services.

Educate the staff to sell the hospital formal plan to build hospital on campus.

Research provision of differently priced services.

Market hospital to university employees.

Improve access to hospital.

Improve intelligence.

Residents to use Medical Center for private practice.

Improve managing of patients for maximum reimbursement.

Create new markets.

Improve efficiency.

Recognize hospital as a business.

Reconcile difference in goals between Foundation and hospital.

Definitive Goals

1. Increase paying patients.
   1.1 Plan for incentive for MDs (Steve).
   1.2 Who are private MDs using hospital? (Pat).
   1.3 Survey private MDs in town (John).
   1.4 Market HMO (internal) (Susie and John).
   1.5 Input from department heads (Brookley meeting).
   1.6 Create new markets and identify opportunities through money arrangements.
      1.6.1 Where are they? (dept. heads).
      1.6.2 Maintain ROA.
      1.6.3 Maintain Keesler arrangement.
      1.6.4 Surrounding counties.
      1.6.5 HHC.
      1.6.6 Public service (plan for industry—Pat).
      1.6.7 Organizations and involvement (clinic and campus).
      1.6.8 Student organizations on campus.
   1.7 Market hospital to university employees.
2. Increase awareness of resources among public.
   2.1 PR plan.
   2.2 Short-term marketing plan of what we sell (identifying what we are selling now).
3. Long-term marketing plan of what we sell.
   3.1 What new products can we sell (or divert)?
   3.2 Formal plan to build hospital on campus.
4. Educate the staff to sell the hospital.
   4.1 Just for the pride of it.
   4.2 Management people in civic organizations.
   4.3 Reference 1.4.
   4.4 Employees identify with PR and marketing people.
   4.5 Recognize hospital as a business
5. Research provision of differently priced services.
   5.1 Innovative ways to bill for services.
6. Improve access to hospital.
   6.1 Parking.
   6.2 Waiting areas.
   6.3 Emergency Department.
7. Improve intelligence (above board).
   7.1 Professional groups.
   7.2 Reference 4.2.
   7.3 Internal network.
8. Residents to use Medical Center for private practice.
9. Improve efficiency.
   9.1 Improve managing of patients for maximum reimbursement.
      9.1.1 Audit bills with charts.
10. Improve cooperative relationship between Foundation (C of M) and Medical Center.

SOURCE: Courtesy of the University of South Alabama Medical Center, Mobile, Alabama.

Figure 3-10 • *Goals of the University of South Alabama Medical Center*

The objectives of this Division of Nursing shall be to provide the patient:

1. Individualized care in a safe environment to meet the patient's total needs as assessed by the professional nurse, utilizing the nursing process. This care covers physical, emotional, spiritual, environmental, social, economic, and rehabilitational needs involved in planning total patient care.

2. An effective teaching program which will include guidance and assistance in the use of medical resources and community agencies.

3. Benefits of effective communication, cooperation, and coordination with all professional and administrative services involved in the planning of total patient care.

4. Benefits of a continuous, flexible program of in-service education for all departments of nursing personnel adapted to orientation, in-service, continuing education, and leadership development.

5. Benefits from nursing services' participation in education of students.

6. With cost-effective care by the timely procurement, effective utilization, and proper handling of equipment and supplies.

7. Benefits through a positive work atmosphere in which nurses' job satisfaction is attained.

8. Benefits from a close association between division of nursing personnel and community nursing organizations and groups to keep abreast of current trends and advancements in nursing.

9. Maximum nursing care hours, by relieving nursing personnel of nonnursing duties.

10. Benefits from the development of a cost-effective balanced budget for the division of nursing.

11. Benefits from close supervision by an RN of all personnel who give patient care, and from continuous evaluation of the care given.

12. Benefits from implementation of the results of nursing research.

SOURCE: Courtesy of the University of South Alabama Medical Center, Mobile, Alabama.

Figure 3–11 • *Objectives of the Division of Nursing*

The objectives of the Sixth Floor shall be to provide the patient, family, and/or significant others:

1. Individualized total patient care based on an assessment by an RN, considering all needs, physical, emotional, and spiritual, of the patient, family, and/or significant others.

2. The nursing process will be the basis of all care given by the professional nurse.

3. To provide quality care in a cost-effective manner to patient and hospital.

4. To coordinate information from all disciplines, to plan for optimum care while hospitalized and after discharge.

5. To involve the patient's family and/or significant others in caring for the patient to meet their needs.

6. To identify problem areas in nursing care through monthly audits to ensure the quality of our nursing care.

7. To provide a variety of in-service training from all departments involved in the care of the patient to increase knowledge and improve nursing care.

SOURCE: Courtesy of the University of South Alabama Medical Center, Mobile, Alabama.

Figure 3–12 • *Objectives of Sixth Floor*

achieve. Major categorical areas for objectives include:

1. Organization and use of all resources—human, financial, and physical.
2. Social responsibility.
3. Staffing.
4. Requisition of supplies and equipment.
5. Planning educational programs.
6. Innovation.
7. Marketing.
8. Evaluation of patient care.
9. Evaluation of personnel performance.

Operational or management plans convert objectives into action and include activities, assignments, deadlines, and provision for accountability. A major strategy of an organization is the planning process and the formulation and use of statements of mission, philosophy, and objectives and organi-

Objective. The client receives skilled nursing services to meet his total individual needs as diagnosed by professional nurses. This process is systematic, beginning with the gathering of base data, and it is planned, implemented, evaluated, and revised continually. It covers physical, emotional, spiritual, environmental, social, economical, and rehabilitational needs and includes health teaching involved in the planning of total client care. Its ultimate goal is to assist clients to, or return them to, optimal health status and independence as quickly as possible.

Actions	Target Dates	Accomplishments
1. Institute primary care nursing.	January 1–June 30	Assigned to Ms. Scott. Decision made to attempt to use self-care concepts of Orem: (1) definition, and (2) nursing systems.
1.1 Assign problem of overall development of a plan.	January 31	
1.2 Assign development of a self-care concept for application using Orem and Kinlein as references.	February 15	Assigned to Ms. Longez, January 19. In discussion with Ms. Scott and Ms. Longez a decision was made to investigate application of self-care using the nursing process as described by Kinlein. The nursing staff were particularly interested in the nursing history process described by Kinlein. Ms. Longez has added this dimension to her assignment. She has requested Mr. Jarmann be assigned to assist her and he has agreed.
1.3 Organize resources.	February 28	February 5: Ms. Scott has just updated me on the project. A good portion of her plan has been developed. They are now doing a staffing plan including job descriptions and job standards. February 27: The plan is completed and has been discussed with me. A few minor adjustments are being made.
1.4 Coordinate plan.	March 31	
1.4.1 Nursing personnel		Done. All want to participate.
1.4.2 Administrator		Done.
1.4.3 Public relations		Announcements made to community through new media.
1.4.4 Physicians		Done and well received.
1.4.5 Others as needed		Presented to board per request of administrator. They want progress reports.
1.5 Select and train staff.	April 30	Assigned to Ms. Finch for training. Will be assisted by Ms. Scott and Ms. Longez. I will select staff with their recommendations.
1.6 Implement.	June 30	Ms. Scott wants to direct implementation and I have concurred.

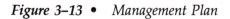

Figure 3–13 • *Management Plan*

1. A written management plan has been developed that operationalizes the objectives of the nursing division, department, service, or unit. It specifies activities or actions, persons responsible for accomplishing them, target dates or time frames, and provides for evaluation of progress. Each activity or action has been listed in problem-solving or decision-making format where appropriate.

2. The management plan is personal to the position occupied by the incumbent who selects the standards for developing, maintaining, and evaluating it. The nurse manager solicits desired input from appropriate nursing persons and others.

3. The actions reflect planning for:

3.1 Nursing care programs to ensure safe and competent nursing services to clients.

3.1.1 The nursing process including data gathering, assessment, diagnosis, goal setting and prescription, intervention and application, evaluation, feedback, change, accountability to the consumer.

3.1.2 Process and outcome audit.

3.1.3 Promotion of self-care practices.

3.2 Establishment of policies and procedures for employing competent nursing personnel: recruitment, selection, assignment, retention, and promotion based on individual qualifications and capabilities without regard to race, national origin, creed, color, sex, or age.

3.3 Integration of nursing care programs into the total program of the health care organization and community through committee participation in professional and service activities, and credentialing of individuals in organizations including nursing.

3.4 A budget that is evaluated and revised as necessary.

3.5 Job descriptions that include standards stated as objectives, outcomes, or results and that are known to the incumbents.

3.6 Detailing utilization of personnel.

3.6.1 According to a staffing plan based on timing nursing activities and on rating patients.

3.6.2 Matches competencies of people to total job requirements.

3.6.3 Places prepared people in practice.

3.6.4 Places prepared people in administration.

3.6.5 Places prepared people in education.

3.6.6 Places prepared people in research.

3.6.7 Fosters identification and assignment of nonnursing tasks to appropriate other departments or to nonnursing persons.

3.6.8 Recognizes excellence in all fields: administration, education, research, and practice.

3.7 Provision of needed supplies and equipment to do nursing activities.

3.8 Provision of input into remodeling and establishing required physical facilities.

3.9 Orientation and continuing education of all nursing personnel.

3.10 Education of students in the health care field according to a written agreement and collaborative implementation between faculty of the educational institutions and personnel of the service organization.

3.11 Nursing research—staff, application of research findings of others, and ongoing research activities.

3.12 Evaluation of all objectives—organizational, divisional, departmental, service, unit, and those stated in the individual's job description and standards.

4. The management plans have mileposts that are reasonable and attainable. There are deadlines.

5. Management plans are based on complete information.

6. You may add to these standards.

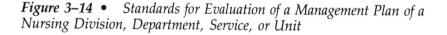

Figure 3–14 • *Standards for Evaluation of a Management Plan of a Nursing Division, Department, Service, or Unit*

zational plans developed with the broadest possible input.

Statements of mission, philosophy, and objectives support each other at different management levels: from the unit up to the service or department, then to the division, and finally to the organization.

EXPERIENTIAL EXERCISES

1. Use the standards for the evaluation of mission or purpose statements of the nursing division, department, service, or unit in Figure 3–15 to evaluate or develop a mission statement of the unit in which you work as a student. Summarize your findings.

2. Use the standards for evaluation of philosophy statement of the nursing division, department, service, or unit in Figure 3–16 to evaluate a philosophy statement of the unit in which you work as a student; or, use the standards to develop a new philosophy statement. First, develop a list of key words or concepts that embody your peer group's beliefs about nursing. Summarize your findings or state your philosophy.

3. Match each categorical area for writing objectives listed in Section I with the appropriate objective from Section II by placing the correct letter in the space provided. The objectives were actually written for various divisions of nursing.

I

   a. Evaluation of patient care
   b. Evaluation of personnel performance
   c. Planning educational programs
   d. Staffing
   e. Requisition of supplies and equipment
   f. Marketing
   g. Innovation

II

____ 3.1 To collaborate and consult with intradepartmental and interdepartmental health team members for maximal effectiveness in promoting health care and disease prevention.

____ 3.2 To influence progressive nursing practices and research training programs in supporting changing trends that improve the quality of patient care.

1. The mission statement tells the reason for the existence of the nursing division, department, service, or unit in relation to the practice of nursing and of self-care as defined by the nursing staff and in relation to the service being provided to the community of clients. Once definitions of nursing and self-care have been developed by the nursing staff and ratified by the nursing administration, they may be quoted in the mission statement.

2. The mission statement supports the mission of the organization, within the nursing division.

3. It indicates that the nursing organization exists to provide a public good.

4. You may add to these standards.

Figure 3–15 • *Standards for the Evaluation of Mission or Purpose Statements of the Nursing Division, Department, Service, or Unit*

____ 3.3 To develop methods of measuring the quality of patient care.

____ 3.4 To supply nursing personnel with adequate resources to facilitate patient care. To anticipate future nursing needs and plan for the acquisition of needed resources.

____ 3.5 To establish a systematic staffing pattern for patient care so that all members of each department can function in accordance with the skill level for the maintenance of continuity of nursing care and management of nursing service.

____ 3.6 The patient benefits from a continuous, flexible program of in-service education for all department of nursing personnel, adapted to orientation, skill training, continuing education, and leadership development.

____ 3.7 The patient benefits from close nursing supervision of all nonprofessional personnel who give patient care and from continuous evaluation of the nursing care given and performances of all nursing personnel based on professional standards.

4. Use the standards for evaluation of statements of objectives for a nursing division, department, service, or unit in Figure 3–17 to evaluate objectives of the unit in which you work as a student; or, use

1. A written statement of philosophy should exist for the nursing division, department, service, or unit.

2. A written statement of philosophy should be developed in collaboration with nursing employees, the consumers, and other health care workers.

3. Nursing personnel share in an annual (or more frequent) review and revision of the written statement of philosophy.

4. The written statement of philosophy should reflect these beliefs or values:

   4.1 The meaning of the clinical practice of nursing.

   4.2 Recognition of rights of individuals and of the responsibility of nursing personnel to serve as advocates for those rights.

   4.3 Selective other statements about humanity, society, health, nursing, nursing process, and self-care relevant to external forces (community, laws, etc.) and internal forces (personnel, clients, material resources, etc.), research, education, and family as are deemed appropriate to accomplishing the mission of the division, department, service, or unit.

5. The nursing philosophy should support the philosophy of the organization as expressed at all levels above it in the nursing division.

6. The statement of philosophy should give direction to the achievement of the mission.

7. You may add to these standards.

Figure 3–16 • *Standards for Evaluation of Philosophy Statement of the Nursing Division, Department, Service, or Unit*

1. The objectives for the nursing division, department, service, or unit should be in written form.

2. The objectives should be developed in collaboration with the nursing personnel who will assist in achieving them.

3. Nursing personnel should share in an annual (or more frequent) review and revision of the written statements of objectives.

4. The written statements of objectives should meet these qualitative and quantitative criteria:

   4.1 They operationalize the statements of mission and philosophy; they can be translated into actions.

   4.2 They can be measured or verified.

   4.3 They exist in a hierarchy or sequence that is by priority.

   4.4 They are clearly stated.

   4.5 They are realistic in terms of human and physical resources and capabilities.

   4.6 They direct the use of resources.

   4.7 They are achievable (practical).

   4.8 They are specific.

   4.9 They indicate results expected of nursing efforts and activities; the ends of management programs.

   4.10 They show a network of desired events and results.

   4.11 They are flexible and allow for adjustment.

   4.12 They are known to the nursing personnel who will use them.

   4.13 They are quantified wherever possible.

   4.14 They exist for all positions.

5. You may add to these standards.

Figure 3–17 • *Standards for Evaluation of Statements of Objectives for a Nursing Division, Department, Service, or Unit*

the standards to develop new objectives. Summarize your findings or state your objectives.

5. Use the standards for evaluation of a management plan of a nursing division, department, service, or unit in Figure 3–14 to evaluate a management plan of a unit in which you work as a student, or develop one from an objective in Figure 3–11.

6. Make each of the following statements true by crossing out the inappropriate words or phrase within parentheses.

6.1 The division of nursing exists (to make a profit; for the good of the people).

6.2 (Like; Unlike) business and industry, the department of nursing has (no impact on society; a social impact on society because it provides health care services).

6.3 The division of nursing (produces an impact; does not produce an impact) on society because of the number of people employed there.

6.4 Used disposables such as syringes and needles, contaminated dressings, and other waste products and pollutants from the division of nursing (have; do not have) an impact on society.

6.5 People may view (business and industry; the division of nursing) as more concerned for the quality of life than (economic institutions of the business world; nursing services).

6.6 It is the business of nurse managers to (satisfy the needs of patients; make a profit for the stockholders and the business).

NOTES

1. For a classic article on purpose, philosophy, and objectives, refer to M. A. Moore, "Philosophy, Purpose, and Objectives: Why Do We Have Them?," *Journal of Nursing Administration*, May-June 1971, 9–14.
2. V. Henderson, *The Nature of Nursing* (New York: Macmillan, 1966), 15.
3. H. Yura and M. B. Walsh, *The Nursing Process*, 5th ed. (New York: Appleton-Century-Crofts, 1988), 1.
4. I. M. King, "A Conceptual Frame of Reference in Nursing," *Nursing Research*, Jan.-Feb. 1968, 27–31.
5. D. E. Orem, *Nursing: Concepts of Practice*, 3d ed. (New York: McGraw-Hill, 1985), 18.
6. M. L. Kinlein, *Independent Nursing Practice with Clients* (Philadelphia: J. B. Lippincott, 1977), 23.
7. S. D. Truskie, "The Driving Force of Successful Organizations," *Business Horizons*, May-June 1984, 43–48.
8. G. E. Sussman, "CEO Perspectives on Mission, Healthcare Systems, and the Environment," *Hospital and Health Services Administration*, Mar./Apr. 1985, 21–34.
9. R. M. Hodgetts, *Management: Theory, Process, and Practice*, 4th ed. (Orlando, FL: Academic Press, 1986), 277–280.
10. Moore, op. cit., 13.
11. P. F. Drucker, *Management: Tasks, Responsibilities, Practice* (New York: Harper & Row, 1978), 99–102.
12. *Report on the Project for the Evaluation of the Quality of Nursing Service* (Ottawa, Ontario: Canadian Nurses Association, 1966), 47–48.
13. R. Cushman, "Norton's Top-Down, Bottom-Up Planning Process," *Planning Review*, Nov. 1979, 3–8, 48.
14. A. P. Meier, "The Planning Process," *Managerial Planning*, July/Aug. 1974, 1–5, 9.

FOR FURTHER REFERENCE

Cavanaugh, D. E., "Gamesmanship: The Art of Strategizing," *Journal of Nursing Administration*, Apr. 1985, 38–41.

Ehrat, K. S., "A Model for Politically Astute Planning and Decision Making," *Journal of Nursing Administration*, Sept. 1983, 29–35.

Sherman, V. C., "Taking Over: Notes to the New Executive," *Journal of Nursing Administration*, May 1982, 21–23.

•4•

Staffing and Scheduling

STAFFING PHILOSOPHY

Staffing is certainly one of the major problems of any nursing organization, whether it be a hospital, nursing home, home health care agency, ambulatory care agency, or another type of facility. Aydelotte has stated, "Nurse staffing methodology should be an orderly, systematic process, based upon sound rationale, applied to determine the number and kind of nursing personnel required to provide nursing care of a predetermined standard to a group of patients in a particular setting. The end result is prediction of the kind and number of staff required to give care to patients."[1]

The staffing process is complex. Components of the staffing process as a control system include a staffing study, a master staffing plan, a scheduling plan, and a nursing management information system (NMIS). The NMIS includes these five elements:

1. Quality of patient care to be delivered and its measurement.
2. Characteristics of the patients and their care requirements.
3. Prediction of the supply of nurse power required for items 1 and 2.
4. Logistics of the staffing program pattern and its control.
5. Evaluation of the quality of care desired, thereby measuring the success of the staffing itself.[2]

West adds a position control plan and a budgeting plan. See Figure 4–1.[3]

Nurse staffing must meet certain regulatory requirements. Among these are legal requirements of Medicare. The Medicare Survey report is excerpted in Figure 4–2.

This legal standard is further supported by other standards such as Nursing Services (NR) Standard NC4 of the *Accreditation Manual for Hospitals, 1991* depicted in Figure 4–3.

Other standards include the ANA *Standards for Organized Nursing Services and Responsibilities of Nurse Administrators across All Settings,* ANA *Standards of Nursing Practice,* and state licensing require-

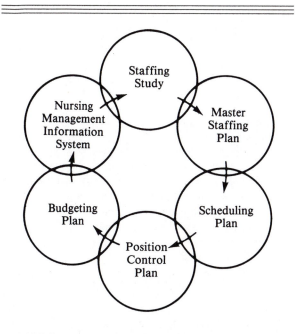

SOURCE: Reprinted from *Topics in Health Care Financing*, Vol. 6, No. 4, p. 15, with permission of Aspen Publishers, Inc., © 1980.

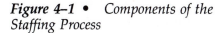

Figure 4–1 • Components of the Staffing Process

ments. From all of these and from the expectations of the community, of nurses, and of physicians, the nurse administrator will develop a staffing philosophy as a basis for a staffing methodology. Community expectations will be related to economic status, to local value and belief systems, and to local standards of culture. Nurses' expectations will be related to the same community standards and in addition to their perceptions of the practice of nursing and its components, to the results desired, and to the workload tolerated.

Nurse managers can discern from the nursing division's existing purpose, philosophy, and objectives various values related to staffing. A staffing philosophy may encompass beliefs about using a patient dependency system or patient classification system (PCS) for identifying patient care needs. It may cover beliefs about use of skilled personnel as a core staff with a float pool for supplemental staffing. It may also specify who will be responsible for hiring.[4]

Objectives of nurse staffing are excellent care and high productivity. Professional nurses can develop a statement of purpose that is comprehensive in stating the quality and quantity of performance it is intended to motivate. Purpose

statements should be quantified.[5] Examine those in Chapter 3.

STAFFING CONSIDERATIONS

A staffing study should gather data about environmental factors within and outside the organization that affect staffing requirements.

Such a study will use techniques drawn from engineering to measure the work of nurses. According to West a cardinal rule for forecasting staffing requirements is to base staffing projections on past staffing history.[6] Figure 4–4 is designed as a data sheet for this purpose. The data can be collected from the patient classification reports and census reports. Such data are readily available in most hospitals; some NMISs, such as Medicus, provide numbers of personnel required, including the mix of RNs, LPNs, and nurse aides. Other data needed are sick time, overtime, holidays, and vacation time. The attrition rate is also important. In some patient classification systems these are built into the staffing formula. For example, at the University of South Alabama Medical Center, the Medicus system provides the following formula for staffing:[7]

$$\frac{\text{Average Census} \times \text{Nursing Hours} \times 1.4 \times 1.14}{7.5}$$

Staffing requires much planning on the part of the nurse manager. Data must be collected and analyzed. These data include facts about the product—patient care. They include diagnostic and therapeutic procedures performed by both physicians and nurses. They include the knowledge elements of professional nursing translated into professional nursing skills of history taking and assessment, nursing diagnosis and prescription, application of care, evaluation, record keeping, and all other actions related to the primary health care of patients.

Basic to planning for staffing of a unit of nursing is the fact that qualified nursing personnel must be provided in sufficient numbers to ensure adequate, safe nursing care for all patients 24 hours a day, 7 days a week, 52 weeks a year. Each staffing plan must be tailored to the needs of the hospital and cannot be arrived at by a simple worker/patient ratio or formula.

Changing, expanding knowledge and technology in the physical and social sciences, in the medical field, and in economics influence planning for

482.23 *Condition of participation: Nursing services.*

The hospital must have an organized nursing service that provides 24-hour nursing services. The nursing services must be furnished or supervised by a registered nurse.

(a) *Standard: Organization.* The hospital must have a well-organized service with a plan of administrative authority and delineation of responsibilities for patient care. The director of nursing service must be a licensed registered nurse. He or she is responsible for the operation of the service, including determining the types and numbers of nursing personnel and staff necessary to provide nursing care for all areas of the hospital.

(b) *Standard: Staffing and delivery of care.* The nursing service must have adequate numbers of licensed registered nurses, licensed practical nurses (vocational), and other personnel to provide nursing care to all patients as needed. There must be supervisory and staff personnel for each department or nursing unit to ensure, when needed, the immediate availability of a registered nurse for bedside care of any patient.

(1) The hospital must provide 24-hour nursing service furnished or supervised by a registered nurse, and have a licensed practical nurse or registered nurse on duty at all times, except for rural hospitals that have in effect a 24-hour nursing waiver granted under §405.1910(c) of this chapter.

(2) The nursing service must have a procedure to ensure that hospital nursing personnel for whom licensure is required have valid and current licensure.

(3) A registered nurse must supervise and evaluate the nursing care for each patient.

(4) The hospital must ensure that the nursing staff develops, and keeps current, a nursing care plan for each patient.

(5) A registered nurse must assign the nursing care of each patient to other nursing personnel in accordance with the patient's needs and the specialized qualifications and competence of the nursing staff available.

(6) Non-employee licensed nurses who are working in the hospital must adhere to the policies and procedures of the hospital. The director of nursing service must provide for adequate supervision and evaluation of the clinical activities of non-employee nursing personnel which occur within the responsibility of the nursing service.

(c) *Standard: Preparation and administration of drugs.* Drugs and biologicals must be prepared and administered in accordance with Federal and State laws, the orders of the practitioner or practitioners responsible for the patient's care as specified under §482.12(c), and accepted standards of practice.

(1) All drugs and biologicals must be administered by, or under supervision of, nursing or other personnel in accordance with Federal and State laws and regulations including applicable licensing requirements, and in accordance with the approved medical staff policies and procedures.

(2) All orders and biologicals must be in writing and signed by the practitioner or practitioners responsible for the care of the patient as specified under §482.12(c). When telephone or oral orders must be used, they must be—

(i) Accepted only by personnel that are authorized to do so by the medical staff policies and procedures, consistent with Federal and State law;

(ii) Signed and initialed by the prescribing practitioner as soon as possible; and

(iii) Used infrequently.

(3) Blood transfusions and intravenous medications must be administered in accordance with State law and approved medical staff policies and procedures. If blood transfusions and intravenous medications are administered by personnel other than doctors of medicine or osteopathy, the personnel must have special training for this duty.

(4) There must be a hospital procedure for reporting transfusion reactions, adverse drug reactions, and errors in administration of drugs.

SOURCE: Commerce Clearing House, Inc., Medicare and Medicaid Regulations. As adopted, 51 F.R. 22010 (June 17, 1986, effective September 15, 1986), 8551-4 to 8551-5.

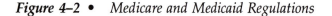

Figure 4–2 • *Medicare and Medicaid Regulations*

Standard

NC.4 The hospital's plan for providing nursing care is designed to support improvement and innovation in nursing practice and is based on both the needs of the patients to be served and the hospital's mission.*   1 2 3 4 5 NA

Required Characteristics

NC.4.1 The plan for nurse staffing and the provision of nursing care is reviewed in detail on an annual basis and receives periodic attention as warranted by changing patient care needs and outcomes.*   1 2 3 4 5 NA

NC.4.1.1 Registered nurses prescribe, delegate, and coordinate the nursing care provided throughout the hospital.*   1 2 3 4 5 NA

NC.4.1.2 Consistent standards for the provision of nursing care within the hospital are used to monitor and evaluate the quality and appropriateness of nursing care provided throughout the hospital.*   1 2 3 4 5 NA

NC.4.2 The appropriateness of the hospital's plan for providing nursing care to meet patient needs is reviewed as part of the established budget review process.*   1 2 3 4 5 NA

NC.4.2.1 The review includes

NC.4.2.1.1 an analysis of actual staffing patterns; and   1 2 3 4 5 NA

NC.4.2.1.2 findings from quality assurance activities.   1 2 3 4 5 NA

NC.4.2.2 The allocation of financial and other resources is assessed to determine whether nursing care is provided appropriately, efficiently, and effectively.   1 2 3 4 5 NA

NC.4.2.2.1 The allocation of financial and other resources is designed to support improvement and innovation in nursing practices.   1 2 3 4 5 NA

*The asterisked items are key factors in the accreditation decision process. For an explanation of the use of the key factors, see "Using the Manual," page ix.

SOURCE: Copyright 1990 by the Joint Commission on Accreditation of Healthcare Organizations, Oakbrook Terrace, IL. Reprinted with permission from the 1991 *Accreditation Manual for Hospitals.*

Figure 4–3 • *Nursing Services (NC) Standard NC.4 JCAHO*

staffing. Health care institutions are treating more clients on an outpatient basis. New drugs, improved diagnostic and therapeutic procedures, and reimbursement charges have decreased the lengths of hospitalization. Standards of the Joint Commission on Accreditation of Healthcare Organizations (JCAHO), the American Nurses' Association (ANA), and other professional and governmental organizations have required upgrading of health care.

Planning for staffing is influenced by changing concepts of nursing roles for clinical nursing practi-

tioners and specialists. Decision making is being delegated to the lowest practical level. Unit clerks and managers have assumed duties formerly done by nursing personnel.

Patient populations are changing as birth rates decline and people live longer. Staffing plans are influenced by institutional missions and objectives related to research, training, and many specialties. They are influenced by personnel policies and practices related to vacations, time off, overtime, holidays, and other factors. They are influenced by policies and practices related to admission and dis-

Year _____   Month _____   Cost Center _____

Day	ADC	Patient Acuity	Personnel				
			Sick Hours	Overtime Hours	Holiday Hours	Vacation Hours	Other
1							
2							
31							
Average							

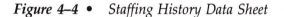

SOURCE: Constructed from M. E. West, "Implementing Effective Nurse Staffing Systems in the Managed Hospitals," *Topics in Health Care Financing,* Summer, 1980, 16.

Figure 4–4 • *Staffing History Data Sheet*

charge times of patients, assignment of patients to wards, and intensive and progressive care practices.

The amount and kind of nursing staff required will be influenced by the degree to which other de-partments carry out their supporting services. This is particularly true during weekends, evenings, nights, and holidays. Plans must be made to staff the requirements for nursing personnel to perform nonnursing duties such as dietary functions, clerical work, messenger and escort activities, and housekeeping. Whether these services should or should not be carried out by nursing personnel is not the point here; the point is that the degree to which the situation exists must be considered in any plan. Nurse managers must avoid assuming responsibility for nonnursing services and plan to encourage the appropriate departments to assume such services. When they do not, nurse managers should have a system of charging the provided services to the appropriate other cost center. This will then become revenue to the nursing cost center.

Staffing plans will be influenced by the number and composition of the medical staff and the medical services offered. Nursing requirements will be affected by characteristics of patient populations determined by the size and capability of the medical staff. Special requirements of individual physicians, time and length of their rounds; time, complexity, and number of tests, medications, and treatments; and kind and amount of surgery will all affect the quality and quantity of nursing personnel required and influence their placement.

Arrangement of the physical plant has a large impact on staffing requirements. Fewer personnel are needed for a modern, compact facility equipped with labor-saving devices and efficient working arrangements than for one that is spread out and has few or no labor-saving devices. Staffing for a facility that is arranged functionally will differ from one that is not so structured. If, for example, the operating suite is not next to the labor and delivery rooms, recovery room, and intensive care units, more staff will be needed to meet acceptable standards of quality and safety. Many other architectural features must be considered, such as location of patient rooms in relation to the nursing stations, the location of specialized units, work rooms, and storage space, and the time required to transport patients to other sections of the hospital for diagnostic or therapeutic services such as radiography and nuclear medicine.

Staffing is further affected by the organization of the division of nursing. Plans must be reviewed and revised to organize the department to operate efficiently and economically with written statements of mission, philosophy, and objectives; sound organizational structure; clearly defined functions and responsibilities; written policies and procedures; effective staff development programs; and planned periodic evaluation. Staffing plans for such a division will be different from those of a loosely organized division with overlapping functions and responsibilities, vague or conflicting policies, and poorly defined standards of nursing practice.

STAFFING ACTIVITIES

Price identified seventeen different staffing activities and suggested that the nurse administrator identify by names the persons responsible for each of the seventeen activities. These seventeen activities are:

1. Recruitment
2. Interviewing and screening
3. Hiring registered nurses
4. Hiring licensed practical nurses
5. Hiring nurse aides
6. Hiring orderlies
7. Assignment to clinical units
8. Assignment to shifts
9. Preparing work schedule in advance
10. Maintaining daily schedule
11. Adjusting: Staff absence, patient needs
12. Calculating turnover
13. Calculating hours of care
14. Checking time cards, payroll
15. Policy development
16. Telephone communication
17. Contract compliance

Price further suggested:

1. The one person ultimately responsible for each activity be identified.
2. The category and position of the person who *should* be responsible for each activity should be identified.
3. The activity should be specified as requiring nursing or nonnursing personnel.
4. The review be performed for the day shift, evening shift, night shift, and weekend and holiday shifts.[9]

Orientation Plan

A main purpose of orientation is to help the nursing worker adjust to a new work situation. This should be a planned program that includes orientation whether through a "buddy" system, a special orientation unit, or other method. Those nursing tasks and skills required of each nursing worker who is not proficient in them should be the focus of this program. Productivity is increased, because fewer personnel are needed when they are fully oriented to the work situation.

Staffing Policies

Written staffing policies should be readily available in at least the following areas:

1. Vacations
2. Holidays
3. Sick leave
4. Weekends off
5. Consecutive days off
6. Rotation to different shifts
7. Overtime
8. Part-time personnel
9. Use of "float" personnel
10. Exchangeability of staff
11. Use of special abilities of individual staff members
12. Exchanging hours
13. Requests of personnel
14. Requests of management
15. The work week

Work Contracts

There should be a work contract between each employee and the institution. The contract should state the date employment is to commence, the job classification, the hours of work, the rate of pay, whether the job is full time or part time, and any other specific points agreed on between employee and institutional representative. Both should sign it. See Figure 4–5.

STAFFING THE UNITS

Each patient care unit should have a master staffing plan. This should include the basic staff needed to staff the unit each shift. Basic staff is the minimum or lowest number of personnel needed to staff a unit. It includes fully oriented, full- and part-time employees. The number may be based on examination of previous staff records and through expert opinion of nurse managers. It includes all categories: registered nurses, licensed practical nurses, and nursing technicians or assistants for each shift. Basic staff may be the minimal number to be provided for determining a core staff per shift. See Figure 4–6 for a formula for determining a core staff per shift.

Next the number of *complementary* personnel are determined. They are scheduled as an addition to the basic group, but the total number in both groups will be controlled by financial resources and the availability of personnel. They provide the flexibility needed to meet short-range and unexpected changes. Complementary personnel are not assured a permanent pattern and are usually scheduled for 4-week periods.

Float personnel are employees who are not permanently assigned to a station. They provide flexibility to meet increased patient loads as well as unexpected personnel absences. The number and kinds of float personnel can be accurately determined from general monthly records that show absence rates, personnel turnover, and fluctuations in patient care workloads. Float personnel may be assigned to a pool.

STAFFING MODULES

Cyclic Scheduling

Cyclic scheduling is one of the best ways to meet the requirements of equitable distribution of hours of work and time off for staff. A basic time pattern for a certain number of weeks is established and then repeated in cycles.

Advantages of cyclic scheduling include the following:

1. Once developed, it is a relatively permanent schedule, requiring only temporary adjustments.
2. Nurses no longer have to live in anticipation of their time off-duty as it may be scheduled for as long as 6 weeks in advance.
3. Personal plans may be made in advance with a reasonable degree of reliability.
4. Requests for special time off are kept to a minimum.
5. It can be used with rotating, permanent, or mixed shifts and can be modified to allow fixed days off and uneven work periods, based on personnel needs and work period preferences.

I accept employment at El Camino Hospital with the following understanding. That I:

1. Must have Health Service clearance prior to hire.

2. Am being hired to work as a Staff Nurse _____ Step _____ at _____ (salary) starting _____ (orientation date). My employee time category will be _____ .

3. Am being assigned to _____ (unit) on _____ (shift) and commit myself to work on this unit and shift for a minimum of ____ months before requesting a transfer or status change.

4. Will float from my assigned area as required.

5. Am being employed on a trial basis for ninety days and that during this period a preceptor will be designated to oversee my orientation and will discuss my progress with me.

6. Will abide by the Job Description for my position, the rules of conduct as stated in the Employees Handbook and the Nursing Department dress code.

7. Understand that because of fluctuating patient census, the hospital cannot guarantee that I will work the full number of hours assigned in my category and that there may be times when it will be necessary for me to reschedule holidays or vacations or take time off without pay.

8. Can obtain information regarding retirement and employee benefits from the Personnel Department.

9. (Optional) We mutually agree to the following: _____

_____

_____

_____

_____

_____

_____

Signature of Applicant _____

Date _____

Original to Personnel
Copy to Employee
PA/hds   10/77

Signature of Head Nurse _____

Date _____

SOURCE: Reprinted from *Nursing Decentralization: The El Camino Experience* by J. N. Althaus et al., p. 50, with permission of Aspen Publishers, Inc., © 1981.

Figure 4–5 • *El Camino Hospital Nursing Service Work Agreement*

6. It can be modified to fit known or anticipated periods of heavy workload and can be temporarily adjusted to meet emergencies or unexpected shortages of personnel.

Because it is relatively inflexible cyclic scheduling only works with a staff that rotates by policy and personal choice. The best use of this type of schedule is as a staffing board indicating shift requirements. Allow personnel to select specific shifts to accommodate their personal needs. An infinite number of basic cyclic patterns can be developed, tailored to suit the needs of each unit. Samples are shown in Figure 4–7. Patterns should reflect policy, workload factors, and staff preferences. Nursing personnel may use a staffing board (Figure 4–8) to develop a pattern and cycle satisfactory to them.

Patterns should be reviewed periodically to see that they meet the purpose, philosophy, and objec-

The average daily census for a 25-bed medical-surgical unit over a 6-month period is 19 patients. The basic average daily hours of care to be provided are 5 hours per patient per 24 hours. How many total hours of care will be needed on the average day to meet these standards? 19 × 5 = 95 hours. If the work day is 8 hours, this means 95 ÷ 8 = 11.9 or 12 full-time equivalents (FTE) staff are needed to staff the unit for 24 hours. An FTE is one person working full time (40 hours a week) or several persons who together work a total of 40 hours a week.

A total of 12 FTE × 7 days per week = 84 shifts per week, will be needed if the staffing is to be the same each day.

If each employee works 5 8-hour shifts per week, 84 divided by 5 = 16.8, the number of FTEs needed as basic staff for this unit.

The number of nursing personnel to cover sick leave, vacations, and holidays or other absences can also be determined and added to the basic staff. This information is determined from a study of personnel policies and use. It is frequently included in patient classification system formulas. Such additional staff may be provided from a float pool.

The next determination to be made is the ratio of RNs to other nursing personnel. If the ratio is determined as 1:1, how many of the basic staff of 16.8 should be RNs? One-half of the total, which would be 8.4 RNs and 8.4 others (LPNs, nurse aides, orderlies, or nursing assistants). A study of staffing patterns in 80 medical/surgical, pediatric, and post-partum units in 12 Salt Lake City community hospitals recommends a mix of 58% RNs, 26% LPNs, and 16% aides.[10]

The final determination is how many personnel are needed for each shift. Warstler recommends proportions of day—47%, evening—35%, and night—17%.[11] This means that for a total staff of 16.8 personnel, 8 would be assigned to days, 6 to evenings, and 2.8 to nights. This is obviously approximate; other patterns could be chosen by the nurse administrator.

The number of complementary nursing personnel would be added to this basic staff. They could be a group of 1 RN, 1 LPN, and 1 other and assigned accordingly. They are entered into the following table as numbers in parentheses added to the figures for basic staff.

In today's reimbursement environment complementary personnel may be budgeted as a pool. They may even exist only as a portion of basic personnel assigned to a pool.

Basic Staffing Plan for 25-Bed Medical-Surgical Unit

	Day	Evening	Night	Totals
RNs	4 + (1)	3	1.4	8.4 + (1)
LPNs	2	2 + (1)	1.4	5.4 + (1)
Others	2	1	0 + (1)	3 + (1)
Totals	8 + (1)	6 + (1)	2.8 + (1)	16.8 + (3)

Figure 4–6 • *Formula for Estimating a Core Staff per Shift*

tives of the organization and the division of nursing, that they are practical with regard to the numbers and qualifications of personnel, that they are satisfactory to nursing personnel, that they are meeting patient needs, and that they are using people effectively.

Scheduling records should be kept for a specific time, probably 1 year. They provide valuable statistical information for staffing planning as well as historical information for questions related to personnel on duty when specific events occurred.

It has been stated previously that staffing policies should be established in specific areas. Policies that may be considered are:

1. Personnel are scheduled to work their preferred shift as much as possible.

2. Personnel choices are balanced to meet the needs of the unit and of other employees.

3. An employee is allowed to make arrangements for special time off or exchange within specific personnel policies.

4. Policies have been established for making schedule changes.

5. Each employee has a copy of the work schedule.

6. Consideration has been given to staffing during hours of clinical experience for students.

7. There is a weekend and holiday schedule policy; it is a common practice in many organizations throughout the United States to plan alternate weekends off for nursing personnel. Weekend coverage can be by "weekends only" employees; staffing levels needed can be influenced by hospital policies on admissions, discharges, and weekend staffing.

week	S	M	T	W	T	F	S	S	M	T	W	T	F	S	S	M	T	W	T	F	S	S	M	T	W	T	F	S
	1							**2**							**3**							**4**						
1	N	N	N	N	N	–	–	–	–	E	E	E	E	E	E	–	–	D	D	D	D	D	D	D	–	–	N	N
2	D	D	D	–	–	N	N	N	N	N	N	–	–	–	–	–	E	E	E	E	E	E	E	–	–	D	D	D
3	E	E	–	–	D	D	D	D	D	D	D	–	–	N	N	N	N	N	N	–	–	–	–	E	E	E	E	E
4	–	–	E	E	E	E	E	E	E	–	–	D	D	D	D	D	D	–	–	N	N	N	N	N	N	N	–	–
charge	–	D	D	D	D	D	–	–	D	D	D	D	D	–	–	D	D	D	D	D	–	–	D	D	D	D	D	–
N	1	1	1	1	1	1	1	1	1	1	1	1	1	1	1	1	1	1	1	1	1	1	1	1	1	1	1	1
D	1	2	2	1	2	2	1	1	2	2	1	2	2	1	1	2	2	1	2	2	1	1	2	2	1	2	2	1
E	1	1	1	1	1	1	1	1	1	1	1	1	1	1	1	1	1	1	1	1	1	1	1	1	1	1	1	1

Minimum Basic Schedule

week		S	M	T	W	T	F	S	S	M	T	W	T	F	S	S	M	T	W	T	F	S	S	M	T	W	T	F	S
		1							**2**							**3**							**4**						
Permanent shifts	1	N	N	N	–	–	N	N	N	N	–	–	N	N	N	N	N	N	–	–	N	N	N	N	–	–	N	N	N
	2	N	N	N	N	N	–	–	–	–	N	N	N	N	N	N	N	N	N	N	–	–	–	–	N	N	N	N	N
	3	E	E	E	E	E	–	–	E	E	E	E	E	–	–	E	E	E	E	E	–	–	E	E	E	E	E	–	–
	4	–	–	E	E	E	E	E	–	–	E	E	E	E	E	–	–	E	E	E	E	E	–	–	E	E	E	E	E
	5	E	E	–	–	D	E	E	E	E	–	–	D	E	E	E	E	–	–	D	E	E	E	E	–	–	D	E	E
	6	D	–	–	N	N	N	N	N	N	N	N	–	–	D	D	D	D	D	D	–	–	–	D	D	D	D	D	–
Rotate	7	–	D	D	D	D	D	–	–	D	D	D	–	D	D	D	–	–	N	N	N	N	N	N	N	N	–	–	D
	8	–	D	D	D	–	D	D	D	D	D	D	D	–	–	–	D	D	D	D	D	–	–	D	D	D	–	D	D
	9	D	D	D	D	D	–	–	–	D	D	D	D	D	–	–	D	D	D	–	D	D	D	D	D	D	D	–	–
Leave relief	10	–	–	D	D	D	D	D	D	D	–	D	D	D	–	–	–	D	D	D	D	D	D	D	–	D	D	D	–
assistant	11																												
charge	12																												

		S	M	T	W	T	F	S	S	M	T	W	T	F	S	S	M	T	W	T	F	S	S	M	T	W	T	F	S
		5							**6**							**7**							**8**						
	1	N	N	N	–	–	N	N	N	N	–	–	N	N	N	N	N	N	–	–	N	N	N	N	–	–	N	N	N
	2	N	N	N	N	N	–	–	–	–	N	N	N	N	N	N	N	N	N	N	–	–	–	–	N	N	N	N	N
	3	E	E	E	E	E	–	–	E	E	E	E	E	–	–	E	E	E	E	E	–	–	E	E	E	E	E	–	–
	4	–	–	E	E	E	E	E	–	–	E	E	E	E	E	–	–	E	E	E	E	E	–	–	E	E	E	E	E
	5	E	E	–	–	D	E	E	E	E	–	–	D	E	E	E	E	–	–	D	E	E	E	E	–	–	D	E	E
	6	–	D	D	D	–	D	D	D	D	D	D	D	–	–	–	D	D	D	D	D	–	–	D	D	D	–	D	D
	7	D	D	D	D	D	–	–	–	D	D	D	D	D	–	–	D	D	D	–	D	D	D	D	D	D	D	–	–
	8	D	–	–	N	N	N	N	N	N	N	N	–	–	D	D	D	D	D	D	–	–	–	D	D	D	D	D	–
	9	–	D	D	D	D	D	–	–	D	D	D	–	D	D	D	–	–	N	N	N	N	N	N	N	N	–	–	D
	10	–	–	D	D	D	D	D	D	D	–	D	D	D	–	–	–	D	D	D	D	D	D	D	–	D	D	D	–
	11																												
	12																												

Eight-Week Cycle—Mixed Shifts

SOURCE: Department of the Air Force, *USAF Hospital Nursing Service Manual* (Washington, D.C.: U.S. Government Printing Office, 1971), 4-4 to 4-14.

Figure 4–7 • *Cyclic Schedules*

(Continued)

Weeks 1–5 (each cell = S M T W T F S)

Team	1	2	3	4	5
1	N N N N N - -	E E E E E - -		- N N N N N -	- E E E
2	- N N N N	N - - E E E E	E -	- N N N N N	
3		- N N N N N -	- E E E E E -		- N N N N N
4	E E -			- N N N N N -	E E E E E -
5	- - E E E E E				- N N N N N -

Weeks 6–10

Team	6	7	8	9	10
1	E E - -			- N N N N N - -	E E E E E -
2	- - E E E E E -			- N N N N N	- - E E E E -
3	N N N N N - -	E E E E E -		- N N N N N - -	E E E
4		- N N N N N - -	E E E E E -	- N N N N N	
5		- N N N N N - -	E E E E E - -		

Weeks 11–15

Team	11	12	13	14	15
1		- N N N N N - -	E E E E E - -		- N N N N N
2		- N N N N N - -	E E E E E - -		- N N N N N -
3	E E -		- N N N N N - -	E E E E E -	
4	- - E E E E E - -			- N N N N N - -	E E E E E -
5	N N N N N - -	E E E E E - -		- N N N N N - -	E E E

Weeks 16–20

Team	16	17	18	19	20
1	- - E E E E E -			- N N N N N - -	E E E E E - -
2	N N N N N - -	E E E E E - -		- N N N N N - -	E E E
3		- N N N N N - -	E E E E E - -		- N N N N N
4			- N N N N N - -	E E E E E -	
5	E E -			- N N N N N - -	E E E E E -

Weeks 21–25

Team	21	22	23	24	25
1		- N N N N N - -	E E E E E -		
2	E E -		- N N N N N - -	E E E E E -	
3	- - E E E E E - -			- N N N N N - -	E E E E E - -
4	N N N N N - -	E E E E E -		- N N N N N - -	E E E
5		- N N N N N - -	E E E E E - -		- N N N N N

Twenty-Five-Week Cycle

Figure 4–7 (Continued)

(Continued)

Cyclic Schedule—Permanent Nights

week	1							2							3							4						
	S	M	T	W	T	F	S	S	M	T	W	T	F	S	S	M	T	W	T	F	S	S	M	T	W	T	F	S
1	N	N	N	N	N	—	—	—	N	N	N	N	N	—	—	N	N	N	N	N	—	—	N	N	N	N	N	—
2	D	D	E	—	—	N	N	N	D	D	—	—	E	N	E	—	D	D	—	N	E	D	—	—	E	N	D	D
3	E	E	—	—	D	D	D	D	E	—	E	D	D	D	D	—	E	—	N	D	E	—	E	N	D	D	E	E
4	—	I	D	E	D	D	D	—	—	D	E	D	D	D	—	D	D	N	—	E	—	E	D	D	N	E	—	—
5	I	—	—	D	D	D	I	—	I	D	D	E	—	—	D	D	N	E	—	—	I	D	D	N	—	—	I	I
charge	—	—	—	—	—	—	—	—	—	—	—	—	—	—	—	—	—	—	—	—	—	—	—	—	—	—	—	—
N	2	2	2	2	2	2	2	2	2	2	2	2	2	2	2	2	2	3	2	2	2	3	2	2	3	3	2	2
D	3	2	3	3	2	2	2	2	3	2	2	3	2	3	2	2	2	2	3	2	2	2	3	3	2	2	3	2
E	—	—	—	—	—	—	—	—	—	—	—	—	—	—	—	—	—	—	—	—	—	—	—	—	—	—	—	—

Seven-Week Rotating Cycle

week	1							2							3							4							5							6							7						
	S	M	T	W	T	F	S	S	M	T	W	T	F	S	S	M	T	W	T	F	S	S	M	T	W	T	F	S	S	M	T	W	T	F	S	S	M	T	W	T	F	S	S	M	T	W	T	F	S
charge	—	—	—	—	—	—	—	—	—	—	—	—	—	—	—	—	—	—	—	—	—	—	—	—	—	—	—	—	—	—	—	—	—	—	—	—	—	—	—	—	—	—	—	—	—	—	—	—	—
N	2	2	3	3	3	2	2	3	3	3	3	3	3	2	3	3	3	2	2	2	2	3	3	3	2	2	3	2	3	3	3	3	3	2	2	3	3	3	3	2	3	2	2	3	3	3	3	3	2
D	2	2	2	2	2	2	2	2	2	2	2	2	2	2	2	2	2	2	2	2	2	2	2	2	2	2	2	2	2	2	2	2	2	2	2	2	2	2	2	2	2	2	2	2	2	2	2	2	2

Figure 4–7 (*Continued*)

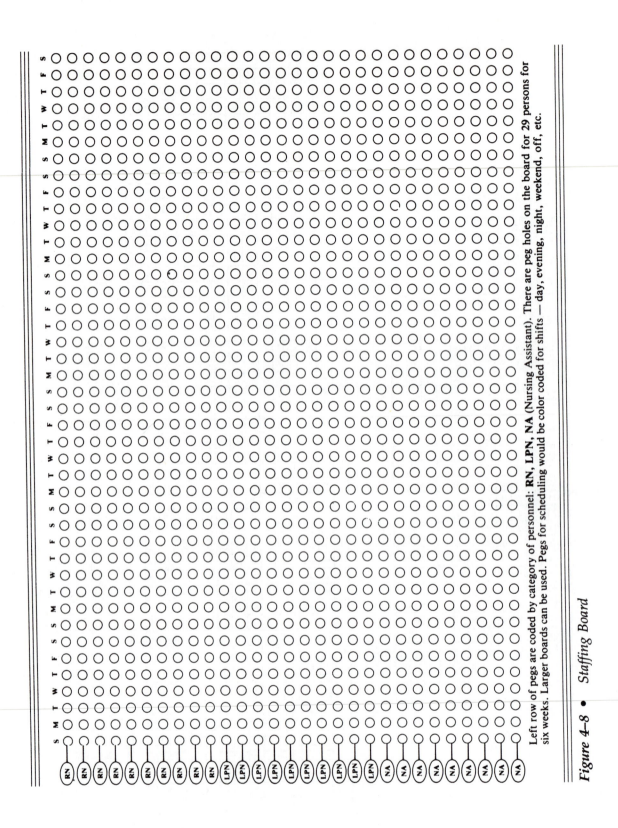

Left row of pegs are coded by category of personnel: **RN, LPN, NA** (Nursing Assistant). There are peg holes on the board for 29 persons for six weeks. Larger boards can be used. Pegs for scheduling would be color coded for shifts — day, evening, night, weekend, off, etc.

Figure 4–8 • *Staffing Board*

PATIENT CLASSIFICATION SYSTEMS

A patient classification system (PCS) is essential to staffing nursing units of hospitals. It quantifies the quality of nursing care. In selecting or implementing a PCS a representative committee of nurse managers and clinical nurses should be used. The committee can include a representative of hospital administration. Inclusion of the latter will decrease skepticism about the PCS.

Purposes

The committee will identify the purposes of the PCS to be purchased or developed. Among these purposes are:

1. Staffing. The system will establish a unit of measure for nursing: *time.* This unit of measure will be used to determine both numbers and kinds of staff needed. Perceived patient needs can be matched with available nursing resources.

2. Budgeting. The predescribed unit of time will be used to determine the actual cost of nursing service. Profits and losses of nursing can then be determined.

3. Tracking changes in patient care needs. A PCS gives nurse managers the ability to moderate and control delivery of care services, adjusting intensity and cost.

4. Determining values for the productivity equation, which is output divided by input. Reducing input costs reduces costs of each output (time unit). In the prospective payment system (PPS) this output measure has been the discharged patient. Outputs become the criteria for measuring nursing productivity, regardless of quality. PCSs provide workload indices as productivity measures.

5. Determining quality. Once a standard time element is established, staffing is adjusted to meet the aggregate times. A nurse manager can elect to staff below the standard time to reduce costs. Thus the nurse manager makes a decision to reduce quality by reducing times and cost. It is best to do this in collaboration with clinical nurses. They are the personnel who are continually present and can assist

with developing and applying more efficient procedures and protocols. This can involve rearrangement of the physical setting and the assembling of equipment and supplies. Their involvement will increase their trust and respect, improve their attendance and work habits, improve work force stability, and reduce errors. Their input into decision making can be through product evaluation and selection, identification of nonnursing tasks to be done by lower-priced workers, increased mechanization, and job evaluation.[12]

Nursing Management Information Systems for PCSs

Nursing Management Information Systems (NMISs) are described in more detail in another chapter. A good one is basic to a sound PCS. It will provide shift reports of personnel needed and assigned, by type. It will provide staffing and productivity data by unit and area. It will provide average data on the intensity of care needed by class of patient. It will provide the cost per time unit of patient care by class of patient.[13]

Characteristics Desired of PCSs

The following characteristics are desirable for PCSs. Such systems should:

1. Differentiate intensity of care among definitive classes.
2. Measure and quantify care to develop a management engineering standard.
3. Match nursing resources to patient care requirements.
4. Relate to time and effort spent on the associated activity.
5. Be economical and convenient to report and use.
6. Be mutually exclusive, counting no item under more than one work unit.
7. Be open to audit.
8. Be understood by those who plan, schedule, and control the work.
9. Be individually standardized as to the procedures needed for accomplishment.
10. Separate requirements for registered nurses and other staff.[14]

MODIFIED APPROACHES TO NURSE STAFFING AND SCHEDULING

Many different approaches to nurse staffing and scheduling are being tried in an effort to satisfy the needs of employees and meet workload demands for patient care. These include game theory, modified work weeks (10- or 12-hour shifts), team rotation, "premium day" weekend nurse staffing, and "premium vacation" night staffing. Such approaches should support the underlying purpose, mission, philosophy, and objectives of the organization and the division of nursing and should be well defined in a staffing philosophy and policies. Nurses are like other workers in one respect: they would like to live as normal a life as possible. Shifts have to be staffed and patient care needs met. The successful nurse executive will try to accommodate both by using the best administrative staffing methodology available. It must be considered from the economic or cost/benefit viewpoint.

Staffing and scheduling are reasons for turnover and retention. Understaffing has a negative effect on staff morale, delivery of quality care, and the nursing practice modality. It can close beds. It causes absenteeism from staff fatigue, burnout, and professional dissatisfaction. On the other hand, nurse managers want to receive value for their money. Economic constraints are further stretched by the costs of recruiting, hiring, and orienting new nurses and for overtime and temporary hires when the environment creates turnovers and absenteeism. However, overstaffing is also expensive and has a negative effect on staff morale and productivity. Staffing and scheduling must balance the personal needs of nurses with economic and productivity needs of organizations.[15]

Modified Work Weeks

Modified work week schedules using 10- and 12-hour shifts and other methods are commonplace. A nurse administrator should be sure they are fulfilling the staffing philosophy and policies, particularly with regard to efficiency. Also, they should not be imposed on the nursing staff, but should show a mutual benefit to employer, employee, and ultimately the clients served.

The 10-Hour Day. One modification of the work week is four 10-hour shifts per week in organized

time increments. A problem of this model is time overlaps of 6 hours per 24-hour day. The overlaps can be used for patient-centered conferences, nursing care assessment and planning, and staff development. Also the overlap can be scheduled to cover peak workload hours. Peak workload demands can be identified by observation, consensus, or self-recording by professional nurses. It can be done by hour or by a block of 3 to 4 hours. The staffing board in Figure 4–8 can be used to solve these problems.

Longer work days can decrease overtime because of overlapping shifts. Absenteeism and turnover are decreased because nurses have more days off. All of these factors decrease costs. Such a system can increase staffing needs if mechanisms are not used to maintain productivity. Some organizations use a 7-days-on, 7-days-off schedule but only pay for 70 hours in 2 weeks.[16]

The 4-day, 10-hour work schedule for night nurses was done in a hospital that had difficulty recruiting qualified nurses to the night shift. It had been perceived that 10-hour shifts had stabilized staffing in intensive care with increased productivity and decreased turnover.

Turnover on the night shift had been 70 percent for an 8-month period. Positions stayed vacant longer than for other shifts and sick time was higher. This increased recruitment and orientation time. Nurses were involved in planning the 4-day 10-hour night shift schedule. Night nurses agreed to use overlap hours to assist with day shift care. The day shift agreed to reduce staff by one FTE. Plans were discussed with and accepted by the union. Assignment of personnel and meeting schedules were addressed and resolved through participatory management.

The results included reduced sick time on the 10-hour shift, reduced turnover, increased incentive, increased requests for night shift, and decreased labor hours.[17] See Figure 4–9.

The 12-Hour Shift. A second scheduling modification is the 12-hour shift in which nurses work seven shifts in 2 weeks: three on, four off; four on, three off. They work a total of 84 hours and are paid 4 hours overtime. Twelve-hour shifts and flexible staffing have been reported to have improved care and saved money because nurses can manage their home and personal life better.[18]

Vik and MacKay report a study of the quality of care by nurses who worked 12-hour versus 8-hour

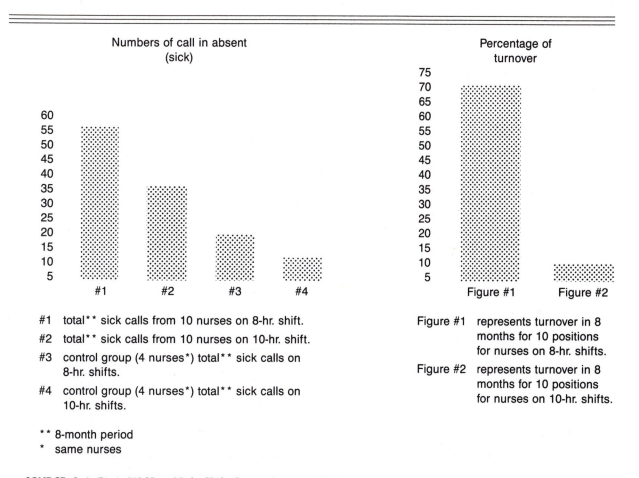

Numbers of call in absent
(sick)

Percentage of
turnover

#1   total** sick calls from 10 nurses on 8-hr. shift.

#2   total** sick calls from 10 nurses on 10-hr. shift.

#3   control group (4 nurses*) total** sick calls on
       8-hr. shifts.

#4   control group (4 nurses*) total** sick calls on
       10-hr. shifts.

Figure #1   represents turnover in 8
                 months for 10 positions
                 for nurses on 8-hr. shifts.

Figure #2   represents turnover in 8
                 months for 10 positions
                 for nurses on 10-hr. shifts.

**   8-month period
*   same nurses

SOURCE: J. A. Ricci, "10-Hour Night Shift: Cost vs Savings," *Nursing Management*,
January, 1984, p. 38. Reprinted with permission.

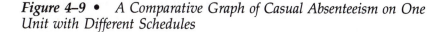

*Figure 4–9 •   A Comparative Graph of Casual Absenteeism on One
Unit with Different Schedules*

shifts. It was a matched study of three units each. The Quality Patient Care Scale was used as the measuring instrument. The "quality of care received by patients on the 8-hour shift units was significantly higher than that received by patients on the 12-hour shift units."[19] Shift patterns worked by nurses do affect the care received by patients. However, recruitment and retention of nurses can balance out reduced quality of care when vacancies are high. This was a limited study needing replication.

There is a break-even point for costs. It is the point at which recruiting, absenteeism, retention, and overtime cost savings equal the shift losses from 12-hour scheduling.[20]

The Weekend Alternative.   Another variation of flexible scheduling is the weekend alternative. Nurses work two 12-hour shifts and are paid for full-time plus benefits. They can use the week days to go to school or for other personal needs. There are several variations of the weekend schedule. Monday through Friday nurses get all weekends off.

Metcalf reports a test of the 12-hour weekend plan of two shifts on Saturday and Sunday, 7:00 A.M. to 7:00 P.M. and 7:00 P.M. to 7:00 A.M. The day shift were paid at rate of 36 hours of pay for 24 hours worked. The night shift were paid at the rate of 40 hours of pay for 24 hours worked.

The sample included RNs, LPNs, and nurses.

Employed staff could volunteer for the shift, and new staff were required to work it, as this was not a "weekends only" schedule. Full-time staff participating in it had two weekends out of three off. Results showed that only 3 percent of the total sample wanted the schedules discontinued, while 75 percent perceived weekend staffing as better.

Although illnesses and absences increased by 19 percent, this negative finding was outweighed by positive ones. Recruiting improved, with vacancy rates dropping from 13 to 7 percent of budgeted positions. Use of agency personnel was cut in half and salary costs did not increase. Staffing and morale both improved. Problems were addressed to improve the plan.[21]

Positive Aspects

Nurses of the 1990s want flexible scheduling to better accommodate their nonworking lives. Flexible time (frequently called *flextime*) schedules have become an increasingly important aspect of employment practices generally with 11.9 percent of all nonfarm wage and salary workers on such schedules in 1980. They have improved attitudes and increased productivity as employees have gained more control over their work environment. There have been adjustments to their own "bioclock" by employees. Transportation has become more efficient and flexible. Employees have better control of work activities.[22]

A study was done by the New York state government to control weaknesses of previous studies. Staggered work hours were compared to fixed work hours. The study showed that:

1. The greatest level of satisfaction and the least dissatisfaction with the workday was expressed by employees in the agency with the greatest flexibility in scheduling.
2. Those in the agency with fixed schedules expressed the strongest dissatisfaction and lowest level of satisfaction.
3. Statistically, there were no significant differences in job satisfaction among these groups.
4. Decreased commuting time may improve satisfaction with flextime.[23]

Flexible scheduling improves recruiting, absenteeism, and retention. There are many flexible scheduling variations available. Before using them nurse managers should establish philosophy and set objectives.

Negative Aspects

Among the disadvantages of 10- and 12-hour days are:

1. Minimum weekend staffing (or excess staff on weekends).
2. Unsafe travel times.
3. Shift overlaps that decrease total number of personnel on duty.
4. Costs for overtime.
5. Fatigue.
6. Strain on family life.
7. If the schedule is not carefully planned, the loss of shifts can require increased staffing.
8. State law may require overtime pay for hours worked in excess of 8 in a day and 40 in a week.
9. Less continuity of care.
10. Less communication among staff.
11. Developing, maintaining, and explaining the master schedule.
12. Modification of primary assessing.[24]

Cross-Training

Cross-training of nursing personnel can improve flexible scheduling. Nurses need to be prepared to function effectively in more than one area of expertise. They can be kept in similar clinical specialties or "families" of clinical specialties. They require complete orientation and ongoing staff development to prevent errors and increase job satisfaction. This can be done for both unit-assigned nurses and pool nurses. There should be policies, job descriptions, and performance evaluations. Pools can be in-house supplemental staffing agencies that use full-time and part-time nurses. Benefits can be prorated or employees can have choice of increased pay instead of benefits.

PRODUCTIVITY

Definition

Productivity is commonly defined as

$$\frac{\text{Outputs}}{\text{Inputs}}$$

Hanson translates this definition into:

$$\frac{\text{Required Staff Hours}}{\text{Provided Staff Hours}} \times 100 = \text{productivity}$$

To illustrate,

$$\frac{380.50 \text{ required staff hours}}{402.00 \text{ provided staff hours}} \times 100$$

$$= 94.7 \text{ percent productivity}$$

Productivity can be increased by decreasing the provided staff hours while holding the required staff hours constant or increasing them. These data become information when related to an objective that indicates variances.[25] Because resources for health care are limited, the nurse manager is faced with the task of motivating clinical nurses to increase productivity.

Productivity in nursing is related to both efficiency of use of clinical nursing in delivering nursing care to avoid waste and the effectiveness of that care relative to its quality and appropriateness. Brown indicates that productivity in the United States has declined. He cites as evidence of this claim increased labor costs without corresponding increases in performance. This is due to such factors as inexperienced workers, technological slowdown due to outdated equipment and lessened research and development, government regulations, a diminished work ethic, increased size and bureaucracy in business and industry, and erosion of the managerial ethic.[26]

Improving Nursing Productivity

Nursing productivity is being improved and the reported knowledge and skills are adding to the theory of nursing management. Rabin indicates that professionals can impose productivity values on themselves. Managers should develop managerial goals and values. They need a standard of performance for themselves. Professionals can commit themselves to fostering innovative attitudes and technologies, stimulating performance by commitment to constructive action and follow-ups, living up to standards of practice, keeping up-to-date, and being receptive to public review. They sometimes revert to protectionism of hierarchical controls rather than self-discipline. Almost any profession can develop measurable standards of performance and productivity.[27]

Employers should measure nursing output objectively and pay for it accordingly in salary, benefits, and promotions. There has been some progress in nursing in the form of standards of practice, clinical ladders, and models of peer review, among others. These need to be supported in the workplace along with respect for the individual dignity of nurses, support for their personal commitment to professional goals, and support for the integrity of their professional judgments.[28]

Productivity can be managed and improved through:

1. Planning that increases the variations between inputs and outputs by:
   1.1 Outputs increasing, inputs decreasing.
   1.2 Outputs increasing, inputs remaining constant.
   1.3 Outputs increasing faster than inputs.
   1.4 Outputs remaining constant, inputs decreasing.
   1.5 Outputs decreasing more slowly than inputs.
2. Soliciting staff's ideas and recommendations.
3. Creating challenges.
4. Managers showing interest in staff's achievement and concerns.
5. Praising and rewarding good performances.
6. Involving staff.
7. Having a meaningful set or family of outcome measures for which data are available or easy to gather and over which workers have some control. Such measures should be easily understood.
8. Selecting measures compatible with white-collar functions and corporate measures.
9. Monitoring workload changes in staffing requirements with established standards.
10. Combining support with employees' understanding, motivation, and recognition.
11. Increasing ratio of professional to nonprofessional staff.
12. Placing admitted patients based on resource availability.
13. Improving skill, energy, and motivation through staff development, books, tuition reimbursement, paid meals, yoga lessons, bonuses and vacation days, and other incentives.

14. Work simplification, work flow analysis, and other approaches.
15. Making an organizational diagnosis of problems, resources, and realities.
16. Setting the climate for productivity by asking nurses what makes them productive and then doing it. Measure before and after.
17. Decreasing waiting and standby time, coffee klatches, social breaks, mealtimes.
18. Stimulating nurse managers and clinical nurses to want to achieve excellence.
19. Setting targets for increasing output on an annual basis without additional capital or employees.
20. Having personnel keep and analyze time diaries to determine personal improvement.
21. Setting personal objectives and measuring performance against them.
22. Making a commitment to improved productivity, effectiveness (doing the right things), and efficiency (doing things right).
23. Seeking new products and services and new methods and ways of producing them.
24. Seeking new and useful approaches to old problems.
25. Improving quality of nursing products, emphasizing such ideas as consistency, longevity, riskiness, perfectibility, and value.
26. Maintaining concern with the process and method of producing nursing care.
27. Improving use of time.
28. Reducing the cost of what nurses do by returning budgeted funds.
29. Improving esthetics: the quality of work life and the pleasantness and beauty of the environment.
30. Applying the ethical policy statements of professional nursing organizations.
31. Gaining the confidence of peers.
32. Recognizing the need to do better.[29]

SUMMARY

Staffing and scheduling are major components of nursing management. Traditional patterns have been slavishly adhered to until recent years. A nursing division needs a practical and written philosophy that guides all staffing and scheduling activities and that is acceptable to the staff.

Staffing studies can be used to determine staffing needs related to personnel skills, numbers of personnel, and time/workload requirements. Staffing can be planned by using computer models that calculate workload requirements from patient classification data or patient classification systems (PCSs). There are many modified approaches to nurse staffing and scheduling, including modified work weeks, team rotation, permanent shifts, and permanent weekends. Although some consultants advise against mixing modified work weeks, they are in practice frequently mixed.

Productivity, the unit of output of nursing, is of increasing interest to nurse managers. It must include observable and measurable quality care indicators. Productivity is commonly defined as the outputs of production, divided by the inputs of production. Research needs to be done to determine the key to increased productivity by professional nurses. Is it money or some other aspect of job satisfaction? One theory is that a combination of work, environment, and rewards will maintain or increase productivity.

EXPERIENTIAL EXERCISES

1. Place a check mark in the blank beside the statement that best summarizes factors related to other departments that have to be considered in staffing the nursing division.

_____ 1.1 Nurse managers do not need to plan staffing requirements for work they do that should be done by other departments.

_____ 1.2 Even though some activities performed by nursing personnel appear to be the primary responsibility of other departments, planning for staffing must include staffing for these activities at the same time the nurse administrator encourages the appropriate departments to assume responsibility for performing them.

_____ 1.3 Nurse managers must not assume responsibility for nonnursing duties that should be performed by other departments and so do not need to plan staffing for them.

2. For each of the following examples, place MS in the blank if the example relates to the medical staff and a PP if it relates to the physical plant.

____ 2.1 In the addition to the hospital, provision was made for all supplies to be placed in pass-through cupboards so that nursing personnel would not have to leave the patient's room for them.

____ 2.2 Separate pass-through cupboards were built to receive soiled linen and used supplies and equipment so that supply personnel could pick them up without entering the patients' rooms.

____ 2.3 Neurology patients are located on the fifth floor and the EEG laboratory in the basement.

____ 2.4 More than twenty-five physicians visited on one ward during an 8-hour period, and each performed a diagnostic test or ordered therapeutic procedures.

____ 2.5 During a 6-month period, hyperalimentation orders have increased from a daily average of two to seventeen.

____ 2.6 A new patient education program for all coronary patients will be done by registered nurses.

3. For each of the following statements, place a + in the blank if the statement is true and a − if it is false.

____ 3.1 A nurse manager of a department that has outdated written statements of mission, philosophy, and objectives will probably be affected adversely in planning for efficient and economical staffing.

____ 3.2 Ms. Robertson is director of nursing in a department that has not developed an operational or management plan for accomplishing the written objectives of the staff development program. Although there are some personnel policies related to preparing time schedules and some written procedures, no evaluation of them has been made for over a year. Job standards are nonexistent. Ms. Robertson will be able to make an efficient and economical staffing plan.

4. *Group Exercise:*

4.1 Form groups of five to eight persons. This can be your permanent seminar group. You may want to consult with a larger representative group of nursing personnel to gain their insights and ideas and to incorporate their beliefs and values into the staffing philosophy.

4.2 Elect a leader to move the group to completion.

4.3 Elect a recorder to keep a written record of the group's accomplishments.

4.4 Prepare to write a staffing philosophy. A philosophy is a statement of beliefs about a subject. It should be representative of the beliefs professional nurses hold about staffing and scheduling. Refer to the figures in Chapter 3 on mission, philosophy, and objectives statements.

4.4.1 Make a list of those key words or statements that you believe should be addressed in a staffing philosophy.

4.4.2 Prepare an outline.

4.4.3 Write a staffing philosophy.

Remember that a hospital or other health care institution exists to provide health care to people—to patients or clients. Also, an institution has to make a profit to stay in business. This applies as well to a not-for-profit institution in which the profits go to improving the facility and its human and material resources. Patients must be cared for 24 hours a day by nurses satisfied with their conditions of work. Prepare a rationale for your final document.

5. Evaluate the staffing policies for the following areas of a health care institution stating whether they need changing and if so, why:

5.1 Vacations

5.2 Holidays

5.3 Sick leave

5.4 Weekends off

5.5 Consecutive days off

5.6 Rotation to different shifts

5.7 Overtime

5.8 Part-time personnel

5.9 Use of "float" personnel

5.10 Exchangeability of staff

5.11 Use of special abilities of individual staff members

5.12 Exchanging hours

5.13 Requests of personnel

5.14 Requests of management

5.15 The work week

Do policies exist? If not, should they? An existing committee representing all levels of nursing personnel will tell you. Members of the committee will also tell you if policies are adequate. They will update or develop policies. Use a management plan. This activity may be done with your student group.

MANAGEMENT PLAN

PROBLEM:

OBJECTIVE:

ACTIONS	TARGET DATES	ASSIGNED TO	ACCOMPLISHMENTS

6. Identify the modified approaches to nurse staffing and scheduling in a division or a department of nursing in which you work. List the advantages and disadvantages. Get input from the staff.

___ *6.1* 10-hour shifts

___ *6.2* 12-hour shifts

___ *6.3* Weekend alternative

___ *6.4* 7 on, 7 off

___ *6.5* Permanent evenings

___ *6.6* Permanent nights

___ *6.7* Others

7. Use Hanson's formula to determine productivity on a nursing unit for a division or department of nursing.[30]

$$\frac{\text{Required Staff Hours}}{\text{Provided Staff Hours}} \times 100 = \text{productivity}$$

8. Identify at least twelve activities that can be done to improve productivity in a division or department of nursing in which you work.

9. Use Figure 4–10 to evaluate the staffing function in the institution in which you work.

	YES	NO

1. Is there a philosophy of staffing that has been developed by staff members of the nursing department?
2. Has the responsibility for the seventeen different staffing activities have identified by name? See page 51.
3. Is there a personal orientation plan for each new employee?
4. Are there consistent staffing policies covering:
   4.1 Vacations
   4.2 Holidays?
   4.3 Sick leave?
   4.4 Weekends off?
   4.5 Consecutive days off?
   4.6 Rotation to different shifts?
   4.7 Overtime?
   4.8 Part-time personnel?
   4.9 Use of "float" personnel?
   4.10 Exchangeability of staff?
   4.11 Special abilities of individual staff members?
   4.12 Changing hours?
   4.13 Requests by personnel?
   4.14 Requests by management?
   4.15 The work week?
5. Is there a written work agreement between each employee and the institution?
6. Is the staffing function centralized?
7. Is the staffing function performed by nonnurse employees?
8. Have staffing patterns for each unit been identified?
   8.1 Basic staff (minimum number and categories for each day of the week)?
   8.2 Complementary personnel (available and budgeted)?
   8.3 "Float" personnel needed?
   8.4 Weekends and holidays?
9. Have work measurement studies been done by the nurse managers?
   9.1 Average census?
   9.2 Average daily hours of care for each patient?
10. Is there at least one RN to every two other workers?
11. Are personnel scheduled to work their preferred shift as much as possible?
12. Are personnel choices balanced to meet the needs of the unit and of other employees?

Figure 4–10 • *Staffing Evaluation Plan*

(Continued)

13. Has a staffing module (staffing board) been developed?

14. Has a cyclical staffing pattern been implemented?

15. Is the staffing schedule posted for a 6-week period?

16. Are employees allowed to make their own arrangements for special time off or exchanges within specific personnel policies?

17. Have policies been established for making schedule changes?

18. Do all employees have a copy of their own work schedules?

19. Has consideration been given to staffing during hours of clinical experience for students?

20. Are records of hours worked accurate?

21. Has a PCS been used and found beneficial to determine nursing hours or assignment of personnel?

22. Have nonnursing tasks been identified and adjustments made between other departments and nursing?

23. Are other approaches to nurse staffing being used?

　23.1 Game theory

　23.2 10-to-12-hour shifts (modified work week)

　23.3 Team rotation

　23.4 "Premium day" weekend nurse staffing

　23.5 "Premium vacation" night staffing

　23.6 Other

Figure 4–10　(*Continued*)

NOTES

1. M. K. Aydelotte, *Nurse Staffing Methodology: A Review and Critique of Selected Literature* (Washington, DC: U.S. Government Printing Office, Jan. 1973), 3.

2. Ibid., p. 26.

3. M. E. West, "Implementing Effective Nurse Staffing Systems in the Managed Hospital," *Topics in Health Care Financing,* Summer 1980, 11–25.

4. J. N. Althaus, N. M. Hardyck, P. B. Pierce, and M. S. Rodgers, "Nurse Staffing in a Decentralized Organization: Part 1," *Journal of Nursing Administration,* Mar. 1982, 34–39.

5. R. C. Minetti, "Computerized Nurse Staffing," *Hospitals,* July 16, 1983, 90, 92; P. P. Shaheen, "Staffing and Scheduling: Reconcile Practical Means with the Real Goal," *Nursing Management,* Oct. 1985, 64–69.

6. West, op. cit., 16.

7. The figure of 1.4 represents 1.4 workweeks of 5 days to cover a 7-day week; 1.14 represents the built-in holidays, sick leave, annual leave; 7.5 represents 7.5 productive hours on an 8-hour shift.

8. West, op. cit. 17.

9. E. M. Price, *Staffing for Patient Care* (New York: Springer, 1970), 12.

10. "Study Questions All-R.N. Staffing," *RN,* Nov. 1983, 15–16.

11. M. E. Warstler, "Some Management Techniques for Nursing Service Administrators," *Journal of Nursing Administration,* Nov.-Dec. 1972, 25–34.

12. T. P. Herzog, "Productivity: Fighting the Battle of the Budget," *Nursing Management,* Jan. 1985, 30–34; T. Porter-O'Grady, "Strategic Planning: Nursing Practice in the PPS," *Nursing Management,* Oct. 1985, 53–56; K. Johnson, "A Practical Approach to Patient Classification," *Nursing Management,* June 1984, 39–41, 44, 46; R. E. Schroeder,

A. M. Rhodes, and R. E. Shields, "Nurse Acuity Systems: CASH versus GRASP," *Nursing Forum,* Feb. 1984, 72–77; R. R. Alward, "Patient Classification Systems: The Ideal versus Reality," *Journal of Nursing Administration,* Feb. 1983, 14–18; J. Nyberg and N. Wolff, "DRG Panic," *Journal of Nursing Administration,* Apr. 1984, 17–21.

13. E. J. Halloran and M. Kiley, "Case Mix Management," *Nursing Management,* Feb. 1984, 39–41, 44–45.

14. Schroeder, Rhodes, and Shields, op. cit.

15. American Hospital Association, "Strategies: Flexible Scheduling," 1985, 12 pp.

16. Ibid.

17. J. A. Ricci, "10-Hour Night Shift: Cost versus Savings," *Nursing Management,* Jan. 1984, 34–35, 38–42.

18. C. M. Fagin, "The Economic Value of Nursing Research," *American Journal of Nursing,* Dec. 1982, 1844–1849.

19. A. G. Vik and R. C. MacKay, "How Does the 12-Hour Shift Affect Patient Care?," *Journal of Nursing Administration,* Jan. 1982, 12.

20. T. W. Lant and D. Gregory, "The Impact of 12-Hour Shift: An Analysis," *Nursing Management,* Oct. 1984, 38A, 38B, 38D–38F, 38H.

21. M. L. Metcalf, "The 12-Hour Weekend Plan—Does the Nursing Staff Really Like It?," *Journal of Nursing Administration,* Oct. 1982, 16–19.

22. J. B. McGuire and J. R. Liro, "Flexible Work Schedules, Work Attitudes, and Perceptions of Productivity," *Public Personnel Management,* Spring 1986, 65–73.

23. Ibid.

24. American Hospital Association, op. cit.; B. Arnold and E. Mills, "Care-12: Implementation of Flexible Scheduling," *Journal of Nursing Administration,* July-Aug. 1983, 9–14; A. Mech, M. E. Mills, and B. Arnold, "Wage and Hour Laws: Their Impact on 12-hour Scheduling," *Journal of Nursing Administration,* Mar. 1984, 24–25; Metcalf, op. cit.

25. R. L. Hanson, "Staffing Statistics: Their Use and Usefulness," *Journal of Nursing Administration,* Nov. 1982, 28–35.

26. D. S. Brown, "The Managerial Ethic and Productivity Improvement," *Public Productivity Review,* Sept. 1983, 223–250.

27. J. Rabin, "Professionalism and Productivity," *Public Productivity Review,* Sept. 1983, 217–222.

28. L. Curtin, "Reconciling Pay with Productivity," *Nursing Management,* Feb. 1984, 7–8.

29. M. F. Fralic, "The Modern Professional and Productivity," Annual Meeting of the Alabama Society for Nursing Service Administrators, Huntsville, AL, 1982; R. L. Hanson, "Managing Human Resources," *Journal of Nursing Administration,* Dec. 1982, 17–23; G. H. Kaye and J. Utenner, "Productivity: Managing for the Long Term," *Nursing Management,* Sept. 1985, 12–13, 15; S. A. W. Haas, "Sorting Out Nursing Productivity," *Nursing Management,* Apr. 1984, 37–40; D. L. Davis, "Assessing and Improving Productivity in the Operating Room," *AORN Journal,* Oct. 1984, 630, 632, 634; D. S. Brown, op. cit.

30. Hanson, "Staffing Statistics," op. cit.

FOR FURTHER REFERENCE

Adams, R., and Duchene, P., "Computerization of Patient Acuity and Nursing Care Planning," *Journal of Nursing Administration,* Apr. 1985, 11–17.

Althaus, J. N., and Hardyck, N. M., "Nurse Staffing in a Decentralized Organization: Part 1," *Journal of Nursing Administration,* Mar. 1982, 34–39.

Althaus, J. N., Hardyck, N. M., Pierce, P. B., and Rodgers, M. S., "Nurse Staffing in a Decentralized Organization: Part 2," *Journal of Nursing Administration,* Apr. 1982, 18–22.

Artinian, B. M., O'Connor, F. D., and Brock, R., "Comparing Past and Present Nursing Productivity," *Nursing Management,* Oct. 1984, 50–53.

Auger, J. A., and Dee, V., "A Patient Classification System Based on the Behavioral System Model of Nursing: Part 1," *Journal of Nursing Administration,* Apr. 1983, 38–43.

Bermas, N. F., and Van Slyck, A., "Patient Classification Systems and the Nursing Department," *Hospitals,* Nov. 16, 1984, 99–100.

Connor, R. J., Flagle, C. D., Hsieh, R. K. C., Preston, R. A., and Singer, S., "Effective Use of Nursing Resources—A Research Report," *Hospitals,* May 1961, 30–39.

Curtin, L., "Reconciling Pay with Productivity," *Nursing Management,* Feb. 1984, 7–8.

Curtin, L. L., and Zurlage, C. L., "Nursing Productivity: From Data to Definition," *Nursing Management,* June 1986, 32–34, 38–41.

Dee, V., and Auger, J. A., "A Patient Classification System Based on the Behavioral System Model of Nursing: Part 2," *Journal of Nursing Administration,* May 1983, 18–23.

Duckett, S., "Nurse Rostering with Game Theory," *Journal of Nursing Administration,* Jan. 1977, 58–59.

Evans, C. L. S., "A Practical Staffing Calculator," *Nursing Management,* Apr. 1984, 68–69.

Fisher, D. W., and Thomas, E., "A 'Premium Day' Approach to Weekend Nurse Staffing," in *Staffing: A Journal of Nursing Administration Reader* (Wakefield, MA: Contemporary Publishing, 1975).

Froebe, D., "Scheduling: By Team or Individually," in *Staffing: A Journal of Nursing Administration Reader* (Wakefield, MA: Contemporary Publishing, 1975).

Gebhardt, A. N., "Computers and Staff Allocation Made Easy," *Nursing Times,* Sept. 1, 1982, 1471–1473.

Giovannetti, P., and Mayer, G. G., "Building Confidence in Patient Classification Systems," *Nursing Management,* Aug. 1984, 31–34.

Grazman, T. E., "Managing Unit Human Resources: A Microcomputer Model," *Nursing Management,* July 1983, 18–22.

Hanson, R. L., "Applying Management Information Systems to Staffing," *Journal of Nursing Administration,* Oct. 1982, 5–9.

Henney, C. R., and Bosworth, R. N., "A Computer-Based System for the Automatic Production of Nursing Workload Data," *Nursing Times,* July 10, 1980, 1212–1217.

Imig, S. I., Powell, J. A., and Thorman, K., "Primary Nursing and Flexi-Staffing: Do They Mix?," *Nursing Management,* Aug. 1984, 39–42.

Jecmen, C., and Stuerke, N. M., "Computerization Helps Solve Staff Scheduling Problems," *Nursing Economics,* Nov.-Dec. 1983, 209–211.

Jelinek, R. C., Zinn, T. K., and Brya, J. R., "Tell the Computer How Sick the Patients Are and It Will Tell How Many Nurses They Need," *Modern Hospital,* Dec. 1973, 81–85.

Malhot, C. B., "Setting OR's Course toward Greater Productivity," *Nursing Management,* Oct. 1985, 42I, 42J, 42L, 42M, 42P.

Moores, B., and Murphy, A., "Planning the Duty Rota, One, Computerized Duty Rotas," *Nursing Times,* July 4, 1984, 47–48.

Price, E., *Simplified Staffing: The Price Plan for Effective Scheduling,* Hospital Workshops, 30951 Cole Grade Road, Valley Center, CA 92082.

Reitz, J. A., "Toward a Comprehensive Nursing Intensity Index: Part 1, Development," *Nursing Management,* Aug. 1985, 21–24, 26, 28–30.

———, "Toward a Comprehensive Nursing Intensity Index: Part 2, Testing," *Nursing Management,* Sept. 1985, 31–32, 34, 36–40, 42.

Smith, J. L., Mackey, M. K. V., and Markham, J., "Productivity Monitoring: A Recovery Room System for Economizing Operations," *Nursing Management,* May 1985, 34A–34D, 34K–34M.

Staffing 1: A Journal of Nursing Administration Reader; Staffing 2: A Journal of Nursing Administration Reader; Staffing 3: A Journal of Nursing Administration Reader (Wakefield, MA: Contemporary Publishing, 1975).

Stuerke, N., "Computers *Can* Advance Nursing Practice," *Nursing Management,* July 1984, 27–28.

Personnel Management

INTRODUCTION

Even though professional nurses' dissatisfactions with work have been widely studied, the long-term solutions have been largely ignored. The theory of nursing management includes knowledge of personnel management related to recruiting, selecting, credentialing, assigning, retaining, promoting, and terminating personnel. Recruiting has two facets, recruiting students into generic programs and recruiting RNs into service institutions and agencies. Credentialing includes licensing.

RECRUITING

Recruiting Students into Nursing

In 1980 the American Hospital Association published a package of materials entitled *Hospital Nurse Recruitment and Retention: A Source Book for Executive Management*. It indicated there was a national shortage of 100,000 hospital nurses.[1] A flood of publicity on this shortage led to the formation of a National Commission on Nursing. This commission listed "eight top themes in descending order of importance" that it considered important in reducing the shortage:

1. Nursing leadership should be an integral part of senior management.
2. Nursing should be more involved in all levels of hospital decision making.
3. Nurses' management skills should be developed and nurses should be provided more opportunities for leadership positions.
4. The organizational structure should be decentralized to facilitate communication and decision making.
5. Collaborative or joint practice programs between nurses and physicians should be established.
6. The nursing educational system needs to be rationalized in terms of entry-level requirements and clinical practice preparation.
7. Career development programs for clinical prac-

tice and administrative positions should continue to be developed and implemented.

8. Nursing leaders should be appointed to key committees to foster and strengthen nurses' interaction with medical staff and the board.[2]

By 1983 the entire situation had changed, with every major nursing journal focusing on a glut of nurses in many (but not all) areas. The reasons were many, varied, and speculative. All related to economics. People did not have health insurance because of its cost and could not be hospitalized short of an emergency. Hospitals were downsizing as occupancy decreased due to diagnosis-related groups (DRGs). A few hospitals reported layoffs of nurses. Nursing publications attempted to analyze the job market and supply the information to nurses.[3]

The 1990s are projected to produce acute shortages of nurses. Enrollments in schools of nursing are declining and the decline is expected to continue. Enrollment in professional (RN) nursing programs dropped 13 percent, falling from a high of 251,000 in 1983 to 218,000 in 1985.[4] The 1987 enrollment was 193,712.[5] Only the part-time RN to BSN student nursing education programs expanded enrollments.[6]

A decline in the number of high school graduates is projected through the mid-1990s. There will be a concurrent increasing growth in persons over 65 years of age, the prime consumers of nursing services.[7] Thus the pool from which nursing students are recruited diminishes at a time when need increases.

There will be other significant changes evinced by the 3.6 million 4-year-olds of 1986, who will be college age in the year 2000. According to Hodgkinson:

1. *Twenty-four percent of them live below the poverty line. In 1984 there were 3,330,000 poor people over 65—but 11,455,000 poor children under 15.*

2. *Far fewer of these 4-year-olds are white, suburban, and middle class than was the case in 1970. (The group with the most rapid decline in birthrate is the group that normally makes up most of the college freshman class.)*

3. *One-third of these 4-year-olds are nonwhite, though minority can no longer be considered synonymous with poor. (Blacks, Hispanics, and Asians have large and growing middle classes and span almost as broad a socioeconomic range as whites. Colleges have yet to realize that they can recruit Blacks from a ghetto, or they can go to Shaker Heights for top-notch minority*

students. Indeed, today many inner-city high schools are turning out excellent students.)

4. *Eighteen percent of today's 4-year-olds were born out of wedlock.*

5. *More than 45 percent of them will be raised by a single parent before they reach 18 years of age.*

6. *A higher percentage of 4-year-olds today than in the past do not speak English. Instead they speak a dazzling array of languages, from Urdu to Mandarin. Spanish is only one of these many languages.*

7. *An increasing number of today's 4-year-olds have physical and emotional handicaps.*

8. *Fifty-four percent of them have mothers who work outside the home, and the children receive some form of day care. By the time they reach school age, two-thirds of their mothers will be working, most of them full time.*

9. *Twenty percent of the girls among today's 4-year-olds will become pregnant during their teen years.*[8]

From the forgoing the implications for nursing can be forecast as:

1. Schools of nursing should now begin to profile their students. Who are they? Where do they come from? What is the level of their achievement in high school?

2. More adults should be recruited into nursing. These include both men and women seeking second careers and women entering a career field after children have entered school.

3. Collaboration with the public schools should be proactive. Nursing educators, managers, researchers, and clinical practitioners should all be part of the recruitment effort. They can advise school counselors on program requirements and support the schools to meet those requirements. Such measures might include financial assistance to keep students in school through graduation and to enable them to enter nursing programs after graduation.

4. Support should be given to potential dropouts in the Black, Hispanic and Asian middle classes to maintain them in high school through graduation and into college. They will require assistance with language, culture, and finances. Schools of nursing will need to make accommodations to the language and customs of these persons. They are the

workers who will be paying Social Security for future retirees.

5. Nurses should give proactive support to public education at all levels. The future of nursing and of our society depends on it, because public school students are potential future nurses and productive workers of all occupations.

6. With more than 14 million immigrants to socialize into U.S. culture, nurses should become a part of the process. Again, they must be proactive in encouraging nursing students to take elective courses in liberal arts that reflect the cultures of these people.

7. Higher education needs to be adapted to assimilate minorities. This is a challenge to nurse educators. They will have to begin the process at high school level by helping to initiate programs of study that prepare minorities to enter nursing programs, including supplemental and remedial programs. Such efforts will need to be continued throughout the nursing education program.

8. Support for high school graduates of lower ability is essential.

9. Attention to retention of college and university students can be of value to schools of nursing. A plan should be made to recruit the 50 percent of 4-year degree candidates who do not graduate. These include students in 24 major academic fields of study with 1300 different academic majors in undergraduate education.

10. Employers will need to prepare minorities, including nurses, for promotion, thus giving them visibility to potential nursing students. The military services have been doing a better job of this than have civilian institutions. One has only to look at the hierarchy of educational institutions, health care institutions, and business and industrial institutions to discern this.

11. Although community colleges handle most students who are outside the mainstream because of their ethnicity, age, and cultural background, this can be changed. Faculty can initiate the changes so that the number of both associate and baccalaureate nursing graduates will increase. Both need to be maintained at levels to meet market demand.

12. Emphasis on research and publication should not diminish. However, faculty should be promoted and tenured based on teaching excellence as well.

13. Teaching methodology should focus on wide use of teaching strategies and less on lectures that keep students passive.[9]

Of late, women have been entering other career fields such as medicine, law, business administration, dentistry, and so forth. These have traditionally been predominantly male fields with higher pay and better working conditions than nursing. Although there are numerous studies of dissatisfaction among nurses, there appears to be only sporadic progress in improving pay and working conditions.

Nurse managers are the people who can change the work environment. They are not the only ones, however. An all-RN staff may not be financially possible. The professional nurse practitioner is highly qualified in terms of knowledge and skills and the decision maker in the nursing process. This nurse can direct the work of others without continual direct involvement in such procedures as bathing, making beds, feeding patients, and other procedures. The professional nurse would do the history, make the nursing diagnosis, direct the application of nursing care, evaluate the results, and make changes as needed. The debate on entry into practice needs to be redesigned and realigned to focus on the professional nurse as the clinical decision maker.

Every major agency or institution employing nurses should have a committee that focuses on the recruitment of students into nursing education programs. Small organizations can form recruitment consortiums. Clinical nurses should be well represented. They will provide ideas that will give an authentic and positive image of professional nursing practice. The focus should be realistic but positive for men and women, for minorities, and for a cross-section of high school students.

A survey of nearly 1,000 hospitals was done by the American Organization of Nurse Executives and the American Hospital Association in December 1986. Participation in high school and college career days was found to be a major recruitment strategy. Most activities were aimed at recruiting student nurses into jobs. A few efforts were directed to junior high school or high school students or guidance personnel.[10]

1. Form committee to make plan.
   1.1 Include clinical nurses.
   1.2 Set goals.
   1.3 Make management plan for each goal.
2. Obtain recruitment materials from organizations.
   2.1 National League for Nursing (NLN).
   2.2 American Nurses' Association (ANA).
   2.3 American Organization of Nurse Executives (AONE)/American Hospital Association (AHA).
   2.4 National Student Nurses' Association (NSNA).
   2.5 American Association of Colleges of Nursing (AACN).
   2.6 State
   2.7 Local
3. Prepare additional recruitment materials.
   3.1 News stories for newspapers, TV, and radio.
   3.2 Posters for schools.
   3.3 Speakers bureau.
   3.4 Model speeches.
   3.5 Tours.
4. Coordinate with other nurse education programs and prospective employers of nurses.
   4.1 Associate degree programs.
   4.2 Diploma programs.
   4.3 BSN programs.
   4.4 Hospitals.
   4.5 Public health.
   4.6 Staffing agencies.
   4.7 Ambulatory care facilities.
   4.8 Nursing homes.
   4.9 LPN programs.
   4.10 Other.
5. Prepare and offer consultation programs for junior and senior high schools.
   5.1 Administrators.
   5.2 Teachers.
   5.3 Guidance counselors.
   5.4 Students.
6. Coordinate activities of recruiters in schools of nursing.
   6.1 Sources of information by telephone and mail.
7. Involve community agencies in recruitment efforts.
   7.1 Professional organizations.
   7.2 Social organizations.
   7.3 Service organizations.
   7.4 Others.
8. Evaluation of results accomplished.
   8.1 Number and locations of programs presented.
   8.2 Number of students counseled.
   8.3 Number of follow-ups.
   8.4 Number of applicants to local or other programs.
   8.5 Home rooms visited.
   8.6 Career days held by high schools.
   8.7 Career days held by schools of nursing.
   8.8 Career days held by employers.
   8.9 Inquiries to source persons by telephone or letter.
9. Work/study programs.
   9.1 High school with employer.
   9.2 High schools with schools of nursing.
   9.3 Schools of nursing with employers.
   9.4 Cooperative education.

Figure 5–1 • *Strategies to Recruit Students into Nursing Education Programs*

Figure 5–1 lists activities to pursue in recruiting students into nursing education programs.

The business of recruiting students into nursing will require long-term strategies for all educators and providers. Recruitment will be more effective if the consumers are activated. The profession tends to lose sight of this source of support.

Professional nurses can work through community organizations to involve the community in changing the image of nursing and in the recruitment effort.

State nurses' associations have geared up to address the nurse shortage. Their efforts should lead to results rather than pronouncements such as resolutions passed at conventions or meetings catalogued in publications.

Efforts should be made to provide education at times convenient to students, most of whom have to work. Little has been done to provide evening and weekend courses for basic or generic students. This should be a major area of breakthrough in recruitment, particularly for older adults. There are no reasons for the lack of evening and weekend courses, including Sundays, except the will and efforts of faculty and clinical facility personnel.

Nurses can do more to obtain financing for student education. Many service organizations would provide scholarships if asked. Minority students should be targeted and marketed, then supported once they are recruited.

Recruiting Nurses into Employment

Employers of registered nurses are competing for available personnel. How do they capture their attention? The channels include newspaper ads, journal ads, professional placement agencies, placement bureaus at universities, and special publications. Professional nurses seeking jobs have personal contacts and obtain information at job fairs, career days, professional meetings and conventions. The business of recruiting clinical nurses into jobs should be managed with planning, organization, direction, and a method of evaluating its effectiveness.

Clinical nurses, the foundation of nursing care of patients, are the sector of nurses in shortest supply. There are few vacancies for top nurse executives. First-line and middle managers are frequently promoted from within—many without management preparation, although this is changing with increased emphasis on development of graduate programs in nursing management. Colleges and universities with baccalaureate programs are fast upgrading their faculty, requiring doctorates rather than master's degrees. Jobs are developing for nursing researchers.

Jobs for nursing managers, educators, and researchers have specific requirements for specialization, education, and experience. Many are filled through search committee procedures that attempt to fit the applicant to the organization. In times of critical shortages, clinical nurses are frequently hired without attempts to achieve such a fit.

The Recruiter. Many large organizations employ a nurse recruiter. This can be a professional nurse or a personnel recruitment specialist. Both should work from a management plan that includes input from clinical nurses working within the organization.

The objective of the recruiter is to induce qualified professional nurses to apply for jobs. First, information about the organization's job openings must be made known to the target population. This is done through advertisements in Sunday newspapers and in issues of nursing journals. The ads should be broad enough to give potential applicants knowledge of particular positions, salaries and fringe benefits, and the organizational climate. Results of studies of factors that attract nurses can be used as a basis for developing job advertisements.

In 1983 an American Academy of Nursing study depicted both nurse administrators and staff nurses as agreeing on what factors attracted nurses to come to hospitals and stay there. Among those factors are "adequate and competent colleagues, flexibility in scheduling, educational programs that allow for professional growth, and recognition as individuals."[11]

During 1985 and 1986 Kramer and Schmalenberg resurveyed 16 of these magnet hospitals comparing them to the best-run corporate communities as described by Peters and Waterman in their book *In Search of Excellence.* Many similarities were found. Magnet hospitals "are infused with values of quality care, nurse autonomy, informal, non-rigid verbal communication, innovation, bringing out the best in each individual, value of education, respect and caring for the individual, and striving for excellence."[12]

A well-thought-out ad can be a successful method of recruiting nurses. It is better to spend money to develop an effective advertisement than to save money on an ineffective one. A successful ad will get attention when it focuses on its subject: the professional nurse. It will obtain results when it piques the interest of the professional nurse in seeking more information. Figure 5–2 lists criteria for developing an effective newspaper or nursing journal advertisement.

Professional nurses should be recruited just like other professionals. If clinical nursing is important, clinical nurses will be recruited, as are nurse managers, educators, and researchers.

In recruiting nurses from outside the community area, efforts should be directed toward those factors that would attract professional nurses to move. These would include geographic attractions: winter sports such as skiing, or sunshine and beaches. They also might include such cultural attractions as museums, symphony orchestras, and operas, or educational opportunities.

1. Target the population.
2. Get the reader's attention.
3. Consider a picture that depicts a professional nurse in action, the kind of action nurses say they want.
4. List several factors that attract nurses.[13] These may include:
   4.1 Opportunity for self-fulfillment.
   4.2 Knowledge of helping others.
   4.3 Intellectual stimulation.
   4.4 Educational opportunity.
   4.5 Fellowship with colleagues.
   4.6 Adequate income.
   4.7 Opportunity for innovation.
   4.8 Opportunity to choose hours.
   4.9 Opportunity for advancement.
   4.10 Chance to be a leader.
   4.11 Adequate support systems.
   4.12 Child care facilities.
   4.13 Good fringe benefits.
5. Involve clinical nurses in developing the advertisement.
6. Test the advertisement on the clinical nurse staff.
7. Run the ad in the Sunday newspapers. Select those that are read by the target population.
8. Run the ad in nursing journals read by the target population.
9. Provide for telephone and mail replies from applicants.
   9.1 Free telephone numbers.
   9.2 Specific address.
10. Provide for effective telephone and mail replies to be returned from organization.
    10.1 The phone answered with positive responses that elicit interviews. It can be effective if clinical nurses make immediate follow-up calls to prospective applicants.
    10.2 Effective packages of recruitment materials mailed to prospective applicants (depict and detail factors listed under number 4).
11. Arrange for interview, including a visit to the organization.
    11.1 Contact person and sponsor.
    11.2 Travel reimbursement.
    11.3 Paid room and meals.
    11.4 Interviews with person doing hiring, personnel specialists including recruiter, and clinical nurses.
12. Follow-up offer in writing.

Figure 5-2 • *Criteria for Developing an Effective Nurse Recruitment Advertisement*

Recruitment Tips. There are a number of important tips for recruiting clinical nurses.

Tip 1. Keep potential applicants and employees from making mistakes when using private employment agencies.

1. Make sure they understand everything they sign and that they agree only to terms they want, including jobs.
2. Be sure they know the employer is paying the finder's fee.

Tip 2. When possible, nurses should talk with nurses already employed and who are involved in the recruitment process. Questions that might come up include:

1. How does management differentiate among associate degree, diploma, and BSN graduates?
2. Can a good salary be negotiated?
3. Are opportunities provided for continuing education, advancement, increased responsibility, and input into the work environment?
4. Is there dissatisfaction among nursing staff?
5. Is the management/administrative staff competent/capable? What are its qualities/abilities?
6. Will nurses be required to rotate shifts or work overtime?
7. Is there a rapid turnover rate in nursing personnel?

Tip 3. Do not use blind ads (those that give a coded box number). They tend to keep applicants from making personal contacts about jobs as names, telephone numbers, and addresses are omitted. Blind ads also slow down the process of making productive contacts.

Tip 4. Use imaginative recruitment procedures. Explore unusual ways of making contacts, for example through the employed nursing staff, service organizations, community organizations, and professional organizations.

It is important to take every opportunity to catch potential applicants' attention. Form a speakers bureau so nurses can give recruitment presentations before special groups: during meetings of service and professional organizations, on talk shows, at community activities such as Friends of the Art Museum or Friends of the Opera, to political action committees, or even at the local political party organization. Brainstorming can generate a list of imaginative procedures for recruiting nurses. It may even be feasible to form a new organization of Friends of Professional Nurses, involving them with the problem of recruiting students into nursing and nurses into the organization.[14]

SELECTING, CREDENTIALING, AND ASSIGNING

Selecting, credentialing, and assigning are all part of the hiring process. Although assigning has sometimes been done after the professional nurse was hired, it is unsatisfactory to applicants. They want to know where they will work before reporting for duty and orientation. They do not want surprises and will begin work dissatisfied if they occur.

Selecting

Selecting includes interviewing, the employer's offer, acceptance by the applicant, and signing of a contract or written offer. The chief nurse executive may interview and hire prospective applicants in small organizations, but it is best for the nurse manager who will directly supervise the employee to do the hiring. This person may want the input of clinical nurses with whom the prospective employee will be working.

The Interview

The nurse recruiter or a personnel specialist will have completed a personnel folder containing a completed application form, a résumé or curriculum vitae, references, and any documents required by policy or law such as a current valid license to practice nursing, transcripts, and loyalty oaths.

The interviewer should be prepared for the interview by reading the information in the applicant's folder. Figure 5–3 is a checklist to use in reviewing this folder.

Notes should be made of questions to be asked about the information contained in the folder.

1. The application form
    1.1 Is completed as directed.
    1.2 Written statements are positive.
    1.3 Contains no blanks.
    1.4 Contains no gaps in employment data.
2. References
    2.1 Are listed.
    2.2 Have been checked.
    2.3 Are satisfactory.
    2.4 Need further checking.
3. RN licensure
    3.1 Has been verified.
    3.2 Is current and valid.
4. Transcripts
    4.1 Have been verified.
    4.2 Are available.
5. Forms signed.
6. Curriculum vitae or résumé
    6.1 Is up-to-date.
    6.2 Lists career goals.
7. Job description provided including blank performance contract.
    7.1 Clinical level established as _____.
    7.2 Years of longevity established as _____.
8. Salary information available.
    8.1 Base salary $ _____.
    8.2 Clinical level pay $ _____.
    8.3 Longevity pay $ _____.
    8.4 Differential $ _____.
    8.5 Total pay $ _____.
    8.6 Pay days made known.

Figure 5–3 • *Checklist for Reviewing Job Applicant's Folder*

Adequate time should be set aside for the interview; it should take place in a private office where there will be no interruptions. An interview guide will be helpful in conducting an interview satisfactory to both nurse manager and the applicant; see Figure 5–4.

Thompson defines an interview as "an equal level, face-to-face discussion between a job seeker and a person with full authority to fill the position under discussion."[15] Nurses are the job seekers and want a face-to-face discussion with the person with hiring authority. They may be looking at several jobs, having narrowed the field down to those that specifically fit their career goals. They know how to make contacts and now want interviews to create opportunities to sell themselves.

The Introduction. The interviewer should prepare for the interview beforehand. The interviewer should seat the candidate for comfort so that she or he will not be blinded by sunlight and will be facing the interviewer. The interviewer should come out from behind the desk, shake hands with the candidate, call the candidate by name, and make introductions. This is done to set the candidate at ease.

Questions. Questions should be prepared beforehand. These may include those listed in Figure 5–4. Those specifically desired by the interviewer should be added. The answers should not be written down as this is distracting and time consuming. Written notes should be made immediately following the interview.

All candidates for nurse jobs should be treated as professionals. They should not be asked illegal questions, such as those listed in Figure 5–5.

Since information about age and date of birth may be necessary for insurance or other fringe benefits, it can be obtained after the candidate is hired.

The candidate will also have questions. If complete information cannot be given at the interview, notes should be made and the information communicated to the candidate as quickly as possible. Figure 5–6 contains possible questions that candidates may ask, which the interviewer should be prepared to answer.

Although it is best not to speculate on the course of a job interview, it is possible to prepare for it in such a way that success will be most likely. An interview is simply a conversation between a potential employer and a candidate. There may be a need to modify the interview if the employer wants to hire the nurse to meet the organization's needs, while the candidate seeks to achieve personal goals.

Candidate: _____

Date and time of interview: _____

1. Arrange seating.
2. Make introductions and establish rapport.
3. Ask prepared questions.
   3.1 Tell me about yourself.
   3.2 What is your present job?
   3.3 What are your three most outstanding accomplishments?
   3.4 What is the extent of your formal education?
   3.5 What three things are most important to you in your job?
   3.6 What is your strongest qualification for this job?
   3.7 What other jobs have you held in this or a similar field?
   3.8 What were your responsibilities?
   3.9 Do you mind irregular working hours? Explain.
   3.10 Would you be willing to relocate? To travel?
   3.11 What minimum salary are you willing to accept?
   3.12 Are you more comfortable working alone or with other people?
4. Answer candidate's questions.
5. Note the following: Candidate was:
   5.1 On time.
   5.2 Well dressed.
   5.3 Well mannered.
   5.4 Positive about self.
6. Maintain eye contact.
7. Note candidate's personal values.
8. Close the interview.
   8.1 Make an offer.
   8.2 Obtain acceptance.
   8.3 Set timetable for making offer or receiving response to offer.

SOURCE: Adapted with permission from R. C. Swansburg and P. W. Swansburg, *Strategic Career Planning and Development for Nurses* (Rockville, MD: Aspen, 1984), 194.

Figure 5–4 • *Interview Guide*

The objective of both interviewer and candidate at the outset of an interview is to create a posi-

Employment interviewers are forbidden by law to ask the following questions:

1. Your age.
2. Your date of birth.
3. The length of time you have resided at your present address.
4. Your previous address.
5. Your religion; the church you attend; your spiritual adviser.
6. Your father's surname.
7. Your maiden name (of women).
8. Your marital status.
9. Your residence mates.
10. The number and ages of your children; who will care for them while you work.
11. How you will get to work, unless a car is a job requirement.
12. Residence of spouse or parent.
13. Whether you own or rent your residence.
14. The name of your bank; information on outstanding loans.
15. Whether wages were ever garnished.
16. Whether you ever declared bankruptcy.
17. Whether you were ever arrested.
18. Whether you were ever convicted, unless this is a job-related necessity. (For example, in jobs requiring a security clearance.)
19. Hobbies, off-duty interests, clubs.
20. Foreign languages you can read, write, or speak, unless this is a job requirement.

SOURCE: Adapted from conference with Paula Andrews, personnel director, University of South Alabama Medical Center, Mobile, AL, 1983. Reprinted with permission.

Figure 5–5 • *Questions That Are Illegal*

1. How much job security does this job have?
2. What previous experience does this type of job require?
3. What is the future of this type of job?
4. What is the growth potential for this particular job?
5. Where will the most significant growth for this type of job in the health care industry occur?
6. What is the starting salary for this job?
7. How do pay raises occur?
8. How does one find out when other job openings occur?
9. What are the fringe benefits of this job?
10. What are the requirements for working shifts and weekends?
11. What are the opportunities for continuing education?
12. What are the opportunities for promotion?
13. What child care facilities are available?
14. What are the staffing and scheduling policies?

SOURCE: Adapted with permission from R. C. Swansburg and P. W. Swansburg, *Strategic Career Planning and Development for Nurses* (Rockville, MD: Aspen, 1984), 196.

Figure 5–6 • *Possible Questions from Candidates*

tive, amicable relationship to the end that a job offer emerges. The interview is the most important factor in gaining this end, as it allows expression of personal ideas, abilities, and accomplishments. It adds individual personality to the résumé and completed application forms. To prepare for a job interview, nurse managers should:

1. Decide beforehand that they want the interview to end in a job offer.

2. Know the specific qualifications needed by the organization. Relating them to the candidate will help to identify a fit between candidate and job.

3. Decide to win the candidate's trust. The interviewer should come across as someone who respects and values employees. It is important for both interviewer and interviewee to be self-confident and exude the personal chemistry of optimism, good manners, charm, and enthusiasm.

4. Gain a feeling for the values of the candidate. Are they compatible with the organization's mission, philosophy, and objectives?

5. Have expectations about the dress, mannerisms, and other personal characteristics of the candidate. A serious candidate will dress conservatively for the interview. If the applicant is a man, he should be clean-shaven, hair neatly cut and styled, be dressed in a business suit and tie, and have appropriate footwear. Beards can be acceptable but should be neatly trimmed. If the applicant is a woman, she should have a neat hairdo, be dressed in a business suit or dress, wear hosiery, and have appropriate jewelry.

The Hiring Executive	The Candidate
1. Gives information about job and institution.	1. Gives information about self.
2. Assesses the competencies the candidate possesses in relation to the job opening.	2. Assesses the opportunity for developing and using competencies on the job.
3. Evaluates the candidate's personal characteristics in relation to the staff members with whom candidate will work (fit to staff).	3. Assesses ability to relate to the employees with whom candidate will work.
4. Assesses candidate's potential to move organization toward its goals.	4. Assesses potential for achieving personal career goals.
5. Assesses candidate's enthusiasm and state of health.	5. Assesses the institution's climate and the morale of the employees.
6. Forms impressions about candidate— behavior, appearance, ability to communicate, confidence, intelligence, personality.	6. Assesses opportunities for promotion and success.
7. Assesses candidate's ability to do the job.	7. Assesses own ability to do the job.
8. Determines facts about candidate.	8. Determines facts about the organization and working conditions.

SOURCE: Adapted with permission from R. C. Swansburg and P. W. Swansburg, *Strategic Career Planning and Development for Nurses* (Rockville, MD: Aspen, 1984), 204.

Figure 5–7 • *What Happens during Interviews*

Makeup should be in good taste and perfume or cologne should be discreet. One's appearance should be interpreted as indicating a person of good judgment and impeccable taste. Candidates thus tell the employer they regard the interview as important. The interviewer should dress, act, look, and smell like the right person to be the candidate's manager.

The candidate should come across as a thoroughly pleasant, cooperative, and competent person, one who can deal with the most difficult people problems tactfully, objectively, and successfully. The candidate should be neither blustery and flamboyant nor mouselike and servile. The interviewer should meet the same personal standards. Candidates who disagree with the interviewer's tastes or values should not be rejected unless the disagreement is unacceptable to the good of the organization. They should not be intimidated.

Interviewers should remember that they are human beings responding to human beings during the interviewing process. Both applicant and interviewer are being assessed. The interviewer is deciding from appearance, conversation, and behavior how the nurse will fit the job. The candidate is deciding from similar observation how he or she will like working for the interviewer.[16] Figure 5–7 summarizes what happens in interviews.

Eye Contact. It is important to maintain good eye contact during an interview. This can be done by following some simple rules. The interviewer should look at the candidate's eyes for about eight seconds, then look away, shifting the body position at the same time. That avoids being thought of as having "shifty" eyes. Also, if eye contact makes one uncomfortable, the focus can be shifted to the bridge of the candidate's nose at a spot between the eyes.

Eye contact tells the candidate the interviewer has trust and credibility.[17]

Establishment of Rapport. At the outset of the interview rapport can be established with the candidate by talking about common friends or interests. This should be kept short as time is important to both sides.[18]

Closing the Interview. Closing the interview means that the session is at a point where the interviewer is ready to make an offer or has all of the information needed. If ready to make an offer, the interviewer should have all of the information related to salary, fringe benefits, assignment, and scheduling ready for presentation and discussion.

If the candidate wants it in writing or wants time to consider the offer, a definite time schedule should be set:

"I want you for this position. I will mail you an offer tomorrow."

"I want you for this position. Please call me and give me your decision between 8 and 10 A.M. Monday."

If the interviewer needs more information, candidates should be so advised and told they will be contacted as soon as the information is available. If there are several candidates for a specific job, all will have to be interviewed and a selection made. Candidates should be notified of their rejection. If possible, reasons for rejection should be stated, but in terms that will not destroy candidate's self-esteem or cause legal problems for the employer.

Credentialing

Credentialing is the process by which selected professionals are granted privileges to practice within an organization. In health care organizations this process has been largely confined to physicians. Limited privileges have been granted to psychologists, social workers, and selected categories of nurses such as nurse anesthetists, surgical nurses, and midwives. Generally these categories have been restricted by physician credentialing policies and fall in the category of allied professional staff.

Requirements of the Joint Commission on Accreditation of Healthcare Organizations (JCAHO) require that hospitals make investigation, develop recommendations, reach conclusions, and be responsible for their actions in credentialing the medical staff. Licensing and certification provide data to consider in the process.

Components of Credentialing. As for physicians the components of a credentialing system for nurses would be:

1. Appointment—Evaluation and selection for nursing staff membership.
2. Clinical Privileges—Delineation of the specific nursing specialties that may be performed and the types of illness or patients that may be managed within the institution for each member of the nursing staff.
3. Periodic Reappraisal—Continuing review and evaluation of each member of the nursing staff to assure that competence is maintained and is consistent with privileges.[19]

Criteria for Appointment. Criteria for appointments and clinical privileges would include proof of licensure, education and training, specialty board certification, previous experience, and recommendations. Clinical privileges criteria would include proof of specialty training and of performance of nursing procedures or specialty care during training and previous appointments.

During the credentialing process the committee should look for "red flags" of high mobility, graduation from foreign schools, professional liability suits, and professional disciplinary actions. Each "red flag" is a reason for exercising extra care in review of the applicant.

Even though professional nurses have mostly been hired through personnel offices, nurse managers should give consideration to increasing the professional status of nursing through the credentialing process.

The American Nurses' Association (ANA). A report of the Committee for the Study of Credentialing in Nursing was made in 1979. It included fourteen principles of credentialing related to:

1. Those credentialed
2. Legitimate interests of involved occupation, institution, and general public
3. Accountability
4. A system of checks and balances
5. Periodic assessments
6. Objective standards and criteria and persons competent in their use
7. Representation of the community of interests
8. Professional identity and responsibility
9. An effective system of role delineation
10. An effective system of program identification
11. Coordination of credentialing mechanisms
12. Geographic mobility
13. Definitions and terminology
14. Communications and understanding[20]

Credentialing in a hospital relates to appointing health professionals to the staff. Credentialing by professional organizations such as the ANA can be a qualification for such appointments.

Assigning

Assigning professional nurses to jobs is the third part of the hiring process following selecting and credentialing. During the assignment period the new nurse is oriented to the job description and its use. Although assignment to a specific position using the job description may not be possible during the selecting and credentialing processes, candidates should know the possible units to which they may be assigned.

If a candidate wants to work in the operating room, but there are no vacant positions, where can that person be assigned? Offer the candidate a choice of vacant positions. Make a verbal or written contract to transfer the individual to a vacated operating room position when one becomes available. If others are waiting, indicate the order in which they will be assigned to the operating room.

Do not give candidates assignment surprises when they arrive for orientation. Assignment policies should be fair, reasonable, and acceptable to candidates. They will then start work with a positive attitude. A principle to follow is to provide necessary orientation and training to nursing employees to ensure competency, job satisfaction, and high productivity in the particular assignments they are accepting.

RETAINING

The retention of competent, professional nurses in jobs is a major problem of the U.S. health care industry particularly for hospitals. Most Americans change jobs about fifteen times by age 35, and nurses are no exception. Nurses change and achieve their major career goals four or five times in their lifetime, including changing their specialty or the role they play in the profession.[21] Many do both. Some even retire from two or more systems.

Career Dissatisfaction versus Job Dissatisfaction

There is a difference between career dissatisfaction and job dissatisfaction. A nurse may make a job change because of job dissatisfaction. If dissatisfied with several jobs a professional nurse looks at the work itself, the tasks involved, and the purposes to be served. If they are all distasteful a professional nurse may make a decision to leave the profession.

Turnover

The turnover rate among hospital nurses nationally appears to be between 20 and 70 percent annually. An organization should determine its turnover rate by unit and by organization. It should be done monthly to keep abreast of trends. Leavers should be profiled and defined to identify characteristics that will give clues that could decrease turnover and increase retention of competent nurses. Nurse managers should also review the performance of the leavers as well as doing exit interviews.

Job Expectations and Satisfactions

The author contends that the high turnover rate in nursing is a result of job dissatisfactions. In a survey of nurses' satisfactions and dissatisfactions with their jobs and careers, 6,277 surveys were mailed to nurses in a five-county area around Jacksonville, Florida. There were 1,921 responses with the following results:

1. One-third of the total reported substantial dissatisfaction with their jobs.
2. One-half of the total reported they felt negative about nursing.
3. One-half of the total were strongly satisfied with their jobs and careers.
4. *Money was the number one concern and the preferred remedy.*
5. Recognition was the second most serious concern; hours and scheduling were third; too much responsibility for the money fourth; and stress fifth.
6. The respondents included 337 nurses who were licensed but unemployed in nursing. They planned to return to nursing but considered hours and pay inadequate.[22]

A study to determine why new graduates select particular settings and why many leave in a short time surveyed 279 nursing seniors in five schools in northern Alabama. The expectations of these new graduates were to:

1. Work full-time.
2. Work days or a desired shift (46 percent of single nurses and 36.5 percent of married nurses would work evenings).
3. Work in a medium-sized to large hospital.
4. Earn a good salary.
5. Have pleasant working conditions.
6. Gain self-fulfillment and a sense of achievement from giving adequate and complete care.
7. Have educational opportunities, intellectual stimulation, and opportunity to develop new skills.
8. Have satisfactory supervision by head nurses.
9. Be recognized and encouraged.
10. Have professional autonomy and power.

11. Work in community that offered higher education opportunities and a good place to raise a family. Factors considered important included good schools, a low crime rate, an economically stable region, a low tax structure, and low cost of living.

In addition, more baccalaureate degree nurses expected to become head nurses, supervisors, and public health nurses than did associate degree nurses. Many would *not* consider working in small hospitals (17.2 percent), Veterans Administration or federally owned hospitals (19.5 percent), investor-owned hospitals (18.8 percent), nursing homes (65.7 percent), doctor's office or clinic (18.6 percent), temporary or private-duty agency (41 percent), or psychiatric or mental health clinic (45.5 percent).[23]

Drucker argues that salaries are not the basic problem with nurse retention and recruitment, a position in opposition to most surveys. He states, "The basic problem is that nurses aren't allowed to do nursing. I've been saying that now for 20 years. The doctors still treat nurses as if they were scullery maids, and that's just not going to work any longer." Drucker believes that hospital administrators must change the attitudes of doctors. Also, focusing nurses' responsibilities on their professional role and increasing their salaries will alleviate the shortage.[24]

Career Planning

Nurse managers will recognize the results of nurse satisfaction surveys. They must now learn to manage professional nurses so they will achieve career and job satisfaction. The first step is to establish a career plan for them within the nursing organization.

To be successful in their careers professional nurses must have a sense of personal fulfillment and job meaningfulness, that they are growing as persons. Nurse managers can create these conditions by determining and correcting the causes of:

- Anxiety and uncertainty
- Inability to meet personal and organizational goals
- Lack of clarity about roles played
- Contradictory demands
- Dissatisfaction with human relations
- Rebellion against rules, policies, and regulations
- The inherent nature of the tasks of the job

- Competition
- Being overworked and underutilized
- Lack of personal and professional growth
- Dissatisfaction with the quality of associates

A professional nurse is a reasonable person and reasonable people can accommodate to reality, accept themselves, be interested in others, learn from experience, and be self-actualized.[25]

Nurse managers should restructure nursing services to link assignments and responsibilities to education, experience, and competence. This should be a part of a career program that provides more promotions and pay for clinical nurses, pay for seniority, and increased participation. It should provide for continuing education to upgrade knowledge and skills. It will provide clinical rotation policies that prevent burnout and it should meet professional nurses' scheduling and salary preferences.[26]

When a career structure has been established it will provide for upward mobility for clinical nurses, nurse managers, nurse teachers and nurse researchers. Professional nurses will decide to take advantage of career advancement opportunities. Jobs for those advancing will be identified and will require advanced knowledge and skills, particularly those related to decision making. Registered nurses who do not want promotion will be rewarded by longevity pay increases (each year during entire employment) and credit for doing their jobs well. Advancing nurses will be rewarded for longevity and for increased responsibility and accountability. Nurses will finally have careers.

The Career Counselor. A career counselor should be part of the grand strategy for establishing a nursing career program.

Even though an organization might not have a career counselor, every nurse should have one in the person of a superior. This person helps nurses clarify their career goals and make a plan for achieving them. The plan includes work experiences related to off-duty time such as courses, workshops, community service, professional activities, and other activities specifically related to goals. It is a total plan that develops individuals professionally to meet their career aspirations. The career counselor facilitates that program. A supervisor who is not the career counselor can be asked to become one or to provide the opportunity to use someone else.

The counselor should help nurses advance their careers in nursing, not just within the organization. There should be at least one counselor who can help individuals assess their interests, skills, and values, who can assist with analyzing all of the options open, and who can aid in making the career plans that will lead to achieving career goals.

That individual could be a supervisor, a nurse administrator, a staff development person, or an expert in the chosen field of nursing. In the final analysis, only the individual nurse can develop and direct a career toward achievement of life goals. All others, be they employers, colleagues, peers, counselors, or whoever, can only form a support group.

Staff Development Career Counselor. One group to contact about career opportunities is the staff development department. There is an awakening notion that staff development can advance the career opportunities of professional nurses. Because such counselors traditionally serve in an organizational relationship that provides a staff service to the line of the nursing hierarchy, their role should be identified by nursing administration. Usually the staff development department fulfills functions of initial orientation and conducts classes in cardiopulmonary resuscitation, intravenous therapy, and the like. On the other hand, some departments are moving toward a career development orientation by involving themselves in such functions as specialty orientation and training and implementing the process of planning, organizing, directing, and evaluating the development of nurses through levels of competency in clinical practice, management, teaching, and research.

Sovie labels the career development functions of the staff development department as professional identification, professional maturation, and professional mastery. These areas can be related to a career ladder program where competencies have been identified for the nurse practicing at one of several rungs or levels of the ladder. The competencies are stated in the form of job descriptions, and increase in complexity. Policies and procedures exist for the process of climbing the ladder. The process is facilitated by a program of staff development for career advancement.

Sovie's model could be used to educate nurses to gain advanced specialized knowledge and skills. This could be achieved through individual plans, with staff development educators acting as counselors and teachers. Nurses could learn to provide the leadership in solving the health care problems of patients and families. They could develop materials for patient and family education. They could learn to be primary nurses in practicing the nursing process, not just within the nursing modality. They could learn to engage in professional nursing dialogue with colleagues. Their training could include the competencies of consulting, participation in quality assurance activities, processing and applying reports of research findings, participation in research, and involvement in committee functions. This learning could be part of a personal career plan.[27]

Efforts outside the Department. In many organizations these maturation skills are shaped outside the staff development department. Professional nurses who select the management ladder enter into a continuous program of staff development. As clinical nurses develop the credentials of mastery in a specialty area, they are assigned to that level of practice. All could be encouraged to produce their own staff development functions, including putting on workshops in which they earn a fee. This income could be used to pay for their own continuing education outside their organization. They could provide nurse-to-nurse consultation in their areas of specialization. They could participate on unit, division, and organization committees. Their mastery is rewarded by higher salaries and additional perquisites related to their professional mastery, because they produce more at the same cost.

Nurses in an organization that has a career development program should be moving up the ladder of their choice. The career development program should also provide an opportunity for moving laterally into clinical practice, management, teaching, or research. It should provide job satisfaction and a salary that increases with development and mastery.

If such a career development program does not exist in the organization, nurses can stimulate it. They can first learn about it through research and study, master the knowledge of career development, and then present it to their supervisors and get their support. If attempts to move up fail, nurses may want to move out, but they should not give up easily.[28]

Career Ladders. Clinical nursing offers the most diverse kinds of opportunities. Clinical nursing was largely a nonpromotable area until recent years. There were numerous interesting clinical areas that had expanded with advanced technology but nurses seldom could be promoted within a clinical area. This is changing fast with the development of clinical career ladders.

A career ladder requires individual effort, assisted by organizational support and reward. It results in career satisfaction to the nurses who participate and in increased productivity for the employer if the program is appropriately conceived and implemented. There must be more results than title changes and increased wages or salaries. The advantages of clinical career ladders are discussed in more detail later.

Among the opportunities are clinical coordinator, clinical specialist, nurse practitioner, primary nurse, patient health educator, and flight nurse. Advertisements in nursing journals and local newspapers identify these and many more opportunities. Those who want to stay in clinical nursing and advance in terms of all rewards, including money, fringe benefits, professional achievement, and satisfaction, will need to be prepared at the highest level of clinical practice. Clinical nurse specialists are professionals with education and experience at the level of the most complicated patient care problems and needs. Examples are clinical nurse specialists in ostomy care, oncology, or cardiovascular care. They should have the experience and education to perform in a consultative nurse capacity. Most clinical nurse specialists have education beyond the bachelor's level, with either an advanced degree or certificate. They also have had the advanced clinical experience to match the knowledge.

A clinical career ladder is a horizontal development system based on specific criteria used to develop, evaluate, and promote nurses desiring and intending to remain at the bedside. Clinical ladders apply to nurses who want to remain in the clinical setting, whereas career ladders are for those who leave the clinical realm in pursuit of a future in administration, teaching, or research.

A clinical career ladder should:

1. Improve quality of patient care.
2. Motivate staff in terms of—
   2.1 Job proficiency/expertise (motivate the individual to reach the highest level of professional competence).
   2.2 Pursuit of education (an important factor in mobility).
   2.3 Development of career goals.
3. Provide methods of objective and measurable performance evaluation and reward clinical competence for the purpose of advancement.
4. Promote retention within clinical area and reduce turnover rate.

Nurses interested in working under this type of system should understand several points. First, most hospitals have a promotion system of some kind and a few are of a clinical ladder type. Unfortunately, many are based on a seniority system or include seniority as the primary criterion for advancement. Some administrators adopt a form of clinical ladder to help alleviate their recruitment and retention problems. Their ladder may look good on paper but the question is whether it provides the nurses with any significant advantages. If the system in which a nurse is working promotes to the next higher level according to a time frame without regard for educational status or job performance, then the individual is at a disadvantage. There is no competition or motivation to improve. Everyone will be promoted when they have served their time—both average and above-average nurses.

If the pay differential between levels is not significant, that also will impede motivation. Salary increases should be enough to further motivate the nurses to improve their skills (competence). Responsibility should increase with promotion. If nurses are still performing the same tasks with the same supervision and no additional responsibility after advancement, then they cannot be said to have really advanced professionally.

Performance criteria in any clinical ladder system should be clearly differentiated and specific at each level. The evaluation process must be measurable. Salary differentials must be significant enough to provide motivation. Any system should involve evaluation of educational and leadership criteria as well as skill performance.

Finally, the evaluation of each individual should include input from the direct supervisor and the individuals themselves. A board or panel of three or more nurses may be assembled to review all eligible personnel for promotion. The advantages of such a system are that it increases job satisfaction, improves clinical skills, offers positive motivation for acceptance of continued leadership and educational responsibility, and provides an opportunity for career advancement while remaining in clinical nursing. The disadvantage is that positions may not always be available at higher levels.

Management promotes the system to the end that productivity will be increased. Also, management must assure the maintenance of quality of nursing care.

The following is a basic clinical ladder model that can be added to or fleshed out by management:

Clinical/Staff Nurse I (beginner/novice)

1. Experience and education
   - Current state licensure with less than 1 year of experience
2. Description
   - Needs close supervision
   - Performs basic nursing skills/routine patient care
   - Begins to develop patient assessment skills/communication skills

Clinical/Staff Nurse II (advanced beginner)

1. Experience and education
   - Current state licensure with more than 1 year of experience
   - BSN with more than 6 months of experience
   - MSN without experience
2. Description
   - Demonstrates adequate/acceptable performance
   - Can differentiate importance of situations and set priorities
   - Requires less supervision
   - Demonstrates interest in continuing education

Clinical/Staff Nurse III (competent)

1. Experience and education
   - Current licensure with 2 or more years of experience
   - BSN with more than 1 year of experience
   - MSN with more than 6 months of experience
2. Description
   - Demonstrates unsupervised competency using nursing process
   - Is able to plan and organize in terms of short-range and long-range goals
   - Demonstrates direction in actions
   - Accepts leadership responsibility readily
   - Demonstrates well-developed communication skills
   - Shares ideas and knowledge with peers

Clinical/Staff Nurse IV (proficient)

1. Experience and education
   - Current licensure with 3 years of clinical experience and pursuit of BSN
   - BSN with more than 2 years of experience (preferred)
   - MSN with more than 1 year of experience
2. Description
   - Demonstrates specialized knowledge and skills
   - Continues professional education
   - Assumes leadership/supervisory responsibility

- Recognizes and adjusts to situations that vary from the norm
- Delegates responsibility appropriately; uses wide range of alternatives in solving problems

Clinical/Staff Nurse V (expert)

1. Experience and education
   - MSN with more than 2 years of appropriate clinical experience
   - BSN required with more than 3 years of experience, pursuing MSN
2. Description
   - Demonstrates expertise in clinical practice
   - Assumes/delegates personnel and management responsibility[29]

Because salary and benefits are the most concrete method of recognizing outstanding performance, valid career ladders should not be undermined with pay practices for certain kinds of nurses such as those who work in critical care areas. Rewards should be given for levels of responsibility, preparation, experience, and performance. General duty nurses share equal responsibility and greater workload variety than specialty care nurses.

Spitzer and Bolton report the results of a staff survey of 956 career-employed RNs. There were 583 respondents who strongly agreed to the following statements on salary and salary equity:

1. *When first hired, staff nurses should be paid according to years of experience, acute care experience, and education.*
2. *Salary adjustments (raises) should be based on clinical performance, additional acquired education, and additional clinical experience (regardless of specialty).*[30]

When redesigning a wage and salary structure, nurse managers need to obtain input from the staff. Clinical ladders should be related to productivity. They can be based on a professional practice model and reward competence, knowledge, and performance. Essential components are:

1. A number of levels of practice
2. Differentiation among levels of practice
3. A job description for performance evaluation
4. Criteria for placement of new hires
5. Methods of communication
6. Identification of development needs of staff
7. Criteria for measuring effectiveness of ladder relative to quality of care, staff satisfaction/retention, and cost effectiveness[31]

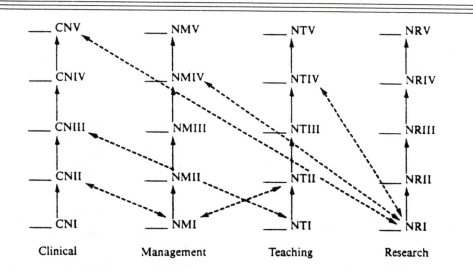

This is a model. Each level would require specific and increasing education, experience and performance accomplishments. The arrows indicate the levels at which nurses from each group could advance laterally. The clinical nurse II (CNII) could advance to nurse manager (NMI) or vice versa. The nurse teacher IV (NTIV) could advance to nurse researcher I (NRI) or vice versa. The blanks in front of each group would have the number of budgeted positions entered. For nurse researchers this could be one position but allow for appointment at, or promotion to higher levels.

Figure 5–8 • *Promotion System*

Master Plan

A master plan for career development should be developed for the nursing organization and for each unit of the organization. It should include objectives, policies on posting of jobs, development of résumés and curriculum vitae, and strategies for moving up in the organization. It should consider lateral transfers, specialty training and cross-training, and plans for nurses who become physically unable to perform the rigors of acute care nursing.

PROMOTING

Professional nurses have had to turn to management, education, or research for promotion. The development of professional nurse clinical ladders is making some headway, albeit not quickly enough. Many professional nurses want to stay in clinical nursing and will do so if they can be rewarded with promotions that increase their pay and standing within the organization.

One way for nurse managers to assure that all professional nurses have promotion opportunities is to develop a promotion system. The system will indicate all promotion categories within the organization; see Figure 5–8.

Nurse managers should develop specific promotion policies with input from all categories of professional nurses and the human resources department. These policies would include the following:

1. All vacant positions will be posted. This should be true even though change in pay and rank do not occur. Some nurses will want to change units, specialty, shifts, and so on.
2. All interested applicants should file applications for promotion in the human resource department.
3. Human resource department personnel should prepare promotion rosters that rank all candidates by education, experience, performance, and other objective criteria. The best qualified candidate should be at the top of the list.
4. Applicants should be interviewed and rated by the same set of criteria.
5. The best qualified candidates should be selected for promotion.
6. The results of the promotion process should be announced. Those not selected should be notified and counseled individually rather than learning they were passed over from hearing about or seeing the list of those promoted.
7. The promotion system must be fair and be perceived as fair by professional nurses.

Darling and McGrath write that nurses experience much trauma when moving upward from clinical to managerial nursing. They are unaware of the transition process involved in a promotion, including the fact that their social and professional ties with other clinical nurses are cut. They take on more responsibilities and burdens and soon feel isolated and alone. Although they gain visibility and prestige, they get complaints instead of appreciation from their staff.[32]

To prevent promotion trauma, supervisors of promotees can plan a transition program. It will alert them to the changes in their relationships. It will help keep them from blaming their difficulties on personal failings. Such a program will include clear role descriptions and expectations, clear job descriptions, and classes to meet their management knowledge and skills needs. Staff development is as essential for nurses promoted to management as it is for those who stay in the clinical domain. They can know what to expect and how to deal with Darling and McGrath's five stages of promotion: uninformed optimism, informed pessimism, hopeful realism, informed optimism, and rewarding completion. A management development program will keep clinical nurses promoted to manager positions from bailing out at the second stage.

TERMINATING

Employees cannot be terminated at will. They are protected by public policy set forth in the National Labor Relations Act, the Civil Rights Act of 1964, the Discrimination in Employment Act, the Vocational Rehabilitation Act, and the Occupational Safety and Health Act. Also, laws protect "whistle blowers."

Employees should be terminated only after all efforts to retain them have been exhausted. The theory of management includes concepts and principles that, when learned and applied by nurse managers, will assist employees to be competent and productive. Punishment or disciplinary action should be a last resort and should be progressive from verbal conference, to a recorded conference, to suspension, to discharge. Such action should be covered by written policies and procedures.

Nurse managers including head nurses should have firing authority. They should consult with superior managers and human resource personnel when terminating staff to make sure the action will stand up in court. All policies must be legal and must be consistently and correctly enforced. Any

employee is entitled to a fair hearing and review. The process must allow for appropriate representatives at investigating interviews. When terminated, employees should be paid all benefits they have accrued.[33]

SUMMARY

A major focus of a theory of nursing management is that personnel should be managed for productivity, for achieving the mission and objectives of the organization. This involves recruiting, selecting, credentialing, and assigning nurses, first into the educational program, then into the division or department of nursing.

Because nursing, a predominantly female occupation, must now compete with all other professions for students, nurse managers should create attractive conditions of work. These include competitive salaries and fringe benefits, flexible schedules, and satisfying conditions of work such as autonomy and recognition.

The population from which all occupations will recruit will change greatly during the next decade. Their demographic makeup will shift causing recruitment goals to change. Nurse managers should plan student recruitment at early stages of the secondary education process. The poor, minorities, children of single parents, and the physically and emotionally handicapped must be prepared now for careers including careers in nursing. It is the promise of America.

Each nurse manager should work with other health care system managers and secondary and high school teachers and counselors to prepare young men and women for careers in nursing. Once nurses are recruited, selected, credentialed, and assigned, nurse managers should develop strategies to retain them.

Nurse managers should consider a credentialing process for professional nurses similar to that used for physicians. It is essential that career planning be a major personnel management program within each nursing organization. Employees desire that they have the opportunity to qualify for promotion to clinical, management, education, and research jobs. They are not motivated by dead-end jobs. There should be clear communication of job vacancies, and they should be filled by the best qualified individuals.

Personnel who do not meet acceptable standards of performance should be counseled, then warned in writing, and then suspended without pay. When all else fails they should be terminated.

EXPERIENTIAL EXERCISES

1. Using Figure 5–1, Strategies to Recruit Students into Nursing Education Programs, prepare a management plan to accomplish those strategies you select. This may be done as a group exercise.

MANAGEMENT PLAN

OBJECTIVE:

ACTIONS	TARGET DATES	ASSIGNED TO	ACCOMPLISHMENTS

2. Using Figure 5–2, Criteria for Developing an Effective Nurse Recruitment Advertisement, prepare a management plan. Prepare the advertisement. This may be done as a group exercise.

MANAGEMENT PLAN

OBJECTIVE:

ACTIONS	TARGET DATES	ASSIGNED TO	ACCOMPLISHMENTS

3. Using Figure 5–4, Interview Guide, simulate interviewing a job applicant by interviewing one of your group members.

4. Do an exit interview using the format of Figure 5–9. Discuss the results with your peer group.

Date _____

Name _____ Date hired _____ Shift _____

Position title _____ Department _____

Supervisor's name _____ Date separated _____

CHECKLIST:
_____ ID card returned to personnel dept.
_____ Final payroll check form completed
_____ State retirement refund form completed
_____ Received insurance conversion information
_____ Locker keys returned

I. REASON FOR SEPARATION (Check appropriate box)

Voluntary resignation
_____ New position
_____ Retirement (voluntary)
_____ Relocation
_____ Illness
_____ Pregnancy
_____ Job dissatisfaction
_____ Return to school
_____ Other (specify)
_____

Involuntary termination
_____ Retirement (mandatory)
_____ Reduction of staff
_____ Other (specify)
_____

II. INTERVIEW

A. SELECTION:
What kind of work have you been doing in our hospital? _____
_____
_____
_____

What kind of work did you do prior to joining our hospital? _____
_____
_____
_____

What type of work do you like best? _____
_____
_____

SOURCE: Courtesy of the University of South Alabama Medical Center, Mobile, Alabama.

Figure 5–9 • *University of South Alabama Medical Center Employee Exit Interview*

(Continued)

What type of work do you like least? _____

_____

Why? _____

_____

B. ORIENTATION:
Who explained your job to you? _____

Describe your orientation: _____

_____

_____

Length of time? _____

What did your orientation lack? _____

_____

_____

Were in-service education programs sufficient for your needs? _____

If not, how could programs be improved? _____

_____

C. SUPERVISION:
How do you feel about your Supervisor? _____

_____

_____

_____

Did you take any complaints to your Supervisor? _____ Yes _____ No

If yes, how were they handled? _____

_____

_____

Have you had any problems with your Supervisor? _____ Yes _____ No

If yes, describe: _____

_____

_____

_____

What kind of working relationship did you have with the staff in your department? _____

_____

_____

Figure 5–9 (Continued)

(Continued)

Was there ample opportunity for communication with co-workers, your Supervisor, and Department Head? _____

_____

How could communication be improved? _____

_____

_____

Have you felt administrative support by Hospital Administrators? _____

_____

_____

D. FINANCIAL:
How do you feel about your pay? _____

_____

_____

How do you feel about your progress within this hospital? _____

_____

_____

E. FOR NURSES:
Was your unit adequately staffed? _____

_____

How do you feel about being pulled to other units? _____

_____

How often were you pulled? _____

_____

F. SUMMARY:
What did you like best about your job? _____

_____

_____

What did you like least about your job? _____

_____

_____

What did you like best about our hospital? _____

_____

_____

Figure 5–9   (Continued)

(Continued)

What did you like least about our hospital? _____

_____

_____

Why are you really leaving? _____

_____

_____

Would you be willing to stay with our hospital under a more satisfactory arrangement?

_____ Yes _____ No

What changes would be required? _____

Would you return to this hospital if the opportunity existed? _____

_____

G. COMPLETE FOR RESIGNATION:

New Employer: _____   Location: _____

Position: _____   Pay: _____

Hours: _____

III. INTERVIEWER COMMENTS: _____

_____

_____

Figure 5-9   (Continued)

5. Use the questionnaire (Figure 5–10) to do a job satisfaction survey of a group of professional nurses. You may elect to add, delete, or modify the items.

Instructions. Read each item carefully and circle the number that best indicates your degree of job satisfaction from 1 (Not at All) to 5 (A Great Deal).

Items	Not at All → A Great Deal
1. Factor: salaries and fringe benefits.	
1.1 Pay is satisfactory.	1 2 3 4 5
1.2 Education and experience are recognized and used.	1 2 3 4 5
1.3 There are opportunities for career advancement.	1 2 3 4 5
1.4 The pay system rewards my years of experience.	1 2 3 4 5

Figure 5-10 •   *Job Satisfaction Questionnaire*

(Continued)

Items	Not at All → A Great Deal
1.5 The pay is adequate for shifts, weekends, and holidays.	1 2 3 4 5
1.6 Fringe benefits are known.	1 2 3 4 5
1.7 Employees are satisfied with fringe benefits.	1 2 3 4 5
1.8 Child care services are satisfactory.	1 2 3 4 5
1.9 The retirement program is a strong one.	1 2 3 4 5
2. Factor: staffing philosophy; clerical work; floating; rotating shifts.	
2.1 The staffing philosophy is fair.	1 2 3 4 5
2.2 A float pool covers absences and supplemental staffing.	1 2 3 4 5
2.3 Clinical nurses have input into staffing policies and procedures.	1 2 3 4 5
2.4 Opportunities for flexible work schedules exist.	1 2 3 4 5
2.5 Clerical duties are performed by clerical personnel.	1 2 3 4 5
2.6 Appropriate activities are performed by other departments such as pharmacy, medical laboratory, and dietary.	1 2 3 4 5
3. Factor: professionalism; interdisciplinary relationships; public relations.	
3.1 Clinical nurses serve on all organizational committees.	1 2 3 4 5
3.2 Administrators promote cooperative interdisciplinary relationships.	1 2 3 4 5
3.3 Clinical nurses spend their time giving care to patients.	1 2 3 4 5
3.4 Clinical nurses make decisions about patient care.	1 2 3 4 5
3.5 Clinical nurses participate in nursing management.	1 2 3 4 5
3.6 Clinical nurses are recognized and rewarded for nursing excellence.	1 2 3 4 5
3.7 Clinical nurses participate in quality assurance.	1 2 3 4 5
3.8 Clinical nurses receive awards for merit.	1 2 3 4 5
3.9 The communication system is informative, provides for clinical nursing input, and gives feedback.	1 2 3 4 5
3.10 Job vacancies are posted.	1 2 3 4 5
3.11 Clinical nurses participate in public relations functions.	1 2 3 4 5
4. Factor: staff development	
4.1 A career development program exists.	1 2 3 4 5

Figure 5–10 (Continued)

(Continued)

Items	Not at All → A Great Deal
4.2 Good opportunities for continuing education are available.	1 2 3 4 5
4.3 A good orientation program is in force.	1 2 3 4 5
4.4 Personnel are reimbursed for staff development activities.	1 2 3 4 5
4.5 Refresher courses are available.	1 2 3 4 5
4.6 Staff development programs are marketed.	1 2 3 4 5
4.7 Incompetent nurses are identified and handled appropriately.	1 2 3 4 5
4.8 Good leadership training courses are available.	1 2 3 4 5
4.9 Clinical nurses participate in staff development planning.	1 2 3 4 5
5. Factor: administration support.	
5.1 Clinical nurses can follow through on beliefs and values.	1 2 3 4 5
5.2 Clinical nurses are not subjected to punitive action by supervisors.	1 2 3 4 5
5.3 Productivity standards are known.	1 2 3 4 5
5.4 Employees have access to senior management.	1 2 3 4 5
5.5 Nursing service and nursing education are in harmony.	1 2 3 4 5
5.6 Patient safety is emphasized.	1 2 3 4 5
5.7 An up-to-date nursing management information system is available.	1 2 3 4 5
5.8 Managers are visible to nursing staff and patients.	1 2 3 4 5

Summarize your findings:

Figure 5–10 (Continued)

6. Make a master plan for self-assessment for your next position. Use the following criteria.

Master Plan for Self-Assessment for Next Position

Action	Date Completed
1. Assessing Personal Goals.	
1.1 Write a career advancement plan.	_____
1.2 Assess your present situation and decide what you like and dislike about your job and lifestyle (or the job and lifestyle you are seeking.) Decide whether you are satisfied with your status or want to change it.	_____
1.3 If you are getting ready for your first job or you decide to change from your present one, write career goals. Do them for this year, for 5 years from now, and for 10 years from now. Do this for the next job you want as a clinician, teacher, administrator, or researcher, or a combination of two.	_____
1.3.1 Write personal goals.	_____

Master Plan for Self-Assessment for Next Position (*Continued*)

Action	Date Completed

    1.3.2 Write family goals. _____

    1.3.3 Write professional goals. _____

  1.4 Obtain information on jobs in the career area to which you want to progress. _____

  1.5 Obtain information on the geographic area in which you want to live. _____

  1.6 Assess your ability to acquire power and status in terms of the personal qualities you now possess. _____

2. Identifying and Obtaining Qualifications Needed.

  2.1 Outline the formal education needed for the job you have chosen as a professional goal. _____

  2.2 Make a plan for obtaining the formal education needed. _____

    2.2.1 Obtain an evaluation from a counselor or adviser at the institution you plan to attend. _____

    2.2.2 Apply for admission. _____

    2.2.3 Register for classes with approval of adviser. _____

  2.3 Outline the experience needed for the job you have chosen as a professional goal. _____

  2.4 Make a plan for obtaining the experiences needed. _____

  2.5 Make a plan for becoming certified in a specialty if this is a career goal. _____

  2.6 Identify the personal characteristics needed for the job you have chosen as a professional goal. _____

    2.6.1 Can deal with restrictions on personal time. _____

    2.6.2 Willing to accept responsibility for own acts. _____

    2.6.3 Able to separate personal and job relationships so as to be perceived as fair. _____

  2.7 Assess your personal characteristics and compare them with those needed. _____

  2.8 Make a plan for modifying any of your personal characteristics that can be modified and that you wish to modify. _____

  2.9 Put your plans into effect. _____

3. Obtaining Information on Availability of Jobs.

  3.1 Do a job search. _____

    3.1.1 Make plan for searching for a job. _____

    3.1.2 Negotiate the support of family and friends. _____

    3.1.3 Review your career objectives and assess your qualifications. _____

    3.1.4 Contact personnel offices of institutions that employ nurses. _____

    3.1.5 Contact people who work in institutions that employ nurses. _____

    3.1.6 Contact faculty of colleges of nursing and the offices of career placement. _____

    3.1.7 Contact area hospitals. _____

    3.1.8 Obtain and read local newspapers. _____

    3.1.9 Contact chambers of commerce. _____

    3.1.10 Contact nursing organizations. _____

    3.1.11 Contact state boards of nursing. _____

    3.1.12 Contact police departments. _____

    3.1.13 Contact employment services. _____

    3.1.14 Make a list of people connections. _____

    3.1.15 Contact investor-owned firms. _____

    3.1.16 Contact nurse staffing agencies. _____

    3.1.17 Contact multiple hospital systems. _____

    3.1.18 Contact employment agencies, public and private. _____

    3.1.19 Check classified advertisements in newspapers and journals. _____

Master Plan for Self-Assessment for Next Position (*Continued*)

Action	Date Completed

3.2 Gather information about jobs in nursing. _____

   3.2.1 Decide whether you want to work full time or part time. _____

   3.2.2 Read job descriptions, philosophy and objective statements, and other information supplied by prospective employers. _____

   3.2.3 Write letters, make phone calls, and talk to people. Complete information. _____

4. Developing a Résumé and Curriculum Vitae.

  4.1 Decide the purpose for which you intend to use your résumé. _____

  4.2 Prepare your résumé for the specific purpose for which you intend to use it. _____

   4.2.1 Use a brief résumé to request an interview. _____

   4.2.2 Use to define past accomplishments and present competencies. _____

   4.2.3 Use a chronological or functional format. _____

   4.2.4 Have your résumé typed neatly and expertly. _____

  4.3 Prepare a personal cover letter for each résumé being mailed. _____

  4.4 Prepare a curriculum vitae. _____

   4.4.1 Name. _____

   4.4.2 Specialties. _____

   4.4.3 Education and training. _____

   4.4.4 Licensure. _____

   4.4.5 Important assignments. _____

   4.4.6 Membership in professional organizations. _____

   4.4.7 Other lectures and courses presented. _____

   4.4.8 Honors. _____

   4.4.9 Published articles, speeches, lectures. _____

   4.4.10 Consulting activities. _____

   4.4.11 Community activities. _____

5. Making Contacts.

  5.1 Develop a support system to ensure professional growth and advancement within nursing. _____

  5.2 Identify all possible contacts. _____

   5.2.1 Develop acquaintances, friends, and business associates as contacts who will refer you to prospective employers or vice versa. _____

   5.2.2 Use a careful strategy in dealing with personnel managers as they do not do the hiring. _____

   5.2.3 Develop a career counselor relationship with someone in your organization. _____

   5.2.4 Initiate or become involved in an organization career development program. _____

   5.2.5 Identify and associate with role models. _____

   5.2.6 Organize a peer pal support group. _____

   5.2.7 Identify and associate with a mentor. _____

   5.2.8 Identify and associate with a sponsor. _____

  5.3 Plan to take on novel assignments and do them well. _____

  5.4 Establish contacts with people in organizations such as honor societies, fraternities, sororities, and through people who know you. _____

  5.5 Make a plan for telephone contacts. _____

  5.6 Write letters that get attention. _____

  5.7 Plan for a network with the purpose of making job contacts or career planning. _____

6. Applying for Specific Positions.

  6.1 Use accurate information to fill out application forms. _____

Master Plan for Self-Assessment for Next Position (*Continued*)

Action	Date Completed
6.2 Type the application.	_____
6.3 Do a previsit of the organization and the area.	_____
6.4 Have enough money to pay relocation expenses. This should be negotiated with the employing institution. They have ways of paying for moves.	_____
6.5 Plan the questions you will ask when requesting an interview by telephone.	_____
6.6 Prepare for search committee interviews.	_____
6.7 Prepare and practice simulated interviews.	_____
6.8 Do information interviews.	_____
7. Negotiating the Contract.	
7.1 Prepare a plan for identifying the conditions of employment you desire including salary and fringe benefits.	_____
7.2 Outline the terms you want included in an individual contract.	_____
7.2.1 Salary based on analysis of complete information.	_____
7.2.2 Expense account.	_____
7.2.3 Relocation expenses.	_____
7.2.4 Company car.	_____
7.2.5 Memberships in professional organizations.	_____
7.2.6 Memberships in social clubs.	_____
7.2.7 Make a list of salary alternatives you are willing to accept.	_____
7.2.8 Others.	_____
7.3 Make a list of fringe benefits you want.	_____
7.4 Make a list of actions you can take to improve your negotiating position.	_____
7.5 Negotiate salary and other perquisites.	_____
7.6 Negotiate further salary revisions.	_____
7.7 Negotiate conditions for termination of contract.	_____
7.8 Evaluate conditions of employment before signing contract.	_____
8. Moving Up.	
8.1 Negotiate a pay raise.	_____
8.1.1 Do self-appraisal.	_____
8.1.2 Compare jobs.	_____
8.1.3 Prepare a written plan that supports a pay raise.	_____
8.1.4 Put the plan into effect.	_____
8.2 Plan for a promotion.	_____
8.2.1 Learn the power structure of the organization.	_____
8.2.2 Learn of upcoming vacancies.	_____
8.2.3 Move up within community organizations.	_____
8.2.4 Expand your competencies.	_____
8.2.5 Increase organizational income.	_____
8.2.6 Reduce organizational expenses.	_____
8.2.7 Be one of the top 10 percent.	_____
8.2.8 Be the best there is.	_____
8.3 Plan for and make an orderly transition when you move up.	_____
8.4 Analyze your job dissatisfactions. Make a plan to deal with them and decide whether to execute it. Do it.	_____
9. Moving On.	
9.1 Assess the pros and cons of staying in your present position.	_____

Master Plan for Self-Assessment for Next Position (Continued)

Action	Date Completed
9.1.1 Work to overcome poor ratings.	_____
9.1.2 Plan to overcome resistance to advanced nursing practice.	_____
9.1.3 Plan to improve an unsatisfactory work area.	_____
9.2 Make a plan for moving on.	_____
9.2.1 Create opportunities for contacts and visibility.	_____
9.2.2 Evaluate better opportunities.	_____
9.2.3 Visit the location.	_____
9.3 Identify your need for growth and make your move to meet it.	_____
9.4 Coordinate career moves with spouse.	_____
9.5 Consider the circumstances of moving down within your organization.	_____
9.6 Decide when to resign rather than be fired.	_____
10. Preventing Burnout.	
10.1 Assess personal potential for burnout.	_____
10.2 Initiate preventive measures.	_____

The position I want is:

_____

_____

The qualifications I need are: _____

_____

_____

_____

_____

_____

_____

_____

_____

SOURCE: R. C. Swansburg and P. W. Swansburg, *Strategic Career Planning and Development for Nurses* (Rockville, MD: 1984), 299–303.

7. The following conditions have been identified by nurses as problems related to nurse shortages.

- Underutilization of knowledge and skills.

- Acceptance by physicians of nurses as colleagues.

- Salaries too low in relation to kind of work performed (job requirements).

- Inflexible management with regard to flexible work schedules and autonomy of nursing practice; want independence, autonomy, responsibility, skill variety, task identity, and feedback.

- Misuse of knowledge and skills.

7.1 Select one of these problems or identify another that your group agrees on as related to the current nurse shortage.

7.2 Use the management plan format to write an objective for solving the problem. List those activities that you would do to accomplish this objective. Choose specific activities and establish time frames. The activities and time frames could be put on a controlling or evaluating chart for purposes of time and budget control. Refer to Chapter 20, Controlling or Evaluating.

7.3 Report

MANAGEMENT PLAN

PROBLEM:

OBJECTIVE:

ACTIONS	PERSON ASSIGNED	TIME FRAME	ACCOMPLISHMENTS

NOTES

1. American Hospital Association, "Background on the National Nursing Shortage," *Hospital Nurse Recruitment and Retention: A Source Book for Executive Management* (Chicago: American Hospital Association, Nov. 1980).
2. National Commission on Nursing, *Nursing in Transition: Models for Successful Organizational Change* (Chicago: American Hospital Association, Hospital Research and Educational Trust and American Hospital Supply Corporation, 1982), 41–42.
3. "Helping Out in Hard Times." *RN* 46, Mar. 1983, 7.
4. N. Miller, *American Organization of Nurse Executives Student Nurse Recruitment Resource Kit* (Chicago: American Hospital Association, 1987), 1.
5. American Nurses' Association, "Fact Sheet: Supply and Demand of Registered Nurses," 1988.
6. Miller, op. cit.
7. Ibid.
8. H. L. Hodgkinson, "Reform? Higher Education? Don't Be Absurd!" *Phi Delta Kappan*, Dec. 1986, 271–274.
9. Ibid. for the statistics.
10. Miller, op. cit.
11. American Academy of Nursing Task Force on Nursing Practice in Hospitals, *Magnet Hospitals: Attraction and Retention of Professional Nurses* (Kansas City, MO: American Nurses' Association, 1983), 99.
12. M. Kramer and C. Schmalenberg, "Magnet Hospitals: Part 2, Institutions of Excellence," *JONA*, Feb. 1988, 17.
13. These are given different priority by nurses in different surveys. L. Donovan, "What Nurses Want (and What They're Getting)," *RN*, Apr. 1980, 22–30; M. A. Wandelt, P. M. Pierce, and R. M. Widdowson, "Why Nurses Leave Nursing and What Can Be Done about It," *American Journal of Nursing*, Jan. 1981, 72–77.
14. R. C. Swansburg and P. W. Swansburg, *Strategic Career Planning and Development for Nurses* (Rockville, MD: Aspen, 1984), 160–162.
15. M. R. Thompson, *Why Should I Hire You?* (New York: Jove Publications, 1975), 94.
16. Swansburg and Swansburg, op. cit., 194–204.
17. Ibid., 205–206.
18. Ibid., 207.
19. H. S. Rowland and B. L. Rowland, *Hospital Legal Forms, Checklists, and Guidelines* (Rockville, MD: Aspen, 1987), 17:1.
20. Committee for the Study of Credentialing in Nursing, "Credentialing in Nursing: A New Approach," *American Journal of Nursing*, Apr. 1979, 674–683.
21. P. E. Norris, *How to Find a Job* (Fairhope, AL: National Job Search Training Laboratories, 1982), 1.
22. E. Ginsberg, J. Patray, M. Ostow, and E. A. Brann, "Nurse Discontent: The Search for Realistic Solutions," *Journal of Nursing Administration*, Nov. 1982, 7–11.
23. C. E. Burton and D. T. Burton, "Job Expectations of Senior Nursing Students," *Journal of Nursing Administration*, Mar. 1982, 11–17.
24. "Peter F. Drucker and Karl D. Bays Discuss the Toughest Job—Running a Hospital, Part 2," *HMQ*, Summer 1982, 2–5.
25. A. Levenstein, "Career Dissatisfaction," *Nursing Management*, Nov. 1985, 61–62.
26. Ginsberg, Patray, Ostow, and Brann, op. cit.
27. M. D. Sovie, "Fostering Professional Nursing Careers in Hospitals: The Role of Staff Development, Part 1," *Journal of Nursing Administration*, Dec. 1982, 5–10.
28. Swansburg and Swansburg, op. cit., 136–138.
29. Ibid., 7–8.
30. R. B. Spitzer and L. B. Bolton, "Attitudes toward Equitable Pay," *Nursing Management*, June 1984, 32, 36–38.
31. Ibid.
32. L. A. W. Darling and L. G. McGrath, "The Causes and Costs of Promotion Trauma," *Journal of Nursing Administration*, Apr. 1983, 29–33.
33. B. C. Rutkowski and A. D. Rutkowski, "Employee Discharge: It Depends . . . ," *Nursing Management*, Dec. 1984, 39–42.

FOR FURTHER REFERENCE

Battle, E. H., Bragg, S., Delaney, J., Gilbert, S., and Roesler, D., "Developing a Rating Interview Guide," *JONA*, Oct. 1985, 39–45.

Colavecchio, R., "Direct Patient Care: A Viable Career Choice," *Journal of Nursing Administration*, July-Aug. 1982, 17–22.

Connelly, J. A., and Strauser, K. S., "Managing Recruitment and Retention Problems: An Application of the Marketing Process," *Journal of Nursing Administration*, Oct. 1983, 17–22.

Duxbury, M. L., and Armstrong, G. D., "Calculating Nurse Turnover Indices," *Journal of Nursing Administration*, Mar. 1982, 18–24.

Hiller, B. R., Okolowski, R. S., O'Driscoll, R. M., Frain, M., and Brady, J. K., "The Search Interview," *Nursing Outlook*, Mar. 1982, 182–185.

Miceli, M. P., "Effects of Realistic Job Previews on Newcomer Affect and Behavior: An Operant Perspective," *Journal of Organizational Behavior Management*, Spring 1986, 73–88.

"Recruitment and Retention: A Positive Approach," *Nursing Management*, Apr. 1984, 15–17.

Reres, M. E., "Academic Courtship Rites," *Nursing Outlook*, Oct. 1970, 42.

Sullivan, E. J., Decker, P. J., and Hailstone, S., "Assessment Center Technology: Selecting Head Nurses," *Journal of Nursing Administration*, May 1985, 14.

Principles of Budgeting

INTRODUCTION

Because the amount and quality of nursing services depend on budgetary plans, nurse managers must become proficient in related procedures. This proficiency will provide them the resources necessary for safe and effective nursing care. With limited resources and a competitive market, personnel and material resources must be wisely and efficiently used. The enlightened nurse manager knows that the control of a budget determines who controls nursing service. The costs of nursing service have been identified for many years, but the income earned from provision of nursing services has been included with the "bed and board." This practice will cease through the efforts of nurse managers who will not only justify the price put on this service, but will institute the program and procedures for charging for direct nursing care. Achieving reimbursement for nursing services will involve changing government regulations and third-party payer policies to allow for direct payment to nursing providers based on the amount of care given and the skills of the persons giving it.

Budgeting is an ongoing activity in which revenues and expenses are managed to maintain fiscal responsibility and fiscal health. The nurse manager has responsibility and accountability for managing the nursing budget. The nurse manager makes all of the decisions about adjustment of the nursing budgets to manage programs and costs. These include adding and dropping programs, expanding and contracting programs, and all modifications of revenues and expenses within the nursing unit.

BASIC PLANNING FOR BUDGETING

Planning, discussed in foregoing chapters, forecasts for a year and for several years. The budget is an annual plan with an intended outcome that will be effective in terms of the use of human and material resources, of products or services, and of managing the environment to improve productivity. Budgetary planning assures the best methods are used in achieving financial objectives. It should be based on valid objectives that will produce a product or service that the community needs and will pay for. In nursing, budgetary planning helps assure that clients or patients will receive the nursing services they want and need from satisfied nursing workers. A good budget should be based on objectives, be simple, have standards, be flexible, be balanced, and use available resources first to avoid increasing cost.

A budget is a best estimate by nurse administrators of nursing revenues and nursing expenses. It should be stated in terms of attainable objectives so as to maintain the motivation of nurse managers at unit or cost center levels. Nurse managers should be encouraged to have objectives that require considerable management expertise in expanding the budget to achieve them. The nursing budget is used for three purposes: (1) to plan the objectives, programs, and activities of nursing service; (2) to motivate nurse managers and nursing workers; and (3) as a standard to evaluate the performance of nurse administrators and managers. Managing the financial end of nursing through an operational budget can obviously create a new dimension for nurse managers. The budget will be a strong support for development and use of written objectives for the nursing division and for each of its units. It will provide strong motivation for effective planning and it will certainly provide standards by which to evaluate the performance of nurse managers. Planning will need to provide for contingencies by indicating what programs or activities can be reduced or eliminated if budget goals are not met.

BUDGETING PROCEDURES

Managing Cost Centers

A cost center is a given area of accountability for both direct and indirect expenditures, for which accountability is assigned. A division of nursing is a cost center as are each of its units, each clinic, in-service education, surgical suites, and any other section with a nursing mission in which nurses provide services to clients. Each cost center is assigned a code. The American Hospital Association (AHA) publishes a Uniform Chart of Accounts and Definitions for Hospitals. An organization may use this coding system, which is usually referred to as the patient care system. There have to be workload measurements, sometimes referred to as performance classifications or units of measure. The unit of measure should be identified for each cost center as a specific, quantitative statistic such as inpatient

days or relative value units (RVUs). RVUs will define the tangible things done as evidence of production and for measuring quantity, quality, and cost.

Each cost center has a manager called the cost center manager or the responsibility center manager. They are responsible for identifying needs for equipment and programs necessary to maintain progress within the current level of technology at the unit level.

Within a cost center budgeted costs are broken down into subcodes. This promotes better budgetary planning and controlling, as items can be more specifically identified as the budget is being planned. Also, each item purchased can be charged against a specific subcode with the balance shown for that subcode.

Many hospitals do not credit nursing units as income-producing (revenue) centers; it is time they did so. The same codes will be used for income-producing centers as for cost centers; in fact, in some organizations they are known as "activity centers." Nurse managers establish systems for (1) determining that work is being performed by the appropriately skilled person and (2) determining the charges for each hour of care a patient receives. Controlling processes determine that an RN is not used continually to perform activities that can be performed by nursing assistants. While minimal downward performance of less skilled activities should be expected as being practical and necessary, upward performance of activities should not be condoned or nurse workers will be performing activities for which they are not educated, skilled, or licensed.

Relationship of Budget to Objectives

One of the chief planning activities is to identify the objectives of the nursing division and each of its units. This includes developing each objective into a management plan. One of the first sources of budgetary information, then, is the nursing objectives. Using these objectives will cause nurse managers to see the benefit of developing pertinent, specific, practical objectives.

Stages of the Budget

For practical purposes there are three stages of development of the nursing budget: (1) the formulation stage, (2) the review and enactment stage, and (3) the execution stage.

Formulation Stage. The formulation stage is usually a set number of months (6 or 7) before the beginning of the fiscal year in which the budget will be executed. During this period procedures are used to obtain an estimate of the funds needed, funds available, expenses, and revenue. These procedures and instructions for performing them should be communicated to nursing administrators and unit or cost center managers by the budget officer.

Financial reports of expenses and revenues will be analyzed by the chief nurse executive, department heads, and cost center managers.

One of the first steps in writing a budget is gathering data for accurate prediction of expenses (costs) and revenues (incomes). This task can be developed into a system. A primary source of data is the objectives for division of nursing and for each cost center, the objectives of that unit. Programs and activities need to have an estimated cost placed on them. If in-service education personnel want new audiovisual equipment, they should not walk into the nurse administrator's office and expect to have it next week or even next year. It should be planned for 6 to 7 months before the budget for the next fiscal or calendar year will begin, and it may be budgeted for any quarter or month within that budgetary year. In surveying the objectives the nurse administrators and managers will evaluate the previous year, review the philosophy, and rewrite the objectives for the future.

Among the cost center reports that will assist the nurse manager are the following:

Daily staffing reports

Monthly staffing reports

Payroll summaries

Daily lists of financial categories of patients

Biometric reports of occupancy

Biometric reports of workload

Monthly financial summaries of revenues and expenses

Review and Enactment Stage. Review and enactment are processes of budget development that put all the pieces together for approval of a final budget. Once the cost center managers present their budgets to the hospital budget council, the chief nurse executive will consolidate the nursing budget. It will then be further consolidated into an organizational budget by the budget officer.

Approval will be made by the chief executive officer of the organization and governing board. During this entire process there will be conferences at which budget adjustments are made.

Preparation of a sound budget by nurse administrators and cost center managers will ensure favorable action by the budget committee. The nurse administrator can defend the budget alone or jointly with each cost center manager. Whichever strategy is used, it should be well planned in advance. When these meetings occur the budget committee will be interested in well-prepared plans. The objective should be clearly stated, the costs should be accurate, and the revenues should be defensible. Although some budget requests can be disallowed, there are generally few setbacks when a reasonable and well-prepared budget is ably defended by informed cost center managers.

Execution Stage. Both the formulation and the review and enactment stages of the budget are planning activities. Execution of the budget involves directing and evaluating activities. The budget is executed by the nurse administrators and managers who planned it. Revisions in execution of the budget may be planned at stated intervals, frequently once or twice during the fiscal year. There will also be procedures for evaluating the budget at cost center levels. Budgets are prepared for either fiscal years or calendar years depending on the policy of the organization. See Figure 6–1, The Budget Calendar.

DEFINITIONS

Budget

According to *Webster's New Twentieth Century Dictionary*, second edition, a budget is "a plan or schedule adjusting expenses during a certain period to the estimated or fixed income for that period."

Herkimer has stated that "an effective budget is the systematic documentation of one or more carefully developed plans for all individually supervised activities, programs, or sections. . . . The budget is a tool which can aid decision makers in evaluating operating performance and projecting what future operations might produce."[1]

A budget is an operational management plan, stated in income and expense terms, covering all phases of activity for a future division of time. It is a financial document that expresses a plan of operation in action. In the division of nursing it sets the

Formulation Stage

1. Develop objectives and management plans.
2. Gather all financial, historical, and statistical data and distribute to cost center managers.
3. Analyze data.

Review and Enactment Stage

4. Prepare unit budgets.
5. Present unit budgets for approval.
6. Revise and combine into organizational budget.
7. Present to budget council.
8. Revise and present to governing board.
9. Revise and distribute to cost center managers.

Execution Stage

10. Direct and evaluate expenses and receipts.
11. Revise budget if indicated.

Figure 6–1 • *The Budget Calendar*

limits of financial support, thereby controlling the extent and quality of nursing programs. The budget will determine the number and kinds of personnel, material, and money resources available to care for patients and to achieve the stated nursing objectives. It is a financial statement of policy.

Unit of Service

The unit of service is a measure for output of hospital service consumed by the patient. In the operating units and recovery room, it will be minutes or hours; in the emergency room, it will be visits; and in the nursing unit, it will be category of acuity of patients and hours per day expressed in RVUs. Measures include procedures, patient days, patient visits, and cases.

Revenue

Revenue is the income from sale of products and services. Traditionally, nursing revenue has been included with room charges. It is increasingly being unbundled from the room rate as a separate charge per patient acuity category and per visit, day, or procedure.

Revenue can include assets such as accounts receivable and income-producing endowments. The latter can be restricted to specific purposes. Buildings, land, and other items can be assets if they produce income or are capable of producing income. Total income is frequently termed gross income, with the excess of revenues over expenses being known as net income.

Revenues also come from research grants, gift shops, donations, gifts, rentals of cots and televisions, parking fees, telephone charges, and vending machines, among other sources.

Revenue Budgeting

Revenue budgeting or rate setting is the process by which a hospital determines revenues required to cover anticipated economic costs and to establish prices sufficient to generate that revenue. Complicating the process is the fact that all patients (purchasers) do not pay an equal share of a hospital's economic costs.

To remain viable any business, including a hospital, must generate sufficient revenue to cover operating costs and profit. These include increases in working capital needs, capital replacement, and inflation adjustment. Nonprofit hospitals are identified as such for tax status only! Profits are used to improve plants and services and cannot go to stockholders or owners.

Fundamental to the rate-setting process are adequate statistical data, historical and projected, for implementing the rate-setting methodology to be used. This includes, on a departmental basis, volume of services, current rate, allocated costs, and rate increase constraints. The goal is to obtain the greatest impact from a minimum cumulative rate increase in today's cost management environment. This is done by increasing rates in high-profit departments while instituting rate reductions in low-profit departments, so that they offset each other. An example of this would be pediatric or rehabilitational services paid by charges versus internal medicine services paid by DRG.

Expenses

Expenses are the costs of providing services to patients. They are frequently called overhead and include wages and salaries, fringe benefits, supplies, food service, utilities, and office and medical supplies. As part of the budget they are a collection or summary of forecasts for each cost center account.

Expense Budgeting

Expense budgeting is the "process of forecasting, recording, and monitoring the manpower, material and supply, and monetary needs of an organization in such a manner that the operation of the various components of the organization can be controlled."[2] The components of expense budgeting are cost centers. Purposes of expense budgeting include:

- Prediction of labor hours, material and supplies, and cash flow needs for future time periods.
- Establishing procedures for making comparative studies.
- Providing a mechanism for determining when changes in procedures need to be made, providing gross information on the kinds of changes needed, and providing evidence that control has been established or reestablished.

Historical trends are the single best inexpensive indicator available to the institution. They are valid for predicting present and future trends most of the time.

Patient Days

Patient days are statistics used to project revenues. They are commonly used as units of service to compute staffing. Patient-day statistics are usually derived from census reports that are done daily at midnight and summarized monthly, for the year to date, and annually. A patient admitted on May 2 and discharged May 10 is charged for 9 patient days. See Table 6–1 for an illustration of patient days per unit for one month (June and July columns).

Fiscal Year (FY)

The fiscal year is the budgetary or financial year. It may be the calendar year in some organizations, beginning on January 1 and ending on December 31. Many organizations use the period of October 1 to September 30 as the fiscal year. Some use the period of July 1 to June 30. This is done to coincide with budget decisions of state legislatures and the U.S. Congress. In the latter examples, the fiscal year obviously overlaps two calendar years.

Year to Date (YTD)

The term "year to date" is used to describe the accumulated units of service at a particular point in the fiscal year. If the fiscal year begins October 1, the year-to-date patient days for December 31 would be the summary for 92 days. See Table 6–1 for an illustration of year-to-date statistics (Current Year and Previous Year columns).

Average Daily Census (ADC)

The census is summarized for a specific number of days and divided by that number of days. As an example, the average daily census for the month of June would be the total patient days for June divided by 30. In Table 6–1 the number of patient days for June was 7,436. When this is divided by 30, the average daily census is 248.

Hours of Care

From the nursing viewpoint, hours of care has traditionally been the number of hours of care allocated per patient per day (24 hours) on a unit. With the use of patient acuity rating systems, hours of care can be determined to the hour or even parts of an hour. Usually patients are determined to fall into one of four or five categories, each assigned a specific number of hours of care per patient day.

Care Giver

Each nurse person who works with patients is labelled a care giver. In nursing there are three commonly used types of care givers: registered nurses, licensed practical nurses, and nurses' aides. Most personnel budgets have a ratio of registered nurses to other care givers. Considerable research supports an all–registered-nurse care giver staff. The current nurse shortage will alter this goal.

Product Line

Hospitals are reorganizing on the basis of product lines. These can include outpatient or ambulatory surgery, home health care, a burn center, a comprehensive cancer center, or other products. As in business or industry, each functions as a profit center within the overall accounting system. Even one DRG can be a product. A product must pay for itself, be paid for through cost shifting, or be deleted.

	July	OCC %	June	Total to Date		
				Current Year	OCC %	Previous Year
Nursing Station						
3rd Floor	1,014	79.8%	833	9,792	78.6%	8,650
4th Floor	811	76.9%	718	7,834	75.8%	7,255
5th Floor North	526	65.3%	524	5,300	67.1%	4,838
5th Floor South	622	77.2%	592	5,587	70.7%	5,603
6th Floor	792	71.0%	866	8,730	79.8%	8,176
7th Floor	850	68.5%	895	9,086	74.7%	8,885
8th Floor	0	0.0%	0	0	0.0%	4,403
8th Floor North	376	60.6%	383	4,624	76.1%	2,393
8th Floor South	303	69.8%	274	3,253	76.4%	1,729
9th Floor	0	0.0%	0	0	0.0%	5,138
9th Floor North	526	84.8%	501	5,332	87.7%	2,690
9th Floor South	481	77.6%	506	5,118	84.2%	2,617
MINU	104	83.9%	89	1,041	85.6%	432
SINU	73	58.9%	84	964	79.3%	471
Burn Unit	173	79.7%	188	1,723	81.0%	1,912
Labor and Delivery	138	37.1%	99	1,228	33.7%	1,258
CCU	206	83.1%	148	1,848	76.0%	1,937
Clinical Research Unit	137	73.7%	132	1,342	73.6%	1,361
EAU	23	0.0%	7	390	0.0%	634
MICU	213	85.9%	191	2,099	86.3%	2,291
PICU	169	54.5%	112	1,612	53.0%	1,834
SICU	229	92.3%	207	2,175	89.4%	2,302
NTICU	209	84.3%	87	1,891	77.9%	2,277
Total	7,975	73.1%	7,436	80,969	75.7%	79,086
Nursery						
Newborn	832	103.2%	632	7,666	97.0%	7,307
Intermediate	577	103.4%	457	4,761	87.0%	3,991
Intensive Care	955	110.0%	716	8,526	100.2%	7,022
Total	2,364	105.9%	1,805	20,953	95.7%	18,320

SOURCE: Courtesy of the University of South Alabama Medical Center, Mobile, Alabama.

Table 6–1 • *University of South Alabama Medical Center Statistics as of July 31*

Cost/Benefit Analysis

Cost/benefit analysis is a planning technique. What are the costs of pursuing a goal, an objective or a program? How do they compare with benefits?

Zero-Base Budgeting

Zero-base budgeting provides no incentive but is rather a method of budgeting that relates to cost control. It ignores the previous budget and the pre-vious historical database. Zero-base budgeting starts from zero and justifies everything. A previous activity can be included in the budget but funding for it must be justified by its relation to the organizational objectives. In theory, each and every function in a zero-base budget is isolated to stand on its own merits. The merit of each function is reviewed annually. All labor power and costs are recalculated and decisions are made as to whether to continue the function and at what levels.

In actual practice, zero-base budgeting seldom

reviews all costs. Much of the previous budget is accepted; a complete analysis could cost more than it saves. With cost studies becoming more prevalent in nursing, the application of zero-base budgeting techniques will increase.

OPERATING OR CASH BUDGETS

The cash budget is the actual operating budget in detail, excluding the capital budget. A cash budget requirement is cash flow that must be adequate to meet debt obligations, including replacement and expansion of facilities, unanticipated requirements, the payroll, payment for supplies and services, and a prudent investment program. Cash receipts come from third-party payers, tuition, endowment fund earnings, and sales of food, gifts, and services.

The cash budget is the day-to-day budget and represents money coming in and going out. It is advisable to have cash reserves so that cash flow, the money coming in, will pay the bills. Otherwise revenues must be speeded up or payment of bills slowed down.

Negative Cash Flow

The magic factors influencing negative cash flow are:

1. Time lag between delivery of services and collection of payments.
2. The difference in cycles between the timing of net income and flow of cash.
3. Lag created by the large up and down cycles of volume during the different seasons (cash deficit during a busy census cycle or surplus during a low census cycle).
4. Labor expense (60 to 70 percent of operating expense) paid out in salary and wages not cycling concurrently with collections.

To maintain solvency, cash flow must be managed carefully and cycles of cash shortage planned for appropriately. The cash budget should plan for the ability to borrow cash during shortfalls, investment of excess cash, and *strict* monitoring and reporting of lost charges and of the billing and collecting process. The cash budget is a part of the total budget and is apportioned to departments based on individual cost center activity.

Developing the Operating Budget

Operating budget information supplied to the chief nurse executive, department head, and cost center managers include a budget worksheet and an adjustment explanation worksheet. The budget work sheet depicts information by cost center account number and subcode. It lists prior year expense, original budget, and annualized expense. Usually this form is provided during a fiscal year (FY) and the annualized expense is the projected total expense if current rates continue to the end of the fiscal year. The columns headed "Budget Detail" and "Budget Pool" are empty so the cost center manager can fill in the budget expenses for the projected fiscal year. Note in Table 6–2 that the annualized expense for the 200–213 subcodes was $8,985 for the current year. The cost center manager projected $10,780 for the fiscal year. This was reduced at the budget council hearings because hospital administration had decided not to project inflation.

Also in Table 6–2, note that subcode 232, office supplies, was increased by $138. This was justified on the adjustment explanation; see Figure 6–2. However, information available to the administrator indicated that $320 had been budgeted and expended in the current year for new chart backs. Since this was a one-time expense it was backed out of the budget. A similar transaction for $53 was backed out of subcode 501 minor equipment. Increases were approved for subcodes 501 minor equipment, and 372 books. The supply and minor equipment budget for the fiscal year for this cost center was approved for $14,595.

In the budget formulation stage described here, the assistant administrator for finance distributes the worksheets to the other assistant administrators and department heads. They develop budgets with their cost center managers and defend them before the budget council.

PERSONNEL BUDGET

Most nursing personnel budgets are based on quantitative workload measurements. Nursing service should have a patient acuity system. It is usually a computer program that produces staffing requirements by shift and by day. It produces an acuity index for each patient, and the formula indicates needed staff by category (RN, LPN, nursing assistant) and by shift. It also compares actual staffing with that required and can be summarized by

Subcode	Description	ABR	Prior Year Expense	Original Budget	Annualized Expense	Budget Detail	Budget Pool
200	Pool-Med/Surg Supply	0	.00	10,975.00		$10,780	$ 8,985
211	Med & Surg Supplies	4	10,893.80	.00	8,790	$ 8,790	
213	Drugs	4	129.59	.00	195	$ 195	
Pool Total			11,023.39	10,975.00	8,985		
220	Pool-General Supply	0	.00	2,705.00			$ 2,848
232	Office Supplies	4	303.34	.00	672	$ 810	– 320
234	Printing	4	37.75	.00	3	$ 3	
240	Housekeeping Supply	4	1,404.06	.00	1,482	$ 1,482	
270	Food Expense	4	913.73	.00	523	$ 523	
Pool Total			2,658.88	2,705.00	2,680		
300	Pool-Travel/Entertain	0	.00	110.00			$ 50
314	Local Travel	4	13.80	.00	18	$ 50	
Pool Total			13.80	110.00	18		
320	Pool-Other Expenses	0	.00	130.00			$ 660
336	Equip Maint & Repair	4	66.60	.00	123	$ 610	
372	Books & Subscription	4	25.00	.00		$ 50	
Pool Total			91.60	130.00	123		
501	Minor Equipment	0	.00	.00	72	– 53	$ 465
Pool Total			.00	.00	72		
Acct Total			13,787.67	13,920.00	11,878		
						Total	$14,968
							– 373
							$14,595

SOURCE: Courtesy of the University of South Alabama Medical Center, Mobile, Alabama.

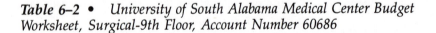

Table 6–2 • University of South Alabama Medical Center Budget Worksheet, Surgical-9th Floor, Account Number 60686

month and year. Each day at a given time a registered nurse enters each patient's acuity rating into a computer terminal. To promote objectivity of the ratings, RNs should be trained to use the same procedures when evaluating each patient. Quality assurance tests can be performed to compare trainer ratings with those done by registered nurses.

Figure 6–3 is a nursing budget that is based on a patient acuity rating system. The average daily census (ADC) is obtained from records produced in the admissions office. It is the result of dividing the total patient days for a unit for one year by 365 days. Census reports are computer generated on a daily, monthly, and annual basis.

Acuity is the result of the sum of all acuities for one year divided by 365 days. This figure is also computer generated daily, monthly, and annually. The nursing hours are generated from the acuity

standard listed in paragraph 1 of Figure 6–3. Application of a staffing formula for preparing the personnel budget for a specific unit is illustrated in Figure 6–4.

In planning the personnel budget, the nurse manager has quantified information related to staffing and can accurately predict the number of full-time equivalents (FTEs) needed for patient care. Other considerations must be made at the same time. Will there be a pay increase next year? If so, it must be calculated and budgeted for. Will fringe benefits increase or decrease? They must also be budgeted for. If new programs are being implemented do they require additional labor power? Will this manpower come from cutbacks in other programs or from added FTEs? See Figure 6–5 for adding new positions to the budget.

Careful planning ensures that the nurse ad-

DEPARTMENT NAME _____ 9th Floor _____

DEPARTMENT NUMBER _____ 60686 _____

Subcode Number	Subcode Description	Adjustment Amount	Adjustment Explanation
		$ 30.00	2 large blue policy binders 15.00 ea
		6.00	1 small blue policy binder
		32.00	2 large red 4″ (8½ × 11) 3-ring binders— normal wear and tear 2 yrs old
232	Office Supplies	$ 25.00	4 black 3-ring binders (MAR & Kardex)— normal wear & tear
		28.00	48″ × 36″ cork & wooden frame bulletin boards—↑ appearance ↓ clutter
		17.00	25″ × 25″ ¼″ thick Plexiglas—↑ appearance
		$138	
		$	
		$ 30.00	*Taber's Medical Dictionary*—ref. book needed to ↑ professionalism
372	Books	$ 20.00	*Webster's Ninth New Collegiate Dictionary*— ↑ learning
		$ 50.00	

SOURCE: Courtesy of the University of South Alabama Medical Center, Mobile, Alabama.

Figure 6–2 • *Adjustment Explanation, Calendar Year*

ministrator will control the nursing budget. It will ensure that the nurse administrator has a handle on the total dollar amount that will be expended on personnel and that personnel will generate income.

In the budgeting process, personnel account for the largest portion of the nursing budget. When one is preparing budgets for clinics, emergency departments, recovery rooms, operating rooms, and delivery rooms, it is important to have quantitative data. These include number of visits, procedures, deliveries, and the like. Samples of

lengths of time required for each can be taken by using management engineering techniques in which visits, procedures, or other activities are charted over a period of time.

Data should be collected over a representative period to show the actual hours worked by shift and by day. These data will indicate fluctuations in the workload by shift and by day of the week. Use of a second data sheet is suggested to determine the total number of patients in the emergency department area at any one time, including those patients in a holding status. Conversion of these data

Nursing Budget

1. The attached budget for all nursing units is based on a patient acuity rating system purchased from Medicus Systems. The standard is:

Acuity	Nursing Hours Per Patient Needed During 24-hour Period
.5	0–2 hours
1.0	2–4 hours
2.5	4–10 hours
5.0	10–24 hours

2. The staffing formula is:

$$\frac{\text{Average Census} \times \text{Nursing Hours} \times 1.4 \times 1.14}{7.5}$$

3. The total nursing personnel needed includes ward clerks and units not using a patient acuity rating system.

Maternal Child

Unit	ADC	Acuity	NSG/HRS	RN	LPN	NA	Other	Total
3rd	31.8	0.9	4	14	9	4	5	32
Peds	22.0	1.3	4.5	16	5	0	4	25
PICU	4.4	3.4	12	11	0	0	2	13
ICN	21.7	2.9	12	41	7	6	4	58
Inter.	11.9	2.3	4.5	6	4	1	1	12
NBN	19.7	1.0	4	9	6	1	3	19
Del. Rm.	—	—	—	20	3	1	4	28
Play Rm.	—	—	—	—	—	—	1	1
Total				117	34	13	24	188

Medical

Unit	ADC	Acuity	NSG/HRS	RN	LPN	NA	Other	Total
5 No.	14.3	1.3	4.5	11	3	0	3	17
5 So.	22.1	1.3	4.5	12	5	4	3	24
CRU	3.6	—	4.5	6	—	1	1	8
8th	25.1	1.7	4.5	15	7	2	3	27
MICU	7.2	4.0	12	18	0	0	3.5	21.5
CCU	6.5	3.0	12	18	0	0	1	17
Telemetry	—	—	—	—	1	5	0	6
Total				78	16	12	14.5	120.5

Surgical

Unit	ADC	Acuity	NSG/HRS	RN	LPN	NA	Other	Total
9th	16.2	1.2	4.5	11	2	2	3	18
6 Surg.	26.5	1.6	4.5	16	6	3	3	28

NOTE: The formulary budget is based on actual ADC for 12 months. All positions above formula calculations are placed in CVICU budgeted cost center and held vacant.

SOURCE: Courtesy of the University of South Alabama Medical Center, Mobile, Alabama.

Figure 6–3 • *Nursing Personnel Budget*

(Continued)

Surgical (Continued)

Unit	ADC	Acuity	NSG/HRS	RN	LPN	NA	Other	Total
6 Ortho.	23.5	1.5	4.5	15	4	4	3	26
SICU	6.4	3.8	12	17	0	0	2	19
B.U.	3.7	2.8	12	8	2	0	1	11
Ortho Tech	—	—	—	—	—	—	1	1
Total				67	14	9	13	103

Psychiatry

Unit	ADC	Acuity	NSG/HRS	RN	LPN	NA	Other	Total
7th	23.5	—	5.5	11	4	11	6	32

OR/RR/EAU/ED

Unit	ADC	Acuity	NSG/HRS	RN	LPN	NA	Other	Total
OR	—	—	—	21	13	4	2	40
RR/EAU	—	—	—	16	0	1	2	19
ED	—	—	—	25	0	7	8	40

Administration

Unit	ADC	Acuity	NSG/HRS	RN	LPN	NA	Other	Total
N/S Adm.	—	—	—	13	0	0	3.5	16.5
Staff Day	—	—	—	8.5	0	0	1	9.5
Health Nurse	—	—	—	1	—	—	—	1
CVICU								
Pool	—	—	—	4.5	12	18	2	36.5
Total				362	93	75	76	606

Figure 6–3 • (Continued)

into graphs provides information to compare staffing with workload. These data will provide the following information:

1. The current nursing hours available per patient visit.
2. Fluctuation in available hours by shift and day.
3. Fluctuation in workload by time of day.
4. Fluctuation in staffing levels to patient load.[3]

In the process of budgeting, the nurse manager knows how much each decision will cost, whether it involves numbers and kinds of personnel or amounts and kinds of supplies and equipment. Few nurse managers will have the luxury of a budget that provides all of the resources that can be used. Hard decisions have to be made. They are easier to substantiate when workloads are quantified. In the personnel area, if the patient dependency or acuity system is reliable and valid and has quality checks on the raters, it will provide data that justifies the personnel budget. When the number of highest acuity level adult patients increases from 24 to 32 per shift and day, the budget must be adjusted. Comparisons must be made to determine whether other levels have decreased. Estimates must be made as to whether the increases and decreases are permanent or temporary. Then the budget decisions are made.

To provide for fluctuations in personnel costs, a personnel pool can be established. This can consist of permanent or temporary FTEs; full-time or part-time workers; persons who work flexible hours; a mixture of RNs, LPNs, nursing assistants, and clerk; and provision for all shifts and days of the week. An effective pool must be well managed by one line manager or staffing director. Its personnel require staff development programs and concern for managing them as a unique work force of human beings. The nurse manager or administrator determines the level of service and then expresses it in financial terms to produce a budget.

The staffing formula is

$$\frac{\text{Average Census} \times \text{Nursing Hours} \times 1.4 \times 1.14}{7.5}$$

Example: 3rd Floor

Average daily census = 31.8

Nursing hours = 4 (per 24 hours)

1.4 is a constant representing 7 days in a week with a full-time worker 5 days in a week:

7 ÷ 5 = 1.4

1.14 is a constant representing an allowance of 0.14 FTE for vacation, illness, etc. for each 1.0 FTE

7.5 represents one work day

$$\frac{31.8 \times 4 \times 1.4 \times 1.14}{7.5} = 27 \text{ FTEs}$$

There are 14 RNs, 9 LPNs, and 4 NAs (27 FTEs) budgeted for 3rd Floor. The "others" column represents ward clerks or other nonnursing personnel not included in the formula. Although quantitative measurements justify a full complement of nursing personnel, the budget committee can reduce this number. Note that ICN has been reduced from the formula calculation by 1.0 FTE.

Figure 6–4 • *Calculating the Nursing Personnel Budget*

SUPPLIES AND EQUIPMENT BUDGET

The supplies and equipment budget is part of the operating or cash budget. It includes all supplies and equipment used in provision of services except capital equipment and supplies charged directly to patients as revenues. Examples of supplies to be budgeted include office supplies, medical/surgical supplies, pharmacy supplies, and others. Refer to Table 6–2 and Figure 6–2.

Minor equipment includes such items as sphygmomanometers, otoscopes, ophthalmoscopes, and the like. It is equipment costing less than the base set for capital equipment. If the base is $500, all equipment under $500 is budgeted under the supplies and equipment budget as minor equipment.

Generally, the director of materials management furnishes information on the total cost of supplies and equipment per cost center to the accounting office. The accounting office generates a cost per patient day for supplies and equipment for each cost center. This is used for budgeting purposes, increases for inflation being a decision of top management. Based on projected patient days and revenues, decisions can be made to increase or decrease the supplies and equipment budget.

Costs can be decreased by controlling the amounts of supplies and equipment kept in inventory. Nurse administrators should look at any inventories they control and reduce them according to usage.

CAPITAL BUDGET

A capital budget is usually separate from the operating budget; see Table 6–3. Each item of a capital budget is defined in terms of dollar value and is an item of equipment that is reused over a period of time. It projects the costs of major purchases. The budget provides for depreciation of each capital budget item, sets aside the amount of this depreciation in an escrow account, and uses this account to finance new capital budgets. See Table 6–4, column headed "Deprn. Expense 07–31." Capital budgets also deal with land (purchase), buildings (maintenance, renovations, remodeling, replacement), fixed equipment (replacement), and so on. In addition, department heads are required to justify and set priorities on capital budget items. See Figure 6–6. The financial manager for nursing is the nurse manager, who should evaluate past decisions and advise the nurse administrator on whether the decisions were good or bad.

All proposals for capital equipment need to be

1. Department _____ Department number _____

2. Position class, title _____ Position FTE _____

3. Minimum starting salary _____ Expected starting date _____

4. Permanent _____ Temporary _____ If temporary, ending date _____

5. Describe briefly the new position responsibilities:

_____

_____

_____

_____

Need for new position:

6. New service _____ Increased volume _____
   If new service, complete question 7.
   If increased volume, complete question 8.

7. Describe the new service to be provided and estimated new revenues.

_____

_____

_____

_____

_____

8. Document increased volume and provide staffing analysis for your department.

_____

_____

_____

_____

(Attach additional pages if necessary)

_____

SOURCE: The University of South Alabama Medical Center, Mobile, Alabama. Reprinted with permission.

Figure 6–5 • *New Position Questionnaire, Budget Year*

fully evaluated for amount of use, payment methodology, safety, replacement, and duplication of service, and every conceivable angle including the need for space, personnel, and renovation. The needs and desires of the medical staff should be included. Their involvement in planning will help to ensure wise purchase of capital equipment.

When the capital budget list has been analyzed and reduced to the amount available, it is again tabulated. It is now ready to present to the board of directors; see Table 6–3. With their approval, the list is distributed to cost center managers who prepare requisitions for purchase. The purchasing department prepares bid specifications, with input from cost center managers. Purchases are finalized on the basis of results of bids submitted by vendors who meet the required specifications. Finally, new equipment purchase prices are entered into a depreciation budget schedule, the rate of depreciation being obtained from the AHA which is

Department	Dept. No.	Item Description	Budget	Paid 06-30	Encumbrances	Total Committed	Budget Balance
Nursing Services Nursing Services—Admin	60601	Software License	$ 0.00	$ 18,135.00	$2,000.00	$ 0.00	$0.00
		External Modem		527.12			
		Electric & Manual Beds—6		31,704.72			
		Cardio System Special Care Beds		13,725.00			
		Telemetry Monitoring System		113,080.12			
		COMPAQ Computer		9,842.70			
		Department Total	189,014.66	187,014.66	2,000.00	189,014.66	0.00
Private U. 6th Floor	60609	Lifepack 7 Defibrillator		5,500.00			
		Facsimile Machine		1,600.00			
		Lifepack 7 Defibrillator		5,208.00			
		Department Total	12,308.00	12,308.00	0.00	12,308.00	0.00
Coronary Care	60615	Lifepack 6 Defibrillator		7,621.32			
		Department Total	7,621.32	7,621.32	0.00	7,621.32	0.00
5th Fl—Shared Supplies	60619	Facsimile Machine		1,550.00			
		Department Total	1,550.00	1,550.00	0.00	1,550.00	0.00
Fifth Floor—North	60622	Lifepack 7 Defibrillator		5,500.00			
		Department Total	5,500.00	5,500.00	0.00	5,500.00	0.00
CCU	60626	Telemetry Transmitters		3,300.00			
		Department Total	3,300.00	3,300.00	0.00	3,300.00	0.00
Pediatric Unit	60630	Lifepack 7 Defibrillator		5,500.00			
		Facsimile Machine		1,550.00			
		Department Total	7,050.00	7,050.00	0.00	7,050.00	0.00

SOURCE: The University of South Alabama Medical Center, Mobile, Alabama. Reprinted with permission.

Table 6–3 • *University of South Alabama Medical Center Capital Budget, Status as of June 30*

Plant assets consisting of land, buildings, and equipment are stated at cost or, if contributed, at fair market value at date of gift. No provision is made in the accounts for depreciation of plant assets. Investment in Plant is reduced for disposal of plant assets.

All Hospital equipment purchases are funded by the Renewals and Replacements Fund. The Hospital also uses plant assets purchased by the University. These assets are not presented in the Hospital's Financial Statements.

Depreciation expense is included in Medicare, Medicaid, and Blue Cross cost reports. This information is presented below.

	Cost	Deprn. Expense 07-31	Accum. Deprn. 07-31	Net Book Value 07-31
Hospital-Designated Funds				
Land	$ 186,096	$ 0	$ 0	$ 186,096
Buildings	8,070,647	184,063	3,942,812	4,127,835
Fixed Equipment	10,386,318	605,671	5,878,008	4,508,310
Major Movable Equipment	15,079,892	1,235,052	8,971,493	6,108,399
Minor Equipment	186,757	0	186,757	0
Construction in Progress	762,874	0	0	762,874
Total	34,672,584	2,024,786	18,979,070	15,693,514
University-Designated Funds				
Buildings	1,544,927	39,481	581,958	962,969
Fixed Equipment	2,564,683	158,533	1,914,366	650,317
Major Movable Equipment	5,315,499	0	5,315,499	0
Total	9,425,109	198,014	7,811,823	1,613,286
Total equipment used for patient care	$44,097,693	$2,222,800	$26,790,893	$17,306,800

SOURCE: Courtesy of the University of South Alabama Medical Center, Mobile, Alabama.

Table 6–4 • University of South Alabama Medical Center Investment in Plant Assets for the Ten Months Ended July 31

considered the standard for the industry. See Figure 6–7.

REVENUES

What are the sources for nursing revenue or for securing a financial base for nursing? They include grants, continuing education, private practice, community visibility, health care for students and staff, health maintenance organizations, city health departments, industries, unions, third-party payments, professional corporations, and nurse-managed centers.

Operating room nursing is an example of a cost center that can be billed as a source of revenue. This can be done by determining the level of care needed for different procedures and the room charges based on use of supplies and equipment, then billing the services separately. In computing the nursing charges, the cost of nursing personnel per case can be determined from the records. To this can be added cost for preparation time for assembling supplies and equipment and setting up the room, visiting the patient preoperatively and postoperatively, nursing administration, and staff development. Room costs would include environmental services and maintenance.[4]

Maryland and Maine have passed legislation requiring hospitals to list nursing as a separate item on patients' bills. As the hospital bill is unbundled, all nursing cost centers will become major revenue-producing centers. Then all payers will be paying for nursing services based on business procedures. This will include allocated return on equity (profit) and proportionate losses due to bad debts.[5]

Using product line strategy, nursing divisions can sell staff development programs, consultation

DEPT. NAME: Operating Room (Orth.)

DEPT. NO.: 660

RETURN TO STEVE SIMMONS BY 2/10

1. LAYMAN'S DESCRIPTION OF EQUIPMENT: Wolf 70 degree Arthroscope and Attachments. Scope used to look in the knee at a different angle

2. EXPECTED USE: 2 times per week

3. TOTAL PRICE: $3,600.00

4. INSTALLATION & RENOVATION COSTS: none

5. SHIPPING COST:

6. TRAINING COST:

7. STAFFING (INCREASE OR DECREASE)

8. EXPECTED USEFUL LIFE: 15 years

QUESTIONS 9. & 10. ASSUMES BUDGET APPROVED 3/1

9. EXPECTED ARRIVAL DATE: April 1

10. EXPECTED DATE OF FIRST PATIENT USE: April 1

11. TRADE IN VALUE OF REPLACED EQUIPMENT:

12. PROCEDURE CHARGE: $100.50

13. EXPECTED ANNUAL PROCEDURES: 104 per year

14. COST OF SUPPLIES PER PROCEDURE:

15. PROFESSIONAL FEES:

16. JUSTIFY PRIORITY: The 70 degree scope is needed to look in the posterior aspect of the knee behind the femoral condyles and this cannot be done with the 30 degree scopes that we own at the present time. With the increasing importance of arthroscopy and the expertise now supplied by Dr. Dondren being on the part-time faculty, this scope is badly needed to update our equipment.

SIGNATURES: DEPARTMENT HEAD   ASSISTANT ADMINISTRATOR

SOURCE: Courtesy of South Alabama Medical Center, Mobile, Alabama.

Figure 6–6 • *University of South Alabama Medical Center Capital Requests*

Item	Years to Depreciate
Land improvements	
Heated pavement	10
Signs	12
Buildings	
Masonry, wood frame	20–25
Boiler house	15–25
Major movable equipment	7–12
Minor movable equipment	2–5

SOURCE: Reprinted, with permission, from *Estimated Useful Lives of Depreciable Hospital Assets*, published by American Hospital Publishing, Inc., copyright 1988.

Figure 6–7 • *Excerpt from Depreciation Schedule*

services, home health care, wellness programs, computer software, and many other product lines.

Many items and services generate revenues for hospitals. These include drugs, supplies, respiratory therapy, and physical therapy. In most instances the charges have been excessive and there have been areas where cost shifting accounted for revenues (and profits) to cover services delivered and charged at a price below costs. As the hospital bill is unbundled, charges will eventually reduce to costs at a 1:1 ratio. Not-for-profit hospitals are not allowed a return on equity or credit for bad debts as a cost of doing business.

Budgeting is a competency of nursing managers indicating responsibility and accountability. A well-prepared unit budget indicates that the best nurse manager has been delegated and has accepted the responsibility for this facet of the job. Management of the budget to keep expenditures and revenues in balance indicates the nurse manager accepts responsibility for it. Within the budgetary plan the nurse manager should be allowed some flexibility in making decisions about the mix of expenditures. This would mean that monies for staff, supplies, education, and other budgeted expenses could be interchanged so long as revenues are not exceeded and the objectives of the unit are being met.

A concept related to budgeting is "value for money." Is the unit or the organization getting full value for the money expended? This question relates to such areas as turnover of personnel, waste of supplies, ineffective use of clinical skills, and inaccurate staffing standards.[6]

THE CONTROLLING PROCESS

Now that the nursing budget has been viewed from its planning and directing aspects, it will be looked at from its controlling or evaluating aspects. The budget establishes financial standards for the division of nursing and through its cost center for each nursing unit. Feedback on a daily, weekly, monthly, and quarterly basis will supply information needed to compare managerial performance with the established standards. The results are used to make adjustments. What kind of feedback is needed by nurse managers relative to their budgets and cost control? They need information to tell whether their goals are being met. Are they exceeding the budget? Is the excess both for cost and revenues? Are the supplies and expenses of the quantity and quality planned? Is the equipment being purchased and installed as scheduled? Are employees being recruited and used effectively to produce the needed quality and quantity of nursing services? Is employee morale good? What adjustments need to be made? Where are the problem areas and who is responsible for them?

Budget processes should be flexible, to allow for increased and decreased volume of business. The business office provides cost center managers with needed biometric information to make adjustments in staffing and in use of supplies.

It should be remembered that a budget is a plan based on the best estimates of running an organization. It cannot be inflexible, but it also cannot hide waste and inefficiency.

The nurse administrator should be sure that nurse managers will not be penalized when the budgetary objectives are not met due to events beyond their control. They are working within the confines of an organizational environment that is affected by both internal and external constraints. One of the external constraints facing them is federally mandated cost control or cost containment, which is seen by some administrators as reimbursement control.

DECENTRALIZATION OF THE BUDGET

Cost center managers, usually head nurses and supervisors of wards or units, are capable of planning and controlling their own budgets. The nurse administrator, assisted by financial managers, should prepare them to do so. Through decentralized budgeting, cost center managers propose innovative objectives. They gather data to defend their objectives and operating plans. The unit budget becomes their responsibility and they guard its integrity with zeal. They sense when adaptations have to be made because of increased costs or decreased revenues. In these instances they make or recommend immediate remedies. Decentralized budgeting provides for internal controls.

MONITORING THE BUDGET

While various techniques have been described and defined for monitoring the budget, all budget objectives should contain procedures for quality review. These techniques include identification of a team to perform such a review. If a program is not successful—is not meeting objectives or is running above predicted costs and below predicted revenues—a decision should be made to cancel it. This is very difficult but is essential to good control. The technique of cancelling budgeted programs is sometimes referred to as "sunsetting." A nurse manager should accept the responsibility for sunsetting programs that are costly and unprofitable.

In developing the nursing budget it is necessary that the unit structures for nursing administration are compatible. This can be ensured by developing and providing financial instructions of policies and guidelines. This approach is most successful when the top administration team works together with the budget monitor in developing such financial policies. The nurse administrator will be part of this team and will bring to its meetings standards of service that are defensible, such as data on workload including numbers and types of procedures, patients, surgical operations, and visits. These policies should reflect the long-range plans of the governing board.

Part of the information furnished to nurse administrators and managers is in the form of reports. These include statistical reports of revenues and expenditures for the current year. Table 6–5 illustrates financial information that is needed by the cost center manager and the nursing service administrator.

Note that the account number is 4-60680. The prefix "4" denotes that the account balance does *not* turn over at the end of the fiscal year. The cost center or department is 60680. Any financial transaction, including purchase orders for supplies and minor equipment as well as the payroll, will be identified with this cost center number and will be charged by purchasing and accounting to this number and to the appropriate subcode, 100 through 501. Horizontal columns indicate the operational budget; the actual expenditures for the current month of July and the fiscal year; any open encumbrances and the balance available. Since 83 percent of the fiscal year (beginning October 1) had elapsed, this has some relationship to the percent used column. Although 103 percent of the budgeted salary has been used, only 78 percent of employee benefits have been used, indicating a use of overtime plus part-time employees working less than the 0.5 FTE required to qualify for fringe benefits. Zero percent of the budgeted monies for minor equipment had been spent to date. The total budget expenses were 96 percent indicating 13 percent overspending. Although this report serves as a control for nurse managers, the expenditure of budgeted monies for any one subcode could cause the total expenses to date to be greater than the percent of fiscal year elapsed without creating an alarm. In this instance overspending should be related to increased census and revenues.

Table 6–6 informs the nurse managers of the specific financial transactions that took place during the month of July. They can be checked against Table 6–5.

Information on revenues is reported similarly. Table 6–7 illustrates the inpatient revenue for the Medical Intensive Care Unit which includes nursing and hotel services. It is all credited to nursing.

The revenue account is 4-30815 while the cost center is the same as for expenses, 60680. The budgeted revenues for the year are listed as were the revenues for the month of July and for the fiscal year. Note that although 83 percent of the fiscal year has elapsed, only 76 percent of the budget revenues have been charged. Also, Table 6–8 indicates that 76 percent of budgeted equipment revenues have been charged.

Because the amount charged is 76 percent, being less than the 83 percent of fiscal year elapsed, the nurse managers can note that revenues are behind expenses, a negative financial report that needs to be analyzed. The goal is to control this kind of financial situation to the end of the fiscal year.

Additional financial information can be furnished each nurse manager. This includes summary reports in whole dollars and for all cost centers supervised. This can be done by subcode

Account statement in whole dollars for 07/31

83% of fiscal year elapsed
Distribution code = 700
Medical intensive Care Unit—8th Floor—Expense

Report Page 6722
User ID 44.2
FAS1029
To: Britten Sandy
USAMC-NRS SVC Admin

Subcode	Description	Budgets		Actual		Open Encumbrances	Balance Available	Perc Used
		Original	Revised	Current Month	Fiscal Year			
100	Pool—Salary & Wages	948,742	901,053				901,053	0
130	Professional Salary			72,533	775,790		775,790 –	***
135	Tech Salary & Wages			4,085	50,947		50,947 –	***
140	Office Salaries			4,347	53,168		53,168 –	***
155	Service Empl Wages			3,936	52,195		52,195 –	***
160	Student Wages		14,898	1,518	14,898			100
166	Accrued Salaries		32,791	11,462	32,791			100
	Salaries	948,742	948,742	97,880	979,789		31,047 –	103
170	Pool—Empl Benefits	254,683	55,722				55,722	0
182	Employers FICA		112		112			100
183	Group Life Ins		2,569	264	2,569			100
184	Disability Ins		4,869	526	4,869			100
185	Teachers Retirement		134		134			100
188	Group Health Ins		59,973	5,887	59,973			100
198	State Paid Retirement		62,158	5,591	62,158			100
199	State Paid FICA		69,146	6,313	69,146			100
	Employee Benefits	254,683	254,683	18,581	198,961		55,722	78
200	Pool—Med/Surg Supply	75,000	23,920				23,920	0
211	Med & Surg Supplies		128,235	14,846	128,235			100
213	Drugs		1,317	140	1,317			100
214	Solutions		36,091	4,389	36,091			100
	Med/Surg Supplies	75,000	189,563	19,375	165,643		23,920	87

SOURCE: The University of South Alabama Medical Center, Mobile, Alabama. Reprinted with permission.

Table 6-5 • *University of South Alabama Medical Center Accounting System Report*

(Continued)

Subcode	Description	Budgets		Actual		Open Encumbrances	Balance Available	Perc Used
		Original	Revised	Current Month	Fiscal Year			
220	Pool–General Supply	5,789	2,553 –			1	2,553 –	0
232	Office Supplies		1,070	19	1,069			100
233	Copying & Binding		36	30	36			100
234	Printing		1,494	115	1,494			100
235	Printing Paper		633	83	633			100
240	Housekeeping Supply		1,880	323	1,880			100
243	Housekeeping Furnish		1,395		1,395			100
244	Linen Replacement		214		214			100
250	Maintenance Supplies		1,001		1,001			100
270	Food Expense		619	49	619			100
	General Supplies	5,789	5,789	620	8,341	1	2,553 –	144
300	Pool–Travel/Entrtain		1,005				1,005	0
316	Workshop & Training		425		425			100
	Travel/Entertainment	1,430	1,430		425		1,005	30
320	Pool–Other Expenses		12,624				12,624	0
324	Contract Service		140,390	16,720	140,390			100
336	Equip Maint & Repair		3,700		2,950	750		100
372	Books & Subscription		286		286			100
	Other Expenses	157,000	157,000	16,720	143,626	750	12,624	92
501	Minor Equipment	4,000	4,000				4,000	0
	Total Expenses	1,446,644	1,561,207	153,176	1,496,785	751	63,671	96
	** Account Total **	1,446,644	1,561,207	153,176	1,496,785	751	63,671	96

Current month detail is shown on the Report of Transactions (AM091)
Questions: University call 460-6241, USAMC call 434-3535

Open Encumbrance Status

Account	P.O. Number	P.O. Date	Description	Original Enc	Liquidating Expenditures	Adjustments	Current Enc	Last Act Date
4-60680-232	H01764	10/06	Waller Brothers	.85			.85	10/18
4-60680-336	H07584	07/24	Scaletronix Inc	750.00			750.00	08/01
			*** Account Total **	750.85			750.85	

Table 6–5   (Continued)

Computer Date 08/03
Time of Day 06:47:57
PGM = AM091
Acct: 4-60680
Dept: 60680

Report Page 6724
User ID 44.2
FAS1030
To: Britten Sandy
USAMC-NRS SVC Admin

Report of transactions for 07/31

Distribution code = 700

Medical Intensive Care Unit—8th Floor—Expense

Subcode	Description	Date	EC	Ref.	2nd Ref.	J.E. Offset Account	Budget Entries	Current Rev/Exp	Encumbrances	Batch Ref.	Batch Date
130	Payroll Expense	07/07	64	900001		0-10080-118CR		35,017.03		PPS584	07/07
130	Payroll Expense	07/21	64	900001		0-10080-118CR		37,516.33		PPS588	07/21
130	CM Total Professional Salry							72,533.36			
135	Payroll Expense	07/07	64	900001		0-10080-118CR		1,630.89		PPS584	07/07
135	Payroll Expense	07/21	64	900001		0-10080-118CR		2,454.11		PPS588	07/21
135	CM Total Tech Salry & Wages							4,085.00			
140	Payroll Expense	07/07	64	900001		0-10080-118CR		2,082.44		PPS584	07/07
140	Payroll Expense	07/21	64	900001		0-10080-118CR		2,264.26		PPS588	07/21
140	CM Total Office Salaries							4,346.70			
155	Payroll Expense	07/07	64	900001		0-10080-118CR		1,884.26		PPS584	07/07
155	Payroll Expense	07/21	64	900001		0-10080-118CR		2,051.29		PPS588	07/21
155	CM Total Service Empl Wages							3,935.55			
160	Payroll Expense	07/07	64	900001		0-10080-118CR		494.83		PPS584	07/07
160	Payroll Expense	07/21	64	900001		0-10080-118CR		1,022.81		PPS588	07/21
160	CM Total Student Wages							1,517.64			
166	Susp Corr/Accr Sal	06/30	60		S01544	0-13000-160CR		65.00		HJV002	07/10
166	Susp Corr/Accr Sal	06/30	60		S01543	0-13000-160CR		45.00		HJV002	07/10
166	RVS Accrd Sal & Wage	07/01	60		075101	0-15300-220DR		40,318.00 –		HJV001	07/10
166	RVS Accrd Sal & Wage	07/01	60		075101	0-15300-220DR		65.00 –		HJV001	07/10
166	RVS Accrd Sal & Wage	07/01	60		075101	0-15300-220DR		45.00 –		HJV001	07/10
166	Accrued Sal & Wages	07/31	60		075100	0-15300-220CR		51,780.00		HJV019	07/31
166	CM Total Accrued Salaries							11,462.00			
183	Payroll Expense	07/21	64	900001		2-77000-180CR		264.04		PPS588	07/21
183	CM Total Group Life Ins							264.04			
184	Payroll Expense	07/21	64	900001		2-77000-180CR		526.48		PPS588	07/21
184	CM Total Disability Ins							526.48			

SOURCE: The University of South Alabama Medical Center, Mobile, Alabama. Reprinted with permission.

Table 6–6 • *University of South Alabama Medical Center Accounting System Report*

123

Subcode	Description	Date	EC	Ref.	2nd Ref.	J.E. Offset Account	Budget Entries	Current Rev/Exp	Encumbrances	Batch Ref.	Batch Date
188	Payroll Expense	07/07	64	900001		2-77000-180CR		65.81		PPS584	07/07
188	Payroll Expense	07/21	64	900001		2-77000-180CR		5,821.12		PPS588	07/21
188	CM Total Group Health Ins							5,886.93			
198	Payroll Expense	07/07	64	900001		2-77000-180CR		2,659.96		PPS584	07/07
198	Payroll Expense	07/21	64	900001		2-77000-180CR		2,930.66		PPS588	07/21
198	CM Total State Paid Retiremnt							5,590.62			
199	Payroll Expense	07/07	64	900001		2-77000-180CR		3,019.55		PPS584	07/07
199	Payroll Expense	07/21	64	900001		2-77000-180CR		3,293.55		PPS588	07/21
199	CM Total State Paid FICA							6,313.10			
211	Inventory Exp Alloc	07/31	60		075264	0-12100-140CR		14,845.75		HJV027	07/31
211	CM Total Med & Surg Supplies							14,485.75			
213	Pharmacy Distrib—Jul	07/31	60		075006	4-60730-213CR		140.34		HJV033	07/31
213	CM Total Drugs							140.34			
214	Inventory Exp Alloc	07/31	60		075264	0-12100-140CR		4,389.27		HJV027	07/31
214	CM Total Solutions							4,389.27			
232	Inventory Exp Alloc	07/31	60		075264	0-12100-140CR		19.49		HJV027	07/31
232	CM Total Office Supplies							19.49			
233	Xerox Expense-J/J	07/31	60		075008	4-60960-965CR		30.21		HJV026	07/31
233	CM Total Copying & Binding							30.21			
234	Print Shop Chrgs—Jul	07/26	60		075011	4-60960-960CR		115.20		HJV013	07/27
234	CM Total Printing							115.20			
235	Inventory Exp Alloc	07/31	60		075264	0-12100-140CR		82.69		HJV027	07/31
235	CM Total Printing Paper							82.69			
240	Inventory Exp Alloc	07/31	60		075264	0-12100-140CR		323.42		HJV027	07/31
240	CM Total Housekeeping Supply							323.42			
270	Inventory Exp Alloc	07/31	60		075264	0-12100-140CR		48.61		HJV027	07/31
270	CM Total Food Expense							48.61			
324	Nephrology Applicati	07/26	68		563631	0-15030-211CR		3,520.00		HPD850	07/26
324	Accure Jly	07/31	60		075259	0-15030-210CR		13,200.00		HJV024	07/31
324	CM Total Contract Service							16,720.00			
336	Scaletronix Inc	07/24	50	H07584					750.00	HEN010	07/31
336	CM Total Equip Maint & Repair								750.00		
	*** Account Total ***							153,176.40	750.00		

Table 6–6   (Continued)

Account statement in whole dollars for 07/31

Computer Date 08/03
Time of Day 06:47:57
PGM = AM090-B1
Acct: 4-30815
Dept. 60680

Report Page 6557
User ID 44.2
FAS1029
To: Asst Admin – Nursing
    USAMC-NRS SVC Admin

83% of fiscal year elapsed
Distribution code = 700
Medical Intensive Care Unit – 8th Floor – Revenue

Tab Code	Description	Budgets		Actual		Open Encumbrances	Balance Available	Perc Used
		Original	Revised	Current Month	Fiscal Year			
040								
0/0	Inpatient Revenue	1,511,400 –	1,511,400 –	115,500 –	1,146,600 –		364,800 –	76
	Total Revenues	1,511,400 –	1,511,400 –	115,500 –	1,146,600 –		364,800 –	76
	** Account Total **	1,511,400 –	1,511,400 –	115,500 –	1,146,600 –		364,800 –	76

Current month detail is shown on the Report of Transactions (AM091)
Questions: University call 460-6241, USAMC call 434-3535

SOURCE: The University of South Alabama Medical Center, Mobile, Alabama. Reprinted with permission.

Table 6–7 • *University of South Alabama Medical Center Accounting System Report*

Account statement in whole dollars for 07/31

Computer Date 08/03
Time of Day 06:47:57
PGM = AM090-B1
Acct: 4-30818
Dept. 60680

83% of fiscal year elapsed
Distribution code = 700
Medical Intensive Care Unit—SP&D—Revenue 8th flr

Report Page 6559
User ID 44.2
FAS1029
To: Asst Admin—Nursing
    USAMC-NRS SVC Admin

Subcode	Description	Budgets		Actual		Open Encumbrances	Balance Available	Perc Used
		Original	Revised	Current Month	Fiscal Year			
040	Inpatient Revenue		1,080,088 –	101,637 –	818,031 –		262,057 –	76
	Total Revenues		1,080,088 –	101,637 –	818,031 –		262,057 –	76
	** Account Total **		1,080,088 –	101,637 –	818,031 –		262,057 –	76

Current month detail is shown on the Report of Transactions (AM091)
Questions: University call 460-6241, USAMC call 434-3535.

SOURCE: The University of South Alabama Medical Center, Mobile, Alabama. Reprinted with permission.

Table 6–8 • *University of South Alabama Medical Center Accounting System Report*

(Table 6–9), by subcode and cost center (Table 6–10) and by any unit or department (Tables 6–11 and 6–12).

"Rollover" funds designated by prefix "3," are also included in the financial reports that can be provided to the chief nurse executive. Balances in these funds are carried over into the next fiscal year to be spent at any future date. An example of a rollover fund is account 3-64155, the maternal child health education fund. Table 6–13 shows activities for this fund for the month of July, and Table 6–14 shows how the debits were spent.

Rollover funds can be managed by the chief nurse executive, a department head, or cost center manager.

MOTIVATIONAL ASPECTS OF BUDGETING

Budgeting can be a motivational force for personnel—if current programs must increase in effectiveness and efficiency to remain in the budget; if decentralization and staff involvement provide an increased sense of responsibility and satisfaction; and if merit increases, promotions, and bonuses are tied to budgetary performance.

Budgeting facilitates communication within interdependent departments, thus increasing knowledge and understanding of other areas. It provides needed learning opportunities for future nurse managers.

The budget can be dysfunctional and fail to facilitate attainment of organizational objectives when it is viewed as an end rather than a means. This happens:

- If it is inflexible and permits no deviation from established plan.
- If it is viewed as being externally imposed by administrators who do not understand patient care.
- If health care providers feel left out of budget decisions.
- If there is overemphasis on staying within the budget, leading to a decrease in interdepartmental communication and cooperation
- If managers are held accountable without being given authority.[7]

CUTTING THE BUDGET

When the budget has to be cut, planning is a vital aspect of the process. This is happening today as hospital admissions and stays decrease and reimbursement takes on a new character. The form and the process of nursing management can determine the course of events when the budget has to be cut.

A nursing administration that delegates decision making to the lowest level and encourages participative management is an effective administration. When clinical nurses are informed at unit level and invited to give their input, they will help with suggestions for cutting costs. They will later implement and support the activities they view as resulting partly from their input. A nursing organization that promotes self-direction at the clinical nurse level, head nurse level, clinical consultant level, and executive nurse level will support direction to reduce cost and to increase productivity and profit. As an example, when a hospital CEO discovered that self-pay patient care was the only category not reviewed for use of resources, a review process was established by a clinical nurse. This process was supported by physicians and other health care professionals.

Nursing budgets are enormous, with budgets for a single unit running hundreds of thousands of dollars a year. Pay awards or increases have to be met by budget cuts (personnel cutbacks), use of cheaper supplies and techniques, or increased productivity. The latter requires more paying patients, shorter stays, and increased sales of all paying services. When personnel cuts are to be made, numbers make nursing vulnerable. Some cuts can come from all services but nursing has greater numbers. The nurse manager who controls these numbers daily, weekly, and yearly will have greater credibility. Many sources indicate that turnover is costly. The cost of turnover of personnel low on the salary scale is sometimes weighed against the higher cost of employees who are at the top of the salary scale. An assumption is made that long-time employees are better satisfied with their jobs and do better work, an assumption that needs to be validated through research. As workload data indicate shifts from one unit to another, resources must be shifted. This can be done by asking for volunteers, moving vacated positions, and using pools. There is a shift today from inpatient procedures in hospitals to outpatient procedures, either in hospitals or ambulatory surgery centers. Also, many more diagnostic procedures are done on an outpatient basis. As a result patients are often a sicker group.

Because nurse administrators control multimillion dollar budgets they are powerful people. They are also vulnerable for personnel cuts. Much of this vulnerability stems from external controls imposed by the state and federal governments and health in-

Computer Date 08/03
Time of Day 05:06:11
PGM = AM095-B1

Report Page 106
User ID 44.2
FAS1033

Summary report in whole dollars for 07/31

Distribution code = 750

Subcode	Description	Budgets		Actual			Open Commitments	Balance Available	Perc Used
		Original	Revised	Current Month	Fiscal Year	Project Year			
001	Prior Year Balance		302,976					302,978	0
002	Transfers								0
010	Income	16,419,272 –	16,419,272 –	1,342,529 –	13,782,618 –	13,782,618 –		2,636,654 –	84
020	Income			13,078 –	127,981 –	127,981 –		127,981	0
023	Interest Income			1,353 –	11,022 –	11,022 –		11,022	0
025	Original Budget	600,000 –	600,000 –	77,740 –	1,236,565 –	1,236,565 –		636,565	206
026				191 –	210 –	210 –		210	0
028	Bad Debt Recovery				169,932	169,923		169,932 –	0
030									0
040	Inpatient Revenue			1,852 –	29,682 –	29,682 –		29,682	0
041	Outpatient RF								0
042	Outpatient ED								0
050	Ded/Gross Revenue	75,009,000	75,009,000	8,904,127	72,586,402	72,586,402		2,422,598	97
099	State Paid Benefits								0
	Total Revenues	57,989,728	58,292,706	7,467,383	57,568,256	57,568,256		724,450	99
100	Pool – Salary & Wages	1,416,748	82,157					82,157	0
110	Exec & Adm Salaries		170,518	23,443	170,518	170,518			100
120	Instruction Salaries								0
130	Professional Salary		210,392	15,839	210,592	210,592 –		200 –	100

SOURCE: The University of South Alabama Medical Center, Mobile, Alabama. Reprinted with permission.

Table 6–9 • *University of South Alabama Medical Center Accounting System Report*

Subcode	Description	Budgets		Actual			Open Commitments	Balance Available	Perc Used
		Original	Revised	Current Month	Fiscal Year	Project Year			
131	Interns Salaries								0
135	Tech Salary & Wages		11,906	1,195	11,906	11,906			100
140	Office Salaries		840,893	79,028	840,893	843,866			100
150	Craft/Trade Wages					2,973		2,973 –	0
155	Service Empl Wages				143	808		808 –	0
159	Temp Craft/Trade Wge					154		154 –	0
160	Student Wages		20,975	2,678	20,975	20,975			100
164						2,431		2,431 –	0
166	Accrued Salaries		41,158	10,264	41,158	41,158			100
167									0
168	Tuition Reimbursemnt		6,971	2,756	6,971	6,971			100
169	Budget Correction								0
	Salaries	1,416,748	1,384,969	135,202	1,303,156	1,309,378		75,591	95
170	Pool—Empl Benefits	340,007	116,982					116,982	0
180	Employee Benefits	187,747	205,413	3,318	421,300	421,300		215,888 –	205
181	Unemployment Ins	41,307	41,307	7,722	22,717	22,717		18,590	55
182	Employers FICA		266	54	266	1,871		1,605 –	703
183	Group Life Ins		91,969 –	435	91,969 –	91,967 –		3 –	100
184	Disability Ins		9,090	1,015	9,106	9,110		20 –	100
185	Teachers Retirement		4		4	4			100
186	Meal Books								0
187	TIAA-CREF Retirement		2,068	259	2,068	2,068			100
188	Group Health Ins		96,262	12,650	116,322	116,342		20,080 –	121
190	Tuition Reimbursemnt	56,911	56,911	7,955	49,916	49,916		6,996	88

Table 6–9 (Continued)

Subcode 001 summary audit report for 07/31

Computer Date 08/03
Time of Day 05:06:11
PGM = AM095-B1

Distribution code = 750

Report Page 111
User ID 44.2
BUS1033

Cost Center	Cost Center Description	Original Budget	Revised Budget	Current Month	Year to Date	Project to Date	Open Commitments	Balance Available
364100	General Hospital Fnd	0.00	30,653.57	0.00	0.00	0.00	0.00	30,653.57
364105	Burn Unit	0.00	22,495.81	0.00	0.00	0.00	0.00	22,495.81
364110	Intensv Care Nursery	0.00	4,438.37	0.00	0.00	0.00	0.00	4,438.37
364120	J Erwin Ped Surgery	0.00	942.96 −	0.00	0.00	0.00	0.00	942.96 −
364127	Heart Statn−Holters	0.00	14,205.00	0.00	0.00	0.00	0.00	14,205.00
364173	Helping Hands/3&4 Fl	0.00	3,618.70	0.00	0.00	0.00	0.00	3,618.70
364174	Telethon−C&W USAMC	0.00	32,797.51	0.00	0.00	0.00	0.00	32,797.51
364175	Heart Fund Donations	0.00	864.10	0.00	0.00	0.00	0.00	864.10
364176	Telethon−C&W	0.00	71,327.96	0.00	0.00	0.00	0.00	71,827.96
364178	WOCD/Palmer Mem Fund	0.00	1,403.81	0.00	0.00	0.00	0.00	1,403.81
364179	Telethon−C&W	0.00	122,923.92	0.00	0.00	0.00	0.00	122,923.92
364197	Payroll Inserter	0.00	1,308.00 −	0.00	0.00	0.00	0.00	1,308.00 −
	Subcode Total	0.00	302,977.79	0.00	0.00	0.00	0.00	302,977.79

SOURCE: The University of South Alabama Medical Center, Mobile, Alabama. Reprinted with permission.

Table 6–10 • *University of South Alabama Medical Center Accounting System Report*

surance companies. Power comes from the ability of nurse administrators to use knowledge and skills in defending their budgets and in directing and controlling them. They learn to hold the line on staffing, on overtime, and on appropriate use of items of supply and equipment.

SUMMARY

It is important for clinical nurses to have a working knowledge of the nursing budget. Every activity that takes place in a hospital costs money. There must be a standard for assigning costs to user departments. The nursing division should pay its user share and no more.

Budgeting operations for the unit include those for personnel, supplies and equipment, and capital budgets. The nursing personnel budget for today's hospital is based on accurately quantified data from a patient acuity rating system. Nurse managers thus need to develop a staffing philoso-

phy and plans that will expand and contract staffing to provide for fluctuations. This can be partially done with part-time personnel, float pools, and the use of historical census data.

Nursing personnel budgets will be ultimately regarded as revenue budgets as laws and regulations change to allow for direct reimbursement for nursing care. Efficient nurse managers will use a budget calendar that covers formulation, review and enactment, and execution stages of the total budget process.

Evaluation is an administrative aspect of budgeting that in itself serves as a controlling process. Decentralization vests control at the lowest competent level of decision making. Good budget feedback information is essential for use of the budget as an effective controlling process. This includes information about revenues and expenses and internal comparisons of projected and actual budgets. The budget can be used to motivate professional nurses.

The belief of clinical nurses that budgets are beyond comprehension can effectively sabotage their effectiveness in a managerial position. Spiral-

Time of Day 05:09:39
PGM = AM047-H1

Cost-Center 9-82301
Reports to: 9-81000
Ledgers: 4

Report Page 11
User ID XX.1
Page 1
To: Britten Sandy

Responsibility roll-up report as of 07/31
Revenue—Britten

Responsibility Units	Budgets		Actual			Open Commitments C	Balance Available A-B-C	Perc Used (B+C)/A
	Original	Revised A	Current Month	Fiscal Year	Project Year B			
Cardiovas Rehab	790 –	790 –		869 –	869 –		79	110
Revenue-Enter Thpy	3,968 –	3,968 –	2,960 –	39,582 –	39,582 –		35,614	997
Chemothrapy-O/P Revn	90,729 –	90,729 –	15,107 –	110,452 –	110,452 –		19,723	121
Clinical Research Un	268,800 –	482,051 –	34,340 –	346,521 –	346,521 –		135,530 –	71
Cardiac ICU	1,524,600 –	3,254,816 –	252,996 –	2,426,084 –	2,426,084 –		828,732 –	74
Orthopedic Cast Room	108,459 –	108,459 –	8,128 –	91,765 –	91,765 –		16,696 –	84
5th Floor North/Reve	31,592 –	31,592 –	4,013 –	39,076 –	39,076 –		7,484 –	123
5th Floor South/Reve	2,054,000 –	2,977,320 –	236,359 –	2,331,656 –	2,331,656 –		645,664 –	78
Psychiatric Unit/Rev	1,701,300 –	1,725,507 –	137,906 –	1,463,792 –	1,463,792 –		261,715 –	84
8th Flr Medical/Reve	2,315,220 –	2,959,584 –	216,324 –	2,456,181 –	2,456,181 –		503,403 –	82
Medical ICU/Revenue	1,773,840 –	2,853,928 –	244,778 –	2,232,035 –	2,232,035 –		621,893 –	78
Coronary Care/Revenu	2,148,888 –	2,148,888 –	167,130 –	1,801,879 –	1,801,879 –		347,010 –	83
6th Flr Surgical/Rev	1,787,100 –	2,409,563 –	172,079 –	1,930,916 –	1,930,916 –		478,648 –	80
Burn Center/Revenue	1,254,000 –	3,090,809 –	193,436 –	2,155,646 –	2,155,646 –		935,163 –	69
9th Flr Surgical/Rev	2,029,260 –	3,122,028 –	230,728 –	2,446,790 –	2,446,790 –		675,238 –	78
Neuro/Trauma ICU/Rev	1,504,800 –	1,504,800 –	111,100 –	1,035,650 –	1,035,650 –		469,150 –	68
Newborn Nursery/Reve	804,600 –	896,817 –	87,603 –	794,535 –	794,535 –		102,282 –	88
Premature Nursy/Reve	615,672 –	615,672 –	71,803 –	596,432 –	596,432 –		19,240 –	96
Neonatal Nursy/Reven	4,692,600 –	5,468,373 –	580,112 –	5,178,067 –	5,178,067 –		290,306 –	94
Obstetric Unit/Reven	1,930,440 –	2,379,997 –	217,489 –	2,091,217 –	2,091,217 –		288,781 –	87
Pediatric Unit/Reven	1,438,080 –	2,013,282 –	171,673 –	1,658,513 –	1,658,513 –		354,769 –	82
Pediatric ICU/Revenu	1,141,800 –	1,915,268 –	115,489 –	1,208,778 –	1,208,778 –		706,490 –	63

SOURCE: The University of South Alabama Medical Center, Mobile, Alabama. Reprinted with permission.

Table 6–11 • *University of South Alabama Medical Center Accounting System Report*

	Budgets		Actual			Open Commitments C	Balance Available A-B-C	Perc Used (B+C)/A
	Original	Revised A	Current Month	Fiscal Year	Project Year B			
Delivery Room/Reven	3,396,552 –	3,396,552 –	410,192 –	3,553,291 –	3,553,291 –		156,738 –	104
Emergency Room	4,922,867 –	4,922,867 –	446,310 –	4,716,353 –	4,716,353 –		206,514 –	95
Total	37,539,957 –	48,373,660 –	4,128,055 –	40,706,080 –	40,706,080 –		7,667,586 –	84
Rev/Exp by Fund								
Operating Revenues	37,539,957 –	48,373,600 –	4,128,055 –	40,706,080 –	40,706,080 –		7,667,586 –	84
Total	37,539,957 –	48,373,660 –	4,128,055 –	40,706,080 –	40,706,080 –		7,667,586 –	84
Rev/Exp by Type								
Revenues	37,539,957	48,373,660	4,128,055	40,706,080	40,706,080		7,667,586	84
Expenses								
Salaries								
Employee Benefits								
Med/Sur Supply								
Office/Other Suply								
Travel/Entertain								
Other Expenses								
Minor Equipment								
Cost Offsets								
Total Expenses								

Table 6–11   (Continued)

Computer Date 08/03
Time of Day 05:09:39
PGM = AM047-H1

Cost-Center 9-82300
Reports to: 9-81000
Ledgers: 4

Report Page 9
User ID XX.1
Page 1

To: Britten Sandy

Responsibility roll-up report as of 07/31

Expense—Britten

| | Budgets | | Actual | | | Open Commitments | Balance Available | Perc Used |
Responsibility Units	Original	Revised A	Current Month	Fiscal Year	Project Year B	C	A-B-C	(B+C)/A
Medical Nursing	1,446,644	1,561,207	153,176	1,496,785	1,496,785	751	63,671	95
Psychiatric Nursing	659,186	661,552	63,520	590,664	590,664	566	70,323	89
Staff Development	274,449	274,748	17,680	295,828	295,828	2	21,082–	107
Nursing Svcs-Admin	869,036	880,078	91,347	779,791	779,791	6,242	94,044	89
Clinical Resch Unit	211,846	222,854	17,962	250,545	250,545	16	27,707–	112
Cardiac ICU	429,808	429,807	3,424	53,440	53,440		376,367	12
Float Nurses Pool			110	2,589	2,589		2,589–	
Orothopedic Cast Room	27,195	27,196		12,461	12,461	1,172	13,563	50
Employee Health Nurs	155,423	155,423	18,779	149,601	149,601	5	5,817	96
9th Floor-North	527,221	527,222	46,442	496,133	496,133	98	30,991	94
9th Floor-South	521,411	521,412	40,785	461,240	461,240	2	60,170	88
8th Floor-Medical	810,508	894,965	109,696	1,131,504	1,131,504	1,557	238,095–	126
5th Floor-Shrd Supp	66,529	157,455	25,770	185,295	185,295	862	28,702–	118
Burn Center	546,449	940,030	77,567	836,022	836,022	3,353	100,656	89
6th Floor-Surgical	1,222,187	1,363,087	117,908	1,278,709	1,278,709	2,101	82,276	93
Surgical ICU	1,074,332	1,332,394	138,564	1,309,157	1,309,157	338	22,899	98
7th Floor-Shrd Supp	626,522	696,032	72,802	833,026	833,026	787	137,781–	119
Newborn Nursery	667,925	939,910	81,197	892,992	892,992	868	46,051	95
Intermediate Nursery	236,612	236,612						
Intensive Care Nursery	1,810,927	1,944,960	202,179	1,749,864	1,749,864	1,241	193,856	90
Obstetric Unit	628,047	668,254	64,748	632,055	632,055	226	35,974	94
Pediatric Unit	923,577	998,643	91,105	895,375	895,375	263	103,005	89

SOURCE: The University of South Alabama Medical Center, Mobile, Alabama. Reprinted with permission.

Table 6-12 • *University of South Alabama Medical Center Accounting System Report*

	Budgets		Actual			Open Commitments C	Balance Available A-B-C	Perc Used (B+C)/A
	Original	Revised A	Current Month	Fiscal Year	Project Year B			
Pediatric ICU	560,288	645,410	48,874	568,314	568,314	50	77,045	88
Delivery Room	1,113,286	1,208,604	134,770	1,107,944	1,107,944	20,154	80,506	93
Emergency Room	1,613,253	1,691,149	160,935	1,524,713	1,524,713	13,885	152,550	90
Patient Transport	220,377	220,377	18,889	186,146	186,146	40	34,191	84
Total	17,243,038	18,962,769	1,798,229	17,720,193	17,720,193	54,579	1,187,999	93
Rev/Exp by Fund								
Nursing Division	17,060,420	18,750,317	1,771,862	17,527,171	17,527,171	53,402	1,169,746	93
Professional Division	27,195	57,029	7,588	43,421	43,421	1,172	12,436	78
Administrative Division	155,423	155,423	18,779	149,601	149,601	5	5,817	96
Total	17,243,038	18,962,769	1,798,229	17,720,193	17,720,193	54,579	1,187,999	93
Rev/Exp by Type								
Revenues								
Expenses								
Salaries	12,382,495	12,461,654	1,256,095	12,391,869	12,391,869		69,785	99
Employee Benefits	3,031,241	3,033,250	239,363	2,487,863	2,487,863		545,387	82
Med/Sur Supply	1,502,492	3,020,154	262,420	2,447,985	2,447,985	30,781	541,387	82
Office/Other Supply		109,306	9,788	107,656	107,656	1,652	100	
Travel/Entertain	43,989	45,788	2,209	27,555	27,555		18,233	60
Other Expenses	212,976	211,676	19,555	196,765	196,765	4,019	10,891	94
Minor Equipment	55,585	66,681	7,590	21,443	21,443	18,127	27,113	59
Cost Offsets	14,060	14,060	1,209	39,057	39,057		24,797 –	273
Total Expenses	17,243,038	18,962,769	1,798,229	17,720,193	17,720,193	54,579	1,187,999	93
Net Revenue/Expense	17,243,038	18,962,769	1,798,229	17,720,193	17,720,193	54,579	1,187,999	93
Total	17,243,038	18,962,769	1,798,229	17,720,193	17,720,193	54,579	1,187,999	93

Table 6–12 (Continued)

Account statement in whole dollars for 07/31

Computer Date 08/03
Time of Day 06:47:57
PGM = AM090-B1

83% of fiscal year elapsed
Distribution code = 700
Maternal Child Health Education Fund

Report Page 6544
User ID 44.2
FAS1029

Acct: 3-64155
Dept: 64155

To: Mair Betty
USAMC—Nursing Svc

Subcode	Description	Budgets		Actual		Open Encumbrances	Balance Available	Perc Used
		Original	Revised	Current Month	Fiscal Year			
001	Prior Year Balance		3,624				3,624	0
020	Income				5,285 –		5,285	***
021	Refunds				55		55 –	***
	Total Revenues		3,624		5,230 –		8,854	144 –
224	Recreation Supplies				60		60 –	***
231	Postage				60		60 –	***
234	Printing				257		257 –	***
	General Supplies				377		377 –	***
311	Travel			459	1,463		1,463 –	***
314	Local Travel				27		27 –	***
316	Workshop & Training			3,338	3,498	2,500	5,998 –	***
	Travel/Entertainment			3,796	4,989	2,500	7,489 –	***
422	Honorarium				425		425 –	***
450	Expense Offset				1,000 –		1,000	***
	Total Expenses			3,796	4,790	2,500	7,290 –	***
	** Account Total **		3,624	3,796	440 –	2,500	1,563	57

Current month is shown on the report of transactions (AM091)
Questions: University call 460-6241. USAMC call 434-3535

Open Encumbrance Status

Account	P.O. Number	P.O. Date	Description	Original Enc	Liquidating Expenditures	Adjustments	Current Enc	Last Act Date
3-64155-316	H04118	01/26	Perdido Hilton Hotel	2,500.00			2,500.00	03/22
			*** Account Total ***	2,500.00			2,500.00	

SOURCE: The University of South Alabama Medical Center, Mobile Alabama.

Table 6–13 • University of South Alabama Medical Center Accounting System Report

ing health care costs, hospital cost-containment efforts, and increasing accountability from individual cost responsibility centers should serve as an impetus to learn the fundamentals of budgets and the budget process. To assume the responsibility of budget work increases the nurse manager's poten-

tial realm of planning, predicting, and reviewing programs within his or her jurisdiction.

Similar to a nursing care plan, the budget is an activity guidance tool. It is a plan expressed in monetary terms, carried out within a time frame. To be effective as a care giver the nurse knows how

Computer Data 08/03
Time of Day 06:47:57
PGM = AM090

Acct: 3-64155
Dept: 64155

Report of transactions for 07/31

Distribution code = 700
Maternal Child Health Education Fund

To: Mair Betty
USAMC—Nursing Svc

Subcode	Description	Date	EC	Ref.	2nd Ref.	J.E. Offset Account	Budget Entries	Current Rev/Exp	Encumbrances	Batch Ref.	Batch Date
311	Dorothy May	07/11	48		218418			458.65		HPC804	07/11
311	CM Total Travel							458.65			
316	Perdido Beach Hilton	07/19	48		220893			3,337.73		HPC832	07/19
316	CM Total Workshop & Training							3,337.73			
	*** Account Total ***							3,796.38			

SOURCE: The University of South Alabama Medical Center, Mobile, Alabama. Reprinted with permission.

Table 6-14 • *University of South Alabama Medical Center Accounting System Report*

to develop and use a nursing care plan; similarly, to be most effective the nurse manager knows how to develop and use a budget.

EXPERIENTIAL EXERCISES

1. For each of the following statements, place a + in the blank if it is true and a − if it is false.

___ 1.1 The nurse manager does not need to plan a budget because most supplies and equipment come from central supply and the personnel authorizations are seldom 100 percent filled.

___ 1.2 The budget is not related to the objectives of the division of nursing.

___ 1.3 In many ways the budget of a health care institution is financed by business and industry.

___ 1.4 Budgeted expenses of the division of nursing are paid for by profits from services rendered to clients.

___ 1.5 Budgets are set for a period of time, usually a year, and cannot be changed.

___ 1.6 Budgets allow nurse managers to accomplish operational or management plans.

___ 1.7 Budgeting is planning.

___ 1.8 A budget predicts or estimates income and expenses, thereby setting limits on quality and quantity of health care services.

2. Create a personnel budget for a unit. To do this you need information from the Patient Classification System (PCS), however, for this exercise, use Figure 6–8 and Figure 6–9.

1. The patient has had a donor nephrectomy and has a spontaneous pneumothorax. A thoracotomy tube has been inserted and attached to chest drainage. She has puffy eyelids and a tingling feeling of her hands and feet. Her temperature is 100.8° F and she is receiving IPPB therapy. Remaining kidney function is being monitored with creatinine clearance, blood urea nitrogen, and serum creatinine levels. She cannot void spontaneously, complains of severe pain, and has nasogastric tubes.

2. The patient is stuporous and responds to repeated vigorous stimuli. When aroused, he is not oriented to person, time, and place. The head of his bed is elevated 30 degrees. He is receiving tube feedings with residual stomach contents being removed before each feeding. Bowel sounds are normal. He has a cuffed endotracheal tube to protect his airway.

3. Case #3 is admitted with a hiatal hernia. She has some gastrointestinal distress but appears reasonably well nourished. She appears high-strung, has little or no esophagitis and minimal symptoms. She is on a bland diet with small frequent feedings, is to avoid coffee, alcohol, and smoking. She receives Gelusil® 45 to 60 minutes after meals and at bedtime. She receives a stool softener, is to avoid tight clothing, and has the head of her bed elevated.

4. The patient has been admitted for chemotherapy. He is able to move from the bed by himself and to perform most of the activities of daily living by himself. He needs some help when getting up with IV running. The professional nurse meets with the patient daily to discuss his care.

5. Case #5 has been admitted with simple (endemic) goiter for radioactive iodine uptake studies and for treatment. She has some discomfort in breathing and swallowing but is able to perform all of her own activities of daily living.

6. Case #6 has an uncomplicated fracture of the femur. He is able to go to the bathroom with assistance and most of his care revolves around physical therapy.

7. Case #7 has acute pancreatitis, abdominal pain, mild cystitis, nausea, and vomiting. She is nervous and worried. Her vital signs are taken every 4 hours and she has a nasogastric tube and an IV.

8. Case #8 has been admitted with venous ulcers of the right leg. She is to have an Unna's boot applied and to be taught self-care.

9. Case #9 has been admitted for cataract surgery. She has diabetes mellitus which is controlled with diet and insulin. Fractional urines are done QID. The patient is being prepared for surgery and is receiving Chloroptic® 0.5 percent eye drops in each eye QID. At night about half an inch of erythromycin ophthalmic ointment is to be squeezed into the lower cul-de-sac of each eye.

10. Case #10 is an 85-year-old man complaining of abdominal pain. He needs help with getting into a bathtub, feeds himself, and has no other problems.

Figure 6–8 • *Cases*

Intensive Care (Red)	Modified Intensive Care (Orange)	Intermediate Care (Brown)	Minimal Care (Blue)	Self-Care (Green)
1. Acutely ill; requires constant or frequent observation; not necessarily terminal.	1. Acutely ill; requires frequent observation; may or may not be a terminal case.	1. Extreme symptoms have subsided or have not yet appeared; usually moderately ill.	1. Mildly ill or convalescent.	1. Usually ambulatory; activities not limited; requires a minimum of observation.
2. Activity must be rigidly controlled.	2. Limited activity; is dependent on others for basic needs.	2. Behavior pattern deviates moderately yet does not require close observation.	2. Activity controlled requiring little treatment or observation.	2. In hospital for x-rays and/or treatment or physical therapy.
3. Requires continuous or very frequent treatment.	3. Requires frequent treatment.	3. Activity must be partially controlled; or requires periodic treatment.	3. Needs very little help with personal hygiene.	

Special Condition: Patients having one or more of the following conditions shall be classified as above but at one higher category of nursing care need.

1. Isolation for communicable or infectious disease.
2. Handicap (blind, deaf, mute, amputee).
3. Senility, confusion, or general debility of age.
4. Incontinent or semicomatose or paraplegic.
5. Conditions: temperature above 102°F or nonstable blood pressure.

SOURCE: M. E. Warstler, "Some Management Techniques for Nursing Service Administrators," *Journal of Nursing Administration*, Nov.-Dec. 1972, 25–34.

Case #	Intensive Care (12 hrs.)	Modified Intensive Care (7.5 hrs.)	Intermediate Care (5.5 hrs.)	Minimal Care (3.5 hrs.)	Self-Care (1.5 hrs.)
1.					
2.					
3.					
4.					
5.					
6.					
7.					
8.					
9.					
10.					

Figure 6–9 • *Categories of Nursing Care Needs of Patients: Medical and Surgical (Adult and Child) Patient*

The procedure provided here may be used to determine staffing needs. Patients may be rated using a scale similar to that developed by Warstler, an up-to-date computerized PCS, or the chief nurse executive may arbitrarily use a specified number of nursing care hours per patient per 24 hours.

1. Bed capacity: 31
2. Bed occupancy rate for previous year: 78.1%
3. Staffing for occupancy = (1) × (2) = 31 × .781 = 24.211 = 25 patients
4. Hours of nursing care per patient per 24 hours = 5
5. Hours of nursing care per 25 patients per 24 hours = (3) × (4) = 25 × 5 = 125
6. Total nursing personnel needed per 24 hours = (5) ÷ productive time = 125 ÷ 7.5 = 16.6 = 17 full-time equivalents (FTEs)
7. To cover a 7-day week requires (7 ÷ 5) × (6) = 1.4 × 17 or a total of 23.8 = 24 FTEs
8. A recommended ratio is 1 RN:2 other nursing personnel. If this ratio were used, 8 of the FTEs would be RNs.
9. A recommended ratio of personnel for days, evenings, and nights is D 47%:E 35%:N 17% which would be D 11:E 9:N 4. Distribution could be as follows:

	Days	Evenings	Nights
RNs	4	3	1
Others	7	6	3

10. It should be noted that

   10.1 Staffing can be done on a monthly basis by using workload data (bed occupancy rates).
   10.2 Data can be used without rounding to next highest whole number.
   10.3 Each FTE is expected to be productive 7.5 hours during 8 hours.
   10.4 Several part-time workers can be used to make 1 FTE.
   10.5 Other hours of nursing care per patient per 24 hours may be used.
   10.6 Other ratios of RNs to other nursing workers may be used.
   10.7 Other ratios for days, evenings, and nights may be used.
   10.8 There are other staffing formulas that may be used.

SOURCE: Russell C. Swansburg, *Staffing* (Hattiesburg, MS: University of Southern Mississippi School of Nursing, 1977), 24–26.

Figure 6–10 • Determining Staffing Needs

2.1 Classify each case from Figure 6–8 and enter the information on Figure 6–9 as hours of care needed under the appropriate category (Intensive Care, Modified Intensive Care, Intermediate Care, Minimal Care, or Self-Care).

2.2 Add the hours of care for the 10 patients. What is the total number of hours of care needed? _____ hours.

2.3 Divide the total hours of care _____ by 10 (the number of cases or patients). The result is _____ hours of care. This is the average hours of care needed by each of these ten cases or patients. The PCS in an institution will do this for you and give you an average for a day, week, month, or year.

Warstler was one of the pioneers in the development of a PCS. You may want to use her criteria to classify actual patients and compare your example with one of the modern PCSs such as Medicus or GRASP to determine whether your data are valid and reliable.

3. Figure 6–10 illustrates determination of staffing needs for a nursing unit with a bed capacity of 31 and an occupancy rate of 78.1 percent.

Pick a unit of your department and prepare a staffing plan. Include basic and complementary staff. Include all of the following steps:

3.1 Average daily census = _____.

3.2 Average daily hours of nursing care to be provided* = _____ hours per 24-hour day.

* You determine this based on experience, records, available personnel, budgeted full-time equivalents (FTEs), or mandated requirements of governmental or other standard-setting agencies.

3.3 Total nursing hours per day needed = (1) ____ × (2) ____ = ____.

3.4 Total full-time equivalent personnel to staff unit for 24 hours = (3) ____ ÷ 7.5 = ____.

3.5 Total shifts per week = (4) ____ × 7 = ____.

3.6 Total full-time equivalent personnel needed to staff unit for 7 days = (5) ____ ÷ 5 = ____.

3.7 Total RNs needed if ratio is 1:2 = (6) ____ ÷ 3 = ____.

3.8 Total LPNs and others needed = (6) ____ − (7) ____ = ____.

3.9 Total RNs needed for days if 47% is portion = (7) ____ × .47 ____ = ____.

3.10 Total LPNs and others needed for days if 47% is portion = (8) ____ × .47 = ____.

3.11 Total RNs needed for evenings if 35% is portion = (7) ____ × .35 = ____.

3.12 Total LPNs and others needed for evenings if 35% is portion = (8) ____ × .35 = ____.

3.13 Total RNs needed for nights if 17% is portion = (7) ____ × .17 = ____.

3.14 Total LPNs and others needed for nights if 17% is portion = (10.8) ____ × .17 = ____.

3.15 Fill in basic staffing plan.

____ **BED** ____ **UNIT**
BASIC STAFFING PLAN

	Date	Evening	Night	Total
RNs				
LPNs				
Others				
Totals				

3.16 Add the complementary staff as + ( ).

NOTES

1. A. G. Herkimer, Jr., *Understanding Hospital Financial Management* (Rockville, MD: Aspen, 1978), 132.
2. R. P. Covert, "Expense Budgeting," *Handbook of Health Care Accounting and Finance,* edited by William O. Cleverly (Rockville, MD: Aspen, 1982), 261–278.

3. L. R. Piper, "Basic Budgeting for ED Nursing Personnel," *Journal of Emergency Nursing,* Nov./Dec. 1982, 285–287.
4. P. N. Palmer, "Why Hide the Revenue Produced by Perioperative Nursing Care?," *AORN Journal,* June 1984, 1122–1123.
5. In business and industry bad debts are considered an expense of doing business. In hospitals bad debt is subtracted from revenue, so it becomes a reduction of revenue rather than a cost of doing business. Profit or return on equity is not allowed by Medicare or Medicaid except for for-profit hospitals. A few third-party payers allow a return on equity.
6. C. Hancock, "Value for Money," *Nursing Focus,* Sept. 1981, 447–449.
7. A. E. Hillestad, "Budgeting: Functional or Dysfunctional?," *Nursing Economics,* Nov.-Dec. 1983, 199–201.

FOR FURTHER REFERENCE

Althaus, J. N., Hardyck, N. M., Pierce, P. B., and Rodgers, M. S. *Nursing Decentralization: The El Camino Experience* (Rockville, MD: Aspen, 1981).

American Hospital Association, *Chart of Accounts for Hospitals* (Chicago: American Hospital Publishing, 1976).

———, *Managerial Cost Accounting for Hospitals* (Chicago: American Hospital Publishing, 1980).

Cochran, Sr. Jeanette, "Refining a Patient-Acuity System over Four Years," *Hospital Progress,* Feb. 1979, 56–60.

Esmond, T. H., Jr., *Budgeting Procedures for Hospitals, 1982 Edition* (Chicago: American Hospital Publishing, 1982).

Goetz, J. F., and Smith, H. L., "Zero-Base Budgeting for Nursing Services: An Opportunity for Cost Containment," *Nursing Forum,* Feb. 1980, 122–137.

Hallows, D. A., "Budget Processes and Budgeting in the New Authorities," *Nursing Times,* Aug. 4, 1982, 1309–1311.

Hancock, C., "The Nursing Budget," *Nursing Mirror,* Oct. 20, 1982, 47–48.

Herzog, T. P., "Productivity: Fighting the Battle of the Budget," *Nursing Management,* Jan. 1985, 30–34.

Hicks, L. L., and Boles, K. E., "Why Health Economics?," *Nursing Economics,* May-June, 1984, 175–180.

Hodgetts, R. M., *Management: Theory, Process, and Practice* (Philadelphia: W. B. Saunders, 1975), 208–209.

Huttman, B., "Taking Charge: Selling Your Budget," *RN,* Apr. 1964, 25–26.

Hutton, J., and Moss, D., "Budgetary Control—The Role of the Director of Nursing Services and Treasurers," *Nursing Times,* Aug. 11, 1982, 1364–1365.

Johnson, K. P., "Revenue Budgeting/Rate Setting," in *Handbook of Health Care Accounting and Finance,* edited by William O. Cleverly (Rockville, MD: Aspen, 1982), 279–311.

La Violette, S., "Classification Systems Remedy Billing Inequity," *Modern Healthcare,* Sept. 1979, 32–33.

Lyne, M., "Grasping the Challenge," *Nursing Times,* Nov. 23, 1983, 11–12.

Marriner, A., "Budgetary Management," *Journal of Continuing Education in Nursing,* Nov./Dec. 1980, 11–14.

McCarty, P., "Nursing Administrators Control Millions," *American Nurse,* Sept. 20, 1979, 1, 8, 19.

McCullers, L. D., and Schroeder, R. G., *Accounting Theory Text and Readings* (New York: John Wiley & Sons, 1982), 18–23.

Nordberg, B., and King, L., "Third-Party Payment for Patient Education," *American Journal of Nursing,* Aug. 1976, 1269–1271.

Orem, D. E., *Nursing Concepts of Practice,* 3d ed. (New York: McGraw-Hill, 1985).

Oszustowizc, R. J., "Financial Management of Department of Nursing Services," NLN Publ. 20-1798 (New York: National League for Nursing, 1979), 1–10.

Rowsell, G., "Economics of Health Care," *AARN Newsletter 37,* No. 7, July/Aug. 1981, 6–8.

Ruskowski, U., "A Budget Orientation Tool for Nurse Managers," *Dimensions in Health Service,* Dec. 1980, 30–31.

Sonberg, V., and Vestal, K. E., "Nursing as a Business," *Nursing Clinics of North America,* Sept. 1983, 491–498.

Suver, J. D., "Zero-Base Budgeting," in *Handbook of Health Care Accounting and Finance,* edited by William O. Cleverly (Rockville, MD: Aspen, 1982), 353–376.

Trofino, J., "Managing the Budget Crunch," *Nursing Management,* Oct. 1984, 42–47.

Vracin, R. A., "Capital Budgeting," in *Handbook of Health Care Accounting and Finance,* edited by William O. Cleverly (Rockville, MD: Aspen, 1982), 323–351.

Managing a Clinical Practice Discipline

INTRODUCTION

Nursing is a clinical practice discipline. Effective nurse managers realize this and treat its practitioners accordingly. This means that nurse managers will facilitate the work of clinical nurses, a difficult goal for supervisor-employee relationships in bureaucratic organizations. Professional nurses want autonomy in their own practice. They want to apply their nursing knowledge and skills without interference from nurse managers, physicians, or persons in other disciplines. This is best done by nurse managers who establish professional peer relationships with practicing professional nurses. Such a relationship does not abrogate the supervisor-employee relationship. Nurse managers develop a relationship that embodies trust. The nurse manager trusts the professional nurse to apply knowledge and skills correctly in caring for a group of patients. In turn, the clinical nurse trusts the nurse manager to coordinate supplies, equipment, and support systems with personnel of other departments.

Nurse managers ask clinical nurses for input on implementation of policies and procedures. Clinical nurses come to respect a human relations management process in which they participate rather than one in which they have rules and regulations imposed on them. They use the body of nursing knowledge (theory) gained in nursing school and maintained through continuing education and staff development to practice nursing as they determine it should be practiced. In doing so they adhere to management policy regarding such things as documentation or quality assurance because these requirements are also part of clinical nursing practice.

USE OF NURSING THEORIES

In developing nursing as a scientific discipline, nursing educators and researchers have developed theoretical frameworks for the clinical practice of nursing. These theoretical frameworks are used by clinical nurses as models for testing and validating applications of nursing knowledge and skills. Their results are added to the body of knowledge now commonly called the theory of nursing. Theory gives practicing nurses a professional identity. It is based on scientific inquiry: nursing research. Each result of nursing research adds tested facts to nursing theory that can be learned by nursing students and active practitioners.

Models and Examples

Models are frequently used in the development of nursing theory. A model usually communicates in graphic format an abstract entity, structure, or process that cannot be directly observed. Models depict behavioral processes that exist in reality but cannot be directly observed except as indirect behaviors of those engaged in the process. They order, clarify, and systematize selected components of the phenomenon they serve to depict. Models illustrate and clarify theories. Because nursing theories have not been widely applied they are frequently described or depicted as models.[1]

Theories of Orem and Kinlein.
Dickson and Lee-Villasenor report testing of Orem's self-care nursing theory as modified by Kinlein. As independent generalist nurses they did their research in a private nursing practice setting. They used grounded theory methodology to systematically obtain data from clients and analyze it. As the clients spoke, they recorded, identifying self-care assets, self-care demand, and self-care measures with their clients.

In performing a content analysis, Dickson and Lee-Villasenor catalogued events as expression of need, self-care assets, self-care demand, and self-care measures. They catalogued events by numbers of expressions of need: a perception of self, an action taken, a want, a wish, or a question; and by perception of self according to mind-body combination. Events were also catalogued according to evidence of patterns of self-care actions that contributed positively to the client's state of health and number of self-care assets: action, motivation, knowledge, and potential.[2]

This model can be duplicated by clinical nursing research in hospital settings, home health care settings, and other areas in which nurses practice. The results will add to the body of nursing theory. Nurse managers will facilitate the practice of clinical nursing by supporting acquisition of new knowledge. This can be done through staff devel-

opment by having unit programs, providing periodicals or journal clubs, or offering release time for library use.

Theory of Roy.
Roy advocates adaptation level theory to nursing intervention. She notes that a person adapts to the environment through four modes: physiologic, self-concept, role mastery, and interdependence.[3] Just as the individual patient adapts to changes in the environment, so does the nurse worker.

According to Roy the goal of nursing is to assist the patient to adapt to illness so as to be able to respond to other stimuli. The patient is assessed for positive or negative behavior in the four adaptive modes. Once the assessment is made at the necessary (first or second) level, intervention is established by a nursing care plan of goals and approaches. The approach is selected to match the goal.[4] Roy's adaptive modes can be applied to develop a theory for nursing management.

According to Mastal and Hammond, Roy's views are "that the developing body of nursing knowledge now contains verifiable theories and general laws related to: (1) persons as holistic beings and (2) the role of nursing in promoting the person's maximum potential health and harmonious interaction with the environment."[5]

Although Roy's theory is directed toward the care of patients as persons, the model has the potential of being adapted to management of the practitioner. Nurse managers then have two options: (1) implementing Roy's theory at the clinical practice level or (2) constructing a management model adapting Roy's theory. The latter may appear as a conceptual model; see Figure 7-1.

A nurse manager could support a clinical nurse in her or his adaptation by substituting "practicing nurse" for "client" in Roy's outline of a six-step nursing process as stated by Mastal and Hammond:

1. *Assess the client's behaviors in each of the modes and determine whether they are adaptive or inefficient.*
2. *Assess the stimuli that influence those behaviors and classify them as to whether they are focal, contextual, or residual. All stimuli (both positive and negative) must be considered if a valid situational assessment is to be achieved.*
3. *Identify and state the adaptation problem.*
4. *Establish goals in terms of desired behaviors.*
5. *Manipulate those stimuli that will promote adaptation. Manipulation refers to removing,*

Roy's Concept	Adapted to Management
1. Person is an adaptive system or biopsychosocial being who functions as a totality in constant interaction with a changing internal or external environment. The cognator adaptive mechanism "identifies, stores and relates environmental stimuli to effect symbolic responses. It acts consciously by thought and decision, and unconsciously through defense mechanisms" (p. 73). The regulator adaptive mechanism responds through the autonomic nervous system with reflex action by approach, attack, or flight.	1. The clinical nurse is the focus of nursing management and is affected by the actions of the nurse manager. These management actions can affect the internal or external environment of the clinical nurse. The cognator mechanism of the clinical nurse responds consciously or unconsciously to stimuli from the nurse manager. A nurse manager who creates an autocratic environment may cause clinical nurse responses varying on a continuum from awareness to resignation from the job and that include suppressed anger, absenteeism, and so on.
2. Environment provides the stimuli that provoke adaptation. Stimuli are stressors.	2. The nurse manager can invoke stressors that impede or facilitate goal achievement by clinical nurses.
3. Adaptation is both a process and an end state. It is a person's responses to environmental stimuli to promote that person's goals of survival, growth, reproduction, and self-actualization.	3. A clinical nurse may feel so harassed by a nurse manager as to go on a permanent shift to survive. If a clinical nurse cannot achieve career goals, this person may transfer, change jobs, or adapt his or her work schedule.
4. Health/illness is a dimension of a person's life that occurs on a continuum: 4.1 peak wellness 4.2 high-level wellness 4.3 good health 4.4 normal health 4.5 poor health 4.6 extreme poor health 4.7 death	4. The health/illness concept applies to all persons but nurse managers need an awareness of its impact on the performance of the clinical nurse.

SOURCE: Adapted from M. F. Mastal and H. Hammond, "Analysis and Expansion of the Roy Adaptation Model: A Contribution to Holistic Nursing," *Advances in Nursing Science*, July 1980, 71–81; Sr. C. Roy, *Introduction to Nursing: An Adaptation Model* (Englewood Cliffs, NJ: Prentice-Hall, 1976).

Figure 7–1 • Adaptation of Roy's Theoretical Concepts to Nursing Management

changing, increasing, or decreasing the stimuli so that adaptive behaviors are reinforced and inefficient ones are modified.

6. Evaluate the person's response to nursing intervention in terms of meeting the established goals.[6]

Theory of Newman.   Engle tested Newman's conceptual framework of health in a sample of older women. She indicates that Newman uses Rogers's concept of the life process and the relationship of the individual within the environment. In this model aging is considered a natural process, the person's individual state being a fusion of health and disease. Movement is a correlation of health measured by a basic time factor or tempo.[7]

Engle defines tempo as the characteristic rate of performing a task. Time is the second correlation of health. Tempo and time occur in a succession of events, rhythmic patterns of temperatures and movement, and patterns within the environment. Time perception and tempo are hypothesized to be altered by age and illness. The patient does self-assessment of his or her health as a criterion measure. Self-assessment and physician assessment of health have been shown to correlate. Self-assessment of health is altered by ability to perform everyday activities, by age self-concept, and by movement and time.[8]

In her study Engle measured personal tempo, time perception, and self-assessment of health by using the Cantril Ladder, in 114 females aged 60 or older. She found no age effect for time perception in this study nor did Newman and Tompkins in similar studies. Nor was there any age effect for personal tempo.[9]

There was a significant relationship between time perception and personal tempo that could have significance for the patient and the clinical nurse. The patient or nurse with a physical or mental condition that alters personal tempo may have an altered perception of time. This could be true in older nurses in whom physical and mental states are more often altered. Further research in this area is needed, particularly as the population ages.

Theory of Levine. Levine indicates that nursing practice has mirrored prevailing theories of health and disease. Nursing has created an environment for healing: cleanliness, safety, and physical and emotional comfort. Nursing enhances the reparative process. Nursing became "disease-oriented" when diseases, not patients, were the focus of treatment. As nurses became concerned with the multiple factors affecting the course of disease, they developed the "total patient care" concept.[10]

People respond to illness in individual ways. Nursing intervention should match the individual response, which is identified from observation and data analysis. Assessment reveals unique needs requiring unique nursing measures. Nursing supports repair and maintenance of a person's integrated self—homeostasis and equilibrium. Equilibrium is maintained by adaptation. The nurse intervenes to support successful adaptation, to achieve a therapeutic or supportive role.[11]

Levine's theory could be applied to nursing management within an organization. The nurse manager wants to maintain the equilibrium of a unit, service, department, or division. When this equilibrium is upset because of staff turnover, nurse managers need to act in concert with clinical nurses to adapt to working with fewer professional nurses. Data are collected and analyzed to make adjustments that can include increased productivity and increased efficiency as well as changes to decrease turnover.

Theory of Johnson. The Johnson Behavioral Systems Model is a theory of nursing practice. Johnson incorporated the nursing process (assessment, planning-diagnosis, intervention, and evaluation) into a general systems model. Rawls applied it to care of a patient for the purpose of testing, evaluating, and determining its utility for predicting the effect of nursing care on a patient. Rawls indicates the model has disadvantages but is a tool that can be used "to accurately predict the results of nursing interventions prior to care, formulate standards of care, and most importantly administer truly holistic empathic nursing care."[12]

The Johnson Behavioral Systems Model could be applied to nursing management. It could be tested as a predictor of the effect of nursing management on clinical nurses.

Theory of Peplau. Although Peplau's theory that nursing "is a significant, therapeutic, interpersonal process" has been applied to clinical nursing, there is merit to its application to nursing management. The nurse manager uses the interpersonal process in relationships with personnel, patients, families, visitors, and other individuals and groups. As a manager of clinical nurses, the nurse manager could use the interpersonal process in assisting employees to manage life situations that cause anxiety, depression, and insecurity.

Peplau's theory involves communication techniques, assessment, definition of problems and goals, direction, role clarification, and other concepts relevant to human resource management. The nurse manager adept in the theory could assist personnel in meeting their needs, thereby preventing or reducing anxiety. Room exists for research in application of Peplau's theory to nursing management. This would include identification of principles that apply.[13]

Theory of Orlando. Orlando's theory of nursing develops three basic concepts:

1. Professional nursing has as its function the identification and meeting of patients' needs for help.
2. Professional nursing has as its outcome or product both verbal and nonverbal improvement in the patient's behavior.
3. Regardless of its form, the patient's presenting or initial behavior may be a plea for help.

Orlando's theory has been implemented in a department of nursing under the leadership of a director of nursing. Thus nursing theory is used by nurse managers to promote clinical nursing.

Schmieding applied Orlando's theory to solving problems in managing the behavior of clinical nurses. She recommends that the work of one theorist be used as the practice model within a given organization. This application of Orlando's model helped nurses apply common concepts and a framework for nursing. They could be adjusted if the nursing staff synthesized the concepts of several theories.[14]

Applications to Nursing Management

Nurse managers use management skills to motivate clinical nurses. Their work rests on a theoretical understanding of communication, motivation, and leadership (directing activities), as well as of planning, organizing, and evaluating. The adaptive aspects of the nurse manager's behavior are multidimensional in response to management problems, just as is clinical nursing behavior in response to the problems of sick patients.

Just as modern clinical nurses have access to theory, so do nurse managers. Scientific management knowledge is as essential to the nurse manager as scientific biological, physical, and social knowledge is to the clinical nurse. The nurse manager is responsible for maintaining the wholeness, integration, and equilibrium of the clinical nurse.

According to Goldstein the tendency to actualize oneself is the only motive by which human activity is set going. If this theory is applied to the nurse manager it has two possible directions: promotion of self-actualization in clinical nurses by nurse managers and development of the self-actualization motive within nurse managers.[15]

Clinical nurses learn theories of nursing in preservice programs. They learn to synthesize knowledge and skills and apply them in clinical practice. Through staff development and personal endeavors they add to their body of nursing theory knowledge as the knowledge is tested and disseminated.

Nurse managers facilitate the process by encouraging learning, research, and excellence of performance. They pursue research in nursing management and draw on the theory of business, management, human relations, and related disciplines as well as the theory of nursing.

Clinical practitioners in any field need to apply some management theory to their work. Structure is always an essential element. Work needs to be planned, goals set, outcome criteria set, organization designed, budget and resources identified, controlling techniques established, and the decision-making process determined. Nurse managers

assist and support applications of management theory in their relationships with clinical nurses. They provide the work processing tasks that include procedures, tools, techniques, harmonious work relationships, problem solving, budget and schedule preparation, communication, and working.

Nurse managers thus facilitate clinical nurses to:

1. Utilize the nursing process.
2. Perform nursing diagnosis and treatment.
3. Accept accountability for nursing activities of other nursing personnel.
4. Accept accountability for nursing outcomes.
5. Control the nursing practice environment.[16]

Participation in the management process by clinical nurses can be fostered by nurse managers in at least five ways:

1. *Upward participation.* Professional nurses become involved in the manager's work. Nurse managers accustomed to autocratic management may not support such a process if they have difficulty giving up control. When they involve the nurses in the structuring process, it is more likely to be successful. Nurse managers should teach employees the skills of upward participation.

2. *Downward participation.* Nursing work is structured by nurse managers who may become involved in it. This can be positive or negative in its effect on employees. If there is mutual agreement that defines the reason for and the scope of the manager's involvement, the result will be positive. Participation can be from the division, department, or service level to any lower level or levels, including unit level.

3. *Lateral participation.* Collaboration among nursing units requires skills in group processes and in managing individual and group differences. Usually the unit or departments will be within a nursing service or the nursing division.

4. *Organizational participation.* Collaboration across divisions or departments corrects isolationism and separation, requiring strong managerial and clinical leadership to breach territorial imperatives. Nurses sometimes want to participate with other professionals and in other departments, but they do not always welcome reciprocal participation.

5. *Personal participation.* The individual uses personal mental and physical capabilities in doing work. Nurse managers should uncover barriers to autonomy of practice. Personal participation enhances self-esteem and feelings of professional and personal worth in nurses.[17]

Many other applications and suggested applications of nursing theory to nursing administration theory, practice, and research have been made. These include cultural care theory (Leininger); systems theory (King); man-living-health theory (Parse); and unitary human beings theory (Rogers).[18]

MODALITIES OF NURSING PRACTICE

Several modalities or methods of nursing practice have evolved during the past 35 years. These include functional nursing, team nursing, primary nursing, case method, joint practice, and case management. All are practiced in various forms in health care institutions in the United States. Although nurse managers frequently decide the method of nursing practice to be used in their organizations, it is best to involve practicing clinical nurses in making this decision. The latter are the ones who will do it; if the choice is theirs they will make it work. Clinical nurses should be provided with sufficient information about the modality and how the institution will support it so they can provide input for a workable decision.

Once the decision is made an ad hoc committee can develop policies and procedures for implementing the modality. There should be adequate resources, including appropriate categories of nursing personnel, to make the modality work. Personnel need to be adequately prepared through staff development programs. These can be supported by staff development instructors in large organizations. Small organizations may need assistance from a consultant, usually available within the larger organizations of the nearest urban area.

Functional Nursing

This is the oldest nursing practice modality. It can best be described as a task-oriented method in which a particular nursing function is assigned to each staff member. One registered nurse is responsible for administering medications, one for treatments, one for managing intravenous admin-

istration; one licensed practical nurse is assigned admissions and discharges, another gives bed baths; a nurse's aide makes beds, passes meal trays, and so on. No nurse is responsible for total care of any patient. The method divides the tasks to be done, with each person being responsible to the nurse manager. It is efficient and may be the best system when confronted with a large patient load and a shortage of professional nurses.

The advantage of functional nursing is that:

- It accomplishes the most work in the shortest amount of time.

Disadvantages of functional nursing are that:

- It fragments nursing care.
- It decreases the nurse's accountability and responsibility.
- It makes the nurse-client relationship difficult to establish, if it is ever achieved.
- It gives professional nursing low status in terms of responsibility for patient care.

Functional nursing was largely a development of the World War II era, when large numbers of nurses entered military service and ancillary personnel were trained to staff many nursing functions of hospitals. It is still alive and well in many institutions.[19]

Team Nursing

Team nursing developed in the early 1950s, when various nursing leaders decided that a team approach could unify the different categories of nurse workers. Under the leadership of a professional nurse, a group of nurses would work together to fulfill the functions of professional nurses. Assignment of patients is made to a team consisting of a registered nurse as a team leader, and other staff RNs, LPNs, and aides as team members.

The team leader has the responsibility for coordinating the total care of a block of patients and is the leadership figure. Team nursing is practiced in many institutions.[20]

The intent of team nursing is to provide patient-centered care. The patient's nursing care needs are identified and met through nursing diagnosis and prescription. Ward clerks and unit managers perform the nonnursing functions of the unit. The process requires planning to meet the objective of taking nursing personnel to the bedside so that they can focus on nursing care of patients.

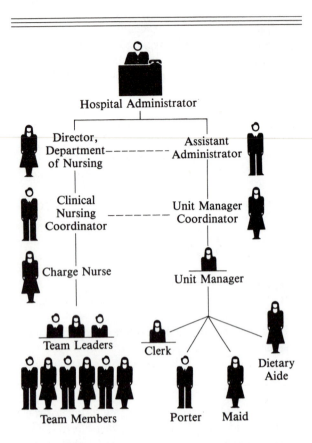

SOURCE: D. P. Newcomb and R. C. Swansburg, *The Team Plan* (New York: G. P. Putnam's Sons, 1953, 1971).

Figure 7–2 • *Team Nursing Organization*

Implementing team nursing requires study of the literature on the team plan, development of a philosophy of team nursing, planning for appropriate use of all categories of nursing workers, planning for team conferences, developing nursing care plans, and development of team leadership. Figure 7–2 depicts an original schema for a team nursing organization. It would be somewhat modified today to depict a less bureaucratic structure, with team members performing different roles.

The following is a summary of the team plan as advocated by Newcomb and Swansburg:

The team plan gives priorities to the development of leadership potential—leadership in the practice of nursing—leadership that is creative and that encourages improvement of communications among team members, patients, and leaders. It gives priority to emphasis on democratic leadership, the nurturing of cooperative effort, and free expression of ideas of all team members. It gives priority to motivation of people to grow to this self-approved or maximum level of performance.

Through the team plan the contributions of all team members in improving patient care are recognized. Priority is given to the strengthening of their weaknesses.

Patient-centered care employs effective supervision and recognizes that personnel are the media by which the objectives are met in a cooperative effort between team leaders and team members. Through supervision the team leader identifies nursing care goals; identifies team members' needs; focuses on fulfilling goals and needs; motivates team members to grow as workers and citizens; guides team members to help set and meet high standards of patient care and job performance—all of them supporting the priority of practicing nursing.[21]

The advantages of team nursing are:

- It involves all team members in planning patients' nursing care, through use of team conferences and writing nursing care plans.
- It provides the best care at the lowest cost, according to some advocates.

Disadvantages of team nursing include:

- It can lead to fragmentation of care if the concept is not implemented totally.
- It can be difficult to find time for team conferences and care plans.
- It allows the RN who is the team leader to have the only significant responsibility and authority.[22]

The disadvantages of team nursing can be overcome by educating competent team leaders in the principles of nursing management.

Primary Nursing

The most touted method of assignment and practice today is that of primary nursing. It is an extension of the principle of decentralization of authority, the primary authority for all decisions about the nursing process being centered in the person of the professional nurse. The primary nurse is assigned to care for the patient's total needs for the duration of the hospital stay.

Responsibility covers a 24-hour period, with associate nurses providing care when the primary nurse is not there. The care given is planned and prescribed totally by the primary nurse.[23]

Marram, Schlegel, and Bevis state, "Primary nursing . . . is the distribution of nursing so that the total care of an individual is the responsibility of one nurse, not many nurses."[24] They indicate autonomy to be the key to the development of professional nursing. Characteristics of the primary nursing modality are:

1. The primary nurse has responsibility for the nursing care of the patient 24 hours a day, from admission through discharge.
2. Assessment of nursing care needs, collaboration with patient and other health professionals, and formulation of the plan of care are all in the hands of the primary nurse.
3. Execution of the nursing care plan is delegated by primary nurse to a secondary nurse during other shifts.
4. The primary nurse consults head nurses and supervisors.
5. Authority, accountability, and autonomy rest with the primary nurse.[25]

Primary nursing parallels decentralized patient education because the nurse becomes the primary provider. In comprehensive patient care the primary nurse is responsible and accountable for patient education.[26]

Since 1974 primary nursing has been implemented in many hospitals and has undergone numerous modifications. Primary nurses frequently do the hands-on nursing care of the patient. Sometimes they direct other care givers while retaining the functions of decision makers.

Fagin states that research studies on primary nursing indicate it reduced hospital stays and complications of renal transplant patients at the University of Michigan Medical Center in Ann Arbor. They saved $51,000 in one year. Primary nursing at Evanston Hospital in Illinois resulted in fewer nursing hours and less salary expense per patient during a 5-year period. Nurse aides had 27 percent unoccupied time per day while RNs had 8 percent at Rush Presbyterian. Also, turnover was decreased in the operating suite with increased RN to operating room technician ratio. Other studies indicate that primary nursing saves money; increases job satisfaction, group adhesion, and patient satisfaction; and decreases costs of overtime, sick time, and compensatory time.[27]

Studies support primary nursing as enhancing patient satisfaction, nurse satisfaction, and cost effectiveness. They also suggest that "individual differences in nurses and nurse competencies may have a greater impact on the quality of care than does the primary nursing structure." It should be noted, however, that when educational backgrounds of nurses were matched, differences in quality of care between team and primary nursing disappeared. The structure for primary nursing is generally a better system for organizing care. Effectiveness of primary nursing differs for types of nurses, patients, hospitals, and even nursing units within a single hospital.[28]

Both primary and team nursing need efficient nursing support systems: communication, distribution, transportation, and unit management. Shukla proposes the contingency theory that primary nursing is more effective when support systems are efficient and patients' dependence on nurses is high. Primary nursing is not better than team nursing for all hospitals, all nursing units within a hospital, or all types of patients.

Decentralized support systems such as those for supplies, linens, and drugs to patients' rooms, are more efficient and improve the benefit of primary nursing over team nursing. When primary nurses have to go to centralized areas for such items they are impeded in providing direct care. Also, modular nursing or modified primary nursing alternatives require performance of more indirect and routine nursing and nonnursing tasks. Patients requiring extensive care benefit more from primary nursing than those capable of self-care. Primary nursing is best for intensive care.[29]

Advantages of primary nursing are the following:

- It provides for increased autonomy on the part of the nurse, thus increasing motivation, responsibility, and accountability.
- It assures more continuity of care as the primary nurse gives or directs care throughout hospitalization.
- It makes available increased knowledge of the patient's psychosocial and physical needs, because the primary nurse does the history and physical assessment, develops the care plan, and acts as liaison between the patient and other health workers.
- It leads to increased rapport and trust between nurse and patient that will allow formation of a therapeutic relationship.
- It improves communication of information to physicians.
- It eliminates nurse aides from the administration of direct patient care.
- It frees the clinical nurse manager to assume the role of operational manager: to deal with staff problems and assignments and to motivate and support the staff.

The main disadvantage of primary nursing is:

- It is said to require the entire staff to be RNs, which increases staffing and costs. However, this has been disputed in cost studies. For example, money is saved when nonnursing duties are performed by other categories of personnel and are not taken over by RNs.[30]

Case Method

The case method of nursing provides for a one-to-one RN-to-client ratio and the provision of constant care for a specified period of time. Examples are private duty, intensive care, and community health nurses. This method is similar to that of primary nursing except that relief nurses on other shifts are not associate RNs.[31]

Joint Practice

Joint practice is more than a modality. It entails nurses and physicians collaborating as colleagues to provide patient care. They work together to define their roles within the joint practice setting, such goals being reciprocal and complementary rather than mutually exclusive. They may use mutually agreed-on protocols to manage care within a primary setting.[32]

The primary nursing modality is preferred for joint practice or collaborative practice. There must be adequate professional nurses freed of nonnursing tasks. Nurse managers facilitate the growth of individual professional nurses. Decision making is decentralized and in-service education and certification are used to upgrade the nurse's scope of practice. Compensation is increased to match increased responsibility and accountability.

Physicians are required to accept responsibility for their part in joint collaborative practice. Administration includes joint practice nurses on every committee within the hospital. It takes as long as a year to establish true functional relationships. Both physicians and nurses have to modify their behaviors.

The elements needed to establish successful joint practice in a hospital setting are:

1. A committee of physicians and nurses with equal representation and equal voice in establishing the objectives and ground rules of operation.
2. An integrated patient record.

3. Primary nursing and case management.
4. Collaborative practice with honest communication and encouragement of clinical decision making by nurses.
5. Joint education of physicians and nurses.
6. Joint nurse-physician evaluation of patient care.
7. Trust.

Results of a joint practice demonstration project at four hospitals concluded that:

- *Patients receive better nursing care and are highly satisfied with their care.*
- *Doctor-nurse communications are better and there is increased mutual respect and trust between nurses and physicians.*
- *Both doctors' and nurses' job satisfaction is increased.*[33]

Case Management

Case management is also more than a modality of nursing. It has been described as

a system of patient care delivery that focuses on the achievement of outcomes within effective and appropriate time frames and resources. Case management focuses on an entire episode of illness, crossing all settings in which the patient receives care. Care is directed by a case manager who ideally is involved in a group practice. Case management incorporates the principles of managed care.[34]

Case management involves collaborative practice that in turn involves groups of professional nurses who collaborate to move the patient through the system. It is episode based rather than unit based. Nurses of various units collaborate to move the patient on a critical path through the hospital stay.[35]

Group practice is

a formal structure for case-based nursing care delivery and management throughout an episode of illness. Membership includes pre-identified primary nurses from serial units (and agencies) who work in partnership with (1) the key physicians for that case type and (2) the patients and their families to facilitate care that meets specific clinical standards within appropriate resource obligation.[36]

Collaborative practice is group practice that includes physicians. At the New England Medical Center group practice is mainly composed of nurses. Joint practice like collaborative practice, implies a joint effort by MDs and RNs. The aims of these practice modalities appear to be similar.

Managed Care

Managed care in its broadest sense goes beyond the health maintenance organization and preferred provider organization or hospital plans. In this book, managed care is case management by nurses as developed by Zander and others and adopted as a system by many hospital nursing organizations.

Managed care is

unit-based care that is organized to achieve specific patient outcomes within fiscally responsible time frames (length of stay) utilizing resources that are appropriate in amounts and sequence to the specific case type and to the individual patient. Care is structured by case management plans and critical paths which are based on knowledge by case type regarding usual length of stay, critical events and their timing, anticipated outcomes, and resource allocation.[37]

Managed care can use any modality of nursing including team nursing, primary nursing, functional nursing, or case management. Tools for managed care include CareMaps™. See Figure 7–3.

At the New England Medical Center critical paths have been developed for over 150 diagnosis-related groups (DRGs) and case management plans for approximately 50 DRGs as of early 1988.

In addition to being cost effective, managed care meets established quality control indicators. It is outcome based and identifies the business of nursing. A professional nurse who practices managed care may be doing primary care nursing, a solo act of case management, or collaborative practice with nurses in other units such as the operating suite or emergency department—or all at the same time.

Managed care develops management skills that include variance identification and analysis, negotiation, consulting, clinical assessment, time management, problem solving, and priority setting. Management development of staff nurses is a factor in managed care.[38]

ETHICAL CONCERNS

Many ethical issues are directly related to the provision of patient care services. These have become more important during the past decade because of the increased sophistication of medical science and technology, concern about practical limits on financial resources for health care, changes in society, and growing emphasis on the autonomy of the individual.[39]

Nurse managers implement the employer's policy concerning the moral responsibility for health care. Nurse managers have responsibility for supervision and review of patient care, meeting quality standards, making certain that decisions about patients are based on sound ethical principles, developing policies and mechanisms that address questions of human values, and responding to social problems and dilemmas that affect the need for health care services.[40]

To fulfill this responsibility the nurse manager supports nurses confronted with ethical dilemmas and helps them think through situations by open dialogue. Nurse managers establish the climate for this. Davis recommends ethics rounds as a means of discussing ethical dilemmas. Such discussions can focus on hypothetical cases, case histories, or a current patient. Ethical reasoning requires participation by a knowledgeable person.

There are many ethical issues that relate to nursing and health care. One of these is the issue of the right to health care. We do not have a law that says society is obliged to provide health care. Other ethical issues are:

1. The rights of individuals and their surrogates versus the rights of the state or society. This issue creates confrontations among consumers and practitioners. As an example, cancer cases frequently lose money under reimbursement mechanisms. This may lead to management efforts to cut costs by cutting services (staff) or closing treatment centers. A survey of the Association of Community Cancer Centers indicated that 84 percent staff oncology units higher than other medical/surgical units.[41]
2. The rights of patients unable to make their own decisions versus the rights of their family versus the rights of institutions.
3. The rights of patients to forego treatment versus the rights of society.
4. Issues related to:
    4.1   Reproductive technology, preselection of desired physical characteristics of children, genetic screening.
    4.2   Organ harvesting and transplants.
    4.3   Research subjects.
    4.4   Confidentiality.

CareMaps™: The Core of Cost/Quality Care

CareMaps(tm) are the newest break-through in cost/quality outcomes management. They have evolved from their longer version, Case Management Plans, and their condensed version, Critical Paths, into "user friendly" documents which:

- **replace nursing care plans** as patient care plans[1]
- describe the contributions of every department
- show standards of care and standards of practice, and the timed, sequenced relationship between the two for a given case type, DRG, ICD9, or **constellation of problems**
- individualize care through analyzing and acting upon variances
- provide a data base for **Continuous Quality Improvement** (CQI)
- integrate with **acuity** systems, **costing** systems, and **research.**

CareMaps(tm) are cause and effect grids, i.e., staff actions should result in patient/family reactions or responses, which over time are "transformed" into desired outcomes. Staff actions are equivalent to Standards of Practice; Patient reactions are equivalent to Standards of Care. CareMaps(tm) are built on a basic formula:

$$\text{Patient/family Problems} \longrightarrow \text{Outcomes}$$
$$\uparrow$$
$$\text{Staff Actions}$$

This basic formula describes very complex practice patterns, which themselves have many sources. **To build a CareMap(tm) requires deep respect for the knowledge, concern and tradition that the clinicians of each discipline use in the care of their patients.** They reflect good practice, and can never replace good judgement.

Format

CareMaps(tm), like their Critical Path predecessors, are simplistic charts which graph phenomena associated with a homogeneous patient population on two axes:

action vs. time. Critical Paths graph multidisciplinary staffs' actions in terms of interventions against the timeline most appropriate for the phase of treatment of a specific population. CareMaps(tm) go an additional step by including patient/family actions in terms of responses to staffs' interventions.

		Time →
Patient/Family Actions	problems	
Multidisciplinary Staff Actions	categories	

(Classic Critical Path)

Patient/Family actions are categorized by problem statements which transform into intermediate goals and, by the last time frame, outcomes. Patient/Family actions are measurable and behavioral, and may include responses in the realms of physiological, selfcare, activities of daily living, followup plans, psychological, and absence of complications often related to their medical diagnoses. In 1987, Stetler and DeZell suggested four generic categories that should always be considered for inclusion in problem outcome statements[2]:

1. Potential for Complications Selfcare: Presence of risk factors that may limit a patient's ability to manage his or her own disease and/or engage in health promoting activities in the home environment.

2. Potential for Injury Unrelated to Treatment: Presence of risk factors related primarily to the person's general state of health, and/or to the specific disease symptom that could lead to physical injury within the institutional setting.

3. Potential for Complications Related to Treatment: Presence of risk factors, at times inherent in the in-hospital treatment, that endanger the health and safety of the patient if (a) appropriate preventive measures are not instituted and maintained and/or (b) on-going observations and

monitoring are not instituted.

4. Potential for Extension of the Disease Process: Presence of a specific condition or pathological process that carries with it a risk that endangers the recovery of the patient; i.e., presence of a risk that will be increased if a treatable extension or sequela are undetected.

Multidisciplinary staff actions can be categorized in a variety of ways. Over the last five years, eight classic categories have emerged:

1) Consults/Assessments
2) Treatments
3) Nutrition
4) Meds (IV, other)
5) Activity/Safety
6) Teaching (Patient, Significant Other)
7) Discharge Planning/Coordination

Additional Categories such as "Chest-tube Management" or "Psychosocial" may be desired depending on the case-type. Some institutions have incorporated their intermediate patient/family goals and outcomes into the traditional (staff action) Critical Path. Others have written the staff's actions into the patient/family outcomes section. Yet others have integrated actions and outcomes into their current data flow sheets. **Anytime both the staff's and patient/families' behaviors are graphed against a timeline, the concept of a CareMap(tm)-by whatever name-is being used.** A sample CareMap(tm) and variance record from Brighton Medical Center in Portland, Maine is included with their permission in this issue.

A CareMap(tm) System

A CareMap(tm) System includes the use of CareMaps(tm) twenty-four hours a day. The heart of the system is the written CareMap(tm) and the variances that arise from the standard interventions

SOURCE: Sally Barney and Barbara Toland. Reprinted with permission of K. Zander, K. Bower, and M. Etheridge, The Center for Nursing Care Management, New England Medical Center, Boston, MA.

Figure 7–3 • *CareMap*™

(Continued)

Brighton Medical Center   Case CareMap™
Profile: Uncomplicated MI

Case Manager:_____

(Addressograph)

Patient Problem/ Nursing Diagnosis	DAY 1	DAY 2	DAY 3	DAY 4	DAY 5	DAY 6
Pain R/T ischemia	Pt. will verbalize pain or discomfort appropriately to RN	Pt. will be pain free	— — —	— — — —	— — — —	Pt. will be pain free at discharge
Activity intolerance R/T ischemia	Pt. will be able to tolerate BSC without chest pain / Pt. can participate in "ADL protocol" without chest pain — — —	Pt. can participate in "PT protocol" without chest pain	— — —	— — — —	— — — —	Pt. will be discharged at anticipated activity tolerance as evidenced by B/P does not change by 20 torr and HR does not change by≥ 20 BPM
Knowledge deficit R/T new MI	Pt. can state why admitted to hospital / Pt. will understand the importance of notifying RN of chest pain	Pt. will demonstrate a readiness to learn / Pt. will begin to read MI packet	— — — / Pt. will be able to state what an MI and angina are and risk factors & use of sublingual nitrates	Pt. demonstrates understanding of diet by making appropriate choices on menu / Pt. can verblize discharge needs	Pt. can verbalize community resources / Pt. can take own pulse	Pt. can verbalize activity restrictions and rationale. Pt. can restate discharge instructions. Pt. will have completed all MI teaching packet goals.
Anxiety R/T hospitalization	Pt. can verbalize fears and concerns related to hospitalization	— — —	Pt. displays appropriate coping skills	— — —	— — — —	Pt. can identify appropriate resources and support systems
Potential for injury R/T bleeding (TPA)	Pt. will verbalize understanding of reasons to notify RN of signs of bleeding	— — —	— — — —		— — —	Pt. can state rationale for risk factors of anticoagulant therapy
Potential for alt. in cardiac output R/T myocardial damage 2° MI	B/P, HR, U/O, clear lung sounds and norm. range other hemodynamic parameter with or without intervention will be maintained	— — —	Maint. B/P — — — without IV vasoactive Rx		— — — —	— — — —

Critical Path

	DAY 1	DAY 2	DAY 3	DAY 4	DAY 5	DAY 6
Consults	Notify ER attending & family physician, Social Services, Quality Review, Case Manager	PT Dietary consultation	Social Services ± home care referral	± Pharmacy consult (coumadin teaching)		
Tests	MCPs q 8° X 3 EKG, routine lab work/coag. CXR, O₂ sat	EKG ±MCP ± 2 D echo ± routine labs ± O₂ sat	± EKG ± schedule Holter monitor	± Holter monitor	± coag. ± routine labs ± schedule stress test	± stress test
Treatments	I & O, weight, IV access, cardiac monitoring, B/P, V/S monitoring	± weight — — — — Same as Day 1	— — — — D/C cardiac monitoring & transfer	IV access — — — Same as Day 3	IV access	D/C IV
Meds	± O₂ ± tPa Ntg ± Reg meds ± Lidocaine ± MS ± Sleeper Heparin ± Tylenol ± Beta Blockers ± Ca channel blockers Anti anxiety agent Stool Softner	Same ± wean Lido ± wean Ntg ± O₂	Same wean Lido wean Ntg	Same Assess anticoag therapy (D/C heparin & consider ASA)		Discharge prescription with completed discharge form
Diet	Cardiac Diet	— — —	— — —	— — — —	— — — —	— — — —
Activity	Bedrest with BSC ADL protocol	PT protocol — — — — — —	— — — — — —	— — — — — —	— — — — — —	— — — — — —
Teaching	Orientation to unit & routine Dietary reading material	MI packet progressive dietary teaching	— — —	Evaluate process & target problem areas, ±coumadin teaching info bracelet	— — —	Discharge instruction review
Discharge Planning		Share CareMap if appropriate	Update to Social Service from QR transfer to general floor	As per Social Service	Consider outpatient needs	Discharge

Figure 7–3   (Continued)

Brighton Medical Center
VARIATIONS TO THE CAREMAP[tm]

Please Initial Variation Entries

	DAY 1	DAY 2	DAY 3	DAY 4	DAY 5	DAY 6
Date						
Variation						
Related To (Code)						
Action						

CODE - VARIANCE SOURCE

1 - Event not applicable
2 - Unpredicted event

A. Patient/Family	B. Care Giver/Clinician	C. Hospital	D. Community
3 - Patient Condition	7 - Physician order	11 - Bed/appt. time availability	16 - Placement/Home
4 - Pt/family decision	8 - Caregiver(s) decision	12 - Information/data availability	care availability
5 - Pt/family availability	9 - Caregiver(s) response time	13 - Supplies/equip. availability	17 - Ambulance delay
6 - Pt/family other	10 - Caregiver other	14 - Dept. overbooked/closed	18 - Community other
		15 - Hospital other	

Key to MI CareMap (tm) on page 2:
R/T = Related to   HR = Hear Rate   UO = Urine Output   PT = Physical Therapy   BPM = Beats per minute
CXR = Chest X-ray   BP = Blood Pressure   2° = Secondary to   MCP = Myocardial Profile   ADL Protocol - Activities of Daily Living
D/C = Discontinue   QR = Quality Review   SL = Sublingual   BSC = Bed side Commode   ≥ = Greater than or equal to

Authors of the Uncomplicated MI CareMap(tm): Linda Madore, RN, RNC, Gail Crocker, BSN, RN, Pat Moore, BSN, RN, Kim Norbert, MS, RD, Debbie Jo Harvery, RPT, Theresa Boulos, BSN, RN, CCRN, Carol Marshall, RN, ONC, Marilyn Young, RN, Howard Glass, DO, Stuart Herrick, MD.

Continued from page 1

and outcomes. In a CareMap(tm) System, variances are not bad, they are real and reflect the way staff are responding to individual patient needs. Variances can be categorized per patient using standard codes, and when aggregated retrospectively for groups of similar patient populations, form a data base for Continuous Quality Improvement.

The ultimate result of a CareMap(tm) system is that unnecessary variance is reduced to a minimum because of an increasingly accurate learning curve that helps clinicians predict, prevent, and manage. It is not unusual for collaborative groups to begin developing CareMaps(tm) for the more straight-forward diagnoses, proceed to several varieties of that map, then combine constellations of problems, and finally map care for the patient populations that were initially felt to be totally unpredictable.

Currently, CareMaps(tm) are used either on paper as references only, on paper as permanent documentation, on personal computers, or on mainframes. As institutions and clinicians become increasingly comfortable with CareMap(tm) development, and as computer systems convert to CareMap(tm) systems, higher percentages

of patients will be managed by them (with daily or per visit screens). Similarly, variances are presently being handled differently depending on each agency's goals for implementing the system in the first place. Minimally, patient/family and community variances are recorded in the medical record. A few institutions have decided to also include clinician and hospital-generated variances in the chart as well.

Summary

A complete CareMap(tm) System includes variance analysis, use of CareMaps(tm) in change-of-shift report, case consultation and health care team meetings for patients at more-than-acceptable variance, and continuous quality improvement. The challenge, of course, is creating a dynamic system of complex care management from a static piece of paper. This can be accomplished with a series of CareMaps(tm) for different phases of treatment (i.e., Acute Myelogenous Leukemia: AML - induction, AML - consolidation, AML - fever and neutropenia, etc.) and the use of blank CareMaps(tm) for anecdotal documentation or for those patients who require a totally

individualized map. Any individualized outcomes and interventions written on a CareMap(tm) are generally outside the variance field. When a patient's reason for remaining in the hospital changes in a major way (such as a patient having a craniotomy who remains on a vent), the CareMap(tm) changes as well.

All professional disciplines should be involved in the formation of CareMaps(tm) and education as to their use. Secretaries, computer and medical records department members, and the "forms" department are all integral to the implementation of a CareMap(tm) System. Our future issues will address physician involvement in CareMap(tm) Systems and Case Management, as well as other key development and maintenance factors.

References:
1. Brider, P. "Who Killed the Nursing Care Plan?" *American Journal of Nursing*. May, 1991. pp. 35 -39.
2. Stetler, C. and DeZell, A. *Case Management Plans: Designs for Transformation*. Boston: New England Medical Center Hospitals. 1987. pp. 26-32.

Figure 7–3   (Continued)

4.5 Restraints.
4.6 Continuity of care.
4.7 Disclosure.
4.8 Informed consent.
4.9 Patient incapacity.
4.10 Court intervention.

The American Nurses' Association Committee on Ethics has published several position statements and guidelines that seek to assist nurses in making ethical decisions in their practice. These guidelines are based on ethical theory and the ANA Code for Nurses, which is an expression of "nursing's moral concerns, goals, and values." They are designed to provide nurses with guidance on a range of ethical issues, including the withdrawing or withholding of food and fluid; risk versus responsibility in providing care; safeguarding client health and safety from illegal, incompetent, or unethical practices; nurses' participation in capital punishment, and nurses' participation and leadership in ethical review practices.[42]

Current dilemmas in nursing are partly due to limitations in nursing management knowledge. Changes are needed that address values and goals. There could be a hierarchy of values in managing practice. Nurse managers need to determine how much decision-making power clinical nurses want and how much they can delegate. A theory of ethics should be meshed with a theory of nursing management. Nurse managers need a theory of ethical conduct that is congruent with one for clinical nurses.

Both clinical nurses and managers use scientific knowledge to determine whether conditions support change. The intrinsic value of the management actions should be given careful thought and should be debated by nurse managers who consciously attempt to practice management that realizes the highest good. The manager is more apt to be successful if scientific management knowledge is applied.

Ethics in management was the topic in an interview with Kenneth Blanchard. His comments are applicable to nurse managers; translated into nursing theory, they can be summed up as follows:

1. Nurse managers can influence the ethical behavior of nursing personnel by treating them ethically.
2. Nurse managers have a code of ethics that peers have agreed on. They enter into ethical dilemmas when they go against that code.
3. Nurse managers fall into moral dilemmas when they go against their internal values.

4. Although ethical and moral dilemmas differ, an ethical nurse manager is a moral nurse manager.
5. Ethical functions can be confronted by three questions:
   5.1 "Is it legal?" Resolves some dilemmas but not nonsensical laws and policies.
   5.2 "Is it balanced?" Nurse managers should aim for a win-win solution.
   5.3 "How will it make me feel about myself?" Nurse managers should consider the impact of each action on their self-respect.
6. Nurse managers with high self-esteem usually have the internal strength to make the ethical decision.
7. An ethical leader is an effective leader.
8. Nurse managers should apply six principles of ethical power:
   8.1 The chief nurse executive promotes and ensures pursuit of the stated mission or purpose of the nursing division, since this statement reflects the vision of its practicing nurses. The mission should be reviewed periodically, but goals or objectives are set for yearly achievement.
   8.2 Nurse managers should build an organization to win, thereby building self-esteem of employees through pride in their organization.
   8.3 Nurse managers should work to sustain patience and continuity through a long-term effect on the organization.
   8.4 Nurse managers should plan for persistence by spending more time following up on education and activities that build commitment of personnel.
   8.5 Nurse managers should promote perspective by giving their staff time to think. They should practice good management for the long term.
   8.6 Nursing service managers should consider developing an organization-specific code of ethics expressed in observable and measurable behaviors.[43]

Ethics should be ingrained in employees to create a strong sense of professionalism. A code of ethics can be developed to do this. Such a code should be the basis of a planned approach to all management functions of planning, organizing, directing, and controlling.

Nursing employees can help develop the code of ethics, can help implement it, and can help determine the rewards and punishment associated with it. A code of ethics should be read and signed by employees. It should be reviewed and revised on a regular schedule.

Contents of a code of ethics include definition of ethical and unethical practices, expected ethical behavior, enforcement of ethical practices, and rewards and punishments. To be objective a code of ethics specifies rules of conduct. It should be applied to all persons to be effective.[44]

Two centers exist to help organizations, including nursing, to establish standards for ethics programs:

Ethics Resource Center. Located in Washington, DC, the Ethics Resource Center is involved with "research on ethics and advising associations, businesses, educational institutions, and government agencies in the development of ethics programs."

Center for the Study of Ethics in the Professions. Located at the Illinois Institute of Technology in Chicago, this organization has concentrated on engineering and science, including nursing.[45]

DISCHARGE PLANNING

by Julie Konkol, BSN, MS, RN

Case Manager
Case Management/Social Services
St. Mary's Hospital and Medical Center
San Francisco, CA 94117

More patients with complex needs are being discharged from acute care settings and as a result discharge planning and coordination of care are becoming more important. Early identification of patients requiring discharge planning may shorten the length of stays, affect hospital expenditures, decrease readmission rates, and provide timely discharge planning intervention. Health industry leaders maintain that Medicare's prospective payment requirements will cause discharge planning to become more important to overall hospital functioning. Hospital administrators view discharge planning as a multidisciplinary link among nurses, physicians, hospital administrators, and those who provide social services, that can effectively shorten the length of stays.[46]

Because of close monitoring of bed use, early referral is crucial to the discharge planning process. The Joint Commission for Accreditation of Healthcare Organizations (JCAHO) states that "to facilitate discharge as soon as an acute level of care is no longer required, discharge planning is initiated as early as a determination of the need for such activity is made."[47] Late referrals for discharge planning may cause patients to assume financial responsibility of nonacute hospital-bed usage commonly not included in insurance or Medicare health benefits.

Inadequate case finding may also increase the frequency of readmissions. Patients who require home health care, health counseling, or teaching and community services but are not assisted in the procurement of the service before discharge often return to the emergency room with minor problems, are frequently readmitted for 24 to 48 hours, and then discharged again.[48] Despite the lack of precise measurements, experience has proven that discharge planning has great cost effectiveness.

Discharge planning is a multidisciplinary concern or interaction. It is the process by which health care professionals, patients, and their families collaborate to provide and arrange for the continuity of care the patient requires. Planning should center on patient concerns, that is, preventive, therapeutic, rehabilitative, and custodial care. It should also include nonmedical needs. Discharge planning is a systematic coordinated program designed to effect a patient's timely discharge to the next appropriate level of care or to his or her normal living situation. The secret is organized planning. It is an ongoing process that needs continual refinement and monitoring to ensure that the most suitable plans are developed to meet the patient's needs. Part of the plan of care for the patient includes the following:

1. Assessing and identifying current and anticipated physiological and psychological needs.
2. Planning appropriate continuing care to meet those needs.
3. Preparing and referring the patient for admission to another organized health care setting or for self-care.

Discharge planning is the mechanism for providing continuous care, information about continuing health requirements after discharge, appointments for follow-up, and self-care instructions. Continuity of care is a series of organized, connected patient-care events or activities that occur, even though the patient's need or desire for care varies and even when health care is given by numerous providers. Ideally, health care systems identify and set up linkages among providers so that each contributes to the general health care plan for the individual. Also, a means of two-way communication, referral, and follow-up must be provided in the continuum of care.

Discharge planning includes a team of people in which the patient and family are central members. Depending on the setting, the team may include the following individuals: nurse, physical therapist, speech therapist, occupational therapist, social worker, dietitian, physician, utilization management nurse, chaplain, discharge planner, pharmacist, and respiratory therapist. It may also include a public health or home health nurse, vocational counselor, government social service worker, volunteer agency support worker, and a meal transportation representative. Since there is no recipe for effectiveness, the more inclusive the input involved in planning, the better the patient is served after discharge.

A case manager can obtain much input through consultation and coordination.

Discharge planning can begin with a prehospital

screening in a clinic setting, admit unit, or by home survey. It should occur from the moment of admission and carry over into discharge with a follow-up survey.

Discharge planning occurs anywhere on a continuum from home to hospital. Some settings could be the home, where the planning can be minimal, intermediate, or intensive, a physician's office or clinic, a social services outpatient clinic, inpatient unit, acute care hospital, intermediate care nursing facility, skilled care nursing facility, or rehabilitation hospital.

Why Do Discharge Planning?

1. Discharge planning is required by regulatory and accrediting bodies such as the Joint Commission on Accreditation of Healthcare Organizations.
2. It is required by state nurse practice acts, and American Nurses' Association Standards for Nursing Practice.
3. It is required by state and national social work guidelines.
4. Anticipatory planning and documentation decrease the number of concurrent and retroactive denials from insurance carriers, Medicare, and Medicaid.
5. It also decreases the number of relapses, hospital readmissions, and unnecessary emergency room visits except for some diagnoses.
6. It ensures the proper use of health care manpower, the optimal use of resources and services, and cuts down on duplication of services.
7. It helps patients understand the need for aftercare and cost of treatment. If meaningfully involved, patient and family may demonstrate increased compliance with the plans.
8. It ensures community resources are mobilized to meet the needs of patient and family.

The discharge planning process includes implementation of the following steps: assessing and diagnosing the discharge-planning needs, identifying major problems, designing a plan and setting goals for the patient, deciding on and testing the plan, measuring results, evaluating the program and making changes as needed, and documenting action and evaluation of the plan. Tasks included in setting up discharge programs are selecting patient groups that require discharge plans and prioritizing their needs by identifying high-risk criteria, developing support and staff member roles in the process, and ensuring the continuous flow of information and communication among aftercare agencies, physicians, and other team members. Tasks may include multidisciplinary planning meetings, quality assurance/use integration, staff development/in-service regarding continuing care, and development of a written policy and procedures to meet accrediting standards.

The success of a discharge planning program depends on six variables:

1. Degree of illness/health on a continuum.
2. Expected outcome of care.
3. Duration of care needed.
4. Types of service required.
5. Addition of complications (i.e., extension of services).
6. Available resources.

All teamwork depends on communication, cooperation, and documentation.

Nurses' input is crucial to all discharge plans. Part of the nurses' role is to take assessments and diagnoses to Step 2, which is to identify real and potential problems to other disciplines involved. The *ANA Standards of Nursing Practice* focus on practice. "They provide a means for determining the quality of nursing which the client/patient receives regardless of whether such services are provided solely by a professional nurse or by a professional nurse and nonprofessional assistants."[49] It uses assessment, diagnosis, prescription, implementation, and evaluation.

Keep in mind the process is multidisciplinary; it is process oriented and interactive. It includes coordinating services, interagency referrals, resource management, staff development and in-service, documentation, quality assurance, and manpower budget mandates. The idea is to provide an efficient comprehensive process whereby the patient and family have maximal benefit from team effort.

One of the best ways to find cases is to screen all admissions for high-risk discharge criteria at the time of history-taking/initial assessment. What characteristics make a patient more prone to discharge planning problems? What prehospital behaviors interfere with discharge plans? How do nurses, despite the setting, identify high-risk indicators? Risk factors or indicators may point to a need for discharge planning intervention. O'Connor stated that a risk factor merely establishes a probability.[50] Combinations of risk factors increase the danger to the patient and may be given a higher priority.[51] Risk theory specific to a particular group is used by multidisciplinary discharge planners.

High-risk screening is not a new concept. Before World War I, Jane Addams and others used screening and case finding mechanisms in the settlement house movement to identify malnourished or poor subjects and those with tuberculosis, mental illness, or social problems. In many hospitals, traditional screening and case finding are physician referred. Berkman, Clark, and Butler found that traditional screening and case finding based on referrals was cause for delayed intervention.[52] Recently, hospitals have begun to incorporate case finding as a form of tertiary intervention where established risk factors are identified earlier, and prospects for alleviation are improved as risk factors can have an effect on hospital stays. Additionally, 1986 Medicare guidelines require documented plans for appropriate follow-up of care or discharge planning with consideration given to physical, emotional, and mental status needs at the time of discharge. Failure to provide and document such plans may result in sanctions against the institution.[53] Risk factors in disease are found to be multifactoral. Three variables—severity of illness, life threatening; severity of illness, physically dysfunctional; and chronic illness—were good predictors of a need for discharge planning.[54] The idea behind identifying high-risk criteria is to "turn on flags" when certain data are assessed. The combination of *social factors*: lives alone, no social support or family, over age 72; *financial factors*: no income because illness interferes with ability to work, no insurance (medically indigent adult), Medicaid beneficiary, multiple resources but still under poverty level, or needs overextending coverage; and *medical/nursing factors*: new or catastrophic diagnosis, inability to perform self-care/ADLS as a result of accident or illness, major life-style changes because of illness such as AIDS, diabetes mellitus, or cancer, may indicate a need for discharge planning intervention. O'Grady reported that the reasons for case finding within 48 hours of admission arises from a variety of resources that include physicians, physician's office personnel, emergency room staff, social services, nursing services, and business office personnel.[55]

Identifying high-risk factors is not difficult for nurses. Cunningham reported that the use of high-risk criteria, mutually developed with the physician staff, has been supported since their initial use.[56] According to Rossen and Coulton, nurses have prioritized discharge with the potential in this area to contribute to the goal of managing a wide scope of continuity of care. A nurse-utilized tool—a grid system for identifying patient's needs, medical/educational, communication, social, and prescriptive factors—was developed for recognizing high-risk patients needing assistance and referral for discharge screens used by nonprofessionals and professional personnel alike. Some institutions use a computer approach that screens all admissions for predetermined criteria specific to the institution, and includes a mechanism for identifying those previously at risk and readmitted.[57] Medicare has mandated that a screening tool be a part of the medical record. Risk factors mean different things to each member of the multidisciplinary team. The assessment of high risk, the diagnosis, and the intervention and coordination of care require nurses' participation in the patients' discharge planning process.

Many governing and accreditation bodies influence how discharge planning programs are designed. Optimal programs meet criteria outlined by the JCAHO, AHA, Medicare (HCFA), and State Title XX services. Institutions are required to designate professional staff members who are cognizant of the various regulations facilitating discharge planning for patients. Realizing that the role of the discharge planner is dependent on the institution's philosophy, the literature supports nurses in psychosocial/physiological management. Because of the same taxonomy, nurse-to-nurse referral is the ticket for smooth transition. In traditional case-finding approaches, discharge planning intervention meant waiting for physician's orders. Now, hospitals have designed systems in which discharge teaching and planning can be initiated by multidisciplinary team members including nurses as needs are determined. The ANA

Statement of Continuing Care and Discharge Planning calls for three necessary elements to be present. The health care system must provide for and identify linkages among health care workers. Its providers must be identified as participants in the plan of care, and planning, coordination, communication, referrals, and follow-up must exist among disciplines to achieve mutually defined goals. Documentation of the process and outcome is mandated by accreditation criteria.[58]

SUMMARY

Nurse managers work with staff or are clinical practitioners. Educated in nursing management they can assist these practitioners to guide their work according to the model of such theorists as Orem, Kinlein, Roy, Newman, Levine, Johnson, Peplau, Orlando, and others.

Several modalities of nursing have evolved during the past 50 years. In the 1940s, functional nursing was predominant as many professional nurses were in the armed forces during World War II and hospitals were thus staffed with auxiliary personnel.

Later, team nursing became the modality of choice for many hospital nursing services. Under the leadership of a professional nurse, a group of nurses work together to provide patient care. Team nursing rests on theoretical knowledge related to philosophy, planning, leadership, interpersonal relationships, and nursing process.

During the past two decades the modality of total patient care through primary nursing has evolved. With primary nursing the total care of a patient and a case load is the responsibility of one primary nurse.

Joint or collaborative practice by a physician-nurse team has developed as a modality of nursing in a very few hospitals. The latest development is case management, a method of practicing nursing that incorporates any modality but in which the knowledgeable nurse becomes the case manager, making or facilitating all clinical nursing decisions about a caseload of patients during an entire episode of illness.

Nurse managers establish the climate for meeting all requirements for professional nursing. They do so with abilities that provide satisfaction to professional nurses, enhance the productivity of nurses, and make nursing care profitable and of high quality.

Discharge planning is an essential element of

the nursing process. It will usually shorten the patient's hospital stay and will provide for continuity of care following discharge.

EXPERIENTIAL EXERCISES

1. Identify the theory of nursing being practiced in the organization in which you are getting clinical experience. Again, you may work with a group of your peers. Examine theory from the global meaning of being a body of knowledge of the principles and methods of nursing. This body of knowledge is drawn from many sources and theorists. To better prepare this assignment you may want to read some of the articles in the reference section of this chapter.

2. Does the theory of nursing as practiced in your institution have gaps? List them.

3. Use your student group or form an ad hoc committee of nurses to plan for needed implementation of nursing theory in a nursing unit. Make a management plan.

MANAGEMENT PLAN

PROBLEM:

OBJECTIVE:

ACTIONS	TARGET DATES	ASSIGNED TO	ACCOMPLISHMENTS

4. Identify the ethical issues related to the providing of patient care services in the organization in which you are gaining clinical experience. It can be from one of the following areas *or* another of your choosing.

- The right to refuse treatment
  Prolongation of life
  Competent versus incompetent person
  Support of suicide
  Withholding and withdrawing of treatment
  Nutritional support (withholding food and fluid)
  Resuscitation
  Living wills
  Involvement of patients and families in consent decisions
  Respect of patients' personal liberties
- Reproductive rights
  Custody of frozen embryos resulting from in vitro fertilization
  Abortion
  Surrogate parenthood
- Distributive justice
  Is justice blind?
  Is it equally available?
- Science versus justice
  Malpractice
  Provider competence
  Patient abuse
  Animal research
- Decision-making ethics
  Laws and courts
  Allocation of scarce medical resources
  Death definitions: brain death versus heart-lung death
  Euthanasia: passive versus active
  Rationing of health care
  Who shall live?
  Who shall receive what level of health care?
  Harvesting of organs. Life state of donors
  Court intervention in patient care decisions

- Health care policy
  Allocation of health care dollars
  Access to health care
- Conflicts of interest
  Maternal-fetal: fetus versus person
  Maternal-fetal: addiction
  Prenatal care
- Mergers, acquisitions, and contracts among health care providers
- Third-party payer fraud
- Confidentiality of patients' records
- Risk versus responsibility of nurse providers
- Safeguarding client health and safety
  Use of restraints
  Continuity of care
- Ethical review procedures

The environmental variables include people, their personal differences and cultures, society, personal opinions, quality of life, law, medicine and health care, money, religion, science, technology, health care policy, diagnoses and testing (AIDS), organ donations, and genetic engineering including selection of desirable traits and mapping of the human genome or genetic code for which the United States will spend three billion dollars in the 1990s. Thus, scientists will be able to replace defective genes (or others) during in vitro fertilization. For further reading on this topic refer to A. J. Koleszar, "The Great Debate," *CWRU,* Feb. 1990, 16–20; and "Biomedical Ethics and the Bill of Rights," *National Forum,* Fall 1989, the entire issue.

4.1 State the issue:

4.2 What are the opposing sides or arguments of the issue?

   For:

   Against:

4.3 Identify legal precedents:

4.4 Make a management plan to include an objective, actions to be taken, persons to be involved, and a timetable.

MANAGEMENT PLAN

PROBLEM:

OBJECTIVE:

ACTIONS	TARGET DATES	ASSIGNED TO	ACCOMPLISHMENTS

Name: _____

Address: _____

Diagnosis: _____

Last readmission: _____

Case screened for high risk by: _____ Date: _____

Screening:

	Yes	No		Yes	No
Lack of obvious family/social support systems			Admitted to ICU		
Diagnosis			From out of Mobile area		
From nursing home/institution			Medicare		
Previous home health services			Data sheet indicator "R"		
Self-pay			Repeated admission		
Other			Previous home care equipment		

Date/Time   Signature

| Social worker/family/discharge planner indicates intervention not necessary at this time. |
| Discharge needs cannot adequately be evaluated at this time, will reassess. |
| Intervention is indicated at this time. |
| Discharge planning in progress. |

Figure 7–4 • Discharge Planning Worksheet

Refer to Figure 7-4 to assist in obtaining answers to questions 5 and 6.

5. Discharge screens and computer grids are examples of systems nurses use for discharge planning. Visit the discharge planning section of the organization in which you are assigned as a student. Compare the information on the discharge screens and computer grids. Figure 7-4 contains information similar to that on these screens and grids. Who uses this information?

6. Discharge screens are best designed by comparing the individual institutional data to the literature and examining readmission and discharge DRGs (diagnosis) and regional data. List the top five indicators found in the setting you visited.

Refer to Figure 7-5 to answer questions 7 through 11.

7. Discuss and prioritize the teaching/learning needs for home management of Mr. O.

8. Describe the nurse involvement and written teaching plans you would provide the Mr. O. caretakers.

9. Describe precautions related to enteral feeds and trach care at home you would teach and expect demonstrated by Mrs. O. before discharge.

10. What would you recommend to keep the peace between care givers in this difficult family situation, and to whom could you refer the family for follow-up and support?

11. Describe the methods the institution in which you work as student requires to document the four nursing process elements of assessment, diagno-

Mr. O. was a twenty-year-old married black male from Florida who sustained a closed head injury from a motor vehicle accident on June 6, 1987. Upon admission he was in a comatose condition, with decerebrate posturing, without response to pain, had positive Doll's sign, and had pinpoint pupils. He underwent the following procedures: a ventricular pressure monitor placement, a lumbar puncture, and a tracheostomy. One week before discharge he was responding by tracking with eyes, had some voluntary squeezing of hands on commands, and had some movement in his lower extremities bilaterally.

Nutrition: An enteral feeding tube was placed and gastric residuals were checked every 2 hours and held 1 hour if over 150 cc. A week before discharge, he had successfully swallowed pureed food but because of insufficient caloric intake, the dietitian and physician preferred to plan for enteral feedings after discharge. He was discharged on Ensure Plus at 75 cc/hr continuously per enteral pump.

Skin: He developed some sacro-coccygeal reddened areas that were being dressed with normal saline wet to dry T.I.D. In addition, a Clinitron bed was used and he wore "Bunny Boots" bilaterally. While hospitalized, he wore pneumatic thromboembolic stockings and had Granulex to heels T.I.D. The head of his bed was elevated 30 degrees continuously with the use of wedges and pillows. He was discharged with TED hose (off twice a day for 1 hour), and an Air Mattress.

Respiratory: He had a tracheostomy size 6 Shiley with disposable inner cannula and required trach care T.I.D. while hospitalized. The inner cannula and trach ties were changed daily and site care to the trach stoma was done T.I.D. He was frequently suctioned using both a Yankeur tonsil suction for oral and pharyngeal secretions and a #14 French suction catheter. He also required oxygen per trach collar while hospitalized. Two days before discharge, he was successfully extubated but still required oral pharyngeal suctioning with a Yankeur suction and a #14 Fr. suction catheter.

Elimination: Elimination was a problem for him as he developed erythematous areas around his penis related to use of a condom catheter to depend on drainage. Floor nurses propped the urinal and began a bowel program before discharge.

Medications: Only two were used at time of discharge: Reglan 10 mg T.I.D. per duo tube and Zantac 150 mg B.I.D. per duo tube.

Social: Mr. O. was a recently married male who had worked construction before this accident. He and his wife, an unemployed 19-year-old, lived at her mother's house and neither had health insurance. Mrs. O. verbalized a desire to take him to her mother's home at time of discharge. During his 35-day hospital stay, however, she was seldom at his bedside, electing to remain at home as she was advised by her OB/GYN physician in Florida. She was 5 months pregnant. Her mother-in-law was in constant attendance at the bedside and elected to stay overnight during his last week of stay to learn everything she could about his nursing needs. The floor nurses had instructed the M-I-L about skin care, dressing changes, enteral feedings residual checking, filling feeding bags, auscultating for tube placement, medication administration, and elimination needs. She verbalized a desire to take her son to her home as she "felt better prepared."

Floor primary nurse concurred that M-I-L was indeed better prepared. Discharge planning nurse was consulted on the case 7 days before discharge at the social worker's request. At this point, a family conference was requested to determine Mr. O.'s discharge destination and describe his care needs. The conference was attended by a medical student of the neurosurgery team, the primary RN from the floor, the social worker, the discharge planning nurse, the wife, the wife's mother, the M-I-L, and the M-I-L's sister. After describing the total situation, no decision was made regarding destination. The social worker recommended that the Florida county Department of Human Resources investigate both homes and home situations for suitability for home care. Wife and M-I-L were distressed and told the social worker about their individual concerns. As the wife is legally next of kin, according to the risk manager, she had the right to decide destination unless the environment was not suitable.

Before discharge, the following list of supplies needed for home care was provided after consulting with the discharge planning team who were present at the meeting. It was decided that the following were suitable for home care:

Air mattress	TED hose
Enteral pump	Disposable respiratory,
Suction machine	enteral feeding
Hospital bed	products, syringes,
Bag with T connection	and Ambu dressing
Stethoscope	supplies

Figure 7–5 • *Discharge Planning: A Multidisciplinary Approach*

(Continued)

His lack of financial support will not prevent his obtaining home care. Because he would qualify for SSI/Medicaid in the future, arrangements were made to procure the necessary supplies and equipment with an initial family deposit paid by the family. Their home town county hospital responded to his heavy care needs by agreeing to take the home care case through their home health agency. The ambulance, also a part of the hospital, agreed to work out a financial agreement with Mrs. O. (wife) for transportation home (some 200 miles away).

A Florida physician who agreed to take his case was called by our physicians and given the complete history. An important point to remember is that once a patient crossed state lines, the discharging doctor's team orders and prescriptions cannot be legally filled unless he/she is licensed in that state. Therefore finding a physician to cover Mr. O.'s case was imperative before discharge.

Finally, the DHR reported to the social worker. The wife's mother's home situation was adequate for Mr. O.'s return home. The M-I-L agreed to visit and assist in every way the wife would allow.

Two days before actual discharge, the discharge planning nurse recommended to the discharge team that Mrs. O. remain overnight and assume total care of her husband, returning a demonstration of every aspect to the nurses. She also advised that the M-I-L return home. The team agreed and the wife stayed. A day before discharge, the equipment was delivered to the house in Florida. The home health orders were called, and the ambulance coordinated for pickup. Wife was allowed to ride home in the ambulance.

Figure 7-5   (Continued)

sis, plan, and evaluation as they relate to discharge planning.

NOTES

1. H. A. Bush, "Models for Nursing," *Advances in Nursing Science,* Jan. 1979, 13–21.
2. G. L. Dickson and H. Lee-Villasenor, "Nursing Theory and Practice: A Self-Care Approach," *Advances in Nursing Science,* Oct. 1982, 29–40.
3. Sr. C. Roy, "Adaptation: A Basis for Nursing Practice," *Nursing Outlook,* Apr. 1971, 254–257.
4. Ibid.
5. M. F. Mastal and H. Hammond, "Analysis and Expansion of the Roy Adaptation Model: A Contribution to Holistic Nursing," *Advances in Nursing Science,* July 1980, 71–81.
6. Ibid.
7. V. F. Engle, "Newman's Conceptual Framework and the Measurement of Older Adults' Health," *Advances in Nursing Science,* Oct. 1984, 24–36.
8. Ibid.
9. Ibid.
10. M. E. Levine, "Adaptation and Assessment: A Rationale for Nursing Intervention," *American Journal of Nursing,* Nov. 1966, 2450–2453.
11. Ibid.
12. A. C. Rawls, "Evaluation of the Johnson Behavioral System Model in Clinical Practice," *Image,* Feb. 1980, 12–16.
13. L. Thompson, "Peplau's Theory: An Application to Short-Term Individual Therapy," *Journal of Psychosocial Nursing,* Aug. 1986, 26–31.
14. N. J. Schmieding, "Putting Orlando's Theory into Practice," *American Journal of Nursing,* June 1984, 759–761; I. J. Orlando, *The Discipline and Teaching of Nursing Process: An Evaluative Study* (New York: G. P. Putnam's Sons, 1972); I. J. Orlando, *Nurse-Patient Relationship: Function, Process, Principles* (New York: G. P. Putnam's Sons, 1961).
15. S. Fredette, "The Art of Applying Theory to Practice," *American Journal of Nursing,* May 1974, 856–859; K. Goldstein, *Human Nature Is the Light of Psychopathology* (New York: Schocken, 1963), 201.
16. "Accountability in Nursing Practice," *Nursing Management,* Nov. 1984, 72.
17. S. R. Hinckley, Jr., "A Closer Look at Participation," *Organizational Dynamics,* Winter 1985, 57–67.
18. B. Henry, C. Arndt, M. DiVincenti, and A. Marriner-Tomey, eds., *Dimensions of Nursing Administration: Theory, Research, Education, Practice* (Boston: Blackwell, 1989).
19. R. C. Swansburg and P. W. Swansburg, *Strategic Career Planning and Development for Nurses* (Rockville, MD: Aspen, 1984), 26–27.
20. Ibid., 27; D. P. Newcomb and R. C. Swansburg, *The Team Plan* (New York: G. P. Putnam's Sons, 1953, 1971); R. C. Swansburg, *Team Nursing: A Programmed Learning Experience,* 4 vols. (New York: G. P. Putnam's Sons, 1968).
21. Newcomb and Swansburg, op. cit., 56.
22. Swansburg and Swansburg, op. cit., 27.
23. Ibid.
24. G. D. Marram, M. W. Schlegel, and E. O. Bevis, *Primary Nursing: A Model for Individualized Care* (St. Louis: Mosby, 1974), 1.
25. Ibid., 16–17.
26. S. Malkin and P. Lauteri, "A Community Hospital's Approach—Decentralized Patient Education," *Nursing Administration Quarterly,* Winter 1980, 101–106.
27. C. M. Fagin, "The Economic Value of Nursing Research," *American Journal of Nursing,* Dec. 1982, 1844–1849.
28. R. K. Shukla, "Primary or Team Nursing? Two Conditions Determine the Choice," *Journal of Nursing Administration,* Nov. 1982, 12–15.
29. Ibid.
30. Swansburg and Swansburg, op. cit., 27–28.
31. Ibid., 28.
32. National Joint Practice Commission, *Guidelines for Establishing Joint or Collaborative Practice in Hospitals* (Chicago, IL: Neely Printing, 1981).

33. Ibid.

34. E. Comeau, K. Zander, K. Bower, M. L. Etheredge, and J. G. Somerville, "Glossary," New England Medical Center Hospital, Department of Nursing, 1987.

35. K. A. Bower and J. G. Somerville, "Managed Care and Case Management Outcome-Based Practice: Creating the Environment," Program at Sheraton Grand Hotel, Tampa, FL, Feb. 15–16, 1988.

36. Comeau et al., op. cit.

37. Ibid.

38. Ibid.

39. "Report of the Special Committee on Biomedical Ethics," *Values in Conflict: Resolving Ethical Issues in Hospital Care* (Chicago: American Hospital Association, 1985).

40. Ibid.

41. L. E. Mortenson, "Are Oncology Nurses Too Expensive?," *Oncology Nursing Forum*, Jan./Feb. 1984, 14–15.

42. Committee on Ethics, American Nurses' Association, *Ethics in Nursing: Position Statements and Guidelines* (Kansas City, MO: American Nurses' Association, 1988).

43. K. C. Fernicola, "Take the Highroad . . . to Ethical Management: An Interview with Kenneth Blanchard," *Association Management*, May 1988, 60–66.

44. M. Mizock, "Ethics—the Guiding Light of Professionalism," *Data Management*, Aug. 1986, 16–18, 29.

45. "Ethics Programs: More Than Lofty Phrases," *Association Management*, May 1988, 66–67.

46. S. Rossen and C. Coulton, "Research Agenda for Discharge Planning," *Social Work in Health Care*, 1985, 10, (4), 55–61.

47. Joint Commission on Accreditation of Healthcare Organizations, Accreditation Manual for Hospitals 1990 (Chicago: JCAHO, 1989), 274.

48. I. Cunningham, "Early Assessment for Discharge Planning," *Quarterly Review Bulletin*, 1981, 7, (10), 11–16.

49. *Standards of Nursing Practice* (Kansas City, MO: American Nurses' Association, 1973).

50. G. O'Connor, "Risk Identification and Management in Clinical Practice," *Physician Assistant*, 1985, 9, (1), 63–88.

51. E. Backett, A. Davies, and A. Petros Bargovian, *The Risk Approach in Health Care* (Public Health Papers, no. 76, WHO, 1984).

52. B. Berkman, E. Clark, and N. Butler, "Regional Profile Data as Basis for Social Work Audit," *Health and Social Work*, 1980, 5, (10), 40–44.

53. Healthcare Financing Administration, General Memorandum, July 1986.

54. B. Berkman, H. Rehr, and G. Rosenberg, "A Social Work Department Develops and Tests a Screening Mechanism to Identify High Social Risk Situations," *Social Work in Health Care*, 1980, 5, (4), 373–385.

55. E. O'Grady, "Discharge Planning—An Expanded Role under Prospective Payment," *Monitor*, 1984, 2, (4), 1–8.

56. Cunningham, op. cit.

57. Rossen and Coulton, op. cit.

58. G. Olsen, E. Cochrane, and S. McSkimming, "OHSU Discharge Planning Program High Risk Screening Grid," *Coordinator*, Apr. 1986, 36–37.

FOR FURTHER REFERENCE

American Academy of Nursing, *Primary Care by Nurses: Sphere of Responsibility and Accountability* (Kansas City, MO: The Academy, 1977).

Berger, K., and Fields, W., *Pocket Guide to Health Assessment* (Reston, VA: Reston Publishing, 1980).

Chinn, P. L., and Jacobs, M. K., *Theory and Nursing: A Systematic Approach* (St. Louis: Mosby, 1987).

Ciske, K. I., "Response to Zander's 'Primary Nursing Won't Work . . . Unless the Head Nurse Lets It,' " *Journal of Nursing Administration*, Jan. 1978, 26, 43, 50.

Clausen, C., "Staff RN: A Discharge Planner for Every Patient," *Nursing Management*, Nov. 1984, 58–61.

Discharge Planning for Hospitals (Chicago: American Hospital Association, 1974).

Felton, G., "Increasing the Quality of Nursing Care by Introducing the Concept of Primary Nursing: A Model Project," *Nursing Research*, Jan.-Feb. 1975, 27–32.

Hartigan, E., and Brown, D., *Discharge Planning for Continuity of Care*, NLN Publ. 20-1977 (New York: National League of Nursing, 1985).

Kitto, J., "Designing a Brief Discharge Planning Screen," *Nursing Management*, Sept. 1985, 28–30.

Little, D. E., and Carnevali, D. L. *Nursing Care Planning*. 2d ed. (Philadelphia: Lippincott, 1976).

McKeehan, K. M., ed., *Continuing Care: A Multidisciplinary Approach to Discharge Planning* (St. Louis: Mosby, 1981).

Mulligan, H. A., "Scruples Not Just Name of a Game," *Augusta Chronicle, Augusta Herald*, Apr. 23, 1989, 1D, 4D.

O'Grady, E., "Discharge Planning—An Expanded Role under Prospective Payment," *Monitor*, 1984, 2 (4), 1–8.

Roy, S. C., "Relating Nursing Theory to Education: A New Era," *Nurse Educator*, Mar.-Apr. 1971, 16–21.

Sandowski, C., "The Role of the Discharge Planner," *Rehabilitative Literature*, Jan.-Feb., 1985, 16–20.

Sherman, J. L., Jr., and Fields, S. K., *Guide to Patient Evaluation*. 3d ed. (Garden City, NY: Medical Examination Publishing, 1978).

Shukla, R. K., "Structure Versus People in Primary Nursing: An Inquiry," *Nursing Research*, July-Aug. 1981, 236–241.

Williams, L. B., and Cancian, D. W., "A Clinical Nurse Specialist in a Line Management Position," *Journal of Nursing Administration*, Jan. 1985, 20–26.

Zander, K., "Nursing Case Management: A Classic," *Definition*, Spring 1987.

8

Nursing Service Policies and Procedures

INTRODUCTION

Policies, procedures, rules, and regulations are the standing plans of the nursing organization. Standing plans are fixed in both nature and content. They apply until reviewed and modified or abandoned.[1] While hospitals and other nurse employers seldom use the terms "rules" or "regulations," they frequently develop and maintain policies and procedures that incorporate the rules and regulations imposed by government agencies such as the Health Care Financing Administration, which administers Medicare and Medicaid.

NURSING SERVICE POLICIES

Nursing service policies exist for standardization and as a source of guidance of the nursing staff. As guidelines they give the nurse manager input into nursing activities of each unit, ward, and clinic in which nursing personnel practice. Generally policies fall into three main categories: those that apply to patients, to personnel, and to the environment in which patients are cared for and in which personnel work. A fourth category could be that of relationships with other disciplines or departments. Nursing management also gives input into institutional policies and policies of other departments sharing in the care of patients. Major administrative policies of the division of nursing are best developed by the chief nurse executive in consultation with representatives of all groups concerned in their implementation, including clinical nurses. Such a process of participatory management assumes that employees will follow and support policies they have helped to develop.

Policy making is a part of the planning function of top nursing management. All policies of lower levels of management supplement and support those of top management. Although any supervisor may set a policy, policy cannot conflict with one enforced by a higher authority; policy may be made by a manager only for the area over which that manager has authority.

Megginson, Mosley, and Pietri define policies as "broad general statements of expected actions that serve as guides to managerial decision making or to supervising the actions of subordinates."[2] Figure 8–1 offers an example. The first and last paragraphs fit the definition of a *policy,* but the guidelines more properly fit the *procedures* category.

Policies are usually developed by a policy committee. At the organizational level the committee will be representative of departments and top management. At the nursing division level the committee will be representative of nursing specialties and top nursing management. The policy development process includes the following steps:

1. Determination that a policy is needed.
2. Assignment of the development of each policy to a committee member or members.
3. Development of policy from appropriate sources of information, such as those for the policy on "no code."[3] Sources for developing such policies can be found through computer search or by using references found from published sources.
4. Review of the draft policy by the committee.
5. Circulation of the draft to appropriate clinical committees of physicians who will write orders and nurses who will carry them out. A "no code" policy, for example, would go to these groups, and other policies would go to other appropriate groups.
6. Review of returned comments.
7. Referral to the organization's attorney for approval when indicated (such as "no code" policy).
8. Final approval by committee and signature of the organization's chief executive officer.
9. Distribution with appropriate communication. In the case of a "no code" policy, all personnel who would respond to a cardiac arrest need to be informed.

A policy is a mechanism that establishes constraints or boundaries for administrative action and sets a course to be followed. Within those boundaries nursing personnel still have latitude for independent action. A clinical nurse working alone can refer to policies to make decisions.

Policies are closely related to departmental and unit mission, philosophy, objectives, and operating plans. Objectives may be expressed through policies, and policies may be used to help achieve objectives.

Policies will not always be written down, be-

A decision not to resuscitate a patient is the responsibility of the attending physician. An order must be written on the physician's order sheet by the attending physician or delegated to a house officer. [Such orders cannot] be accepted verbally.

The following guidelines will be adhered to by the physician when writing "no code" orders and documented in the progress notes:

1. Assess for viability of the patient, quality of life of the patient, and competency of the patient.
2. Discuss with the patient and/or family the results of this assessment and the writing of a "no code" order by this physician.
3. This order for "no code" will be reviewed by the physician daily and updated weekly. Changes will then be made as needed.

The hospital nursing procedure for "code 1" will be immediately implemented on all patients without a "no code" order.

SOURCE: Courtesy of the University of South Alabama Medical Center, Mobile, Alabama.

Figure 8–1 • Subject: "No Code"

cause a consistent pattern of administrative decisions and actions related to specific problems also indicates policy. An example of unwritten policy in an organization is that an employee who is within two years of retirement is not promoted, even though her record may be better than employees with less service. Such covert policies are sometimes precedent-setting policies. Employees make decisions and act on their own without comment or action by supervisors. Thus they set a precedent for other clinical nurses. Also, supervisors sometimes act in such a way as to imply policy. Policies established by precedent or implied action are the covert or unwritten policies of nursing.

Policies are formal or informal, covert or written. Formal policies are those that apply to:

1. Organizations as a whole
2. A functional entity such as a division or department
3. A basic unit such as a ward, floor, special care unit, or clinic

Policies impact nursing at each of these levels.

Policies that define an organization's philosophy or position on philosophical issues such as ethics or religion are apt to be developed at top management level. Those that enforce legal rules or government regulations are the responsibility of top management. Policies must be in harmony with legal aspects of organizational operations.

Policies have value because of their effect in promoting consistency of action and stability. They provide guidance from top management to lower levels, and in so doing they transfer and thus speed up some decision making. Absence of policy creates situations in which similar problems are addressed over and over again, sometimes within several sections at one time, without establishing a management position. Policies conserve time by setting standards, discipline problems being an example. If there are no policies, one manager can terminate an employee for the same act for which another manager gives counsel, written warning, or suspension. Uniformity of policies prevents conflict and promotes fairness.

Too much imposition of policies is frequently perceived by professionals as authoritative and bureaucratic. Administrative directives in any form, including policies, should be kept to a minimum. They should be pertinent, concise, and comprehensive and should state their underlying reasons. When policies are written for every eventuality, they stifle independent thought and action.

Standards

Some written policies are required by the Joint Commission on Accreditation of Healthcare Organizations (JCAHO). Implementation of standards implies that policies will be developed for carrying them out. Many will affect administrative areas: these should be reviewed by the nurse administrator, who provides recommendations for policy development, revision, and implementation as it relates to the care of patients and the activities of nursing personnel. Policies will need to include standards applicable to the practicing nurse, particularly with regard to clinical privileges and standards of professional ethical practices. These clinical privileges will be covered by the state nursing practice act and will be based on education, experience, and demonstrated competence and judgment. They will include policies related to assignments; diagnostic and therapeutic orders of medical staff members; medication administration; confidentiality of information and the role of the nursing staff in discharge planning and in patient and family education; the maintenance of required records, reports, and statistical information; cardiopulmonary resuscitation; patient, employee, and visitor safety; and the scope of activity of volunteers or paid attendants.[4]

The American Nurses' Association (ANA) *Standards for Organized Nursing Services and Responsibilities of Nurse Administrators Across All Settings* imply nursing policies related to:

1. Philosophy
2. Objectives
3. Organizational plan
4. Recognition of patients' cultural, economic, and social differences and their value systems
5. Collaborative planning with patients, their families, and the interdisciplinary team
6. Fiscal resource management
7. Staffing
8. Assignments
9. Clinical nursing privileges
10. Advancement in clinical practice
11. Quality assurance
12. Support services
13. Orientation
14. Education
15. Ethics
16. Research

In addition, ANA standards state that nurses will be involved in policy making.[5]

Specific written hospital policies are required for management of patient care services. Since nursing personnel are frequently responsible for implementing these policies, the nurse administrator should be involved in their development and revision. It has been the experience of many nurse administrators that these policies have to be totally developed, revised, and implemented by the nursing staff. Other areas related to JCAHO standards for which nurse managers will have to assist in developing, revising, or implementing policies are diagnostic radiology services, hospital-based home care services, hospital-sponsored ambulatory care services, pharmaceutical services, anesthesia services, dietetic services, emergency services, infection control, medical record services, nuclear medicine services, plant technology and safety management, professional library services, quality assurance, radiology oncology services, rehabilitation services, respiratory care services, social work services, and special care units.

Specific policies and procedures for the ambulatory care services and special care units are of particular import to nursing personnel. In the standards for special care units it is required that each special care unit have specific written policies and procedures that supplement the basic hospital policies and procedures. An administrator or manager of a division of nursing knows the standards of the JCAHO and develops policies and procedures for all areas in which nursing personnel perform services. A practical way of doing this is to make a checklist of these standards and involve appropriate nurse managers and clinical nurses in developing policies that will be workable and helpful to all who have need to refer to them.

Continuing education has become a condition of employment written into some personnel policies. It is required by the employer for clinical advancement and may or may not be a fringe benefit. Policies also cover the organization of committees, including purposes, membership, and operating procedures. Other areas frequently covered by policies include:

1. Personnel policies reflecting goals of an affirmative action program to maintain equal employment practices while maintaining an efficient, productive work force
2. Moving and travel costs
3. Sabbaticals
4. Pay
5. Programs to recognize outstanding performances and achievements
6. Suggestion programs
7. Orientation programs that foster creativity
8. Provisions that make jobs meaningful
9. Four-day workweek
10. Flexible hours in workweek
11. Drug and alcohol abuse
12. Handicapped employees
13. Performance appraisal
14. Management by objectives

Most of these fourteen areas would be covered by organizational policies. In large organizations entire staff positions may be devoted to policy and procedure writing.

These policies will usually be written and available as manuals and used by appropriate personnel. There will be provision for their periodic review and revision. For this reason it is practical to have them in a loose-leaf notebook.

Policies may be combined with procedures, with policy stated first. Policies may stand alone or require many procedures to be implemented.

NURSING SERVICE PROCEDURES

In addition to policies, a written and current nursing procedures manual should be available to all nursing personnel. Procedures outline a standard technique or method for performing duties and serve as a guide for action. Procedures are detailed plans for nursing skills that include steps in proper sequence. See Figure 8–2.

Purposes

Procedures are used for communication, understanding, standardization, and coordination. They are referred to for review when an employee has not done a procedure for some time. They are used to teach and evaluate students and new employees, to orient new employees to distinguishing characteristics of an institution's procedures, and to update employees in developing technologies.

Patient care procedures should inform, teach, and reduce errors. They should relate new and changing equipment to patient care practices. They should tell where to order, call, or send for something, how to perform tasks, and why. Procedures are updated by a committee of professional nurses representing those who use them, relate to them, and contribute theoretical insights. The following is a recommended sequence of events to follow in developing a new procedure:

1. A task or title is stated.
2. A need is identified (purpose stated).
3. A draft is made by a user (an outline on paper of all possible steps and substeps).
4. References and experts, including manufacturers, are consulted.
5. The committee member responsible for development of the specific procedure drafts it in standard format, including related policies, equipment needed, line drawings, location of equipment, and ordering procedure. The draft provides step-by-step instructions in performance, brief theory statements, and supporting documents.
6. The draft is edited.
7. An index code number is assigned.
8. The procedure is typed and distributed to reviewers (labelled "draft") with a deadline for feedback.
9. Returned drafts are used to revise the procedure.
10. The revised manuscript is submitted to approval authorities.

I. Policy Statement. Patient care assignments for nursing personnel will be made by a qualified professional registered nurse/charge nurse according to the University of South Alabama Medical Center standards of care.

II. Purpose. To guarantee the best possible nursing care for the patient, based on the patient's care needs and the staff competencies.

III. General Information. Patient assignments will be made at the beginning of each shift. Each patient's care will be directed by a written management plan. Patient care will be supervised by an RN.

IV. Equipment.
  Management plan
  Patient Kardex
  Assignment sheets

V. Procedures.

Nursing Action	Basis for Nursing Intervention
1. Have written assignment for staff members.	1. Allows staff to see duties required on that shift.
2. Receive a verbal report on the patients.	2. Allows nurse to communicate any changes in plans of care or patient status.
3. Take orders from management plan and doctors' orders.	3. Allows for review of management plan and current physician orders.
4. Review patient assignment with staff members.	4. Allows RN to direct other staff members and clarify care orders.

VI. Documentation. Write assignments on assignment sheet and update as needed. Include patient acuity on assignment sheet.

SOURCE: Courtesy of the University of South Alabama Medical Center, Mobile, Alabama.

Figure 8–2 • Nursing Policy and Procedures on Patient Care Assignments

11. When approved, the procedure is printed and distributed.
12. In-service training on the procedure is given to all appropriate personnel.[6]

Policies and procedures are reviewed, revised as necessary, and dated to indicate the time of the most recent review. They must be abandoned when obsolete.

Advantages

Six major advantages of procedures are that they:

1. Conserve management effort
2. Facilitate delegation of authority
3. Lead to more efficient methods of operation
4. Permit significant economy in personnel
5. Facilitate control
6. Aid in coordination of activities[7]

Disadvantages

Policies and procedures do not always encourage participatory management. They provide a "party line," thereby limiting individual discretion and decision making. For this reason their review should include such questions as, "Is this policy (or procedure) really needed?" and, "Can this policy (or procedure) be modified to give more leeway to clinical and managerial decision making throughout the division?"[8]

Nurse administrators can review commercially produced nursing skills books with the object in mind of adopting one that meets most needs. It can be supplemented with only those procedures absolutely necessary for organizational fit. Nurses are thus saved untold hours of procedure meetings.

Rules and Regulations

Most rules and regulations are included in policy and procedure manuals. They describe what can or cannot be done under specified circumstances. They permit no variations. As previously stated, flexibility should be written into the document itself. Figure 8–3 shows how rules are spelled out in hospital policy.

OTHER MANUALS

Policy and procedure manuals are only two of the possible manuals developed for use in hospitals or other health care institutions. Depending on the size of the institution there may be manuals on

Policy. Body substance precautions will be used by all departments in this institution and are to be used for *any* contact with *all* patient blood or body secretions.

Purpose. The purpose of these guidelines is to prevent the transmission of infectious diseases within this institution.

General Information. Use body substance precautions on all patients and for all patient care at *All Times.*

Some of the steps to be taken for *All* contact with patient substance and/or fluids are:

1. Wash your hands for at least 15 seconds both before and after any patient contact.

2. Wear gloves when touching *any* body substance or mucous membrane.

3. Wear gowns when clothing or uniform is likely to be soiled.

4. Place soiled linen in a laundry bag.

5. Place used needles or sharps in needle disposal containers. *Do not recap needles!!*

6. Inform Infection Control Nurse if patient has an infectious disease for appropriate isolation.

7. Wear goggles when splashing of body fluids is possible.

Remember: Gloves should be worn for all contact with mucous membranes, nonintact skin, and moist body substances, for all patients at all times.

Note: Direct all inquiries to the Infection Control Department.

SOURCE: Courtesy of the University of South Alabama Medical Center, Mobile, Alabama.

Figure 8–3 • University of South Alabama Medical Center—Body Substance Precautions

safety, disaster preparedness, nutrition and food service, pharmacy, and others.

Grubb recommends the following process for developing manuals:

1. *Initiating*
2. *Proposing*
3. *Gathering data*
4. *Analyzing data*
5. *Setting content priorities*
6. *Delegating responsibilities*
7. *Selecting format*
8. *Organizing materials*
9. *Outlining topics*
10. *Writing*
11. *Checking facts*
12. *Reviewing rough draft*
13. *Rewriting*
14. *Evaluating*
15. *Typing final draft*
16. *Proofreading*
17. *Numbering pages*
18. *Indexing*
19. *Printing*
20. *Binding*
21. *Distributing*
22. *Utilizing*
23. *Maintaining*
24. *Revising*[9]

These steps can be applied to procedures also.

This process is more likely to be followed if one person is responsible for it. That person will advise the committee and implement its work. Bylaws of a policy and procedure committee are presented in the chapter on committees, as is an example of policy and procedure minutes.

Manuals may be used in many ways, including conferences, meetings, and procedure demonstration days or through exercises and games, demonstrations, videotapes, case studies, and group learning sessions. A predetermined and coded distribution list should be a part of each policy.

SUMMARY

In developing a theory of nursing management, nursing service policies and procedures are conceptual plans translated into physical entities, usually called manuals. Both should be developed with input from clinical nurses who will be led to view them as one source of nursing standards.

Lower-level policies support upper-level ones. All are developed from appropriate sources of information and are updated periodically. It is important for nurses to note that policies and procedures set standards and hold the profession to meeting them.

Although many policies come from external sources and are mandated, nurse managers should work with clinical nurses to determine the necessity for each policy.

All policies and procedures are communicated to users, making it essential that nurse managers have such a communication plan and exercise it periodically.

Some policies and procedures cover topics so extensively as to be developed into separate manuals. These include disaster plans and safety manuals. Including representatives of all categories of professional nurses on policy and procedure committees helps them to accept responsibility for activities in which they participate.

EXPERIENTIAL EXERCISES

1. For each of the following statements, place a + in the blank if it is true and a − if it is false.

____ 1.1 A director of nursing has effective plans when personnel of nursing units are confused, working without planned assignments of individuals, and written policies are not evident, but the director states they are "understood."

____ 1.2 A unit policy can be written to counteract one of the division or institution.

____ 1.3 Policies set limits within which personnel are to function and within which they should be encouraged to be creative.

____ 1.4 Policies should be used to achieve stated objectives.

2. For each of the following statements, place a + in the blank if it is true and a − if it is false.

____ 2.1 A nurse administrator who issues a written policy, letter, or memorandum for every situation that arises will promote creative activity on the part of the staff at the patient care level.

____ 2.2 If the nursing process is poor in terms of nursing history taking, diagnosis, prescription, and action, a written policy on the subject giving active interest by the nurse manager will probably create interest and activity in this area by nursing personnel.

____ 2.3 A nurse administrator should not consult her supervisors and charge nurses in developing and revising policies.

____ 2.4 Policies are helpful to new employees, because they provide them with knowledge of the position of administration and the boundaries or parameters within which they will work.

____ 2.5 A policy that is placed in each ward's policy book and not discussed with personnel will be effective.

____ 2.6 Personnel have a right to an explanation for the policy of the nurse manager.

3. For each of the following statements, place a + in the blank if it is true and a − if it is false.

____ 3.1 Goals of nursing service should be made known to selected nurses.

____ 3.2 Goals of nursing service will be achieved by written administrative and care policies that define realistic and attainable objectives that will be made known to all nursing personnel.

____ 3.3 Standards of the JCAHO may be used in lieu of professional standards of nursing practice and the nurse practice act of the state.

____ 3.4 All nursing practice and administrative policies should be based on scientific knowledge.

____ 3.5 The JCAHO standards require policy for charting by nursing personnel.

____ 3.6 A policy for patient safety is not required by the JCAHO standards for nursing services.

4. For each of the following statements, cross out the word or phrase in parentheses to leave the statement a true one.

4.1 A division of nursing should have (a procedure book; a policy book) that outlines standardized methods of performing selected nursing duties.

4.2 A director of nursing should have direct input into (all organizational policies; all policies that will be implemented by nursing personnel).

4.3 A director of nursing should be involved in making and revising policies (for the nursing service only; for many areas, including environmental services and outpatient services).

4.4 Specific policies and procedures for the special care units should be developed by (the director of nursing; a committee of people responsible for patient care in these units).

5. Although there is no written policy, every nurse working in the intensive care units is given a proficiency test annually. This test covers up-to-date knowledge related to physiology of shock, use of

arterial lines, monitoring of all vital signs and functions, including arterial blood gas determinations, drugs, including hyperalimentation therapy, and other subjects. Is a policy existent here? Why?

6. For each of the following statements, place a + in the blank if the statement is true and a − if it is false.

_____ 6.1 A clinical nurse manager of a unit is practicing sound management when she modifies a policy of the institution because she believes it to be outdated.

_____ 6.2 Absence of management policy may cause duplication of effort.

_____ 6.3 Policies should be written for every eventuality so as to promote creativity.

_____ 6.4 The value placed on policies is evident from the manner in which they are distributed and made known to employees.

_____ 6.5 A director of nursing writes a policy for nursing personnel working in the cardiopulmonary lab without coordinating it with the physician-in-charge of that laboratory. Since it pertains to their treatment of inpatients, her action is sound administrative practice.

_____ 6.6 The director of nursing decided that the critical care units should have policies that defined those emergency procedures that would be performed by nurses. She requested an emergency meeting of the critical care committee and asked that her proposed policy be reviewed, revised as needed, and implemented. The proposed implementation included a training conference with personnel of the units. Her action indicated sound management practice.

7. Attend a meeting of a policy and/or procedures committee meeting for the purpose of determining:

7.1 The purpose of the committee

7.2 Its work

8. From the text, use the sequence of events to follow in developing a new procedure to evaluate the work of the procedure committee.

8.1 How did the committee differ from the textbook?

9. Review the indices of a hospital or nursing division policy and procedure manuals. Pick one of each and decide whether it is obsolete and outdated and why. Make a management plan to update it or get rid of it. You may want to work with a peer group.

MANAGEMENT PLAN

OBJECTIVE:

ACTIONS	PERSON RESPONSIBLE	TARGET DATES	ACCOMPLISHMENTS

NOTES

1. L. C. Megginson, D. C. Mosley, and P. H. Pietri, Jr., *Management: Concepts and Applications,* 2d ed. (New York: Harper & Row, 1986), 129–134.

2. Ibid., 130.

3. M. Cushing, " 'No Code' Orders: Current Developments and the Nursing Director's Role," *Journal of Nursing Administration,* Apr. 1981, 22–29.

4. JCAHO, *Accreditation Manual for Hospitals, 1990* (Chicago: American Hospital Association, 1989), 133–143.

5. ANA Task Force on Standards for Organized Nursing Services and Responsibilities of Nurse Administrators, *Standards for Organized Nursing Services and Responsibilities of Nurse Administrators Across All Settings* (Kansas City, MO: ANA, 1988).

6. M. A. Grindol, "A Manager's Guide to Procedure Manuals," *Nursing Management,* Jan. 1984, 12–14; J. Griffith and D. Ignatavicius, "Procedure Development: A Simplified Approach," *Journal of Nursing Administration,* Sept. 1984, 27–31.

7. Megginson, Mosley, and Pietri, op. cit., 132–134.

8. C. W. Clegg and T. D. Wall, "The Lateral Dimension of Employee Participation," *Journal of Management Studies,* Oct. 1984, 429–442.

9. R. D. Grubb, *Hospital Manuals: A Guide to Development and Maintenance* (Rockville, MD: Aspen, 1981).

FOR FURTHER REFERENCE

Henry, K. H., *The Health Care Supervisor's Legal Guide* (Rockville, MD: Aspen, 1984).

Jellinek, R. C., Zinn, T. K., and Brya, J. R., "Tell the Computer How Sick the Patients Are and It Will Tell How Many Nurses They Need," *Modern Hospital,* Dec. 1973, 81–85.

Rowland, H. S., and Rowland, B. L., eds., *Hospital Administration Handbook* (Rockville, MD: Aspen, 1984).

Swansburg, R. C., *Management of Patient Care Services* (St. Louis, MO: Mosby, 1976).

9

Decision Making and Problem Solving

CLAUDETTE COLEMAN, EdD, RN

Assistant Professor, School of Nursing
Auburn University at Montgomery
Montgomery, Alabama

INTRODUCTION

Decision making is essential to problem solving. It is doubtful that anyone would argue with that statement. Nurses already know how to do this, don't they? Nurses have been making decisions since they were small children. Certainly these decisions were not always made after careful deliberation, by consciously following specified steps in a process. Nurses may not have known how they did it; they just did. Thus a nurse might be thinking "I wouldn't be where I am professionally if I didn't know how to do this—so I'll go to the next chapter."

Wait! How often have nurses made bad decisions? Why were they bad? How do they prevent making similar errors in future decisions? How do they deal with indecision?

The answers to these questions are explored in this chapter. Complex decision making is a part of any level of nursing management. To function successfully the nurse manager must consistently demonstrate problem-solving skills in rapidly changing and uncertain situations in which indecisiveness or poor decisions are costly. Ability to foster organizational decision making and problem solving are personal skills essential to the nurse manager. This chapter deals with models and strategies that can be used by the nurse manager to successfully strengthen personal skills and further develop the decision-making and problem-solving abilities of staff members.

The theory of decision making is an essential component of the nursing process and of the management process. It is a required competency for all professional nurses.

THE DECISION-MAKING PROCESS

Definition

Because everyone is involved at some time in making decisions, it may be assumed that innate abilities, past experience, and intuition form the basis for successful decisions. Decisions are often made by choosing among known alternatives. But what about unknown alternatives? Making a choice is not the only element of decision making. The process involves a systematic approach of sequenced steps, and it should be adaptable to the environment in which it is used. Lancaster and Lancaster defined decision making as a systematic, sequential process of choosing among alternatives and putting the choice into action. This definition does not eliminate natural and learned abilities, yet provides orderliness and continuity to the process of decision making.[1]

Models

A review of the literature yields a number of models of decision making. Three models are covered in this chapter.

The Normative Model. This model is at least 200 years old. It is assumed to maximize satisfaction and fulfills the "perfect knowledge assumption" that "in any given situation calling for a decision, all possible choices and the consequences and potential outcome of each are known."[2] Seven steps are identified in this analytically precise model:

1. Define and analyze problem.
2. Identify all available alternatives.
3. Evaluate the pros and cons of each alternative.
4. Rank the alternatives.
5. Select the alternative that maximizes satisfaction.
6. Implement.
7. Follow up.

The normative model for decision making is unrealistic because of its assumption of clear-cut choices among identified alternatives.

The Decision Tree Model. Various adaptations of decision tree analysis are found in the literature; the essential elements described in the 1960s are standard. All factors considered important to a decision can be represented on a decision tree. Vroom used answers to seven diagnostic questions in the form of a decision tree to identify types of leadership style used in management decision-making models. The questions focus on protecting the quality and acceptance of the decision and deal with adequacy of information, goal congruence, structure of the problem, acceptance by subordinates, conflict, fairness, and priority for implementation.[3] Magee and Brown depict decision trees as starting with a basic problem and making "event forks" and "action forks" represented as branches. The number of branches at each fork correspond to the number of identified alternatives. Every path through the tree equates to a possible sequence of actions and events, each with its own separate consequence. Probabilities of both positive and negative consequences of each act and event are estimated and recorded on the appropriate branch. Additional options (for example, delaying the decision) and consequences of each action/event sequence can be depicted on the decision tree. Computer simulations of decision trees are now available and are adaptable to a limited or highly complex number of "branches" involved in the decision-making process. Normal analysis of the tree is conducted by computing predicted consequences of all event forks (the right hand edge of the tree), substituting that value for the actual event fork and its consequences, and selecting the action fork with the highest expected consequences. Both the optimum strategy and its expected consequences will be determined. Quantitative analysis in the form of decision trees can be used for any type of problem but may be unnecessary in simple problems involving limited consequences.[4]

Descriptive Model. Simon developed the descriptive model based on the assumption that the decision maker is a rational person looking for acceptable solutions based on known information. This model allows for the fact that many decisions are made with incomplete information because of time, money, or people limitations and the fact that people do not always make the best choices. Simon wrote that few decisions would ever be made if we always sought optimal solutions. Instead, he contended, we identify acceptable alternatives. Steps in the descriptive model (Figure 9–1) include:

1. Establish acceptable goal.
2. Define subjective perceptions of the problem.
3. Identify acceptable alternatives.
4. Evaluate each alternative.
5. Select alternative.
6. Implement decision.
7. Follow up.[5]

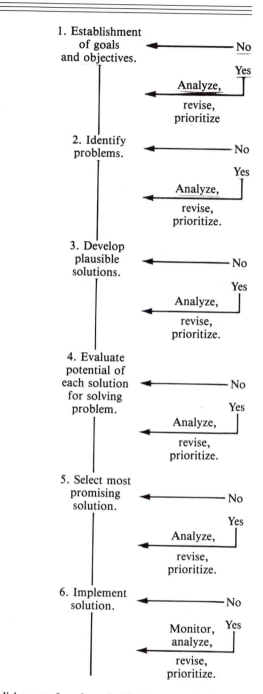

1. Establishment of goals and objectives.
— No
Yes
Analyze, revise, prioritize

2. Identify problems.
— No
Yes
Analyze, revise, prioritize.

3. Develop plausible solutions.
— No
Yes
Analyze, revise, prioritize.

4. Evaluate potential of each solution for solving problem.
— No
Yes
Analyze, revise, prioritize.

5. Select most promising solution.
— No
Yes
Analyze, revise, prioritize.

6. Implement solution.
— No
Yes
Monitor, analyze, revise, prioritize.

The establishment of goals and objectives requires that decisions be made as to how they will be achieved. A first decision may be the priority in which they will be carried out. Decisions do not relate only to problems. They relate to development of plans and programs to accomplish nursing goals and objectives. A best alternative that does not work requires making a decision whether to start over from Step 1 if other alternatives have less chance of success.

Figure 9–1 • *The Decision-Making Process*

This descriptive model may lend itself well to nurse managers faced with daily decision making that must be completed rapidly and with significant consequences. Steps in the model are not unlike those in the familiar nursing process, although the sequence is different. Readers may readily identify conditions in their own environments similar to those described by Simon and see immediate applicability.[6] Lancaster and Lancaster illustrated use of this model for nursing administrators.[7]

Steps in the Process

From these and other models of decision making, five general steps of the process are identified.

First, the problem must be identified. Although this step may seem simple, recognizing and defining the problem is complex because of the diversity of individual perceptions. Because all individuals affected by the problem should be involved in discussing it, authority for decision making should be delegated to individuals at the level of impact. When this is impossible, representatives of various affected groups may provide input. Each may have a different perspective as to what the outcome should be. Nurse managers should make certain that the identified problem actually requires their attention and cannot be handled alone by those involved. Collecting factual data in addition to subjective perceptions is essential. Logical and systematic fact finding includes questioning all sources for divergent opinions and objective data. When the difference between desired and present situations or outcomes is significant, problem recognition may occur.

Once the problem has been identified, the nurse manager must then evaluate the potential for a solution and determine the priority of the problem. Reitz suggests three approaches to prioritizing problems:

1. Deal with problems in the order in which they appear.
2. Solve the easiest problems first.
3. Solve crisis problems before all others.

A decision will depend on the time and energy that can be devoted at that time. When a high-priority problem is identified with limited potential for resolution, the decision maker may be forced to give it lower priority until more information is collected and acceptable alternatives can be found.

The fact that needed information is missing may help define the real problem underlying the perceived one.[8]

The second step in decision making is gathering and analyzing information related to the solution. This step involves defining the specifications to be met by the solution through a series of activities. A thorough information search may be essential for validating the correct identification of a problem. This search should include knowledge of organizational policy, prior personal experience or training, or experiences of others. Externally, the nurse manager begins to identify alternatives comparing the potential alternatives with the desired outcome and desired outcome with available resources. In organizational settings, database information systems may provide this information quickly. Establishing goals with measurable objectives for attainment helps focus the search for alternatives. Certainly when comparing potential alternatives, consider the cost involved for implementing, the time required and available, and the capabilities of those who will be involved for implementation. Once again, it is essential to involve in discussions of alternatives those individuals who are or will be affected by the choice. Irrelevant, insignificant, and extraneous factors must be eliminated from consideration. Gaining a commitment to implement a decision before the choice is made supports the process. It is possible to reach a point of information overload when the searcher has received information too quickly to process or in too great a quantity. Research indicates that the quantity of information sought has a direct positive correlation with the degree of anticipated risk in the decision to be made. Personal confidence of the decision maker also affects the amount of information required for support of choices in decision making. Less searching is required by the manager who recognizes patterns or similarities to previously encountered problems and confidently makes a choice of alternatives.

The third step in decision making is evaluating all alternatives and selecting one for implementation. In the evaluation of alternatives, possible positive and negative consequences of each choice are identified with probability of each estimated. A common approach involves identifying the best and worst possible outcomes to an alternative and then the outcomes that fall between the two extremes. As each alternative is evaluated, additional options may become apparent. Disagreement may stimulate the imagination and produce better solutions. The effects of taking no decision must be weighed against the effects of each proposed solu-

tion. Each alternative must be systematically evaluated for its efficiency and effectiveness in accomplishing the desired outcome as well as the likelihood of achievement with available or obtainable resources. The advantages and disadvantages of each alternative are identified to determine risk factors in possible outcomes. Identifying the solution that best satisfies specifications should receive attention before any compromises, concessions, or revisions are made between involved parties. An alternative that provides the greatest probability of an acceptable desired outcome using available resources is most likely to be selected.

A fourth step in the decision-making process is to act on or implement the selected alternative. Knowledge and skills of the decision maker transform the alternative into action by completing any necessary plans involving sequencing of necessary steps and preparing individuals to implement the solution, effectively communicating the process with all involved.

Orton suggests asking oneself seven questions to increase the success of one's decision choice:

1. Does the quality of the decision really make a difference?
2. Do I have all the information I need to make the decision alone?
3. Do I know what I'm missing? Do I know where to find the information? Will I know what to do with the information I'm given?
4. Do I need anybody's commitment to make sure this succeeds?
5. Can I gain commitments without offering participation in the decision?
6. Do those involved in the decision share the organization's goals?
7. Is there likely to be conflict about the available alternatives?[9]

A final step in the process of decision making is to monitor the implementation and evaluate outcomes. The nursing manager compares actual results with anticipated outcomes and makes modifications as needed to accomplish the desired outcome. Evaluation criteria obtained from measurable objectives provide feedback for testing the validity and effectiveness of the decision against the actual sequence of events in the process. Determination of flaws or gaps in the process may assist the decision maker to monitor the process more closely in the future and preventing the reoccurrence of such problems. The effective decision maker consciously follows these five steps in a logical sequence.

PITFALLS OF DECISION MAKING

Even though information technology is increasing its effect on decision making, pitfalls in the process stem more from the individual than from computers. Individual managers still are resistant to change involving risk and new ideas, often lacking trust in others who will test new areas. Such attitudes stifle not only individuals but groups. When nurse managers find themselves resisting needed change they should analyze their behavior toward the goal of becoming more imaginative and creative managers. It is important to move away from being authoritarian, controlling managers. If the manager chooses to control decision making and omit those affected by the decision from the process, less commitment to implementing the decision is a natural result. When feasible, the nurse manager may use a team approach to decision making, as in a matrix organization. Group decision making usually produces greater commitment to putting the selected alternative into action and working for success.

Other pitfalls of decision making include:

- Inadequate fact finding. Decisions should be based on accurate information. For this reason, information should be obtained from wide and varied sources who are authorities on the subject. They do not have to be contacted personally; instead their publications can be reviewed.
- Time constraints. Collection and analysis of facts, opinions, assumptions, and feelings of those directly involved should be completed in a timely fashion. Pressures of time, resources, and priorities make the decision-making process more complex. It is not always possible to obtain all the necessary facts. This produces a degree of uncertainty, especially when multiple alternatives are identified.
- Poor communication. Communicating the decision to appropriate individuals is as essential as following up to determine if results are as expected.
- Failing to systematically follow the steps of the decision-making process will likely result in unanticipated results.

IMPROVING DECISION MAKING

Basic precepts are identified in the literature for improved decision making. In addition to those already mentioned they include: educate people so they know how to make decisions; seeking support of top management for decision making at the lowest possible level; establishing decision-making checkpoints with appropriate time limits; keeping informed of progress by establishing means of getting firsthand information; using statistical analysis when possible to pinpoint problems for solution;[10] and staying open to use of new ideas or technologies in analyzing problems and identifying alternatives. Numerous strategies and tools are available to improve our decision-making abilities.

Successful managers stay informed about decisions being made at different levels of the organization after appropriately delegating these responsibilities, deal only with those decisions requiring their level of expertise, support implementation of decisions, and credit the decision maker. McKenzie states that managers who make all the decisions themselves convey a lack of trust in the ability or loyalty of their subordinates. Delegation of decision making on a selective basis gains the support of the staff and raises their self-esteem. They gain a sense of belonging and develop loyalty. Delegation leads to leadership. Leaders share authority and power rather than impose it. This is not to say that leaders do not ever make decisions without input from subordinates. This may be necessary on occasion and is acceptable by subordinates who know they participate in decisions that rely on their level of knowledge and experience.[11] Wrapp wrote that good managers don't make policy decisions. Instead they concentrate on a limited number of significant issues, identify areas where they can make a difference, judge how hard to force the issue, give a sense of direction to the organization through open-ended objectives, and spot opportunities that permit others to "own" their ideas and plans for implementation. Wrapp's description of the successful manager portrays a motivator who is knowledgeable and skilled in both decision making and problem solving and serves as a role model for others.[12]

THE PROBLEM-SOLVING PROCESS

At this point one may be wondering about the relationship between decision making and problem solving. The first step in decision making was to identify the problem. But problem solving may involve multiple incidents of decision making. The best way to define their relationship is to define the steps of problem solving.

Steps in the Process

In reality, the steps of the problem-solving process are the same as the steps of the nursing process: assess and analyze, plan, implement, and evaluate. Assessment includes systematic collection, organization, and analysis of data into related information that may be associated with a specific problem or need. It involves logical fact finding, questioning all sources, and differentiating between objective facts and subjective feelings, opinions, and assumptions. Knowledge and experience guide in data collection and analysis. Assessments should also include whether a commitment exists to implement a decision/action before the process goes any further.[13] Making certain there is no readily apparent solution is also a time saver in consideration of the number of people who may become involved in problem solving. Once the problem is identified, it must be determined if it requires other than routine handling—that is, whether it is a rare or unique situation, not a recurrent one. This will lead into the second step of problem solving: planning.

Planning involves several phases. In nursing terms we determine priorities, set goals and measurable objectives, and plan interventions. Management literature essentially says the same: break the problem down into components and establish priorities, develop alternative courses of action, determine probable outcomes for each alternative, decide which course is best in relation to resources, goals, risks, and the like, and decide on a plan of action with a timetable for implementation.[14]

Nurse managers should relate the problem to the corporate mission when determining priorities. Decisions involve a selection among alternative courses of action. Decisions must have an acceptable effect on those directly involved, other areas affected, and the entire organization. Plans should include when and how to alter a course of action when undesired results occur.

The third step is implementation of the plan. Managers should keep informed of the status of the process because it is unlikely they will be directly involved. This is the step in the process most likely to be delegated to subordinates. Implementation requires knowledge and skills appropriate to specific selected alternatives. Evaluation, the final step in problem solving, includes determining how closely goals and objectives were met, the success or failure of actions taken in resolving the problem, and whether the plan should be terminated because the problem is resolved or continued, with or without modification.

Group Problem Solving

Although each step of the problem-solving process can be approached by the individual, input from all affected individuals or areas promotes the probability of more complete data collection, creative planning, successful implementation, and evaluation indicating problem resolution. Managerial problem-solving groups are often formed in organizations with the expectation that the group's effect will prove to be greater than the sum of its parts. Brightman and Verhoeven state that a

team of problem solvers has greater potential resources than an individual, can have a higher motivation to complete the job, can force members to examine their own beliefs more carefully, and can develop creative solutions.[15]

Two types of group techniques that may prove successful in problem solving have been identified—Delphi and nominal group techniques. In the Delphi group technique, only the group leader knows the identity of members. Questionnaires are completed by each member, consolidated, and recirculated until a consensus emerges. The Delphi technique is especially useful when group members are experts physically separated from each other. Electronic mail has eliminated the primary limitation of this technique by reducing the amount of time required for sending and tabulating the questionnaires.

The nominal group technique avoids development of a self-proclaimed expert by combining independent activity with interacting group structures at specific points in the problem-solving process. Individuals first generate solutions for a problem independently, then present and defend the alternatives individually. Each person may be questioned for clarification but not criticized. The group leader collects the written ideas; after group members interact to reach agreement, each member ranks each option silently and independently. Group size of five to ten members is suggested.

Scharf suggests a problem-solving team of five to ten persons plus a facilitator to be most effective because each is assigned a specific responsibility. His effective team has a person who has a real interest in the problem, one who will be implementing the selected alternative, one who will receive output from the alternative, a decision maker with sufficient power to implement, a needed technical expert, a resource controller, an "integrator" or uninvolved party, and a trained workshop team facilitator. Perhaps the success of such a group lies in individual autonomy for a specific task and a facilitator who motivates and monitors the group function.[16]

If group problem solving has so many advantages, why would the failure rate be high? Brightman and Verhoeven cite a number of reasons for failure of managerial problem-solving groups. Among them are the group leader's ineffective leadership skills and lack of a game plan, a homogeneous group using similar styles of problem solving, use of improper group structure (for example, interacting), and developing counterproductive norms such as "group-think" in which consensus is sought at the expense of critical thinking and realistic consideration of alternative ideas.[17]

Effective groups need varied perspectives and values. That means members are needed who use their senses to evaluate hard facts as well as members who use intuition to imagine. People are needed who use their feelings as well as people who think logically and analytically. Effective group leaders comprehend group dynamics and use appropriate intragroup intervention skills and techniques to promote open sharing, constructive conflict, minority opinion, and clarification of all ideas and feelings.

Whether functioning essentially as an individual or participating with a group, the nurse manager must daily make decisions related to problems encountered by and with individual patients, their families, nursing staff, and the organization in which they function. Systematic use of the decision-making and problem-solving processes described in this chapter should enhance professional growth and consistency in making sound decisions and resolving problems.

SUMMARY

Decision making and problem solving occur concurrently with all major functions of nursing management. Three models of the cognitive thinking skills involved in decision making are presented: the normative model, the decision tree model, and the descriptive model.

Decision making involves having an objective, gathering data pertaining to the objective, analyzing the data, identifying and evaluating alternative courses of action that will achieve the objective, selecting an alternative (the decision), implementing it, and evaluating the results. Nurse managers make the best decisions through knowledge and use of the theory of decision making combined with intuitive ability developed over years of experience.

Problem solving is not the exact equivalent of decision making, but it involves a similar thinking process. Decision making is different from problem solving in that the objective does not have to obtain to a problem. It can be an objective that relates to change, to progress, to research, and to implementation of any operational or management plan.

EXPERIENTIAL EXERCISES

1. Delegation is a key responsibility of nurse managers in decision making. Match each rule listed in Section I with the correct example or examples in Section II.

I

a. Delegate decision making to the lowest possible level.
b. A decision has to be made at director of nursing level.
c. A decision can be made at the clinical nurse manager level.

II

_____ 1.1 The objective is to bring all hospital courses into the state nurses' association continuing education program so that all nurses will be eligible for continuing education units.

_____ 1.2 The objective is to set up a planned clinical experience for nurses interested in chemotherapy for cancer patients. Content has not been decided. A qualified, experienced nurse is assigned full time to this activity.

_____ 1.3 A procedure book needs to be developed for each of the special care units. Each will cover only the special procedures peculiar to the unit. All units have well-trained and competent clinical nurse managers and nursing personnel.

2. For each of the following statements, place a + in the blank if it is true and a − in the blank if it is false.

_____ 2.1 A practical way to define a problem that requires a decision is to have all people who will be affected by the problem discuss it.

_____ 2.2 It is important to have consensus rather than dissent in making decisions.

_____ 2.3 The best decision has been made when the entire group is in complete agreement.

_____ 2.4 People will usually support a decision if they have participated in making it even if they do not totally agree with the decision.

_____ 2.5 Before a clinical nurse manager puts a decision into effect she must educate those who will need new knowledge, skills, and attitudes.

3. _Case Study_: You are Ms. Carrie Platt. You have been director of nursing services of Mason General Hospital for one and a half years. Mason General is a 500-bed general hospital in a metropolitan area serving a population of 700,000. The city also has four other hospitals and a University Medical Center. A local ADN nursing program affiliates with your hospital. Today is Monday, March 20th. During the past week on Thursday (March 16th) and Friday (March 17th) you were away from the hospital to conduct a two-day workshop. You have just arrived at 8:00 A.M. and you must leave the hospital at 8:50 A.M. in order to be at the airport at 9:10 A.M. You have had an unexpected death in the family and must be gone the entire week. You notice that the In-Basket contains several items. You should make decisions about these things before leaving.

Instructions: Ten decision-making exercises follow. Each exercise is composed of a memorandum or other message-carrying device and a decision worksheet. On the worksheet list ideas for action and arrive at a decision. If the information given lacks essential detail, make any assumptions necessary. Use the steps of problem solving and decision making. Possible examples of decisions include:

1. Take immediate action and state what the action is.
2. Delegate the action to another person and state who the person is.
3. Postpone the action; state to what time.
4. Other course; please specify.

3.1 *MEMORANDUM*

TO: Mrs. Platt

FROM: Kay Campbell, Head Nurse—5 N

SUBJECT: Poor charting of I & O

DATE: March 17

The I & O record on Mrs. East in 517 is incomplete for evening and night shifts for her postoperative period. She went into shock in the recovery room and is in renal failure. Dr. Blake is *extremely* upset about the lack of thorough charting of I & O. One of the evening aides heard Mr. East call his lawyer about the possibility of a law suit. We thought you needed to be aware of this situation.

Decision Worksheet

Subject	Decision Alternatives	Decision Analysis	Decision Selected

3.2

```
┌─────────────────────────────────────┐
│  ( IMPORTANT MESSAGE )              │
│                                      │
│  FOR  Ms. Platt                      │
│  DATE  March 17      TIME 10 15  A.M.│
│                                  P.M.│
│  MS  Tonia Cole, M.S.N.              │
│  OF  Chicago                         │
│  PHONE _____   │
│        AREA CODE   NUMBER   EXTENSION│
│  ┌──────────────┬───┬──────────────┬─┐│
│  │ TELEPHONED   │ X │ PLEASE CALL  │ ││
│  ├──────────────┼───┼──────────────┼─┤│
│  │ CAME TO SEE  │   │ WILL CALL    │ ││
│  │ YOU          │   │ AGAIN        │ ││
│  ├──────────────┼───┼──────────────┼─┤│
│  │ WANTS TO SEE │ X │ RUSH         │ ││
│  │ YOU          │   │              │ ││
│  ├──────────────┼───┼──────────────┼─┤│
│  │ RETURNED     │   │ SPECIAL      │ ││
│  │ YOUR CALL    │   │ ATTENTION    │ ││
│  └──────────────┴───┴──────────────┴─┘│
│                                      │
│  MESSAGE  Called in reference        │
│  to ad for clinical                  │
│  specialist. Will be in area         │
│  Wed. & Thurs. next week             │
│  and would like appt.                │
│                                      │
│  SIGNED _____     │
└─────────────────────────────────────┘
```

Decision Worksheet

Subject	Decision Alternatives	Decision Analysis	Decision Selected

3.3 MEMORANDUM

TO: Mrs. Platt

FROM: Mrs. Back, In-service Director

SUBJECT: Uniform Regulations

DATE: March 17

The meeting with the nursing assistants regarding uniform regulations has been scheduled for March 21, 10:00 A.M. in In-service Room 406. We appreciate your offer to discuss this matter with the nursing assistants.

Decision Worksheet

Subject	Decision Alternatives	Decision Analysis	Decision Selected

3.4 *MEMORANDUM*

TO: Mrs. Platt

FROM: Michelle Black, RN, Head Nurse—4 East

SUBJECT: Linen Shortage

In the past two weeks we have not had enough sheets and towels to change beds and bathe our patients. I have had to call the linen room again and again for more linen. Their personnel have been very rude and refused to bring any. They say there is none down there.

This interferes with patient care and wastes time. I am sick of this!!!

Decision Worksheet

Subject	Decision Alternatives	Decision Analysis	Decision Selected

3.5 *MEMORANDUM*

TO: Mrs. Platt

FROM: Mrs. Back, In-service Director

SUBJECT: In-service Education

DATE: March 17

The six in-service meetings scheduled regarding the new emergency crash carts were very poorly attended, even though time was allotted for all individuals to attend. As this is vital for patient safety, how can we motivate physicians and personnel to attend?

Decision Worksheet

Subject	Decision Alternatives	Decision Analysis	Decision Selected

3.6

```
┌─────────────────────────────────────────┐
│  ( IMPORTANT MESSAGE )                   │
│                                          │
│  FOR  Ms. Platt                          │
│  DATE  March 17      TIME 3:40 A.M/P.M   │
│  M/D  Sullivan, Director                 │
│  OF  School of Nursing                   │
│  PHONE _____ 272      │
│        AREA CODE    NUMBER    EXTENSION  │
│  ┌─────────────────┬───┬────────────────┐│
│  │ TELEPHONED      │ X │ PLEASE CALL    ││
│  ├─────────────────┼───┼────────────────┤│
│  │ CAME TO SEE YOU │   │ WILL CALL AGAIN││
│  ├─────────────────┼───┼────────────────┤│
│  │ WANTS TO SEE YOU│   │ RUSH           ││
│  ├─────────────────┼───┼────────────────┤│
│  │ RETURNED YOUR   │   │ SPECIAL        ││
│  │ CALL            │   │ ATTENTION      ││
│  └─────────────────┴───┴────────────────┘│
│                                          │
│  MESSAGE                                 │
│    The following GNs                     │
│    failed NCLEX:                         │
│       Katie Bryan                        │
│       Deborah Meeks                      │
│       Judy Purvis                        │
│                                          │
│  SIGNED _____         │
└─────────────────────────────────────────┘
```

Decision Worksheet

Subject	Decision Alternatives	Decision Analysis	Decision Selected

3.7 *MEMORANDUM*

TO: Mrs. Platt

FROM: June Bugg, Nursing Assistant on 5 West

SUBJECT: Uniforms for NA

This request is being made by the nursing assistants to discuss with you the possibility of our wearing white uniforms instead of the pink ones.

A representative group would like to meet with you this week if possible.

Decision Worksheet

Subject	Decision Alternatives	Decision Analysis	Decision Selected

3.8

```
┌─────────────────────────────────────┐
│  ( IMPORTANT MESSAGE )              │
│                                     │
│  FOR  Mo. Platt                     │
│  DATE  March 18      TIME 10:30 A.M.│
│                                P.M. │
│  M S.  Janet Bright                 │
│  OF  Graduate School (S.O.N.)       │
│  PHONE           205-5773           │
│       AREA CODE  NUMBER   EXTENSION │
│                                     │
│  TELEPHONED      │X│ PLEASE CALL    │
│  CAME TO SEE YOU │ │ WILL CALL AGAIN│
│  WANTS TO SEE YOU│X│ RUSH           │
│  RETURNED YOUR CALL│ │SPECIAL ATTENTION│
│                                     │
│  MESSAGE  Wants appt. to            │
│  discuss permission to do           │
│  physical assessment with           │
│  tape recorder on Gyn               │
│  unit.                              │
│                                     │
│  SIGNED                             │
└─────────────────────────────────────┘
```

Decision Worksheet

Subject	Decision Alternatives	Decision Analysis	Decision Selected

3.9

1113 South Short Street
Mason City, Arkansas
March 16

Mrs. Platt
Director of Nurses
Mason General Hospital
Mason City, Arkansas

Dear Mrs Platt:

I was a patient at your hospital from February 10 through February 25. When I was admitted all of my personal belongings were taken from me and they put a hospital gown on me. Two days before I was to go home I started looking for my stuff—my stuff could not be found. This is what I lost:

1 blue knit suit	$75.00
1 pr. black patent shoes	25.00
1 pr. black panty hose	4.75
1 full blue nylon slip	10.00
1 blue girdle	8.00
1 black patent pocketbook	10.00
1 Buxton change purse	11.00
1 pr. eyeglasses (white)	70.00
1 gold chain necklace	70.00
1 gold bracelet	28.00
$250.75	TOTAL

I expect my belongings to be returned to me by March 23 or a check for the above amount. I know you will attend to this matter immediately.

Most sincerely,

Marie Adams

Marie Adams

Decision Worksheet

Subject	Decision Alternatives	Decision Analysis	Decision Selected

3.10

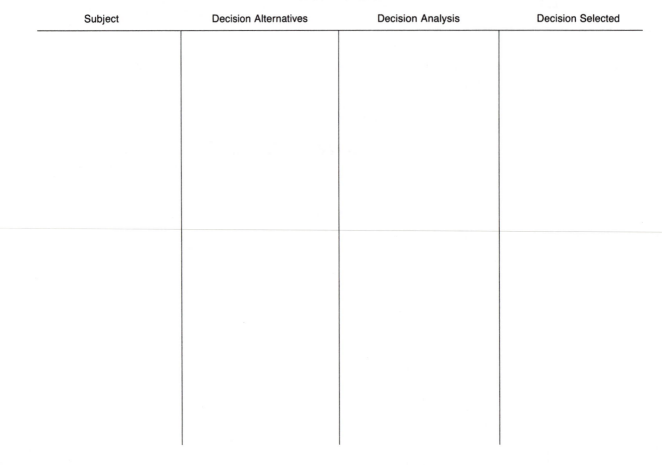

IMPORTANT MESSAGE

FOR *Ms. Platt*

DATE *March 18*   TIME *10:00* A.M.

M S. *Allie Lockler*

OF *Former LPN on 2 East*

PHONE *871-1882*
AREA CODE   NUMBER   EXTENSION

TELEPHONED	X	PLEASE CALL	
CAME TO SEE YOU		WILL CALL AGAIN	
WANTS TO SEE YOU		RUSH	
RETURNED YOUR CALL		SPECIAL ATTENTION	

MESSAGE *Requests recommendation for L.P.N. position at Arthur Memorial Nursing Home.*

NOTE: Was dismissed for excessive absences.

SIGNED _____

Decision Worksheet

Subject	Decision Alternatives	Decision Analysis	Decision Selected

NOTES

1. W. Lancaster and J. Lancaster, "Rational Decision Making: Managing Uncertainty," *Journal of Nursing Administration,* Sept. 1982, 23–28.
2. Ibid., 23.
3. V. H. Vroom, "A New Look at Managerial Decision Making, Organizational Decision Making," *Organizational Dynamics,* Spring 1973, 66–80.
4. R. V. Brown, "Do Managers Find Decision Theory Useful?," *Harvard Business Review,* May-June 1970, 78–89; J. Magee, "Decision Trees for Decision Making," *Harvard Business Review,* July-Aug. 1964, 126; J. Magee, "How to Use Decision Trees in Capital Investment," *Harvard Business Review,* Sept.-Oct. 1964, 79.
5. H. A. Simon, *Administrative Behavior,* 3d ed. (New York: The Free Press, 1976).
6. Ibid.
7. Lancaster and Lancaster, op. cit.
8. J. H. Reitz, *Behavior in Organizations* (Homewood, IL: Richard D. Irwin, 1977), 154–199.
9. A. Orton, "Leadership: New Thoughts on an Old Problem," *Training,* June 1984, 28, 31–33.
10. D. Graham and D. Reese, "There's Power in Numbers," *Nursing Management,* Sept. 1984, 48–51.
11. M. E. McKenzie, "Decisions: How You Reach Them Makes a Difference," *Nursing Management,* June 1985, 48–49.
12. H. E. Wrapp, "Good Managers Don't Make Policy Decisions," *Harvard Business Review,* Sept.-Oct. 1967, 91–99.
13. A. Scharf, "Secrets of Problem Solving," *Industrial Management,* Sept.-Oct. 1985, 7–11.
14. B. Blai, Jr., "Eight Steps to Successful Problem Solving," *Supervisory Management,* Jan. 1986, 7–9.
15. H. J. Brightman and P. Verhoeven, "Why Managerial Problem Solving Groups Fail," *Business,* Jan.-Mar. 1986, 24–29.
16. Scharf, op. cit.
17. Brightman and Verhoeven, op. cit.

FOR FURTHER REFERENCE

Agor, W. H., "The Logic of Intuition: How Top Executives Make Important Decisions," *Organizational Dynamics,* Winter, 1986, 5–18.

American Hospital Association, *Strategies: Nurse Involvement in Decision Making and Policy Development,* 1984, 1–10.

Argyris, C., "How Tomorrow's Executives Will Make Decisions," Reprint from *THINK Magazine,* IBM, 1967.

———, *Reasoning, Learning and Action* (San Francisco: Jossey-Bass, 1982), 87, 102.

Barnard, C., and Beyers, M., "The Environment of Decision," *Journal of Nursing Administration,* Mar. 1982, 25–29.

Denton, D. K. "Problem Solving by Keeping in Touch," *Business,* July-Sept. 1986, 40–42.

Galbraith, J. K., *The New Industrial State* (Boston: Houghton Mifflin, 1967).

Goldstein, M., Scholthaver, D. and Kleiner, B. B. "Management on the Right Side of the Brain," *Personnel Journal,* Nov. 1985, 40–45.

Grandori, A., "Prescriptive Contingency View of Organizational Decision Making," *Administrative Science Quarterly,* June 1984, 192–209.

Greiner, L. E., Leitch, D. P., and Barnes, D. P., "Putting Judgment Back into Decisions," *Harvard Business Review,* Mar.-Apr. 1970, 59–67.

Holland, H. K., "Decision Making and Personality," *Personnel Administration,* May-June 1968, 24–29.

Kersey, J. H. Jr., "Responsibility Accounting: Making Decisions Efficiently," *Nursing Management,* May 1985, 14, 16–17.

Leo, M., "Avoiding the Pitfalls of ManagemenThink," *Business Horizons,* May-June 1984, 44–47.

Locke, E. A., Schweiger, D. M., and Latham, G. P., "Participation in Decision Making: When Should It Be Used?" *Organizational Dynamics,* Winter 1986, 65–79.

McKay, P. S., "Interdependent Decision Making: Redefining Professional Autonomy," *Nursing Administration Quarterly,* Summer 1983, 21–30.

Miller, M. "Putting More Power into Management Decisions," *Management Review,* Sept. 1984, 12–16.

Southern Council on Collegiate Education for Nursing, *Preparing Nurses for Decision Making in Clinical Practice: A White Paper* (Atlanta: SCCEN, 1985).

Suding, M. J., "Decision Making Controlling the Computer Input," *Nursing Management,* July 1984, 44, 46, 48–52.

Swansburg, R. C., *Management of Patient Care Services* (St. Louis: C. V. Mosby, 1976), 149–170.

Implementing Planned Change

INTRODUCTION

As a catalyst, the nurse manager causes or accelerates changes by using knowledge and skills that are *not* permanently affected by the reaction. In essence, the nurse manager may be considered a change agent. Let us first consider the philosophy embodied in the theories of human resource management, theories based on adequate assumptions about human nature and motivation. Has the nurse manager organized money, materials, equipment, and personnel in the interest of providing quality services to patients and thereby giving them their money's worth? Have nursing employees had experiences of supervision that have made them passive and resistant to organizational needs? Or do nursing employees work under conditions that inspire them to develop their potential, assume increased responsibility, and work to achieve their personal goals as well as those of the organization? Are clinical nurses able to direct their own efforts?

Nurse managers should start looking for ways to inspire nursing personnel to use their capabilities, to encourage them to accept responsibility, and to encourage them to be active and to seek real meaning in their work. Autonomy and self-direction are traits that people desire. These traits, when freed, satisfy people's ego needs. Nurse managers can show nurses how to accomplish these goals by gaining knowledge and skills that will satisfy their desires to control their own destinies.[1]

Machiavelli said, "There is nothing more difficult to take in hand, more perilous to conduct, or more uncertain in its success, than to take the lead in the introduction of a new order of things."[2] With a few notable exceptions (such as the weather), most of the change that takes place in our society is planned change. This means that nurse managers can plan with clinical nurses to implement change. It must first be decided that a new skill or technique using a new apparatus or technology is needed to improve patient care and ability to deliver that care. Then nurse managers and clinical nurses can plan and carry out the changes they want to make.

Spradley defines planned change as "a purposeful, designed effort to bring about improvements in a system, with the assistance of a change agent."[3] Change occurs whether one wants it to or not. New technology is developed; new treatments result, causing personnel and organizational adjustments. These changes need to be controlled or managed. Hence we refer to the process as "planned change."

THE NEED FOR CHANGE

Four general reasons for designing orderly change have been defined by Williams:

1. To improve the means of satisfying somebody's economic wants.
2. To increase profitability.
3. To promote human work for human beings.
4. To contribute to individual satisfaction and social well-being.[4]

The basic motivation for change could be that orderly change needs to be designed to improve patient care while lowering costs and increasing nursing's economic status. It could be that the organization should profit by being able to do more for less or at the same cost or by improving its reputation for quality care. The goal could be making the work situation or environment better for the employees. Or it could be improvement of individual satisfaction and social well-being of both patients and staff members.

Implementation of planned change will alter the status quo. New programs of patient care will modify existing relationships among nursing personnel and between them and other members of the health care team.

Change can help achieve organizational objectives as well as individual ones. Individual nurses and the institution of nursing will grow and prosper if they change with improved technology, especially if that technology will cure disease, save infant lives, prolong life without increasing suffering, and in general promote social improvement.

What are the common types of change with which nurses must deal? One obvious type is technological. A few years ago a 200-watt-per-second defibrillator was considered satisfactory. Now 400 watts per second is desirable. Changes also occur in methods and procedures related to machinery and equipment, electronic thermometers and ventilatory equipment being two examples. Changing work standards delineate up-to-date competencies for both nurse managers and clinical nurses.

Other changes include personnel and organizational adjustments, for example, constant turnover of personnel or changes in organizational structure. Nurses are certainly aware of their changing relationships with those who hold authority and power, changes in responsibility and status, and changes in organizational, departmental, and unit objectives. Some employees resist change, but others welcome it as an opportunity to make adjustments in existing work situations, alter their relationships with their associates, and achieve personal goals.

During the past 25 years, there have been significant changes in the nature of health care organizations, the demands placed on nurse managers, and the needs and motivations of nursing personnel. Successful nurse managers have learned to manage change and have publicly related the role of nursing as being an involved and concerned element of society. They recognize the growing complexity of the health care organization, particularly today's division of nursing, and they recognize the changing values of nurses within the profession. Nurses want opportunities for advancement or promotion, recognition for their work, and more help from their peers and supervisors to improve their job skills. One dramatic change has been the impetus of nurses to develop their professional standards to higher levels to which they must raise their credentials, particularly with regard to education. They have also recognized the need for continuing education to deliver up-to-date services. A glance at a nursing journal shows nurses' awareness of society's current problems and their increasing involvement in them. These include problems of health, environmental pollution, poverty, social equality, education, civil rights, religion, and many others. Nurse managers see themselves as agents of change functioning within a profession that draws its basic support from society.

Evidence suggests that technological innovation can cause scientists' and engineers' knowledge to be obsolete in 10 years if they do not pursue further education. Parallel evidence could be developed to support the same conclusion about nursing. Today's nurses are more committed to task, job, and profession than they are loyal to the organization. They look at the kind of services provided (short-term versus critical versus chronic), management's philosophy (participative versus authoritarian), experimental outlook, and physical and geographical location. Nurses want control over their work environments and are dissatisfied otherwise. For these reasons nursing management philosophies and assumptions are changing. Nurse managers are changing their management styles, policies, procedures, relationships with subordinates, and employment and compensation practices. Hospital managers are looking at the kinds of health services they offer. Nurse managers are seeking knowledge of community, state, and national affairs, government trends, individual needs, and group motivations. They are learning to function in a computerized world of business systems.

No longer is the nursing worker bound down by threat and ritual. Nurses are still in great demand in the job market and are highly mobile. The professional nurse looks forward to moving and frequently has the next move planned while still at the present job. This nurse is willing to work but desires an environment where there is humor and opportunity to use imagination. Nurse managers have to change their behavior to suit the changing profile of this new breed of worker. Nurse managers need to learn how to provide avenues for need satisfaction of clinical nurses. They need to look at their own style of management and how it affects others and learn to be more flexible and individualized in dealing with their employees. They must learn to be candid and to confront conflict so that each can express feelings, thoughts, and reactions to others. The change in management in nursing aims to promote ideas of all people, to encourage attentive listening, and to reward people for becoming personally involved and committed to their work.

Adaptation to change has always been a job requirement for nursing. Nursing personnel work for numerous bosses, including individual patients, physicians, the head nurse, and a different clinical nurse manager each change of shift. Nursing practitioners will find their roles changed many times in a day, sometimes being a manager, sometimes a clinical nurse, sometimes a consultant, and always in multiple roles.

Among the reasons for change is evidence that something needs changing. The nurse manager needs to recognize the symptoms. They can be glaring or subtle. An example of the subtle would be offhand comments of float personnel such as "I'd rather work anywhere than unit 3F" or "Could you send me someplace else?"

The health care system is constantly changing. Changes include a labor force that wants wages comparable to other professions, hours of work that fit their personal needs, and the power to make their own professional decisions about patient care. Many times the change focuses on technology without consideration for human relationships and political sensitivities. A case in point is the American Medical Association's 1988 push to solve the nursing shortage by proposing a new health care technician.

Nurse managers require extensive knowledge of community affairs, government trends and constraints, world affairs, international practices and procedures, the changing nature of individual needs, and group motivation. Even the supply and demand of nurses relates to these many areas. Within nursing, needs change with new systems of computers, planning, business, accounting, control, and marketing.[5]

Younger nurses, like other younger professionals, are mobile and have salable skills. They want to use all of their skills and to be collaborative and democratic.[6]

Change is the key to progress and to the future.

CHANGE THEORY

Lewin's Theory

One of the most widely used change theories is that of Kurt Lewin. Lewin's theory involves three stages:

1. *The unfreezing stage.* The nurse manager or other change agent is motivated to create change. Affected nurses are made aware of this need. The problem is identified or diagnosed, and the best solution is selected. Three possible mechanisms giving inputs to the initial change are: individual expectations are not being met (lack of confirmation); the individual feels uncomfortable about some action or lack of action (guilt/anxiety); or, a former obstacle to change no longer exists (psychologic safety). The unfreezing stage occurs when disequilibrium is introduced into the system, creating a need for change.[7]

2. *The moving stage.* The nurse manager gathers information. A knowledgeable, respected, or powerful person influences the change agent in solving the problems (identification). This person can be an influential nurse manager, peer, or superior. A

variety of sources give a variety of solutions (scanning), and a detailed plan is made. People examine, accept, and try out the innovation.[8]

3. *The refreezing stage.* Changes are integrated and stabilized as part of the value system. Forces are at work to facilitate the change (driving forces). Other forces are at work to impede change (restraining forces). The change agent identifies and deals with these forces, and change is established with homeostasis and equilibrium.[9]

Lippitt's Theory

Although Lewin's theory was modified by others, Lippitt added other phases to Lewin's original theory. The seven phases of his theory of the change process are as follows:

Phase 1: Diagnosing the Problem. During this phase the nurse manager as change agent looks at all possible ramifications and who will be affected. People who will be affected are involved in the change process. The nurse manager holds group meetings to involve others and win their commitment. The change agent also motivates key people in top management and policy-making roles to ensure success.

Phase 2: Assessment of the Motivation and Capacity for Change. Possible solutions are determined, and the pros and cons of each are forecast. Consideration is given to implementation methods, roadblocks, factors motivating people, driving forces, and facilitating forces.

Assessment considers financial aspects, organizational aspects, structure, rules and regulations, organizational culture, personalities, power, authority, and the nature of the organization. During this phase, the change agent would coordinate activities among a number of small groups.

Phase 3: Assessment of the Change Agent's Motivation and Resources. The change agent can be external or internal to the organization or division. An external change agent may have fewer bases but must have expert credentials. An internal change agent, on the other hand, knows the people. There may be both. The change agent needs a genuine desire to improve the situation, a knowledge of interpersonal and organizational approaches, experience, dedication, and a personality to suit the situation. The change agent should be objective, flexible, and accepted by all.

	Lippitt	Lewin
	1. Diagnosing the problem	1. Unfreezing
	2. Assessment of the motivation and capacity for change	
	3. Assessment of the change agent's motivation and resources	
	4. Selecting progressive change objective	2. Moving
	5. Choosing the appropriate role of the change agent	
	6. Maintenance of the change	3. Refreezing
	7. Termination of the helping relationship	

Figure 10–1 • *Comparison of Change Theories*

Phase 4: Selecting Progressive Change Objectives. The change process is defined, a detailed plan is made, timetables and deadlines are set, and responsibility is assigned. The change is implemented for a trial period and evaluated.

Phase 5: Choosing the Appropriate Role for the Change Agent. The change agent will be active in the change process, particularly in handling personnel and facilitating the change. Conflict and confrontation will be dealt with by the change agent.

Phase 6: Maintenance of the Change. During this phase, emphasis is on communication, with feedback on progress. The change is extended in time. A large change may require a new power structure.

Phase 7: Termination of the Helping Relationship. The change agent withdraws at a specified date after setting a written procedure or policy for perpetuation. The agent remains available for advice and reinforcement.[10] Figure 10–1 offers a comparison of these theories.

It should be noted that change theories are similar to the problem-solving process, indicating that the latter could be used to implement planned change. Nurse managers should select the theory they feel most comfortable with after identifying the change to be made. A management plan is then made to cover the phases of making the change. The planning phase requires gathering data to support a decision for change. The nurse manager would work with the nursing staff who will be affected by the change to set objectives. Thus the entire group become aware of the need for change and interested in it. A relationship is built between the nurse manager and nursing employees. The plan can be made cooperatively, implemented by an enthusiastic group, and evaluated and maintained by the group.

The Change Agent

As one reads change theory one notes that the applications tend to mimic the problem-solving process. The nurse manager operating as change agent uses change theory to identify and solve problems. Also, this nurse manager learns to anticipate impending change, including that from interdependent systems, responds to change, and takes direct action to direct its course.

Nurses can compete successfully in the world of health care by doing things in new ways. Nursing executives are expected to have the vision to change things, to be change agents.[11] Outsiders are resisted as change agents. Clinical nurse managers can plan change by establishing procedures to evaluate obsolescence and estimate the best time for replacement of equipment and procedures, which in turn engenders a need for updating their cognitive, affective, and psychomotor skills.

RESISTANCE TO CHANGE

Resistance to change, or attempting to maintain the status quo when efforts are being made to alter it, is a common response to change. Change evokes stress that in turn evokes resistance.

Resistance to change is often based on a threat to the security of the individual because it upsets an established pattern of behavior. Questions that should be answered if the problem-solving approach is used will fall under the area of workability of the solution. They include the following: Will the change affect the work standard and subsequent employment, promotion, and raises? Will it mean an increased workload at an accelerated pace? Do employees visualize how they will fit into the picture if this change occurs? In-service education is part of the answer, continuing education may help meet the goal.

Factors that stimulate resistance to change include: habits, complacency, fear of disorganization, set patterns of response to change, conservatism,

perceived loss of power, ego involvement, insecurity, perceived loss of current or meaningful personal relationships, and perceived lack of rewards.[12]

People are afraid of change because of lack of knowledge, prejudices resulting from a lifetime of personal experience and exposure to others, and fear of the need for greater effort or of a higher degree of difficulty.

People have developed fears, biases, and social inhibitions from the cultural environment in which they live. They cannot be employed devoid of these cultural barriers, so it is necessary to find ways of managing them within a system.

Barriers to change include a perception of implied criticism: "You are changing the system because you don't like the way I do it." Employees perceive that machines and systems are replacing them or making their jobs less interesting. As an example, a programmed system could be developed for patients to take their own nursing histories.

Change may necessitate the investment of a great deal of time and effort in relearning. If nurses are to be independent practitioners, what happens to those who are not prepared? "Probably the greatest single personal barrier is that individuals do not understand or refuse to accept the reasons for the change or the need for it. Unfortunately, it is not always easy to equate the reasons and the needs and to communicate them in meaningful and compelling language."[13]

People are members of a social system in a community and will resist change if it affects that social system. Social changes that threaten social customs, values, self-esteem, and security are resisted more than technical changes. One member of the social system may influence others even if they are unaffected by the change.

Values and Beliefs

Cognitive frameworks are based on values and beliefs about effective means of achieving these values. Nurse managers who value the chain of command, policies, and procedures, and who believe their management experience does not need input from clinical nurses may not look for problems needing change. So long as they are successful they are strengthened by success that builds their self-respect. This success fosters resistance to change that threatens the integrity of the framework. People resist discarding their own ideas. Accepting another's idea reduces their self-esteem. They may consider a good idea a unique event to be preserved. Ideas should have life cycles. They shine and then dim and need to be replaced. Ideas should be put on a depreciable basis.[14]

Change is affected by the crucial differences between geographical regions. Some regions are more open to fast change while others accept slow change. Culture changes are affected by religious or political beliefs. People hold fast to meaningful beliefs.[15]

Other Causes of Resistance to Change

Success leads to imprinting and resistance to change. Remember the saying, "If it works, don't fix it"? Units within a division of nursing change at different paces, but in a complex organization many problems require their interaction. The nurse manager as effective change agent must orchestrate this interaction. Time perspectives differ among nursing units. When personnel transfer they have to adjust to the changed pace. Different generations of nurses also have different rates of change.

Sometime nurse managers want to change things at too fast a pace. Excessive changes make a nurse manager and the organizers unpredictable and distrusted.

An Example

Niland describes the failure of change in an attempt to convert an acute care unit into a swing unit of patients awaiting transfer to a nursing home. The reasons given for the failure illustrate the importance of change theory:

1. The unit's goals were not made known to the staff or clinical manager.
2. The workload was too demanding.
3. There was poor communication and planning.
4. The managers were not aware of these staff perceptions:
   4.1 They were being used as work horses.
   4.2 The unit was a waiting area for patient placement.
   4.3 The reason was fiscal.
   4.4 There was no nursing home bed shortage.
   4.5 The unit had become a geriatric unit in which they did not choose to work.
   4.6 They were doing the work of nurse aides.

These problems could have been avoided through careful planning using change theory.[16]

It should be remembered that both individuals and organizations need continuity in policies and procedures so that recurring needs can be dealt with routinely and problems do not have to be resolved anew each time they appear. Hierarchical, bureaucratic frameworks with rules achieve stability, one reason for resistance to change.

The major symptoms of resistance to change are refusal; confrontation; covert resistance such as nonpreparation for meetings or misunderstanding of the place or time; incomplete reports; refusal to accept responsibility; uncooperative employees; passive aggressiveness; absenteeism; and tardiness.[17]

STRATEGIES FOR OVERCOMING OBSTACLES TO CHANGE

Managed Change

Change can be managed, with nurse managers acting as change agents. One of the strategies a nurse manager can use is to request the services of a consultant to make the managerial diagnosis and recommend programs that will improve the productivity of nursing personnel while giving them job satisfaction. Such measures can include educational programs to improve those areas where there are problems.

There is ample evidence that modified forms of management by objectives are an effective strategy for change. The nurse administrators will be the change agents for its success.

Effective managed change leads to improvement of patient care services, raised morale, increased productivity, and meeting of patient and staff needs. Change is an art, the mastery of which can be exhilarating, refreshing, challenging, and exciting, because change represents opportunity. Change is facilitated when nursing employees are matched to demands for adaptability to jobs.

Collection and Development of Data

Nurse managers need to gather data about their work that can be discussed, analyzed, and used to effect change when indicated. Personnel, particularly managers, can be educated to make and manage change. They will learn about labor power planning and use rather than considering this to be the specialized area of the human resources department. They will learn about financial management rather than depending on the accounting office to take care of them. Effective strategies can be developed in these areas for external cooperative efforts among chief nurse executives of similar institutions within a community. Such concepts can be expanded to clinical services. If a division of nursing cannot afford to use such a specialist as a full-time mental health nurse practitioner, several organizations can collectively contract for the services of one. Change thus becomes a cooperative venture.

Integration of computers and automated equipment is essential to the change process. This is particularly true when managers are competing for professional nurses as well as for health care dollars. Within this domain nurse managers can elicit the advice and skills of nursing management information system personnel as impartial third-party critics of the change being effected. Thus these personnel will give nurse managers effective feedback while providing management information support systems.

Preparation or Planning

Preplanning will help to overcome many of the obstacles to change. Planning will keep interpersonal relationships from being disrupted if persons with common frames of reference are brought together. The planner can assist people to meet their goals while minimizing fear and anxiety. Fear is stimulated by the external threat of change. Anxiety is internally stimulated; it is self-induced dread. Planning will help people accept the change without fear or anxiety.

In making changes nurse managers should plan to have people unlearn the old (unfreeze) and use the new (refreeze). Implementation of nursing management information systems can refine much unfreezing and refreezing. Other nurse managers help their staff learn the new without having them unlearn the old. This is a major problem in nursing today because of how the role of nurses is changing. As an example, nurse managers are not helping nurses unlearn the nonnursing routines. This is a big challenge for nurse managers and staff development personnel.

To prepare a plan carefully, share information and decision making, work for common perception and understanding, and support and reinforce the nursing staff's effort to effect change. Clear statements of philosophy, goals, and objectives are needed in preparation for change. Chapter 3, which discusses mission, philosophy, objectives, and management plans, offers guidelines for evaluation.

Beyers recommends that nursing executives be involved in the following elements of strategy planning:

1. Product/market planning
2. Business unit planning
3. Shared resource planning
4. Shared concern planning
5. Corporate level planning[18]

Nursing in all areas, both clinical and managerial, must consider competition. The patient will go where there is higher-quality nursing care. High-quality nursing care results from effectively planned and managed change. Nurse managers should perform market surveys to determine nursing products and services wanted by consumers.[19] This activity itself will constitute change and will also result in changes.

In preparation for change, nurse managers should envision the future so as to create better systems. They should develop a long-range view of nursing as a basis for strategic planning. As an additional preparation for change, nurse managers can voluntarily rotate their own assignments among units and departments to develop their capacity for dealing with a fast pace of change. In this way they can expand their managerial experience and perceptions.

Plans should list everyone on whom the change depends and their level of involvement. Who will oppose and who will support the change? The dominant coalition in the organization and the forces that will stimulate change should be identified and their support enlisted. Appropriate current events should be noted through reading and through meetings, highlighting those that will enhance the mission of the organization and for which the clinical nurses will claim or share ownership.[20] This activity brings new ideas and new knowledge to stimulate and justify the need for change.

Planning will also require thinking in multiple time frames: the changes to be effected in 6 months, in 1 year, and so on. Identify the trade-offs between nursing and other departments, between clinical and management staffs, and within the change process itself. List ways to enlist support.[21]

Be careful not to overplan. Leave some room for people who will implement the change to exercise intelligent initiative. Be sure the rewards or benefits to individuals and to the group are carefully communicated. If people want a change to work, they will make it happen.

Training and Education

Many factors play a part in new learning, including getting the people's attention and stimulating their desire to learn. The staff development instructor and the nurse manager have to find the cues that trigger the desired behavior. This may necessitate working backward from desired behavior to cues. Next they must determine the values that will personally satisfy the learner. When a match is made that satisfies both individual and employer, a new system can be implemented.

The frequency of training and education should match frequency of change. Nursing personnel will require constant staff development programs to keep from depreciating in knowledge and competence. From initial hiring and orientation, change should be portrayed as an integral part of nurses' jobs.[22]

Rewards

Rewards for old behavior patterns should be removed after the individuals have been helped to see the reasons for the proposed change. They need to see the necessity for the new behaviors, and real incentives, financial or nonfinancial, should be provided. Here is where job standards come in. The job standards should incorporate the new methods or skills and phase out the old ones. To provide an incentive, performance appraisals could be based on the new standards. Time must be allowed and opportunity provided for retraining.

Employees affected by change should receive sympathetic understanding from the nurse manager. Also, compensation programs need to be changed for the benefit of more people in the division of nursing rather than being concentrated on the top level. Some effective programs have rewarded outstanding performance with special certificates and ceremonies that cited the behavior earning the award. Rewards should be increased legitimately and should be consistent throughout the organization. There should be a fair arrangement for employees who stand to lose from change.

Other forms of nonfinancial rewards include enriching jobs and encouraging self-development.

These activities can provide satisfaction of individual needs.

Using Groups as Change Agents

Groups in themselves are often effective change agents. When the group appears to work in harmony and to have well-understood goals, it may be used to institute the change. If the idea can be planned in the group, it will be implemented more successfully. A group is more willing to assume risk than most individuals. Planning should make clear the need for change and provide an environment in which group members identify with such needs. Objectives should be stated in clear, concise, and qualitative terms. Administrative policy should contain broad guidelines for achieving the objectives. They should be communicated to the group. The procedures they contain need to be understood.

As agents of change, nurse managers need to use the talents of their staff through use of temporary work teams to solve specific problems and effect change. They need to participate on interdisciplinary task forces. They need to prepare people for job mobility through planned experiences that will facilitate it. Third-party critics may help diagnose and solve problems.

The informal group can promote and support change. It can be formed by enlisting the help of a strong leader and by forming a strong group that will communicate their perception of needed change to nurse managers.[23]

Nurse managers assume multiple managerial roles in matrix organizations. They perform for several bosses and perform several tasks at a time. Improving group teamwork is essential to managed change. In the new work of nursing management no social group or set dominates.

Communications

Too often change is announced by rumor when it should be clearly introduced. Announcements should be factual and comprehensive and should state the objectives, nature, methods, benefits, and drawbacks of the change. If the announcement can be face-to-face, it will be better received.

Discussion of implementation should give people maximum information. The discussion should cover the rate and method of implementation, including the first steps that will be taken and the rate, sequence, and people involved in each element.

Ceremonies may be effective in various aspects of the change. They are useful for retirements; promotion; introduction of a new co-worker, superior, or subordinate; a move to a new job; start of a new system; and reorganization. When used well, ceremonies focus on the importance of the ongoing institution and underline the importance of individual loyalty to that institution and its positions. They convey that the organization and the employees are both needed.

The nurse manager as change agent discusses reasons for resisting change with people. When people understand their real reasons for it, they are not as resistant. They should be encouraged to sound off.

Planned change needs to be successfully communicated to all employees even if they are not directly or immediately involved. Verbal announcements can be followed up with written ones and progress reports. Change occurs smoothly in direct proportion to the positive and democratic behavior that demonstrates management's philosophy and practice at all levels from the top down.

The Organizational Environment

Nurse managers could be more successful if they paid attention to the organizational environment into which change is introduced and the manner in which it is done. Managers need to be committed to a change and to support it by their actions, which express their attitudes. When the nurse administrator attempts to impose change on people in an authoritarian manner, they often resist it.

Managers can establish an environment for change when they:

1. Stress relationships with and between groups.
2. Bring out mutual trust and confidence.
3. Emphasize interdependence and shared responsibility.
4. Contain multigroup membership and responsibility by limiting individuals from belonging to too many groups and ensuring the same responsibilities are not given to several groups.
5. Have a wide sharing of control and responsibility.
6. Resolve conflict through bargaining or problem-solving discussions.[24]

Concern for employees is as important as concern for patients.

Other aspects of the organizational environment that support change include:

1. Permitting job movement to facilitate careers.
2. Anticipating and rewarding change, thus institutionalizing it.[25]
3. Modifying the nursing organizational structure to accommodate changes that provide growth and development.
4. Promoting a "can-do" attitude.

When the organizational climate changes, employees change behaviors. A desired organizational climate fosters high-quality patient care.[26]

THE RELATIONSHIP OF NURSING RESEARCH TO CHANGE

The Need for Nursing Research

Even though there are many predictions of the future directions of health care, it will probably be different from all of them. Nursing research is essential to preparation for the future and for competition within the health care system. Nurse managers must have good information to keep nursing competitive with other care givers in providing patient care. They must also have the knowledge to be competitive among employers and in a global economy. This requires the development and employment of nurse scientists who are researchers. Employment of these nursing researchers will commit nurse managers to developing research in managing humans beings to their full potential. It is an investment that keeps people, the future human capital, from depreciating.[27]

Nursing research improves practice. A profession grounds practice in scholarly inquiry. Nurse managers will improve the quality of nursing practice when they promote nursing research and the application of the findings of nursing research. Nursing administration research will validate the discipline of nursing administration.[28]

Nurse managers, clinical nurses, instructors, and others are often eager to effect change. They like to try something new, to apply the latest technologies; they can do so through the nursing research process. There are two kinds of research activities—those in which nurses are the subjects and those in which they develop their own nursing research program. Real research requires preparation and time.

Nursing Research in the Service Setting

It follows, then, if there is to be research in nursing, and if it is to be part of the organizational goals, there must be planning. Plans incorporate a budget, a staff, and defined problems for research. Staff nurses working in clinical jobs and management personnel usually do not have time for this kind of research. However, they can use the results of such research and apply it to their situation so as to build better health care delivery systems.[29]

A nursing management position filled by a scholar will enhance the chances of a nursing research program being successful. A scholar will have the knowledge to increase nursing administration research of a high intellectual and professional caliber. A nurse researcher can promote the reunification model of nursing education and nursing service through joint appointments and joint nursing research endeavors, supporting cooperation between service and education. Nursing faculty tend to disengage from practice because of the numerous demands of their teaching roles. One reason that faculty focus on wellness may be their disengagement from practice in the service area. Because nursing faculty are often well-prepared scientists, nursing managers should find ways to budget for released time for practice and arrange to pay the school for their work. A coalition will benefit all nurses, because faculty will be recognized for research activities that keep them up to date, and managers will benefit from improved patient care.[30]

Nursing administration scholars will allow clinicians adequate time to develop their projects. They will provide a resource link to help clinicians find research partners with whom they can practice relevant nursing research.[31]

SUMMARY

Ability to manage planned change is a necessary competency of all nurse managers in that it represents viability of the nursing organization. Because planned change is a necessity, nurse managers create the climate for its receptivity by nursing personnel. Change, the key to innovation and the future, has its basis in change theory.

Lewin's change theory is widely used by managers and involves three stages: unfreezing, moving, and refreezing. In the unfreezing stage, employees are made aware of needed changes. A plan for change is made and tested in the moving stage. During the refreezing stage the change becomes a part of the system, establishing homeostasis and equilibrium. Lippitt modified Lewin's original change theory.

Resistance to change is evoked by stress from threatened security of affected employees. It can be overcome by planning that involves those to be affected, particularly if they can see a benefit. Established values and beliefs, imprinting, and time perspectives all stiffen resistance to change.

The nurse manager as change agent is the manager of change and thus requires knowledge of the theory of change. Education and training are necessary for nursing personnel who will be affected. Intrinsic and extrinsic rewards are another management tool. Using groups to effect change will help absorb the risks of change, because risks are part of the process.

Nursing managers can promote change through nursing research, thus committing nursing to a clinical practice based on scholarly inquiry. Promotion of nursing research effects change through application of research findings. Nursing research can be income producing when it produces more effective and efficient nursing prescriptions.

Change involves nurse managers in many functions of nursing. It requires planning. The organization is adapted to accommodate the changes. The nurse manager uses communication, leadership, and motivation theory to overcome resistance and gain support in making the change work. The implemented change is continually evaluated to keep it working and effective.

EXPERIENTIAL EXERCISES

1. Match each reason for designing orderly change in Section I with the correct example from Section II.

I

a. To improve the means of satisfying a person's economic want.

b. To increase profit.

c. To promote human work for people.

d. To help people achieve satisfaction and social well-being.

II

_____ 1.1 A director of nursing has a goal of reducing the amount of time registered nurses spend giving physical care to patients and doing clerical work, because registered nurses are the highest paid members of the staff.

_____ 1.2 Through reorganization of nursing duties, registered nurses will be able to achieve their desire to perform primary patient care—to gather data, make nursing diagnosis and prescription, and supervise the application of medical and nursing care plans.

_____ 1.3 Achievement of the goal should result in more licensed vocational nurses and fewer registered nurses, and increased salaries for both groups.

_____ 1.4 It is a goal to purchase typing equipment that will store original typewritten materials so that, when needed, the materials will have only to be corrected, not retyped.

2. For each of the following statements, place a + in the blank if the statement is true and a − if it is false. Rewrite false statements to make them true.

_____ 2.1 Most changes occurring in nursing relate to methods and procedures in operating machinery and equipment rather than to standards concerning organizational structure and work relationships of employees.

_____ 2.2 Most nursing employees work in environments in which they learn to welcome change as a means of achieving their personal goals.

_____ 2.3 Nursing personnel are apt to resist change when they experience or view it as a threat to their established patterns of behavior.

_____ 2.4 Most nursing employees may view changes in policy, procedure, or work environment as affecting their employment contract in some way, such as more work, changes in pay and other benefits, and changes in the expectations of their employers.

_____ 2.5 People welcome change because they know how it will affect them, and they have had previous pleasurable experiences resulting from change.

_____ 2.6 People fear change because they believe their jobs will be more difficult and require that they do things about which they are ignorant.

_____ 2.7 Culture is important to the management of change.

3. Match each technique for accomplishing change listed in Section I with the correct example from Section II.

I

a. Diagnosis
b. Mutual objective setting
c. Group emphasis
d. Maximum information
e. Discussion of implementation
f. Use of ceremony and ritual
g. Resistance interpretation

II

_____ 3.1 An open house will be held to show the new extended care facility to the people of the community it will serve.

_____ 3.2 When the nursing staff heard that part of the hospital would be closed and renovated into an extended care facility, staff members decided that they would be out of jobs and that they should be looking for new ones. Interviews by the director of nursing when the first resignations came caused her to consult with the administrator. The administrator and director of nursing decided that the entire hospital staff needed to be told about the planned changes so as to avert further rumors and resignations.

_____ 3.3 Some employees were already telling people in the community that their hospital was being closed. The director of nursing decided to meet with the entire nursing staff and discuss the reasons for undermining the plans for the extended care facility. It was long past time to let the staff express its fears and concerns about the change.

_____ 3.4 At this meeting, a group was appointed to represent the nursing staff and to develop objectives for their roles in the changeover. These objectives would be submitted to the director of nursing and the administrator for approval.

_____ 3.5 Several members of the nursing committee would work with other representatives of the hospital staff in making plans to close part of the hospital and open the new facility. One of their objectives was to provide as many services as possible during the construction period. The staff would be educated to provide the new ambulatory care services, particularly those in the rehabilitative and physical medicine area.

_____ 3.6 Because they needed community support, the administrator asked the hospital representatives to submit a list of citizens who could help them to refine the objectives so that they would be seen as meeting needs of both community and institution.

_____ 3.7 Part of the objective setting and planning included preparation of newspaper articles and announcements for use of radio and television media. Progress reports would be issued to the media on a scheduled basis. Speakers would be made available from the citizen-staff planning group.

4. Make each statement true by crossing out the inappropriate word or phrase in parentheses:

_____ 4.1 Knowledge of nurses who do not pursue continuing education within a minimum of (1; 10; 20) years may become obsolete due to technological innovation.

_____ 4.2 Practicing nurses may be more committed to (loyalty to the organization for which they work; task, job, and profession).

_____ 4.3 Nurses gain satisfaction from (being told how they will practice nursing; acting as change agents in deciding how nursing will be practiced).

_____ 4.4 Nurse managers are (holding fast to their authoritarian management practices; changing their management practices to involve their employees in formulating policies and procedures).

_____ 4.5 (Humor and opportunity to be creative; Ritual and job security) represent the environment desired by today's professional nurses.

_____ 4.6 A major change in nursing management activities is to (ignore the needs and goals of the worker while focusing on those of the organization; bring conflict, feelings of dissatisfaction with management practices out into the open).

5. *Scenario:* It was obvious to the entire nursing staff of a community hospital that the workload was decreasing. There were empty beds on every unit. Deliveries on the obstetrical unit were down to an average of one a day, and the daily census of the postpartum unit and newborn nursery was four to six patients. Workload and patient census on the pediatric unit were likewise low. Rumors were rampant. One was that the pediatric and obstetrical units would be combined. Another was that they would both be closed and the patients combined with medical-surgical patients on other units. A third rumor was that the other community hospital was having similar problems and that negotiations were under way to combine several specialty services between the two institutions. It was even rumored that one would become an extended care facility and that the management would be combined. Worries of nursing staff gave way to gossip among various groups in corridors, at coffee breaks, in the dining room and everywhere employees chanced to meet, including areas to which patients were transported such as the x-ray clinic, the physical therapy room, and the medical laboratory. Employees were concerned most about job security and institutional stability—whether there would be jobs for all of them and whether the job benefits would be the same if they worked at either hospital. At a clinical nurse managers' meeting, the director of nursing was asked if any of the rumors were true. She stated that the administrator would make an announcement at the appropriate time, and until then the staff should continue with its work. That afternoon the local newspaper announced a merger of the two hospitals describing in detail the missions and services each would provide to the community. No reference was made to the plans for employees.

Answer the following questions. If the actions taken by the director of nursing and other top managers would create a negative activity, state what that would be.

5.1 What evidence was there that the merger of the two hospitals would harm employees or benefit them and meet their needs?

5.2 What evidence was there that the change would be done in a democratic or an authoritarian manner?

5.3 What evidence was there that the director of nursing promoted harmony or apprehension within her nursing staff?

5.4 What evidence was there that the director of nursing promoted mutual trust and confidence or distrust and lack of confidence between top management and her nursing staff?

5.5 What evidence was there that the director of nursing promoted interdependence and shared responsibility between top management and her staff?

5.6 What evidence was there that the director of nursing acted to contain multigroup membership and responsibility within the hospital staff?

5.7 What evidence was there that top managers acted to share control and responsibility?

5.8 What evidence was there of prevention of conflict through bargaining or problem-solving discussion?

5.9 What evidence was there that concern for employees was as important as concern for patients?

5.10 What evidence was there to demonstrate top management's philosophy and practice?

6. Scan the previous year's issues of *Nursing Research, Journal of Nursing Administration,* and *Nursing Management.* How many articles report

Research in management or administration?
____

Teaching? ____
Practice? ____

7. *Group Exercise:* Change Process

7.1 Organize into groups of approximately five to eight persons. Identify a nursing problem related to work.

7.2 Follow these steps:

7.2.1 What is the problem? What is the single most important activity that requires change?

7.2.2 How is it a problem? What goals of nursing care does it prevent being accomplished?

7.2.3 Why do anything about it? What are the harmful or beneficial effects to patients and/or personnel?

7.2.4 What facts are needed to solve the problem?

7.2.5 What do these facts mean?

7.2.6 What are possible solutions?

7.2.7 What are the probable outcomes?

7.2.8 Put the solution into effect.

NOTES

1. D. McGregor, *Leadership and Motivation* (Cambridge, MA: MIT Press, 1966), 15–16.
2. W. J. Reddin, "How to Change Things," *Executive,* June, 1969, 22–26.
3. B. W. Spradley, "Managing Change Creatively," *Journal of Nursing Administration,* May 1980, 32–37.
4. E. G. Williams, "Changing Systems and Behavior," *Business Horizons,* Aug. 1969, 53–58.
5. R. D. Brynildsen and T. A. Wickes, "Agents of Changes," *Automation,* Oct. 1970. Reprint.
6. Ibid.
7. Spradley, op. cit.; L. B. Welch, "Planned Change in Nursing: The Theory," *Nursing Clinics of North America,* June 1979, 307–321.
8. Ibid.
9. Ibid.
10. Ibid.
11. J. V. Roach, "U.S. Business: Time to Seize the Day," *Newsweek,* Apr. 4, 1988, 10; M. Beyers, "Getting on Top of Organizational Change: Part 1. Process and Development," *Journal of Nursing Administration,* Oct. 1984, 32–39.
12. Williams, op. cit.
13. M. J. Ward and S. G. Moran, "Resistance to Change: Recognize, Respond, Overcome," *Nursing Management,* Jan. 1984, 30–33.
14. R. E. Hunt and M. K. Rigby, "Easing the Pain of Change," *Management Review,* Sept. 1984, 41–45.
15. Ibid.
16. D. Niland, "Managing Change: Same Staff, Same Unit— New Role," *Nursing Management,* Dec. 1985, 31–32.
17. Ward and Moran, op. cit.
18. Beyers, op. cit.
19. Ibid.
20. Ibid.; D. J. Gillen, "Harvesting the Energy from Change Anxiety," *Supervisory Management,* Mar. 1986, 40–43.
21. Gillen, op. cit.
22. Hunt and Rigby, op. cit.
23. Ward and Moran, op. cit.
24. R. E. Endres, "Successful Management of Change," *Notes & Quotes,* Nov. 1972, 3.
25. Hunt and Rigby, op. cit.
26. Beyers, op. cit.
27. T. R. Horton, "Poised for Tomorrow," *Newsweek,* Oct. 5, 1987, S–4.
28. M. L. McClure, "Promoting Practice-Based Research: A Critical Need," *Journal of Nursing Administration,* Nov.-Dec. 1981, 66–70; American Hospital Association, *Strategies: Integration of Nursing Research into the Practice Setting* (Chicago: AHA Nurse Executive Management Strategies, 1985).
29. R. C. Swansburg, *Management of Patient Care Services* (St. Louis, MO: C. V. Mosby, 1968), 334.
30. McClure, op. cit.
31. K. P. Krone and M. E. Loomis, "Developing Practice-Relevant Research: A Model That Worked," *Journal of Nursing Administration,* Apr. 1982, 38–41.

FOR FURTHER REFERENCE

Beyers, M., "Getting on Top of Organizational Change: Part 2. Trends in Nursing Service," *Journal of Nursing Administration,* Nov. 1984, 31–37.

Comella, T., "Understanding Creativity," *Notes & Quotes,* reprint from *Automation,* Apr. 1966 (Hartford: Connecticut General Life Insurance Company, Sept. 1966).

Drucker, P. F., "Creating Strategies of Innovation," *Planning Review,* Nov. 1985, 8–11, 45.

Feldman, J., and Daly-Gawenda, D., "Retrenchment: How Nurse Executives Cope," *Journal of Nursing Administration,* June 1985, 31–37.

Glucksberg, S., "Some Ways to Turn on New Ideas," *Think* (IBM), Mar.-Apr. 1968, 24–28.

Godfrey, R. R., "Tapping Employees' Creativity," *Supervisory Management*, Feb. 1986, 16–20.

Gordon, J., and Zemke, R, "Making Them More Creative," *Training*, May 1986, 30ff.

Hefferin, E. A., Horsley, J. A., and Ventura, M. R., "Promoting Research-Based Nursing: The Nurse Administrator's Role," *Journal of Nursing Administration*, May 1982, 34–41.

Henry, B. M., Moody, L. E., O'Donnell, J., Pendergust, J., and Hutchinson, S., *National Nursing Administration Research Priorities Study*, Division of Nursing, Bureau of Health Professionals, Health Resources and Services Administration, US PHS (R01 NU 01085), Oct. 30, 1985, 19.

Kanter, R. M., *The Change Masters* (New York: Simon & Schuster, 1983). Material from workshop presented by Dr. Kanter.

Lattimer, R. L., and Winitsky, M. L., "Unleashing Creativity," *Management World*, Apr. 1984, 22–24.

Levinson, H., "What an Executive Should Know about Scientists," *Notes & Quotes*, reprint (Hartford: Connecticut General Life Insurance Company, Nov. 1965), 1.

Lindeman, C. A., and Schantz, D., "The Research Question," *Journal of Nursing Administration*, Jan. 1982, 6–10.

"Managing to Improve Value," *Managing Change* (Travenol Management Services, Spring 1985).

Newcomb, D. P., and Swansburg, R. C., *The Team Plan: A Manual for Nursing Service Administrators*, 2d ed. (New York: G. P. Putnam's Sons, 1971): 136–172.

"Peter Drucker—On Managing the New," *Newsweek*, Oct. 1988, S6–S7.

Reinkemeyer, Sr. M. H., "A Nursing Paradox," *Nursing Research*, Jan.-Feb. 1968, 8.

Rutigliano, A. J., "An Interview with Peter Drucker: Managing the New," *Management Review*, Jan. 1986, 38–41.

Schantz, D., and Lindeman, C. A., "Reading a Research Article," *Journal of Nursing Administration*, Mar. 1982, 30–33.

Schantz, D., and Lindeman, C. A., "The Research Design," *Journal of Nursing Administration*, Feb. 1982, 35–38.

Van Gundy, A. G., "How to Establish a Creative Climate in the Work Group," *Management Review*, Aug. 1984, 24–25, 28, 37–38.

· 11 ·

Organizing Nursing Services

ORGANIZATIONAL THEORY

Introduction

Once plans are made, the mission, purpose, or business for which the organization exists has been established, the philosophy has been developed and adopted, and the objectives have been formulated, resources are organized to sustain the philosophy and to accomplish the mission and objectives. Organizations develop as goals become too complex for the individual and have to be divided into units that individuals can manage.[1]

Fayol referred to the organizing element of management as the form of the body corporate and stated that the organization takes on form when the number of workers rises to the level requiring a supervisor. It is necessary to group people, distribute duties, and adapt the organic whole to requirements by putting essential employees where they will be most useful. An intermediate executive is the generator of power and ideas.[2] The body corporate of the nursing organization includes executive management and its staff, departmental managers (middle managers), technical managers (first line managers), and practicing professional and technical nursing personnel. Professional nursing personnel manage the performance of technical nursing personnel. In a theory of nursing management, nurse managers have as their object the development of a nursing organization that facilitates the work of clinical nurses.

Definitions of Organizing

Urwick referred to organizing as the process of designing the machine. It should allow for personal adjustments, but these will be minimal if a design is followed. It should show the part each person will play in the general social pattern, as well as the responsibilities, relationships, and standards of performance. Jobs should be put together along lines of functional specializations to facilitate the training of replacements. The organizational structure must be based on sound principles, including that of continuity, to provide for the future.[3]

Organizing is the grouping of activities for the

purpose of achieving objectives, the assignment of such groupings to a manager with authority for supervising each group, and the defined means of coordinating appropriate activities with other units, horizontally and vertically, that are responsible for accomplishing organizational objectives. Organizing involves the process of deciding the necessary levels of organization needed to accomplish the objectives of a nursing division, department or service, and unit. For the unit it would involve the type of work to be accomplished in terms of direct patient care, the kinds of nursing personnel needed to accomplish this work, and the span of management or supervision needed.

Principles of Organizing

The Principle of Chain of Command. The chain-of-command principle states that to be satisfying to members, economically effective, and successful in achieving their goals, organizations are established with hierarchical relationships within which authority flows from top to bottom. This principle supports a mechanistic structure with a centralized authority that aligns authority and responsibility. Communication flows through the chain of command and tends to be one way—downward. In a modern nursing organization the chain of command is flat, with line managers and a technical and clerical staff that support the clinical nurse staff.

The Principle of Unity of Command. The unity-of-command principle states that an employee has one supervisor and there is one leader and one plan for a group of activities with the same objective. This principle is still followed in most nursing organizations but is increasingly modified by emerging organizational theory. Primary nursing and case management support the principle of unity of command, as does joint practice.

The Principle of Span of Control. The span-of-control principle states that a person should be a supervisor of a group that he or she can effectively supervise in terms of numbers, functions, and geography. This original principle has become an elastic one—the more highly trained the employee, the less supervision is needed. Employees in training need more supervision to prevent blunders. When different levels of nursing employees are used, the nurse manager must coordinate more.

The Principle of Specialization. The principle of specialization is that each person should perform a single leading function. Thus there is a division of labor: a differentiation among kinds of duties. Specialization is thought by many to be the best way to use individuals and groups. The chain of command joins groups by specialty leading to functional departmentalization.

The hierarchy or scalar chain is a natural result of these principles of organizing. It is the order of rank, from top to bottom in an organization. These principles of organizing are interdependent and dynamic when used by nurse managers to create a stimulating environment in which to practice clinical nursing.

Bureaucracy

Bureaucracy evolved from the early principles of administration including those of organizing. It is a term coined by Max Weber. Bureaucracy is highly structured and usually includes no participation by the governed. The principles of chain of command, unity of command, span of control, and specialization support bureaucratic structures. These structures do not work in their pure form and have been greatly adapted in today's organizations.

Among the historically strong points of bureaucratic organizations is their ability to produce employees who are competent and responsible. They perform by uniform rules and conventions, are accountable to one manager who is an authority, maintain social distance with supervisors and clients, thereby reducing favoritism and promoting impersonality, and receive rewards based on technical qualifications, seniority, and achievement.

The characteristics of bureaucracy include formality, low autonomy, a climate of rules and conventionality, division of labor, specialization, standardized procedures, written specifications, memos and minutes, centralization, controls, and emphasis on a high level of efficiency and production. These characteristics frequently lead to complaints about red tape, and to procedural delays and general frustration.[4]

A conclusion could be that the less bureaucratic the organization the more nurses will perceive themselves as professionals.

Role Theory. Role theory indicates that when employees face inconsistent expectations and lack of information they will experience role conflict, leading to stress, dissatisfaction, and ineffective performance. Role theory supports the chain-of-command and unity-of-command principles. Multiple lines of authority are disruptive, divide authority between profession and organization, and create stress. They force employees to make choices between formal authority and professional colleagues. The result is role conflict and dissatisfaction for employees and reduced efficiency and effectiveness for the organization. Role conflict reduces trust, personal liking, and esteem for the person in authority; reduces communication; and decreases employee effectiveness. Rizzo, House, and Lirtzman indicate that role conflict and ambiguity can be reduced by management that provides for:

1. Certainty about duties, authority, allocation of time, and relationship with others
2. Guides, directives, policies, and the ability to predict sanctions as outcomes of behavior
3. Increased need fulfillment
4. Structure and standards
5. Facilitation of teamwork
6. Toleration of freedom
7. Upward influence
8. Consistency
9. Prompt decisions
10. Good, prompt communication and information
11. Using the chain of command
12. Personal development
13. Formalization
14. Planning
15. Receptiveness to ideas by top management
16. Coordinating work plans
17. Adapting to change
18. Adequacy of authority

The implications for nurse managers are obvious. Role conflict and role ambiguity are separate dimensions, role conflict being more dysfunctional. Some employees find stress rewarding.[5]

Organizational Development

Organizational development (OD) deals with changing the work environment to make it more conducive to worker satisfaction and productivity. An underlining premise is that "people planning" is as important as technical and financial planning. OD allows managers to attend to the psychological as well as the physical aspects of organizations. Change is the terrain in which OD applies.

OD can sustain the favorable or desirable aspects of bureaucracy. Change can be used to modify the undesirable aspects of bureaucracy. There is room for directive as well as nondirective leadership within organizations. Nurse managers have to be strong and tough in supporting the values of clinical nurses. They have to be proactive in planning, designing, and implementing new organizational structures and work environments. The object is to develop people, not to exploit them. OD emphasizes personal growth and interpersonal competence.[6]

Autonomy and Accountability. Among the psychological and personality attributes of OD are autonomy and accountability, crucial elements of nursing professionalism. A professional nurse is obligated to answer for decisions and actions. According to Johnson and Luciano this would be achieved using a management by results (MBR) approach. They developed a performance management program for unit supervisors that defined performance standards, incorporating acceptable behavior and results. It included tracking for progress, performance feedback, making adjustments, and personnel accountability.[7]

Characteristics of professional autonomy include self-definition, self-regulation, and self-governance. Professional nurses respond to demographic changes in society to define and reshape the content of nursing practice. They address society's needs, including the need for increased care for the elderly and the control of resources. Autonomy will be strengthened by unbundling the hospital bill and by direct reimbursement for nursing services by third-party payers.

Self-governance for nursing includes a nursing administrator hired or elected with input from nurses, self-employment for nurses, approval of nursing staff privileges by peer review with privileges revoked by the nursing staff organization, and case management.[8]

Culture. Organizational culture is the sum total of an organization's beliefs, norms, values, philosophies, traditions, and sacred cows. It is a social system that is a subsystem of the total organization. Organizational cultures have artifacts, perspectives, values, assumptions, symbols, language, and behaviors that have been effective.

Organizational cultures include communication networks, both formal and informal. They include a status/role structure that relates to characteristics of employees and customers or clients. Such structures also relate to management style, whether authoritarian or participatory. Management style impacts individual behavior greatly. In a health care setting these structures promote either individuality or teamwork. They relate to classes of people and could be identified through demographic surveys of both employees and patients.

The basic mission of the organization is part of its culture: employment, service, learning, and research. There is a technical or *operational system* for getting the work done. Also, there is an *administrative system* of wages and salaries, of hiring, firing, and promoting, of report making and quality control, of fringe benefits, and of budgeting.

The artifacts of an organizational culture may be physical, behavioral (rituals), or verbal (language, stories, myths). Verbal artifacts result from shared values and beliefs. They include traditions, heroes, and the party line, and result in ceremonies that embody rituals. They include ceremonies to reward years of service, the annual picnic, the Christmas party, and the wearing of badges and insignia.[9]

Perspectives are shared ideas and actions. They relate to decision-making methods. For example, social, technical, and managerial systems or subsystems will either support innovation or demand conformity.[10]

Dress, personal appearance, social decorum, and the physical environment are all part of the organizational culture. They will require strict compliance through written or implied rules.

Values are the general principles, ideals, standards, and sins of the organization. Basic assumptions are the core of the culture. They include the beliefs groups have about themselves, others, and the world.

Culture and the Manager.

When output or productivity decreases in amount or kind, managers look at the social, technical, and managerial systems that are part of the organization culture. They know that people behave in accordance with their understanding of the organization's norms and values. If they want to be successful they identify these norms and values and apply their efforts in conformity with them.

A successful manager identifies and accepts the prevailing culture before making changes. It is more difficult to change a culture at the level of basic beliefs, values, and perspectives. It is easier to change technical and administrative systems.

Research indicates that a strong culture that encourages participation and involvement of employees in shared decision making affects an organization's performance positively. Such organizations outperform competitors two to one in return on investments and sales. The organizational culture can be influenced by the CEO.[11]

Climate.

Organizational climate is the emotional state shared by members of the system. It can be formal, relaxed, defensive, cautious, accepting, trusting, and so on. It is employees' subjective impression or perception of their organization. The employees of major concern to nurse managers are the practicing nurses. Practicing nurses create, or at the very least contribute to the creation of, the climate perceived by patients. The work climate set by nurse managers determines the behavior of the practicing nurses in setting the work climate.

Practicing nurses want a climate that will give them job satisfaction. They achieve job satisfaction when they are challenged and their achievements recognized and appreciated by managers and patients. They achieve satisfaction from a climate of collegiality with managers and other health care providers, in which they participate in decision making.

Many studies have been done to determine work climate within business, industry, and health care organizations. One head nurse designed and implemented a project to motivate the nursing staff of a medical unit to better service and greater self-satisfaction. She designed an "employee of the month" motivational strategy that included measurable performance criteria. Although the staff were initially disinterested, they eventually increased their interest and participation. Productivity also increased, as did emergence of talents. The strategy culminated in a recognition ceremony, a free lunch or dinner, and the employee's picture on the bulletin board. By the end of 6 months 25 out of 144 employees had earned the title, their voluntary participation indicating that it met some of their needs.[12]

Activities to Promote a Positive Organizational Climate.

1. Develop the organization's mission, goals, and objectives with input from practicing nurses. Include their personal goals.
2. Establish trust and openness through communication that includes prompt and frequent feedback and stimulates motivation.
3. Provide opportunities for growth and develop-

ment, including career development and continuing education programs.

4. Promote teamwork.
5. Ask practicing nurses to state their satisfactions and dissatisfactions during meetings and conferences and through surveys.
6. Market the nursing organization to the practicing nurses, other employees, and the public.
7. Follow through on activities involving practicing nurses.
8. Analyze the compensation system for the entire nursing organization and structure it to reward competence, longevity, and productivity.
9. Promote self-esteem, autonomy, and self-fulfillment for practicing nurses, including feelings that their work experiences are of high quality.
10. Emphasize programs to recognize practicing nurses' contributions to the organization.
11. Assess unneeded threats and punishments and eliminate them.
12. Provide job security with an environment that enables free expression of ideas and exchange of opinions without threat of recrimination, which may occur as negative performance reports, negative counseling, confrontation, conflict, or job loss.
13. Be inclusive in all relationships with practicing nurses.
14. Help practicing nurses to overcome their shortcomings and develop their strengths.
15. Encourage and support loyalty, friendliness, and civic consciousness.
16. Develop strategic plans that include decentralization of decision making and participation by practicing nurses.
17. Be a role model of performance desired of practicing nurses.

Team Building. The commonly used terms related to the state of "feelings" of an organizational climate are "good morale" or "poor morale." Morale is a state of mind that refers to the zeal or enthusiasm with which someone works. A person who works courageously and confidently, with discipline and willingness to endure hardship would be manifesting a high or good morale. Poor morale is evident in the person who is timid, cowardly, devious, fearful, diffident, disorderly, unruly, rebellious, turbulent, or indifferent as a result of job dissatisfaction and organizational milieu.

Morale is a motivation factor related to productivity and product or service quality outcomes. Firms want high morale among employees and actively promote it.

A team is a group of two or more workers striving for a common purpose or mission. They depend on each other. The leader will emerge (if not appointed) as the person sustaining the confidence of the group. Confidence will be sustained by the leader's expertise in their purpose or mission and the enthusiasm expressed by the leader's verbal and nonverbal behavior. High enthusiasm by the leader will spark high enthusiasm within the group, thereby boosting group morale and stimulating their esprit de corps, their spirit and sense of pride and honor.

One continually hears such remarks as, "This organization does not care about the employees!" or, "This organization really cares about its employees!" It goes without saying that nurse managers want to hear the positive statement. People who have low morale are not satisfied with their work. Dissatisfied workers will not contribute positively to esprit de corps.

Nurses who have high self-esteem are energetic, confident, take pride in their work, have genuine respect and concern for patients, visitors, colleagues, and others. Their self-worth is evident in their behavior including their language. They are committed to excellence in patient care. These nurses have high morale. They work with esprit de corps.

The objective of team building is to establish an environment of cohesiveness among shift personnel and among different shifts in a unit. This is extended to other units, the department, and division. The first step in team building is to find out why nursing employees are unhappy or dissatisfied. This can be accomplished through a questionnaire although an open meeting is probably best. The meeting will be more productive if it is held away from the unit, to eliminate interruptions and the shadow of the organization.

The head nurse or other manager can assume the leadership or allow the group to select a leader. In any event, the nurse manager will have to explain what the effort is all about and what the group is supposed to accomplish. Begin with identification of satisfactions if possible, to set a positive note.

Next, the leader must focus on identifying problems and prioritizing them for action. If the nurse manager can assume the role of facilitator rather than leader, the group will probably proceed at a faster pace.

Once problems or dissatisfactions are identified, a calendar should be established for addressing them. It is important to make a schedule of meetings and attendees for all phases of teambuilding activities. Meetings should be held at times most of the staff can be there. They should be short and focused on the problems, in priority sequence. It is best to make a brief management plan that includes the problem, objectives, actions the team can accomplish on its own authority, actions needing management support, persons assigned specific responsibilities, target dates, and a list of accomplishments.

As the plan is put into effect it should be communicated to the entire staff of the unit, department, or division. Evaluation should occur on a continuous basis to keep the momentum going. Each person can be encouraged to fulfill commitments, and everyone's accomplishments should be recognized. Although each shift can work on their own plans, an occasional open forum of personnel on all three shifts is essential for intershift problems.

Recognition of the individual worth of the individual nurse is an important morale builder. It gives the individual self-esteem. Managers can stimulate self-esteem with praise that promotes a sense of competence, success, and worth. Nurse managers have to feel worthy before they can nurture that feeling in subordinates. Each nurtures the other. Managers who have self-esteem are not afraid to explore their personal feelings with colleagues or subordinates.

Those professional nurses who think highly of themselves and believe that others do too, take risks in their personal relationships. They give and seek praise, love, support, and participation. All grow stronger and feel more worthy.

Many professional women depend on their jobs as a major source of self-esteem. For this reason nurse managers should aspire to building a milieu to develop and enhance the self-esteem of all nurses. Such a milieu promotes outstanding performance.

Praise is even more important when the environment is beset with shortages and stresses. Managers gain self-esteem from the success of their employees. They must supplement it with outside activities such as sports, hobbies, recreation, volunteer work, and work in service and professional organizations.[13]

Recognition can be made with a special plaque, commendation in a local paper or other medium, group social activities, gifts, and group service activities. Consider the benefits of scheduled versus surprise recognition activities. Nave and Thomas suggest fifty specific techniques to boost employee morale.[14] See Figure 11–1.

Many simple things can be done to improve the working environment. Involving the best workers in the decision-making process rewards the best performers and alerts others. One group had a monthly "warm fluffy day" when they complimented each employee and gave them a cotton ball on a pin. It produced spirit![15]

Though people will participate in team building they still want to retain their individuality. Nurse managers provide leadership that is flexible, fair, mindful of tasks and people, inspires, and models the role of professional nurse.[16]

DEVELOPING AN ORGANIZATIONAL STRUCTURE

An organizational structure for a division of nursing must meet the needs of that division as written in the statements of mission, philosophy, and objectives. Most existing institutions already have an organizational structure. Before it is changed, the nurse manager(s) should engage in a systematic analysis as well as some sound thinking about altering its design and structure, starting with objectives and strategy.

Objectives have already been discussed. Strategy covers the key activities of nursing that determine the purpose of the organizational structure. Nursing strategy will indicate the present business of nursing, its future business, and what its business should actually be. The organizational structure allows, supports, and promotes nursing functions consistent with organizational mission, philosophy, and objectives.

Work Activities and Functions

Work activities and functions that will be analyzed and encompassed in identifying the building blocks of organization include:

1. Operating work at the unit level, including primary nursing care (the basic mission, not the method or modality of nursing); operational nursing management, commonly referred to as head nurse and/or clinical nurse manager activities; and support activities essential to the application of primary nursing care, such as training, clerical work, and others. Management at the unit level includes management of the clinical component of direct nursing care and management of nonnursing or indirect activities.

Listed below are fifty of the techniques identified. In reviewing them, remember that there is no best answer for anyone. That is best which best suits your organization.

1. Supervisors greet employees with a handshake as the employees begin their shifts.

2. Supervisors write personal notes such as "Thank You" or "Happy Birthday" on payroll checks.

3. Members of employee groups meet regularly with management representatives to promote understanding, and carry out activities of mutual interest.

4. Employees and management work side by side once a year on a community help project.

5. Employers are personally congratulated by supervisors when they exceed their goals.

6. Supervisors personally introduce new hires to each employee.

7. An employee's years of service are noted each year on the anniversary date of employment in a plaque or poster in the lobby.

8. When department supervisors enter the employee lounge, they treat all employees who happen to be there to a cup of coffee.

9. Supervisors personally hand employees in their department a silver dollar at Christmas as a "little something extra."

10. Relations with retired employees are maintained by means of an annual breakfast and personal delivery by the supervisors of a box of Christmas candy each year.

11. A cash reward is given each month to the employee with the "best idea" for the firm.

12. Part-time employees are invited to all social events.

13. The chief executive officer periodically has "brown bag" luncheon discussions with employees at which their concerns are addressed.

14. Employees are allowed to accept telephone calls at any time.

15. Letters of commendation are sent to employees for performance above and beyond normal expectations. Copies of the letter are included in the employees' personnel files.

16. The plant manager cooks at the supervisor's picnic. At another firm, supervisors serve the food at a company picnic.

17. Birthday cards are signed by the president of the firm or immediate supervisor and are sent to the employees' homes.

18. Free popcorn is always available to employees and customers.

19. Employee birthdays are celebrated with cake and by singing "Happy Birthday."

20. The safety department issues a monthly "safety for the family" newsletter that is mailed directly to the employees' home.

21. Free meals are provided in the company cafeteria for employees working on special days such as Christmas, Thanksgiving, and the like.

22. At irregular intervals managers provide food for employees to munch in the break area.

23. Softdrinks, coffee, and/or snacks are provided for staff at departmental meetings.

24. Flexible working hours are permitted during slow work times.

25. Morale-building meetings are held at which management informs employees of the firm's successes.

26. Brief meetings are scheduled for all new employees with staff from the business office, security, facilities management, and the like to familiarize new hires with policies and procedures.

27. A worker is recognized by being named "Employee of the Week" or "Employee of the Month." The recognition takes many forms, including presentation of a plaque, lunch with the president or supervisor, gifts, and mention in the company newsletter.

28. An activities committee has been established to plan social events, and new employees are introduced to a member of this committee so they become aware of company activities.

29. Snacks are available during employees' first break each day.

30. Employees missing one day or less due to illness or injury during the year receive a gift.

Figure 11–1 • *Fifty Specific Techniques to Boost Employee Morale*

(Continued)

31. Factory eating areas are decorated on special occasions.

32. Free coffee is provided on special days.

33. Once a quarter, ten to twelve employees selected by random drawing are taken on a guided tour of all plant facilities and have lunch on the house in the plant cafeteria.

34. A Halloween costume contest is held each year, employees wear their costumes the work day, and the winner receives one day off with pay.

35. Receptions are given for every employee who retires.

36. In each month that new accounts exceed an established figure, all employees are taken out for dinner.

37. An annual awards banquet is held for employees on the last working day before a holiday.

38. Annual parties for occasions such as Christmas are given by the company.

39. An appropriate gift is distributed to all employees daily, weekly, or monthly, when a production record is established.

40. A cash drawing is held each month that there is no employee time lost due to accident. Variation: A drawing is held each

month for employees who have not missed time due to injury or illness.

41. An annual employee appreciation dinner is given by the company.

42. Lunch and entertainment are provided "on the grounds" for all employees two or three times each year.

43. Some food for snacking is supplied by the company on a daily basis.

44. Positive comments on an employee by a customer result in the employee receiving a silver pin. Three such compliments during the year earn a gold pin.

45. Special food items are given to all employees on occasions such as Thanksgiving or Christmas.

46. Occasional boat rides on a cruiser are made available to all employees.

47. Company-wide potluck luncheons are held.

48. One firm sponsors a daily 15-minute radio program on which one of the employees is recognized/spotlighted.

49. When a new safety record is reached, employees receive a small memento and attend a "cook-out" hosted by management.

50. Lunch is provided for all employees on the last working day before a holiday.

Figure 11–1   (*Continued*)

2. In a fair-sized or big-business type of nursing organization there may be a need for middle managers, commonly referred to as supervisors or clinical coordinators. This would occur in a large university health care complex or a medical center complex. The division of nursing may even be big enough to require a management team for clinical services, organized as departments, such as medical and pediatric nursing. The functions identified will determine the design, the structure, and determination of how many people are needed for top management or middle management jobs. An assistant chairman may be part of the top management group.

3. In any health care institution, top management functions must be performed. In a small division the nurse manager will be top manager of the department and a member of top management of the institution. Within a large division with multiple missions and objectives there will likely exist enough functions and activities for a top manage-

ment team in the division of nursing. The chair will still be a member of top management of the institution, functioning at the strategic planning level in both instances.

4. A technostructure of staff of varying size, depending on the size of the institution, will support the management and clinical components of the nursing organization. These will include experts in infection control, staff development, oncology nursing, quality assurance, and others. In some organizations they are labelled consultants.

5. A need for innovative work would be identified and planned for in designing the organizational structure. It could be assigned to operating level, top management level, or a staff function, the latter being a support activity not in the direct line of authority. It will need top management support but a strategy separate from the management strategy with its own mission, objectives, operational plans, and measurements.

Forms of Organizational Structure

There are two common forms of organizational structures, hierarchical and free-form. A mixture of both is needed in nursing.

Hierarchical Structures. A hierarchical structure is commonly called a line structure. It is the oldest and simplest form and is associated with the principle of chain of command, bureaucracy and a multi-tiered hierarchy, vertical control and coordination, levels differentiated by function and authority, and downward communications. These structures have all of the advantages and disadvantages of a bureaucracy. Most line structures have added a staff component. In nursing organizations both line and staff personnel will usually be professional nurses.

Free-Form Structures. Free-form organizational structures are called *matrix* organizations. The matrix organization design enables timely response to external competition and facilitates efficiency and effectiveness internally through cooperation among disciplines.

Characteristics of a matrix organization include:

1. Maintenance of old-line authority structures.
2. Specialist resources obtained from functional areas.
3. Promotion of formation of new organizational units.
4. Occurrence of decision making at the organizational level of group consensus, the middle management level.
5. The matrix manager exercising authority over the functional manager.
6. Cooperative planning of program development and allocation of resources to accomplish program objectives.
7. Assignment of functional managers to teams that respond to the chief of the functional disipline and matrix manager.[17]

Advantages of matrix nursing organizational structures include:

1. Improved communication through vertical and horizontal control and coordination of interdisciplinary patient care teams.
2. Increased organizational adaptability and fluidity to respond to environmental changes.
3. Increased efficiency of resource use with fewer organizational levels and decision making closer to primary care operations.

4. Improved human resource management because of increased job satisfaction with achievement and fulfillment, improved communication, improved interpersonal skills, and improved collegial relationships.[18]

Disadvantages of matrix nursing organizational structures include:

1. Potential conflict because of dual or multiple lines of authority, responsibility, and accountability relationships.
2. Role ambiguity.
3. Loss of control over functional discipline due to multidisciplinary team approach.[19]

Adhocracy. "Adhocracy" models of organization are like matrix models. There are simple teams or task forces that exist on an ad hoc basis. They are formed, complete their goals, and are disbanded; new groups are then formed to meet changing and dynamic mission and objectives.[20]

Matrix and adhocracy models employ participatory management. Xerox is an example of a company that has successfully used self-managing work teams. They once exceeded cost reduction targets of $3.7 million by $1 million. The expert is the authority that leads the team. They are consultative organizations that delegate rather than tell. They encourage maverick behavior and reward results. Of 360 manufacturing companies studied, the forty-one that were most successful had fewer employees per sale; encouraged risk taking; had fewer headquarters staff; had decentralized decision making; and had self-contained units or cost centers.[21]

Line functions are those that have direct responsibility for accomplishing the objectives of a nursing department (or service or unit). For the most part, they include registered nurses, licensed practical nurses, and nursing technicians. Staff functions are those that assist the line in accomplishing the primary objectives of nursing. These include clerical, personnel, budgeting and finance, staff development, research, and specialized clinical consultants. The relationships between line and staff are a matter of authority. Line has authority for direct supervision of employees, while staff provide advice and counsel. There may be line authority within a staff section.

Line sections may act in a staff capacity when they give advice or consultation to another line section. Authority for decision making may be based on staff recommendations but is a line function.

To make staff effective, top management assures that line and staff authority relationships are clearly defined. Personnel of both must work to make their relationships effective; they attempt to minimize friction by increasing mutual trust and respect.

Functional authority occurs when an individual or department is delegated authority over functions in one or more other departments. This has occurred in the development of infection control and quality assurance systems where professional nurses have line authority to hospital management and staff authority to nursing management, or line authority to nursing management and staff authority to other divisions. They do this through delegated authority to consult and prescribe procedures and sometimes policies, for the function as it is to be carried out in the other departments. These delegated authority functions are clearly defined and carefully restricted. They are usually limited to procedures and time frames and do not include personnel or content. They should not weaken or destroy the authority, and thus the effectiveness, of line managers. For example, staff personnel might be assigned to recruit nurses with line managers retaining final authority over hiring. The nurse administrator should assure effective use of staff functions by line managers so as to use effective use of the advice of experts and reduce duplication of effort of line managers. Staff give information that will facilitate the solution of problems. Such information is sought by line managers in an effective and cooperative relationship.

Figure 11–2 shows a set of standards for evaluating the effectiveness of line and staff relationships within a nursing division, department, or unit.

ANALYZING ORGANIZATIONAL STRUCTURE IN A DIVISION OF NURSING

There are six main steps in analyzing the organizational structure of a division of nursing. They should be used when major organizational problems occur, such as friction among department heads over authority, staffing problems, and the like. These steps also apply to organizing a new corporation, division, or unit, and to reorganizing.

Step 1. Compile a list of the key activities determined by the mission and objectives of patient care. The written philosophy will help by indicating important values to be considered. Once this list is completed it must be analyzed. Group simi-

Standards

1. Line authority relationships are clearly delineated and defined by the organizational and/or functional charts and policies.
2. Staff authority relationships are clearly delineated and defined by the organizational and/or functional charts and policies.
3. Functional authority relationships are clearly delineated and defined by the organizational and/or functional charts and policies.
4. Staff personnel are providing consultation, advice, and counsel to line personnel.
5. Service personnel functions are clearly understood by line and staff personnel.
6. Line personnel seek and effectively use staff services.
7. Appropriate staff services are being provided for line nursing personnel and other organizational departments or services.
8. Services are not being duplicated due to line and staff authority relationships.

Figure 11–2 • Standards for Evaluation of the Effectiveness of Line and Staff Relationships within a Nursing Division, Department, or Unit

lar activities together. What are the central load-carrying elements? Most will be related to primary care; philosophy will usually dictate that excellence of patient care is a requirement for the accomplishment of objectives.

Whenever the strategy changes, the organizational structure should be reviewed and analyzed. This includes changes in mission, philosophy, objectives, and the operational plan for accomplishing the objectives. The analysis of key activities can be done according to the kinds of contributions made. These will include the following:

1. Results-producing activities related to direct patient care, such as the nursing process.
2. Support activities, which may include audit, advice, and teaching.
3. Hygiene and housekeeping activities.
4. Top management activities, including "conscience" activities such as vision, values, standards, and audit as well as managing people, marketing, and innovation.

Service staffs such as those performing advisory and training support should be limited. They should be required to abandon an old activity before starting a new one. Prevent them from building empires as a career. Informational activities are the responsibility of top management though they stem from support activities such as controller and treasurer. There must be a system for disseminating information. Hygiene and housekeeping need the attention of nurses if they are to be done well and cheaply. This does not mean that nurses will do these tasks; rather nurses should recognize their importance and support and facilitate their being done by the appropriate departments. Contract services are the answer in some instances.

Step 2. Based on the work functions to be performed, decide on the units of the organization. Decision analysis will be important here, because it must be decided which kinds of decisions will be required and who will make them. Decisions involving functions of future commitments may have to be a top management function, depending on the degree of futurity of a decision and the speed with which it can be reversed. It will be necessary to analyze the impact of decisions on other functions, the number of functions involved being an important factor. Qualitative factors such as decisions involving ethical values, principles of conduct, and social and political beliefs will have to be analyzed. The frequency of the decision will influence its placement: Is it recurrent, or is it rare?

In principle, all decisions should be placed at the lowest level and as close to the operational scene as possible.

Step 3. Decide which units or components will be joined and which separated. Join activities that make the same kind of contribution. This will require relations analysis and will be related to the sequence of key activities or functions.

Step 4. Decide on the size and shape of the units or components.

Step 5. Decide on appropriate placement and relationships of different units or components. This will result from the relations analysis. There should be the smallest possible number of relationships, with each being made to count.

Step 6. Draw or diagram the design and put it in operation. This will result in an organizational chart or schema.

Steps 3, 4, and 5 involve *departmentation*, the grouping of personnel according to some charac-

teristic. Departmentation is an organizing process. Functional departmentation includes grouping units with similar goals such as medical, surgical, pediatric, and obstetric. Time departmentation includes grouping by shift. Territory departmentation is grouping of activities according to geography or physical plant. This is more common in organizations with geographically separated units. Product departmentation includes weight control, behavior modification (such as to stop smoking), and women's health care, among others.

ORGANIZATION CHARTS

Most nursing organizations have made graphic representations of the organizing process in the form of organization charts. These charts usually show reporting relationships and communication channels. Line charts show supervisor and supervisee relationships from top to bottom of the nursing organization. These are hierarchical relationships on which communication channels follow the line of authority to and through the chief nurse executive. Figure 11–3 is an example.

Staff charts show the advisory relationship of specialists or experts who are extensions of the nurse administrators. These types of charts usually depict the title or rank of each line and staff officer position in the authority relationship structure. They denote the delegation of authority and responsibility as well as the direction of accountability for the goals of the nursing division. Figure 11–4 illustrates a staff chart.

Some organization charts depict dual reporting relationships of functional staff as shown in Figure 11–5.

Figure 11–6 depicts a matrix organizational chart.

Organization charts distribute the nursing responsibilities. These responsibilities may be divided according to one or a combination of functions: contiguous geography, similar techniques, similar objectives, or like clientele.

Organization charts are sometimes referred to as schemas. Decentralized schemas are flatter since there are fewer levels of control or management. Managers have more freedom to act and the emphasis is placed on results.

Figure 11–7 shows how to evaluate an organization chart of a nursing division or department or unit.

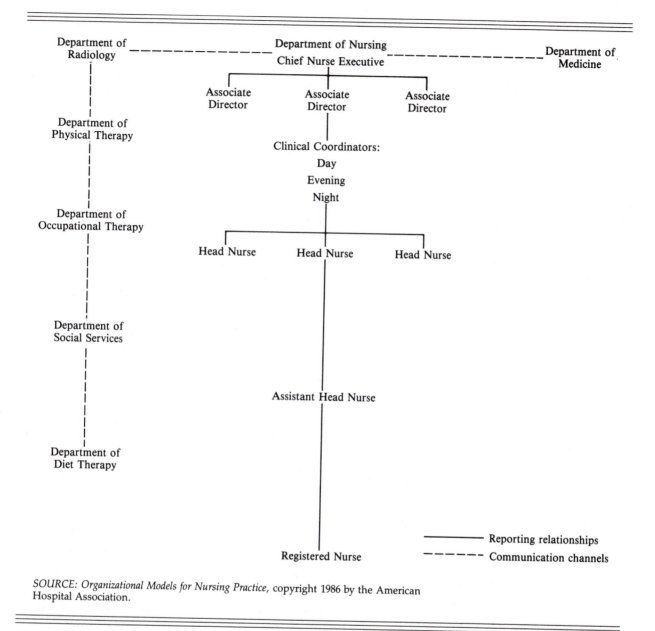

Figure 11–3 • Line

THE INFORMAL ORGANIZATION

Every formal organization has an informal one. The informal organization meets the needs of individuals with similar backgrounds, values, hobbies, interests, and physical proximity. It meets their needs for gregariousness—for sharing experiences and feelings. Some administrators try to hinder the effects of informal organizations because they do not want to facilitate the uncontrolled passing of information such as rumors. However, the best way to combat rumor is by free flow of truthful information. Only information that might violate individual privacy or the survival and health of the enterprise should be kept from subordinates. The informal organization can help to serve the goals of the formal organization if it is not made the servant of administration. It should not be controlled. A major shortcoming in its use is that not all employees are part of the informal organization.[22]

Nurse managers should encourage and nurture informal organizations that:

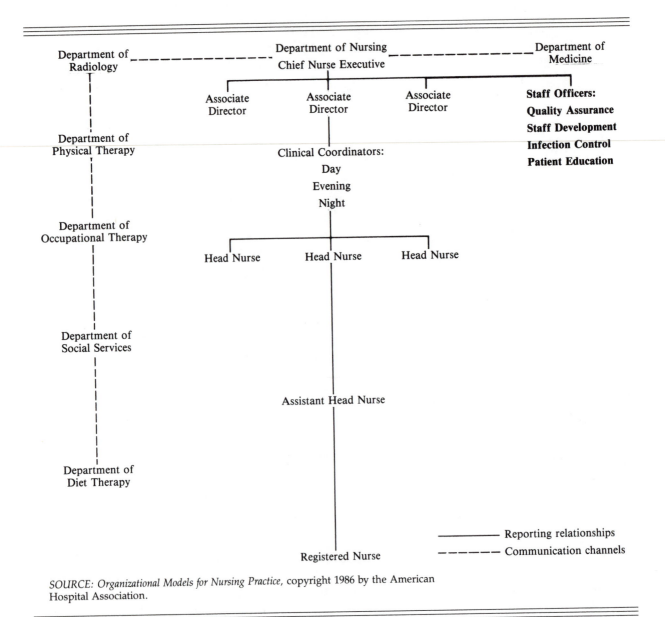

SOURCE: *Organizational Models for Nursing Practice*, copyright 1986 by the American Hospital Association.

Figure 11–4 • *Line and Staff*

1. Provide a sense of belonging, security, and recognition.
2. Provide methods for friendly and open discussion of concerns.
3. Maintain feelings of personal integrity, self-respect, and independent choice.
4. Provide an informal and accurate communication link.
5. Provide opportunities for social interaction.
6. Provide a source of practical information for managerial decision making.
7. Are sources of future leaders.

Problems can include creation of conflicting loyalties, restricted productivity, and resistance to change and management's plans.[23]

SYMPTOMS OF MALORGANIZATION

A symptom of malorganization is recurring problems. They indicate the focus is on the wrong elements of the business when it should emphasize key activities, major business decisions, perfor-

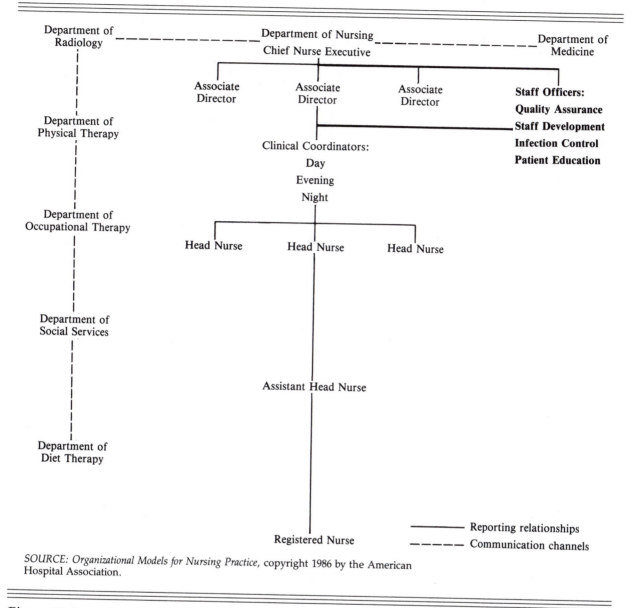

SOURCE: *Organizational Models for Nursing Practice,* copyright 1986 by the American Hospital Association.

Figure 11–5 •   Functional

mance, and results rather than secondary problems. Another symptom of malorganization is too many meetings attended by too many people. Such meetings are poor tools for accomplishing work. An alternative is to give individual assignments and only meet to report and avoid duplication. Committees are instruments of participation and communication and must be made productive. Too many management levels is another symptom of malorganization.

Principle: Build the least possible number of management levels and forge the shortest possible chain of command. This eliminates stresses and levels of friction, slack, and inertia.

If people always have to worry about other people's feelings, there is overstaffing. If the organization is put together to get the job done, layers of coordinators are not needed. Fit the chart to the organization and its needs rather than drawing a chart and building the organization to support it.

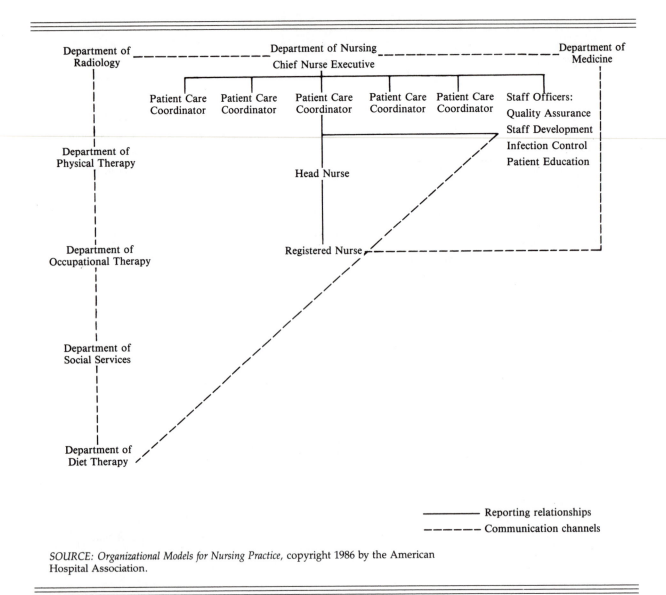

Reporting relationships
Communication channels

SOURCE: *Organizational Models for Nursing Practice,* copyright 1986 by the American Hospital Association.

Figure 11–6 • Matrix

SUMMARY

There is no best design for a nursing organization, nor are there universal design principles. Nurse managers need to work for an ideal organizational structure, and they need to be pragmatic. They should build, test, concede, compromise, and accept. They should design the simplest organization for getting the job done. They should focus on key activities to produce key results. The organization is productive when the people are performing care that meets client needs and for which employees have a sense of accomplishment.

The nursing management function of organizing is an evolving one. It evolves as nurse managers learn and apply the knowledge gained from research and experience in business and industry. They further develop the organizing function through nursing research and experience in nursing management.

1. An organization chart or schema exists for the nursing division or service or unit.

2. The chart is up to date.

3. The chart clearly depicts line and staff authority relationships within the nursing division, service, or unit.

4. The chart serves as a reference for delegation of authority, for specifying responsibility and accountability, for supervision, and for channels of communication.

5. The chart is familiar to all employees of the nursing division or service or unit.

6. There are organization charts available that depict coordination and communication relationships between the nursing division and other departments or units of the overall organization.

Figure 11–7 • Standards for Evaluation of an Organization Chart

EXPERIENTIAL EXERCISES

1. Scenario. A newly appointed Chair of the Division of Nursing in a medical center noted that the management system was unrealistic, unmanageable, and ineffective. Lines of authority were unclear at top management level, and the problem was compounded at lower levels. Two medical/surgical supervisors were managing all units; however, each unit had a clinical nurse manager. There was no input from the Division of Nursing into the outpatient services and no authority regarding nursing practices. There was no system of accountability, because there was little or no planning and no one with enough time to do it. The philosophy and objectives had no real significance.

   1.1 Why was the organizational structure poor?

   1.2 What evidence was there that the Chair of the Division of Nursing was doing a systematic analysis and sound thinking before altering the design and structure of the organization?

   1.3 What will the Chair's next steps be?

2. For each of the following statements, place a + in the blank if the statement is true and a − if it is false.

____ 2.1 Philosophy is a key activity to be analyzed in developing a nursing organization.

____ 2.2 A group of central, load-carrying key activities will center around primary patient care.

____ 2.3 A first step toward organizing a nursing service is to identify, analyze, and group key activities in achieving the mission and objectives of patient care.

____ 2.4 Philosophy does not contribute to the achievement of the mission and objectives of patient care.

3. Match each of the four categories of key activities listed in Section I with an appropriate example in Section II.

I

   a. Result-producing activities related to direct patient care

   b. Support activities

   c. Hygiene and housekeeping activities

   d. Top management activities

II

____ 3.1 Application of data from analysis of nurse epidemiologist's results to determine whether the cause of hospital-acquired infections is poor cleaning techniques, poor nursing practices, or poor equipment.

____ 3.2 Decisions related to changes in wages and salaries of employees.

____ 3.3 Developing and teaching in-service education workshops and classes.

____ 3.4 Transfer of IV admixture to pharmacy.

4. Scenario: Mr. Bishop is a hospital administrator of a 1000-bed university medical center. He insists that supervisors meet the responsibilities for counseling their workers. They must keep records of performance counseling, recommend for promotions and awards, and recommend that unsatisfactory employees be fired. Their recommendations must always be fully documented. In addition, he insists that department heads will not make deals with each other. To control this, all actions between departments must be done through an associate administrator.

   4.1 How does Mr. Bishop support the principle of placing all decisions at the lowest level and as close to the scene as possible?

4.2 What evidence is there to show that he does not support this principle?

5. Place a check in the space before each statement that characterizes a team.

____ 5.1 A team is usually large.

____ 5.2 A team is composed of people with different backgrounds, skills, and knowledge.

____ 5.3 Members on a management team come from the same area of an organization.

____ 5.4 Members of a team work cooperatively on a specific and defined task.

____ 5.5 A team has a leader or captain.

6. *Scenario:* A Chair of a Division of Nursing noted that some problems kept recurring over and over. They never seemed to get solved. One of the recurring problems was incorrect entries on narcotics registers. The Chair decided that the reason for incorrect entries was that nurses did not know how to make them correctly. She discussed it with the supervisors and in-service coordinator. The solution they decided on was to correct each person who made an incorrect entry and to include the teaching as part of the orientation course for newly employed nurses. Within 6 months the entries were being made correctly.

The Chair also noted that endless committee meetings were being held, and few objectives were being achieved. There were twice-monthly meetings with clinical nurse managers, meetings of four standing committees, meetings of intermediate supervisors, and numerous institutional meetings. After discussing the problem with senior level managers, the managers were given responsibility for redefining objectives of all nursing committees, developing procedures for agendas, developing procedures for evaluating effectiveness, and getting needed information to employees without having them attend extra meetings. Within 3 months, the minutes of meetings had been cut in half, and productivity was visible. Some committees had been combined.

The Chair also examined the supervisory levels in her organizational structure and realigned them to focus on the production of primary nursing care of patients. Several positions were eliminated because they duplicated the work of clinical nurse managers. Several nurse positions were absorbed by sections performing like activities. The result was fewer complaints about interference with jobs at the patient-care levels of operation.

List examples of the symptoms of malorganization.

7. Use the list entitled "Activities to Promote a Positive Organizational Climate" in this chapter as a point of discussion for a group of your peers. Assess the organizational climate in the organization in which you are a student.

7.1 Summarize the positive attributes of the organizational climate.

7.2 Summarize the negative attributes of the organizational climate.

7.3 Make a management plan for effecting positive change in the organizational climate for the one attribute you consider most in need of management change.

MANAGEMENT PLAN

OBJECTIVE:

ACTIVITIES	PERSONS RESPONSIBLE	TARGET DATES	ACCOMPLISHMENTS

8. Refer to Figure 11–1, "Fifty Specific Techniques to Boost Employee Morale."

    8.1 Make a list of similar activities found in the organization in which you work as a student.

    8.2 Make an appointment with the chief nurse executive and discuss the practicality of initiating new techniques. Plan this so you will be well prepared.

9. Use Figure 11–2, "Standards for Evaluation of the Effectiveness of Line and Staff Relationships," to evaluate the nursing unit in which you work as a student. Involve your colleagues.

    9.1 Summarize your findings.

    9.2 If basic defects or deficiencies exist, use a problem-solving methodology to plan for changes in line and staff relationships.

    9.3 Make a management plan to correct the defects or deficiencies.

MANAGEMENT PLAN

OBJECTIVE:

ACTIVITIES	PERSONS RESPONSIBLE	TARGET DATES	ACCOMPLISHMENTS

10. Use Figure 11-7, "Standards for Evaluation of an Organization Chart," to evaluate the nursing organization chart of the organization in which you work as a student.

 10.1 Summarize your findings.

10.2 If basic defects or deficiencies exist, use a problem-solving methodology to plan for changes in the organization chart.

10.3 Make a management plan to correct the basic defects or deficiencies.

MANAGEMENT PLAN

OBJECTIVE:

ACTIVITIES	PERSONS RESPONSIBLE	TARGET DATES	ACCOMPLISHMENTS

11. Figure 11–8 is a checklist for evaluation of the organizing function within a nursing division, department, service, or unit. Use it to evaluate the organizing function within the nursing unit in which you work as a student.

11.1 Summarize your findings.

11.2 If basic defects or deficiencies exist, use a problem-solving methodology to plan for changes in organizing.

11.3 Make a management plan to correct the basic defects or deficiencies.

By way of a final evaluation of your organizing function within a department or unit, answer the following questions. For those checked "No," plan the changes so that they will result in effective organizing. Then implement the management plan.

	Yes	No
1. Is there evidence that organizing is an intentional and ongoing function of the division, department, service or unit?		
2. Is there evidence that organizing changes as plans, goals, or objectives change?		
3. Is there evidence that managers are developed or replaced to fit organizational changes emerging from changed plans and objectives?		
4. Are organizational managerial relationships clearly structured to give security to individual managers?		
5. Has authority been delegated to appropriate levels of managers?		
6. Is there evidence that delegation of authority has been balanced to retain control of appropriate administrative functions by the chief nurse executive (CNE)?		
7. Is information dissemination clearly separated from decision making?		
8. Is the authority delegated commensurate with the responsibility?		
9. Is there evidence of acceptance of responsibility and authority by subordinate managers?		
10. Is there evidence that subordinate managers have the power to accomplish the results expected of them?		

	Yes	No
11. Is there evidence that authority and responsibility have been confined within divisional, departmental, service, or unit boundaries?		
12. Is there evidence of balance in support and use of staff functions?		
13. Is there evidence of balance in support and use of functional authority?		
14. Is there evidence of maintenance of the principle of unity of command?		
15. Is there evidence of efficient and effective use of service departments?		
16. Is there evidence of too many levels of managers (overorganization)?		
17. Is there evidence of unneeded line assistants to managers (overorganization)?		
18. Is there evidence that the nursing division, department, service, or unit is organized to facilitate accomplishment of its specified objectives by its personnel?		
19. Is there evidence that the nursing division, department, service, or unit structure has been modified to fit human factors after being organized to accomplish its specified objectives?		
20. Is there evidence that the nursing division, department, service, or unit is organized to accomplish planning for recruiting and training to meet present and future personnel needs?		
21. Is there evidence that the organizational process is flexible to adapt to changes in its external and internal environment?		

Figure 11–8 • *Evaluation of Organizational Function*

(Continued)

	Yes	No
22. Are changes in organization justified, based on deficiencies, experience, objectives, purpose, and plans?		
23. Is there evidence that the organizing process is balanced between inertia and continual change?		
24. Is there evidence that all nursing personnel know the organizational structure and understand their assignments and those of their coworkers?		
25. Is there evidence that the nursing organizational charts are widely used?		
26. Is there evidence that nursing organizational charts provide comprehensive information to all workers?		
27. Is there evidence that there are job descriptions and job standards for every job and that they are widely used by nursing managers?		
28. Is there evidence that nursing		

	Yes	No
employees are all oriented to the nature of the nursing organizing process?		
29. Is there evidence that the organizing process within the nursing division, department, service, or unit prevents waste or unplanned costs?		
30. Is there evidence that the nursing organization has an effective span of control by managers?		
31. Are the lines of authority within the nursing organization clear?		
32. Is there evidence that the management information system is effective?		
33. Is there evidence that each employee has only one supervisor?		
34. Is there evidence that the CNE has absolute responsibility for subordinate nursing managers?		
35. Is there evidence that all nursing managers are able to effect their leadership abilities?		

Figure 11–8 • (*Continued*)

MANAGEMENT PLAN

OBJECTIVE:

ACTIVITIES	PERSONS RESPONSIBLE	TARGET DATES	ACCOMPLISHMENTS

NOTES

1. C. Argyris, "Personality and Organization Theory Revisited," *Administrative Science Quarterly*, v. 18, 1973, 141–167.
2. H. Fayol, *General and Industrial Management*, trans. by C. Storrs (London: Sir Isaac Pittman & Sons, 1949), 53–61.
3. L. Urwick, *The Elements of Administration* (New York: Harper & Row, 1944), 37–39.
4. J. L. Gibson, J. M. Ivancevich, and J. H. Donnelly, Jr., *Organizations: Behavior, Structures, Processes*, 5th ed. (Plano, TX: Business Publications, 1985), 488–491.
5. J. R. Rizzo, R. J. House, and S. I. Lirtzman, "Role Conflict and Ambiguity in Complex Organizations," *Administrative Science Quarterly*, v. 15, 1970, 150–162.
6. D. Dunphy, "Personal and Organizational Change—Status and Future Direction," *Work and People*, Feb. 1983, 3–6.
7. J. Johnson and K. Luciano, "Managing by Behavior and Results—Linking Supervisory Accountability to Effective Organizational Control," *Journal of Nursing Administration*, Dec. 1983, 19–26.
8. E. C. Dayani, "Professional and Economic Self-Governance in Nursing," *Nursing Economics*, Jul.-Aug. 1983, 20–23.
9. D. J. del Bueno and P. M. Vincent, "Organizational Culture: How Important Is It?," *Journal of Nursing Administration*, Oct. 1986, 15–20.
10. W. G. Dyer and W. G. Dyer, Jr., "Organizational Development: System Change or Culture Change?," *Personnel*, Feb. 1986, 14–22.
11. R. L. Desatnick, "Management Climate Surveys: A Way to Uncover an Organization's Culture," *Personnel*, May 1986, 49–54.
12. M. Holt Ashley, "Motivation: Getting the Medical Units Going Again," *Nursing Management*, June 1985, 28–30.
13. C. Logan, "Praise: The Powerhouse of Self-Esteem," *Nursing Management*, June 1985, 36, 38.
14. J. L. Nave and B. Thomas, "How Companies Boost Morale," *Supervisory Management*, Oct. 1983, 29–33.
15. P. Cornett-Cooke and K. Dias, "Teambuilding: Getting It All Together," *Nursing Management*, May 1984, 16–17.
16. J. W. Frederickson, "The Strategic Decision Process and Organizational Structure," *Academy of Management Review*, Apr. 1986, 280–297.
17. M. L. McClure, "Managing the Professional Nurse: Part I. The Organizational Theories," *Journal of Nursing Administration*, Feb. 1984, 15–21; M. M. Timm, and M. G. Wavetik, "Matrix Organization: Design and Development for a Hospital Organization," *Hospital & Health Services Administration*, Nov./Dec. 1983, 46–58; American Organization of Nurse Executives, *Organizational Models for Nursing Practice* (Chicago: American Hospital Association, 1984).
18. Ibid.
19. Ibid.
20. B. Fuszard, " 'Adhocracy' in Health-Care Institutions," *Journal of Nursing Administration*, Jan. 1983, 14–19.
21. R. H. Guest, "Management Imperatives for the Year 2000," *California Management Review*, Summer 1986, 62–70.
22. R. C. Swansburg, *The Organizing Function of Nursing Service Administration* (Hattiesburg, MS: University of Southern Mississippi School of Nursing, 1977); R. C. Swansburg, *Management of Patient Care Services* (St. Louis: Mosby, 1976).
23. P. E. Han, "The Informal Organization You've Got to Live With," *Supervisory Management*, Oct. 1983, 25–28.

FOR FURTHER REFERENCE

American Nurses' Association, *Standards for Organized Nursing Services and Responsibilities of Nurse Administrators across All Settings* (Kansas City, MO: American Nurses' Association, 1988).

———, *Standards of Nursing Practice* (Kansas City, MO: American Nurses' Association, 1973–1977).

Beyers, M., "Getting On Top of Organizational Change: Part 3. The Corporate Nurse Executive," *Journal of Nursing Administration*, Dec. 1984, 32–37.

Brown, D. S., "Shaping the Organization to Fit People," *Management of Personnel Quarterly*, Summer 1966.

Cameron, K., "A Study of Organizational Effectiveness and Its Predictors," *Management Science*, Jan. 1986, 87–112.

Campbell, L. R., "What Satisfies . . . and Doesn't?," *Nursing Management*, Aug. 1986, 78.

Clegg, C. W., and Wall, T. D., "The Lateral Dimension to Employee Participation," *Journal of Management Studies*, Oct. 1984, 429–442.

Cohen, M. H., and Ross, M. E., "Team Building: A Strategy for Unit Cohesiveness," *Journal of Nursing Administration*, Jan. 1982, 29–34.

Crout, T. K., and Crout, J. C., "Care Plan for Retaining the New Nurse," *Nursing Management*, Dec. 1984, 30–33.

Dennis, K. E., "Nursing's Power in the Organization: What Research Has Shown," *Nursing Administration Quarterly*, Fall 1983, 47–57.

Donovan, H. M., *Nursing Service Administration: Managing the Enterprise* (St. Louis, MO: Mosby, 1975).

Drucker, P. F., *Management: Tasks, Responsibilities, Practice* (New York: Harper & Row, 1973), 564.

George, J. R., and Bishop, L. K., "Relationship of Organizational Structure and Teacher Personality Characteristics to Organizational Climate," *Administrative Science Quarterly*, 1971, 467–475.

Guthrie, M. B., Mauer, G., Zawacki, R. A., and Conger, J. D., "Productivity: How Much Does This Job Mean?," *Nursing Management*, Feb. 1985, 16–20.

Hall, R. H., "The Concept of Bureaucracy: An Empirical Assessment," *American Journal of Sociology*, July 1963, 32–40.

———, "Professionalization and Bureaucratization," *American Sociological Review*, Feb. 1968, 92–104.

Heilriegel, D., and Slocum, J. W., "Organizational Climate: Measures Research and Contingencies," *Academy of Management Journal*, June 1972, 255–280.

Hodgetts, R. M., *Management: Theory, Process, and Practice*, 4th ed. (Orlando, FL: Academic Press, 1986), 138–231.

———, and Howe, R. L., *Workbook to Accompany Management, Theory, Process, and Practice* (Philadelphia: W. B. Saunders, 1975).

Jablin, F. M., "Formal Structural Characteristics of Organizations and Superior-Subordinate Communication," *Human Communication Research*, Summer 1982, 338–347.

Jacobsen-Webb, M., "Team Building: Key to Executive Success," *Journal of Nursing Administration*, Jan.-Feb. 1985, 16–20.

Jenkins, R. L., and Henderson, R. L., "Motivating the Staff: What Nurses Expect from Their Supervisors," *Nursing Management*, Feb. 1984, 13–14.

Joiner, C., Johnson, V., Chapman, J. B., and Corkrean, M., "The Motivating Potential in Nursing Specialties," *Journal of Nursing Administration*, Feb. 1982, 26–30.

Joyce, W. F., and Slocum, J., "Climate Discrepancy: Refining the Concepts of Psychological and Organizational Climate," *Human Relations, 11*, 1982, 951–972.

Kamerschen, D. R., Pool, R. J., and Dilts, D. A., "Ownership and Management of the Firm—Another Look," *Business and Society*, Spring 1986, 8–1.

Kanter, R. M., and Seggerman, T. K., "Managing Mergers, Acquisitions and Divestitures," *Newsweek*, Oct. 5, 1987, S–14, S–16.

Krampitz, S. D., and Williams, M., "Organizational Climates: A Measure of Faculty and Nurse Administrator Perception," *Journal of Nursing Education*, May 1983, 200–206.

Lawler, E. E., III, Hall, D. T., and Oldham, G. R., "Organizational Climate: Relationship to Organizational Structure, Process, and Performance," *Organizational Behavior and Human Performance*, Nov. 1974, 139–155.

Leatt, P., and Schneck, R., "Technology, Size, Environment, and Structure in Nursing Subunits," *Organizational Studies*, v. 3, no. 3, 1982, 221–242.

Locke, E. A., Schweiger, D. M., and Latham, G. P., "Participation in Decision Making: When Should It Be Used?," *Organizational Dynamics*, Winter 1986, 65–79.

Mills, P. K., and Posner, B. Z., "The Relationships among Self-Supervision, Structure, and Technology in Professional Service Organizations," *Academy of Management Journal*, June 1982, 437–443.

Niehouse, D. L., "Job Satisfaction: How to Motivate Today's Workers," *Supervisory Management*, Feb. 1986, 8–11.

Payne, R. L., and Mansfield, R., "Relationships of Perceptions of Organizational Climate to Organizational Structure, Context, and Hierarchical Position," *Administrative Science Quarterly*, v. 18, 1973, 515–526.

Pheysey, D. C., Payne, R. L., and Pugh, D. S., "Influence of Structure at Organizational and Group Levels," *Administration Science Quarterly*, v. 16, 1971, 61–73.

Porter, L. W., and Lawler, E. E., III, "The Effects of 'Tall' versus 'Flat' Organization Structure on Managerial Job Satisfaction," *Personnel Psychology*, Summer 1964, 135–148.

Pritchard, R. D., and Karasick, B. W., "The Effects of Organizational Climate on Managerial Job Performance and Job Satisfaction," *Organizational Behavior and Human Performance, 9*, 1973, 126–143.

Pugh, D. S., Hickson, D. J., Hinings, C. R., and Turner, C., "The Context of Organization Structures," *Administrative Science Quarterly*, Mar. 1969, 91–114.

Ridderheim, D. S., "The Anatomy of Change," *Hospital & Health Services Administration*, May/June 1986, 7–21.

Roznowski, M., and Hulin, C. L., "Influences of Functional Specialty and Job Technology on Employee's Perceptual and Affective Responses to Their Jobs," *Organizational Behavior and Human Decision Processes*, Oct. 1985, 186–208.

Schneider, B., "The Preceptor of Organizational Climate: The Customer's View," *Journal of Applied Psychology*, Mar. 1973, 248–256.

———, and Hall, D. T., "Toward Specifying the Concept of Work Climate: A Study of Roman Catholic Diocesan Priests," *Journal of Applied Psychology*, June 1972, 447–455.

Stevens, B. J., *First-Line Patient Care Management* (Wakefield, MA: Contemporary Publishing, 1976).

Swansburg, R. C., *Nurses and Patients: An Introduction to Nursing Management* (Hattiesburg, MS: Impact III, 1978).

Taylor, B. A., "Understanding the Social System in the Work Environment," *Nursing Administration Quarterly*, Fall 1983, 26–29.

Tushman, M., and Nadler, D., "Organizing for Innovation," *California Management Review*, Spring 1986, 74–92.

·12·

Committees

COMMITTEES DEFINED

A committee is a group form that evolves out of a formal organization structure. Committees are formed to make collective use of knowledge, skills, and ideas. They blend the good characteristics of several to many individuals, a reason for making careful appointments or selections. The principle of synergy underlies committee activity: putting the thinking power of a selected group together for the most effective outcome. What is the optimum number of people to produce the desired outcome of synergy? The answer is difficult and depends on the goals to be addressed, the characteristics of committee members, and the environment within which they function. Aim for the best combination of skills and energies.[1]

COMMITTEES AS GROUPS

Because the work of organizations is accomplished by groups, many persons have studied the dynamics of group function. Although all groups are not committees, the management of a group of employees to accomplish the objectives of an enterprise is similar to the leadership and management of a committee in order to accomplish selective objectives. Already in the 1920s researchers at the Harvard Business School found that worker morale and productivity were positively influenced by small, informal work groups.[2]

In the world of the nurse manager, work is performed by individuals and by groups. Primary nursing has become a much used modality or method of practicing nursing because it gives professional nurses more autonomy than other modalities. It adds accountability through continuous responsibility of nurses for patients from admission through discharge. Case management adds group dynamics to the autonomy, because the case manager is responsible for functioning in a collaborative practice with other professional nurses and physicians. Case management also uses managed care as a medium to keep the patient on the critical path from admission through discharge and can extend through the illness episode to include home care.

Committees are formal groups that can serve useful functions in the organizing process of nursing and organizational administration. In addition to being an organizational entity, committees are planned for and in turn make plans. They are directed by leaders appointed by management or elected by constituents as determined by management. Because professional nurses want autonomy but most are employed by organizations, formal groups, including committees, are a medium for promoting autonomy by giving them a voice in managing the organization. Their effectiveness can be controlled internally and externally. If committees do not serve a useful function they should be evaluated and restructured. When no longer needed they should be selectively abandoned.

There are usually two types of committees, *standing* and *ad hoc* or *special*. Standing committees are advisory in authority, although some may have collective authority to make and implement decisions. They have continuity as organizational entities. Ad hoc committees are formed to fulfill a specific purpose and are disbanded when the purpose is achieved.

Stevens advocated the use of groups for management and stated that they can greatly increase productivity when used effectively. Nurse managers need to be able to function in groups for the purpose of promoting problem solving and acceptance of responsibility among other group members. The nonmanager group members can function within an administrative council and demonstrate ability to manage themselves by preparing agendas, reviewing status of agenda topics, obtaining and using learning aids, and handling meetings. In short, nurse managers should be able to structure the business of groups and direct and control the behavior of group members.[3]

Fuszard and Bishop use the term "adhocracy" to refer to the use of ad hoc committees in nursing organizations. They credit Toffler with origination of the term. Applying adhocracy to nursing, a group would be formed to accomplish a specified mission and it would then be dissolved. It could be called a task force, a project team, or an ad hoc committee. Team members would be those nurses with the special qualifications needed to accomplish the task.[4]

BENEFITS OF COMMITTEES

What are the benefits of committees? Committees can transmit useful information in two directions—toward administrators or managers and toward employees. They encourage and involve participation of interested or affected employees in the management of the nursing enterprise. Their advice can be helpful, and they can promote understanding of objectives and programs by other employees. They can promote loyalty. Some of the new ideas that keep nursing an open sociotechnical system come from committees. They provide face-to-face meeting of individuals for purposes of gathering information, seeking advice, decision making, negotiation, coordination, and creative thinking to resolve operational problems and improve the quality of services rendered by the organization.

Committees provide a pooling of people with specific skills and knowledge that can be assimilated into plans of action. They can bridge gaps between departments or units. They can use the pooled expertise of specialists and people with special talents and leadership abilities. They give people an opportunity to participate in the social process of group dynamics. They can help reduce resistance to change. Supervision, control, and discipline can be reduced through committee activities. Care quality can be improved, personnel turnover reduced, and harmony promoted through committee work.

All of the positive or beneficial outcomes of committees can be achieved if they are appropriately organized and led. Otherwise they can become liabilities to the organizing process. They can waste time and money; they can defer decisions or provide wrong information for the making of decisions; they can promote too many compromises and stagnation; they can be used to avoid decision making by administrators.

ORGANIZATION OF COMMITTEES

Every committee should have a purpose and short-range objectives, and every standing committee should also have long-range objectives. Objectives need to be translated into plans of action with time frames and precise responsibility. Assignments should be given ahead of meeting times so they can be presented during these times. Committee chairpersons are accountable to a specific administrator who provides guidance to them through consultation. Composition of committees should be addressed to ensure appropriate choice of members for expertise and representativeness. They should be of manageable size for discussion and disagreement. They should have prepared agendas

1. The committee has been established by appropriate authority: bylaws, executive appointment, or other.
2. There are a stated purpose, objectives, and operational procedures for each committee.
3. There is a mechanism for consultation between chairs and persons to whom they report.
4. There is a published agenda for each committee meeting.
5. Committee members are surveyed beforehand to obtain agenda items, including problems, plans, and sharing of news.
6. There is an effective chair for each committee.
7. Recorded minutes of each committee are used to evaluate its effectiveness in meeting stated objectives.
8. Committee membership is manageable and representative of the expertise needed and the people they affect.
9. Nurses are adequately represented on all appropriate institutional committees.

Figure 12–1 • *Standards for Evaluation of Nursing Committees*

and effective chairs. Figure 12–1 contains standards for evaluating nursing committees.

Nursing should be represented on most health care institution committees and always on those whose activities will affect nursing. They should have representation that will be effective in determining the outcomes of a health team approach to patient care services. In effect, nurses should determine how they will practice nursing.

GROUP DYNAMICS

Each member of a group plays a role in achieving the work of the group. Because each member has a unique personality and individual abilities, the group leader needs to know how groups function so as to facilitate their effectiveness. Original studies of group dynamics were done through observations of informal groups. The Hawthorne studies of 1924–1932 were conducted in four phases designed to discover what would make workers increase their output. Employees respond to identification with groups and to the interpersonal relationships with members of small groups.

Group members perform task roles, group

building and maintenance roles, and individual roles. They do this through interpersonal relationships. In the performance of these roles the group members share the power of the organization and its management.

Group Task Roles

Each member of a group performs one or more roles related to the task of the group or committee. The purpose is to arrive cooperatively at a definition of and solution to a common problem. These roles may include making proposals or suggestions for new group goals or redefining the problem; seeking a factual basis for the group's work; seeking opinions that reflect or clarify the values of group members' suggestions; giving an opinion indicating what the group's view of pertinent values should be; clarifying and coordinating ideas, suggestions and activities of the group members or subgroups; evaluating; summarizing decisions or actions; prodding the group to act; arranging the environment; and recording the group's activities and accomplishments.[5]

Group Building and Maintenance Roles

Individual members of the group work to build and maintain group functioning. Again, each may be performed by a group member or by the leader and, one person may perform several roles. These roles may include accepting and praising the contributions, the viewpoints, ideas, and suggestions of all group members with warmth and solidarity; mediating, harmonizing, and resolving conflicts; yielding a position within a conflict situation; promoting open communication and facilitating participation to involve all group members; listening; evaluating; and recording.[6]

Individual Roles

Group members also play roles to serve their individual needs. To keep individual roles from disrupting the group's activities in meeting their objectives, selected group members are frequently trained in group dynamics. This training is particularly important for the group leader. These individual roles are not suppressed but are managed by the leader and the others trained in group dynamics. These roles may include expressing disapproval of the values or feelings of other members; expressing negative points of view and resurrecting issues; focusing positive attention on oneself;

using the group setting as a forum for personal expression; remaining uninvolved and demonstrating cynicism, nonchalance, or horseplay; evoking members to sympathize with expression of personal insecurity, confusion, or depreciation; and cloaking personal prejudices or biases in speaking for others.[7]

Phases of Groups

Groups have a natural history of development. The following are five generally accepted phases of groups:

1. *Forming or orientation phase.* In this phase group members are discovering themselves. They want uniqueness: to belong while maintaining personal identity. They test each other for appropriate and acceptable behavior. It is the time to exchange information, to discover ground rules, to size up each other, determine fit.

2. *Conflict or storming phase.* During this phase group members jockey for position, control, and influence. There is leadership struggle and increased competition. The leader helps members through this phase, assisting with roles and assignments.

3. *Cohesion or norming phase.* Roles and norms are established with a move toward consensus and objectives. Members reach a common understanding of the true nature of the opportunity. They will diagnose the root cause of the problem, the deviation from expected performance. They will be open to alternative definitions with multiple views. Morale and trust improve and the negative is suppressed. The leader guides and directs as needed.

4. *Working or performing phase.* Members work with deeper involvement, greater disclosure, and unity. They complete the work. The leader may intervene as needed.

5. *Termination phase.* Once goals are fulfilled the group terminates. The leader guides the members to summarize discussions, express feelings, and make closing statements. There is reluctance to break up. A celebration can help.[8]

Group Leaders

Group leaders may be formal, informal, or specialized. Formal leaders are appointed by management or elected by management directives and carry line authority or power to discipline and control group members. Informal leaders emerge from the group process. Their influence inspires cooperation and mediation, and helps group members reach consensus about their contributions to effective functioning in quest of goals. Specialized leaders are often temporary leaders who have a special skill or ability needed by the group at a particular point in time.

Participatory management requires alignment for individuals to work toward shared goals as well as profitability. A dynamic leader inspires people to put spirit into working for a shared goal. The leader can use symbols, posters, slogans, T-shirts, and memorable events. The leader must believe in people and support McGregor's Theory Y that espouses self-direction, self-control, commitment, responsibility, imagination, ingenuity, creativity, and effort. How the leader behaves toward peer group members will exhibit these beliefs.[9] Leaders can make committees and meetings effective by having an extensive knowledge of group dynamics. They will keep the group on course by convincing each member of the genuine need for input and personal sensitivity to group processes. They will draw in the shy and the quiet. They will politely cut off the garrulous and protect the weak. While controlling the squashing reflex in themselves, they will encourage a clash of ideas by mediating domination by cliques. They will refrain from being judgmental. Being a group leader requires a thinking, skilled performance based on knowledge and ability acquired through management education and training.[10]

MAKING COMMITTEES EFFECTIVE

Improving Committee Effectiveness

Nurse managers can improve the effectiveness of standing and ad hoc committees by establishing minimal ground rules, including:

1. Establish clearly stated objectives. For ad hoc or specialized meetings discuss the goals before planning the meeting. Base the goals on advancing the clinical and business goals of nursing.
2. Establish a committee structure to support the clearly stated objectives.
3. Plan all meetings and events to meet the goals and objectives.
   3.1 Keep the committee or event to a manageable size. Define membership. *Assemblies*

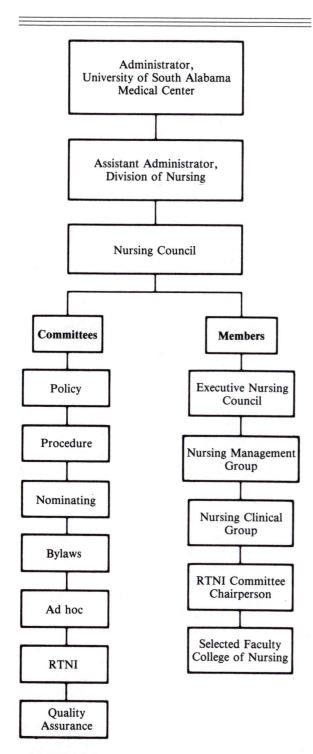

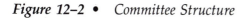

Figure 12–2 • *Committee Structure*

begin at one hundred and increase in size. They see and hear. *Councils* can be forty to fifty persons who listen or comment. *Committees* should be around ten to twelve persons who all participate on an equal footing.

3.2 Draw up a point-by-point agenda and send it to the attendees. Include the purpose of the meeting. Because the sequence of the agenda is important, the following points are helpful:

   3.2.1 Put dull items early and "star" items last.

   3.2.2 Decide whether to place divisive items early or late.

   3.2.3 Plan a time for starting important items.

   3.2.4 Limit committee meetings to 2 hours or less.

   3.2.5 Schedule meetings to begin 1 hour before lunch or 1 hour before the end of work day.

   3.2.6 Avoid extraneous business on the agenda.

   3.2.7 Read the agenda and write in comments before the meeting.

3.3 Tailor the meeting room to the group and prepare it beforehand.

3.4 Prepare for the meeting by learning the subject matter and preparing audiovisual materials to support it. Bring input from people who do not attend via videotaped interviews. Make events memorable.

3.5 Time the agenda items. New or controversial subjects usually take more time. Attention spans diminish after the first hour. Use time efficiently, including mealtimes.

3.6 Referee and set the pace of the meeting. Summarize and clarify as needed.

3.7 Promote lively participation by involving attendees in the program with a warm-up "getting acquainted" phase, a conflict phase, and a total collaboration phase. Bring out the personal goals of the individuals.

3.8 Listen to what others say so there will be a sharing of knowledge, experience, judgments, and folklore.

3.9 Bring the meeting to a definite conclusion by obtaining decisions and commitments.

3.10 Follow up as necessary to eliminate loose ends. Evaluate whether the meeting's purpose was achieved.

3.11 Circulate useful information with the minutes. Keep them brief, listing time, date, place, chair, attendance, agenda items and action, time ended, and time, date, and place of the next meeting.[11]

A meeting should never be held without a solid reason and an interesting subject on which the attendees will exchange ideas. This subject should meet the needs of the attendees. Leaders of meetings should know how to make them successful.

QUALITY CIRCLES

Quality circles are a participatory management technique that involves statistical analyses of activities to maintain quality products. The technique was initiated in Japan through the teaching of Dr. W. Edwards Deming, an American, after World War II. The concept is to use statistical analysis to make quality improvements. Workers are taught the statistical concepts and use them through trained, organized, structured groups of four to fifteen employees called *quality circles*. Group members share common interests and problems and meet on a regular basis, usually an hour a week. They represent other employees from whom they gather and bring information to the meetings.[12]

The quality circle process has become widespread in Japan, raising the quality of Japanese manufacturing to worldwide eminence. It involves workers in the decision-making process. Quality circles have spread to major manufacturing companies and to some health care institutions in the United States.

Quality circles are similar to other elements of participatory management. Employees are trained to identify, analyze, and solve problems. Involved in the process, they make solutions work because they identify with ownership. From being recognized they develop good will toward their employers.

Quality circles are effective when facilitators, leaders, and members are trained in group dynamics and quality circle techniques. Leaders act as peers to generate ideas for operational improvements and problem elimination. In the process all quality circle members reach consensus before decisions are recommended or implemented. Training occurs during regular quality circle meetings and continues during subsequent meetings.[13]

Because quality circles contribute to the knowledge base of human behavior and motivation, the process is important to the development of nursing management theory. This theory will be learned and used by nurse managers concerned with developing job satisfaction of professional nurses to deliver quality nursing care. The objects of quality circles are participation, involvement, recognition, and self-actualization among clinical nurses caring for patients.

Research indicates that productivity and morale are strongly improved when employees participate in decision making and in planning for change. It is important that participation include goal setting, as participation will lead to higher goals and higher levels of acceptance and performance. Research also shows that highly nonparticipatory jobs cause psychological and physical harm. *It is an ethical imperative to prevent harm by enabling employees to participate in work decisions.* Mental health is positively influenced by feelings of interest, a sense of accomplishment, personal growth, and self respect.[14] Nurse managers will use this knowledge in managing clinical professional nurses.

SUMMARY

Synergy—putting the thinking power of a selected group together for the most effective outcome—defines a committee's primary function. Committees provide employees a representative voice in the management of organizations.

A standing committee has continuity as an organizational entity, while an ad hoc committee is formed for a purpose and disbanded when that purpose is fulfilled.

"Adhocracy" is a system in which project teams exist for a single patient and disband when their purpose is accomplished.

Committees can facilitate communication, promote loyalty, pool special human resources, reduce resistance to change, and give people opportunities to work together. They should have purposes, objectives, and operational procedures.

Chairs of committees need knowledge and skills of group dynamics. This can be provided through staff development programs and to all nurses desiring it.

Groups work in five phases:

1. Forming or orientation phase
2. Conflict or storming phase
3. Cohesion or norming phase

Standards	Yes	No		Standards	Yes	No
1. The meeting started on time.				6.7 The chair referees, paces, summarizes, and clarifies discussion.		
2. A quorum existed.				6.8 The meeting concludes with definite decisions and commitment to them.		
3. The meeting agenda is on a schedule.				6.9 The chair follows up on necessary items.		
4. The agenda for the meeting reflects the purpose of the committee.				6.10 Useful information is circulated with the minutes.		
5. The chair acts as an equal member of the group taking no special considerations.				7. The chair allows adequate time for discussion.		
6. The chair follows the agenda.				8. The chair facilitates participation by all members.		
6.1 Dull items are scheduled early, star items last.				9. Items requiring further study are referred to smaller groups as projects. Timetables for results are established.		
6.2 Divisive items are strategically placed.				10. Managers attend meetings when needed to assure support.		
6.3 Important items have a starting time.				11. Managers plan absences from selected meetings to encourage discussion.		
6.4 The agenda avoids "any other business."				12. Technical assistance is provided to facilitate meeting success.		
6.5 Meetings are scheduled for 1 hour before lunch or 1 hour before end of work day.						
6.6 The chair is well prepared for the meeting.						

Figure 12–3 • *Checklist for Evaluating Meeting Effectiveness*

4. Working or performing phase
5. Termination phase

Committees can waste time if they make a premature decision or do not accomplish their objectives. They can be made effective by application of the management functions of planning, organizing, directing (leading), and controlling (evaluating).

Quality circles have emerged as a participatory management technique using statistical analysis of activities to maintain quality products. Quality circles have the characteristics of groups and use group dynamics but are a regular part of the organization whose members are mature work groups.

Committees can lead to improved productivity.

EXPERIENTIAL EXERCISES

1. Figure 12–3 is a checklist for evaluating the effectiveness of meetings. Use it and Figure 12–1 to evaluate the minutes of a nursing meeting in the organization in which you work as a student.

2. When the minutes of the same meeting have been printed and distributed, use the same checklists to evaluate them. Is there a difference between the actual meeting and the minutes? What is it? How can the process be improved? Make a management plan to improve the committee's meetings and/or the minutes. Be tactful and use a positive approach in your planning.

MANAGEMENT PLAN

OBJECTIVE:

ACTIONS	TARGET DATES	ASSIGNED TO	ACCOMPLISHMENTS

4. Examine the files of minutes of a committee covering a period of 1 year. Identify the phases of the committee for each meeting.

5. *Group Exercise*

   5.1 Use your student or peer group.

   5.2 Elect a chair and a recorder.

   5.3 Evaluate the effectiveness of the committee structure of the organization in which you work as a student. Use the Figure 12–1, "Standards for Evaluation of Nursing Committees," and samples of minutes. You will need to have a copy of the committee structure of all hospital, medical staff, nursing, and other committees. These can be distributed among student groups.

   5.4 Which committees need new leadership to meet their purpose? Why?

   5.5 Which committees have overlapping purposes? Which should be abolished? Which redirected? Why?

   5.6 Which committees should have nurse representation but do not? List reasons why nurses should be members.

   5.7 Use the following format to prepare a management plan to implement your recommendations.

MANAGEMENT PLAN

OBJECTIVE:

ACTIONS	TARGET DATES	ASSIGNED TO	ACCOMPLISHMENTS

6. *Scenario:* A director of nursing has a monthly clinical nurse managers' meeting. One of the major objectives of this meeting is to give information to the clinical nurse managers from management. Another objective is to provide them with an opportunity to voice their problems to the Director of Nursing. Usually, the Director of Nursing draws up a definitive agenda; however, it is never distributed to the clinical nurse managers. She has her secretary and clerk-typist prepare the room beforehand. When she plans to use training aids, she has them prepared by staff development personnel. She always learns the subject matter for the meetings. Although the meetings are planned for 1 hour, they frequently extend to 2 hours and are terminated only when another group appears to use the meeting room. Sometimes arguments ensue between attendees, and she does not interrupt them. She listens to what they have to say. Few matters are ever settled at these meetings, and they are seldom evaluated in terms of the stated purposes.

6.1 What evidence is there that an agenda is prepared and sent to the attendees?

6.2 What evidence is there that the meeting room is prepared for the clinical nurse manager group beforehand?

6.3 What evidence is there that the Director of Nursing learns the subject matter for the meeting?

6.4 What evidence is there that the agenda items are timed?

6.5 What evidence is there that the Director of Nursing referees and sets the pace of the meetings?

6.6 What evidence is there that she promotes lively participation?

6.7 What evidence is there that she listens to the clinical nurse managers?

6.8 What evidence is there that the meetings are brought to a definite conclusion by obtaining decisions?

6.9 What evidence is there of follow-up of loose ends with evaluation of achievement of the purposes?

7. Develop a Quality Control Circle program to identify and solve:

- In-class problems
- Clinical experience problems
- Unit management problems

The following references may be helpful:

H. J. Brightman and P. Verhoeven, "Running Successful Problem-Solving Groups," *Business*, Apr.-June 1986, 15–23.

R. A. Golde, "Are Your Meetings Like This One?" *Harvard Business Review,* Jan.-Feb. 1973, 68–77.

S. Johnson, "Quality Control Circles: Negotiating an Efficient Work Environment," *Nursing Management*, July 1985, 34A–34B, 34D–34G.

Remember, meetings should not be "time killers." Executives spend approximately 21 weeks a year in meetings, many of which are a waste of time. They can be improved by:

- Having goals
- Preparing agendas
- Preparing audio visual materials and the physical settings to support the agenda
- Setting time limits
- Inviting the right people
- Assigning responsibility
- Following through[15]
- Making a videotape of a meeting and evaluating the results.

NOTES

1. R. M. Fulmer and S. G. Franklin, *Supervision: Principles of Professional Management*, 2d ed. (New York: Macmillan, 1982), 246–247.

2. E. Mayo, *The Human Problems of Industrial Civilization* (Boston: Harvard Business School, 1946).

3. B. J. Stevens, "Use of Groups for Management," *Journal of Nursing Administration*, Jan. 1975, 14–22.

4. B. Fuszard and J. K. Bishop, " 'Adhocracy' in Health Care Institutions," in B. Fuszard, *Self-Actualization for Nurses* (Rockville, MD: Aspen, 1984), 90–99.

5. K. D. Benne and P. Sheats, "Functional Roles of Group Members," *Journal of Social Studies*, Winter 1948.

6. Ibid.

7. Ibid.

8. L. L. Northouse and P. G. Northouse, *Health Communication: A Handbook for Health Professionals* (Englewood Cliffs, NJ: Prentice-Hall, 1985); H. J. Brightman and P. Verhoeven, "Running Successful Problem Solving Groups," *Business,* Apr.-June 1986, 15–23.

9. N. Dixon, "Participative Management: It's Not as Simple as It Seems," *Supervisory Management*, Dec. 1984, 2–8.

10. L. Caramanica, "What? Another Committee?," *Nursing Management*, Sept. 1984, 12–14; A. Jay, "How to Run a Meeting," *Journal of Nursing Administration*, Jan. 1982, 22–28.

11. Jay, op. cit.; B. Y. Auger, "How to Run an Effective Meeting," *Commerce*, Oct. 1967; R. C. Swansburg, *Management of Patient Care Services* (St. Louis: Mosby, 1976), 273–276; R. M.

Kanter, "Toward the World's Best Corporate Conference," *Management Review,* May 1986, 7–9; Stevens, op. cit.; B. J. Stevens, *The Nurse as Executive,* 2d ed. (Wakefield, MA: Nursing Resources, 1980); H. S. Rowland and B. L. Rowland, eds., *Nursing Administration Handbook,* 2d ed. (Rockville, MD: Aspen, 1985), 39–40.

12. The theory of quality circles was actually developed by Frederick Herzberg and W. Edwards Deming of the United States approximately 50 years ago. S. Johnson, "Quality Control Circles: Negotiating an Efficient Work Environment," *Nursing Management,* July 1985, 34A–34B, 34D–34G; A. M. Goldberg and C. C. Pegels, *Quality Circles in Health Care Facilities* (Rockville, MD: Aspen, 1984).

13. Ibid.

14. M. Sashkin, "Participative Management Remains an Ethical Imperative," *Organizational Dynamics,* Spring 1986, 62–75.

15. N. Alexander, "Meetings Too Often Time Killers," *Augusta Chronicle,* Sept. 10, 1989, 1 E.

FOR FURTHER REFERENCE

Baker, K. G., "Application of a Group Theory in Nursing Practice," *Supervisor Nurse,* Mar. 1980, 22–4.

Blau, P. M., "Cooperation and Competition in a Bureaucracy," *American Journal of Sociology,* May 1984, 530–535.

Ertl, N., "Choosing Successful Managers: Participative Selection Can Help," *Journal of Nursing Administration,* Apr. 1984, 27–33.

Ganong, W. L., and Ganong, J. M., "Reducing Organizational Conflict through Working Committees," *Journal of Nursing Administration,* Jan.-Feb. 1972, 12–19.

Golde, R. A., "Are Your Meetings Like This One?," *Harvard Business Review,* Jan.-Feb. 1972, 68–77.

Hodgetts, R. M., *Management: Theory, Process and Practice,* 4th ed. (Orlando, FL: Academic Press, 1986), 294–300.

Leebov, W., "Problems, Plans, and Sharing: A Format for Productive Meetings," *Supervisory Management,* June 1984, 35–37.

Leo, M., "Avoiding the Pitfalls of Management Think," *Business Horizons,* May-June 1984, 44–47.

Llewelyn, S., and Fielding, G., "Forming, Storming, Norming, and Performing," *Nursing Mirror,* July 21, 1982, 14–16.

Llewelyn, S., and Fielding, G., "Under the Influence," *Nursing Mirror,* July 28, 1982, 37–39.

Mohrman, S. A., and Ledford, G. E., Jr., "The Design and Use of Effective Employee Participation Groups: Implication for Human Resource Management," *Human Resource Management,* Winter 1985, 413–428.

Roberts, V., "The Head Nurse Meeting: Who, What, When, and Where," *Nursing Management,* Aug. 1985, 10, 12.

Rosenblum, E. H., "Groupthink: The Peril of Group Cohesiveness," *Journal of Nursing Administration,* Apr. 1982, 27–31.

Rubin, I. M., Fry, R. E., and Plovnick, M. S., *Managing Human Resources in Health Care Organizations* (Reston, VA: Reston Publishing, 1978).

Swansburg, R. C., *The Organizing Function of Nursing Service Administration* (Hattiesburg, MS: University of Southern Mississippi School of Nursing, 1977).

Veninga, R. L., "Benefits and Costs of Group Meetings," *Journal of Nursing Administration,* June 1984, 42–46.

Webber, J. B., and Dula, M. A., "Effective Planning Committees for Hospitals," *Harvard Business Review,* May-June 1974, 133–142.

·13·

Decentralization and Participatory Management

DECENTRALIZATION

Description

Decentralization refers to the degree to which authority is disbursed downward within an organization to its divisions, branches, services, and units. Decentralization of authority includes dispersal of all the management components of planning, organizing, directing or leading, and controlling or evaluating. It involves the delegation of decision-making power, authority, responsibility, and accountability. Decentralization of these functions represents a management philosophy and reflects the management style of the chief executive officer (CEO) and the chief nurse executive (CNE). Decentralization within an organization varies in degree but is never total. Top management must bear ultimate responsibility for the success of an organization, achievement of goals and objectives, outcomes, and profit or loss.[1]

The United States Compared with Japan and Europe

In Japan, when workers are asked, Who is in charge? they respond, "I am!" Japanese management is a present-day fad. It must be remembered that Japan has an entirely different culture. The Japanese have learned to manage complex organizations. They do it through Theory Z, developed by Dr. William Ouchi after studying Japanese systems and similar management approaches in the United States. Basic management principles of Theory Z are:

- *Long-term employment*
- *Relatively slow process of evaluation and promotion*
- *Broad career paths*
- *Consensus decision making*
- *Implicit controls with explicit measurements*
- *High levels of trust and egalitarianism*
- *Holistic concern for people*[2]

The Japanese studied U.S. management and modified it to fit their culture.

Decentralization is a U.S. business strategy that was instituted in the 1960s to aid in the penetration of European markets. It is considered necessary for the successful management of large firms. The Japanese are still constrained from decentralizing into the United States. Both Europe and Japan have more family-held firms. Japanese firms retain collective, centralized, and strongly hierarchical organizational structures. Managerial reward systems in the United States usually emphasize individual rather than group performance.[3]

The United States has more formal business education schools than Europe and Japan. European firms tend to provide management education and training in-house. Although U.S. colleges and universities graduate more than 60,000 MBAs annually, Japan graduates very few, Great Britain around 1,500, and Germany even fewer.

The United States produces professional managers who switch firms. Japan has strong patterns of corporate loyalty and long-term employment. The United States has professional associations for managers; management is more tolerant of mergers, organizational development, and new ideas such as corporate cultures; U.S. firms hire more outside consultants and adopt external management ideas such as worker representation on corporate boards of directors, flextime work schedules, and worker participation in job design. Organized labor is weaker in the United States.[4]

Reasons for Decentralization

Health care organizations are among the most complex organizations in the world. Their complexity increases with size; thus decisions are better managed at the specific site from which they originate. Communication does not have to travel up and down an organizational hierarchy. Sound decisions can be made and action taken more promptly when decision making is decentralized.

The variety and depth of nursing management problems have increased. Patient care must keep moving; a delay in a diagnostic procedure or treatment can delay progress toward recovery and discharge, thereby increasing expense. Staffing is a complicated process that must account for many variables: physician absences due to education, vacation, or illness; seasonal fluctuations due to such factors as vacations for children; the random nature of tertiary care for heart attacks, strokes,

trauma, cancer, and other conditions; third-party payer requirements; government rules and regulations related to patients and employees; coordination of multiple activities; increased technology with increased specialization leading to environmentally induced human stress; the complexity of managing human beings, including those with dual careers as nurses and homemakers; complaints; quality assurance; staff development; and much more.

The object of decentralizing nursing is to manage decisions in their specific area of origin, thereby facilitating communication and effectiveness. Decentralization also supports role clarification to prevent overlapping and duplication of individual work.[5]

Studies have shown that decentralized decision making increases productivity, improves morale, increases favorable attitudes, and decreases absenteeism. One could conclude that decentralized decision making is good for health care institutions because it is good for nursing personnel. Research on the decentralization of decision making confirms the hypothesis that it enhances job enrichment and job enlargement.[6]

Decentralization embodies the concept of participatory management, including shared governance.

PARTICIPATORY MANAGEMENT

When top management implements a philosophy of decentralized decision making, the stage is set for involving more people—perhaps even all staff—in making decisions at the level at which the action occurs. Both decentralized management and participatory management delegate authority from top managers downward to the people who report to them. In doing so, objectives or duties are assigned, authority is granted, and an obligation or responsibility is created by acceptance. The employee is accountable for results.[7]

In nursing, as in other organizations, delegation fosters participation. A first line manager with delegated authority will contact another department to solve a problem in providing a service. The first line manager does not need to go to a department head, who contacts the department head of that service, creating a communication bottleneck. The people closest to the problem solve it. This is efficient and cost-effective management. The following sections detail some of the characteristics of participatory management.

Trust

Participatory management is based on a philosophy of trust. The employee is trusted to complete the task, with periodic progress reports and a final review with management. The time and rate of participation should be managed to control stress. The entire task or decision should be delegated as much as possible. More and more professional nurses want to control their nursing practice; the manager can facilitate this by teaching them to make complete operational plans, including structuring priorities and setting deadlines. Such plans provide a documented standard for joint review. Managers who empower and facilitate employee performance communicate trust. This process will demonstrate the employee's capabilities and reveal shortcomings.

Commitment

Personal involvement in managing a nursing service requires commitment from the chief nurse executive and other nurse managers. Managers should be highly visible to the staff, supporting and nurturing them in the process. In turn, the staff should also be committed, a characteristic they will develop from association with the committed managers. They gain this commitment from seeing their bosses out at the production level, where patients are being treated, from cooperating with their colleagues and managers in a spirit of teamwork, and from feelings of accomplishment. Nursing commitment comes from knowing that the purpose of the organization is patient care and the managers are working with them to produce that care. Staff share in making decisions and in consensus with the bosses. This experience in participation turns them on and tunes them in, and they do not want to be lazy and mediocre or to featherbed. Commitment inspires staff to be industrious, outstanding, and productive. Under participatory management, commitment is elicited, not imposed.

Professional nurses are motivated to develop their human skills resulting in increased individual self-esteem. They have a sense of accomplishment and feel that their accomplishment has been supported by management. They feel they are expanding their worth through their work.

Professional nurses demand professional courtesies. When these are not extended they may resort to deviant behavior. They tend to align themselves with colleagues and professional associations for recognition and evaluation rather than with the organization.[8]

Goals and Objectives

Conflict resolution is a major requirement or goal of participatory management. Conflict is inevitable when human beings work together. It is nonproductive during process and in outcomes. In nursing as in other occupations, it produces stress and results in turnover and absenteeism. Employees can be sensitized to deal with potential and real conflict and to take action to reduce its destructive consequences of fear, anger, distrust, jealousy, and resentment. This can be accomplished through establishment of a climate of openness with established procedures for problem solving, persuasion, bargaining, and politicizing. The goal is reduced adversarial relations. It is accomplished through joint planning and problem solving, and facilitation of employee consultation.[9] Refer to chapter 19 on conflict management.

A key goal for a nursing organization is to keep itself healthy. A healthy work environment is encouraged by participatory management. Participation will make maximum use of employees' abilities without relinquishing the ultimate authority and responsibility of management. Professional nurses want input into decisions but do not want to do the jobs of managers. They want the support of managers, to be able to talk with them, to be informed. Without this support they develop anger and hostility that results in absenteeism and lower productivity.

Goal-setting activities can occur with reasonably frequent performance review and feedback. Nursing personnel bring their goals and objectives to the conferences. The process is reciprocal, with the manager and employee together developing goals and objectives that are challenging, clear, consistent, and specific. They will both be motivated. Healthy stress will be increased and undesirable stress reduced.

Autonomy

Autonomy is the state of being independent, of having responsibility, authority, and accountability for one's work as well as one's personal time. Professional employees indicate they want autonomy for practicing their profession, for making decisions about their work. They do not want their decisions made for them by hospital administrators, physicians, or others. They want to be treated as equal partners and colleagues in the health care delivery system. This desire for autonomy has increased as nurses have become increasingly sophisticated in knowledge and skills and have used them with effective results.

Professional nurses want autonomy over the conditions under which they work, including pace and content. These decisions are often in conflict with management's coordination roles, a conflict that can be mediated by involving professional nurses in delegated activities of coordination.[10]

Professional nurses are willing to assume and accept responsibility, to be held accountable for a charge. They want the authority, the rightful and legitimate power to fulfill the charge. This authority comes from their expert knowledge and skill, their license, their position, and their peers.[11]

Professional nurses are accountable for the consequences of their acts. Accountability is the "fulfillment of the formal obligation to disclose to referent others the purposes, principles, procedures, relationships, results, income, and expenditures for which one has authority."[12] The relationships among responsibility, authority, autonomy, and accountability are depicted in Figure 13–1.

To have autonomy, nursing employees should be allowed to determine their own means of accomplishing their goals. They should be involved in setting their own goals. This principle applies to all nursing employees. When professional nurses work with other nursing employees they should facilitate participation and input from these groups. This approach promotes these persons' interest, trust, and commitment.[13]

Concept	Key Aspects
Responsibility	The charge
Authority	The rightful power to act on the charge
Autonomy	Freedom to decide and to act
Accountability	Disclosure regarding the charge

SOURCE: Reprinted from "Clarifying Autonomy and Accountability in Nursing Service: Part 2" by F. M. Lewis and M. V. Batey, with permission of *Journal of Nursing Administration*, Oct. 1982.

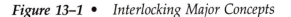

Figure 13–1 • *Interlocking Major Concepts*

Other Characteristics

Participation in management should be inclusive rather than exclusive, but it should be voluntary. The climate of the organization, as set by the philosophy of its managers, will motivate (or fail to motivate) professional nurses to participate at a level consistent with their goals and desires. Participation is increased by facilitators who are enthusiastic and expert.

STRUCTURE OF DECENTRALIZED AND PARTICIPATORY ORGANIZATIONS

Flat organizational structures are characteristic of decentralized management. Traditional hierarchical structures with increasingly authoritative levels of management frighten employees, threaten their security, and make them uncomfortable. Economic events of the past decade favor horizontal organizational structures with no rank, no boss, and no seniority. Flat organizational structures are flourishing, increasing management/employee association and commitment, and deemphasizing numbers of managers and manuals ("M&Ms"), titles, and executive suites.[14]

In nursing there are reports of the elimination of head nurse positions, with committees of professional nurses elected by unit staff to manage unit activities. Their efforts are facilitated by the new breed of leaders who are democratic, participative, and laissez faire or free rein, involving their followers in the decision process, in setting objectives, in establishing strategies, and in determining job assignments. These leaders put emphasis on people, employees, and followers and their participation in the management process. They are employee centered and relationship centered.

Decentralized organizational structures are compatible with primary nursing. Decisions are made, goals are set, there is peer review and evaluation, schedules are made, and conflicts are resolved by primary nurses. Levels of practice are built into staffing.[15]

Top Management

What is the role of top management under a decentralized system with participatory management? Their role is directed toward results. They share in the planning and implementation of the program.

Since effective controls are needed to monitor performance of lower level units, they use computers to assist in making their decisions and in developing controlling techniques for decentralization.

With the dynamics of decentralization, each unit works with its own budget; job descriptions are clear, concise, flexible, and current; in-service training is effective; performance standards are clear; employee recognition occurs; and accountability is enforced at all times.

Vertical versus Horizontal Integration

Vertical integration combines decentralization with integration. Even though businesses and industries decentralize their operations into product lines and subsidiaries, they maintain their partnership and identity within the corporate structure. Before the advent of the prospective payment system (PPS) and competition among hospitals, the industry was largely characterized by horizontal integration of departments within divisions, examples being nursing; operations related to patient care services such as pharmacy, physical therapy, occupational therapy, and others; operations related to plant management including housekeeping and others; and finance.

As competition among hospitals increased they began the quest to diversify into new markets. New corporate structures were formed that included umbrella corporate management with subsidiary companies.

THE PROCESS OF PARTICIPATORY MANAGEMENT

In the process of participatory management, professional nurses are involved in decisions that affect them and in setting their own work standards. This process involves training, changed roles for supervisors, changed roles for unions, and communication. It also involves preparation of managers for changed organizational structures. Participation involves understanding and support of many levels of people in the organization.

As organizations grow they are frequently geographically dispersed. In hospitals this can occur as new services or products are added. Home health care is an example. When this mission is established it is frequently housed in another building and sometimes in another part of the community. Geographic dispersion tends to result from vertical integration and to increase decentralization.

Health care organizations grow as they establish new missions for wellness, sports medicine, outpatient surgery, free-standing emergency centers and surgical centers, birthing centers, and auxiliary services and clinics of many kinds. The diversity of specialization as well as the geographic distribution encourage decentralization and delegation of decision making authority, responsibility, and accountability. Decentralization tends to increase if organizational growth is internal rather than external. As these products and services grow it is more difficult to manage them effectively from a central office. It is important to have well-qualified product and unit managers, particularly when there is a great diversity of products and services.

Hospitals are highly differentiated entities, as are many functions within them. Political differences emerge as each department or function recruits their own experts. Separate functions produce uncertainty, with output for one phase being input for another. Examples of this dynamic are pharmacy and nursing, or the operating room versus other nursing departments. Matrix management and project management are systems aimed at the improvement of lateral coordination and cooperation.

Within a hierarchy, participation based on interaction and influence will succeed to the extent it can operate independently of other parts of the organization. Product management will be done across organizational functions, so managers must attend to the quality of lateral arrangements. This includes integration of line and staff functions such as production and marketing or production and education.[16]

Training

Managers at all levels of nursing should subscribe to the philosophy of participatory management if it is to be successful. All managers and employees must unfreeze the present system of attitudes and values. This unfreezing process will require a comprehensive, well-planned training program. Training will promote a sense of job security as it will prepare everyone for changed roles. Staff at every level learn the reasons for participatory management, the advantages, the disadvantages, and the roles they will play.

Changed Roles of Supervisors

Decentralization with participatory management changes roles which thus have to be redefined and coordinated to prevent conflict. Head nurses, clinical nurse managers, and primary nurses have increased management responsibility. For some nurses this will mean decreased hands-on clinical responsibility. Supervisors of head nurses have decreased responsibility for unit management. They become mentors, role models, and facilitators. With a flattened organizational structure some may lose jobs, while others have the overall scope of their responsibility increased.[17]

As supervisors learn to delegate authority, they modify the climate that promotes obstructive behavior by giving professional nurses what they want, the authority to manage themselves. Because this gives them initiative in performing their jobs and freedom to question managers, the latter should expect loyalty in return. The profession of nursing does not employ nurses; organizations do. Participatory management is a process in which there must be dialogue with constraints. The nurses will control their profession; management uses its input to set objectives and priorities, and to review output. Nurse employees cannot control the enterprise, and management cannot compromise the professional or ethical standards of professional nurses.[18]

In participatory management the supervisor facilitates rather than directs the work force. Traditional supervisory functions are delegated downward. There must be clear delineation of managers' basic responsibilities, as opposed to their behavioral or management style. Managers can gain satisfaction from their ability to make clinical nurses successful and satisfied. The interpersonal skills and conceptual abilities demanded of supervisors will increase. They should be challenged and should have a future. They promote implementation of committee decisions, listen, and offer assistance.[19]

Because there will be fewer supervisors, career development programs for college educated nurses must provide promotional opportunities as clinical practitioners, managers, teachers, or researchers.

Supervisors are important to the success of decentralization of decision making and employee involvement in the management of nursing and the health care system. They should be taught to manage under employee involvement programs. They need to learn that they will have more time to plan and organize work, to be creative. Their jobs can be expanded upward, but they should keep contact with employees, encouraging participation by everyone.

Changed Roles of Unions

Decentralized decision making and participatory management are not processes that give comfort to unions. Unions may view them as threats to their survival and to membership, and as a prelude to efforts to decertify. Plans should include union membership participation that emphasizes the common interests of union and management. Both entities want mutual trust, quality of work life, and employee involvement. Both want job security for their employees and members; successful participatory management programs give security a high priority.

The union's role will have to be redefined. The goal is good labor-management relations. If they are to play a role, union shop stewards will be trained with supervisors. There will need to be a memorandum of understanding for keeping grievance and contractual issues outside the employee involvement program.[20]

Communication

Good communication within the nursing organization is essential to an effective employee participation program. Good communication is effective communication, evident in employees who are informed about the business of nursing. They know what management is saying and what management's intentions are. Management knows what employees are saying and how it squares with perceptions management is working to develop. Broken communication contributes to stress and leads to direct economic losses through low productivity, grievances, absenteeism, turnover, and work slowdowns or strikes.

ADVANTAGES OF PARTICIPATORY MANAGEMENT

The following is a list of advantages of participatory management as cited by writers in business, industry, and health care, including nursing:

1. High trust and mutual support.
2. Eliminated full-time-equivalent positions; fewer levels of management; fewer specialized departments.

3. Increased accountability of managers and employees.

4. Reduced ambiguity in work requirements for practitioners and employees with improved communication.

5. Enhanced role for clinical nurse; self-supervision; active involvement of employees in identifying and solving problems, encouragement of employee contributions; career development.

6. Increased independence of the nursing division.

7. Legal clarity.

8. Increased efficiency of nurse/patient ratio.

9. Teamwork: people become cooperative and independent with increased motivation and initiative.

10. Improved organizational communication, with nurses being briefed on all phases of the nursing business including revenues, costs, and strategic plans, thereby increasing employee understanding of the organization.

11. Decreased absenteeism.

12. Increased effectiveness and productivity. Quality of work done improves; higher level of mastery.

13. Uplifted morale and motivation at work. Increased excitement from fluctuating participation. Participation makes work and values visible.

14. Fresh ideas for management decision making and problem solving.

15. Identification of potential leaders.

16. Fostering within professionals of a strong sense of identification with employer's goals and objectives.

17. Decreased turnover and increased stability of work force.

18. Increased commitment as attitudes become positive.

19. Less overtime.

20. Lower cost.

21. Better use of professional nurses as participants have their skills and talents enhanced and discovered.

22. Increased job satisfaction.

23. Recognition of contribution because participation increases individual and organizational capacities to learn, adapt, and develop toward higher levels of excellence.[21]

Involvement of employees in the decision-making process creates favorable attitudes and behavior. Employees want to be productive and to learn. Decision-making skills raise their competency levels, preparing them for future opportunities. One way of measuring attitude changes is to survey attitudes before and after implementing an employee involvement program. This can be done on an experimental unit basis before being applied to the entire nursing organization. Research findings support the positive results or advantages of employee involvement in management processes.[22]

Participatory management reduces the potential frustration and loss of significance of the individual nurse. Employees have evidence that their suggestions count.

In the Motorola participatory management program, factory-level employees of Plan I belong to groups of 50 to 250 people who set targets and valid standards that measure current cost, in-process quality, product deliveries, inventory levels, housekeeping, and safety. Representatives belong to working committees that review ideas, recommendations, waste, and quality. The committees solve problems and send recommendations to a representative steering committee for review. Committee involvement of workers improves communication. Improved product quality or customer satisfaction is evident in increased sales and profits and results in financial bonuses to employees. In this process, each employee can see the effect of his or her contribution on the group and feels a sense of accomplishment. In one instance, as a result of the participatory management process at Motorola, a 4 percent loss of gold went to zero in 2 months. Volume of production at one plant went up 33 percent with fewer employees. They had team spirit and a sense of cooperation between management and employees, and they worked with less supervision.[23]

Research studies have reported greater motivation and satisfaction when subordinates participate in performance appraisal. Research indicates that mutual goal setting improves performances and increases productivity. It satisfies employees' need for fulfillment and self-actualization, and then contributes to the well-being of the organization. Participatory management develops mature, healthy, self-directed personalities among employees.[24]

DISADVANTAGES OF PARTICIPATORY MANAGEMENT

Some of the disadvantages of participatory management include:

1. There will be occasional failures.
2. Initiation of programs takes time and money.
3. Policies and procedures have to be changed.
4. It is sometimes difficult to determine which responsibilities are whose, even though other ambiguities are reduced.
5. The budget office and other offices or departments have to deal with several units in nursing service rather than a single department.
6. Lacking knowledge of the process, employers do not want it imposed on them. They give such excuses as that employees have too little attachment to the organization, employees are not interested in work and have a weak commitment to the work ethic, employees and managers do not get along, employees have a poor assessment of their supervisors, and employees have low regard for organization-wide openness.
7. It is difficult to change management style to true participation.
8. Employees who view management as being autocratic perceive participatory performance appraisal as being insincere, patronizing, and manipulative. The person who initiates it has gone "soft."
9. Self-evaluation is threatening as the employee feels exposed to the view of others.[25]

All of these disadvantages will be overcome by a committed chief nurse executive (CNE) who prepares and implements a plan with supervisors who are prepared psychologically, politically, and technically. The CNE selects and develops key people who are the human beings developing human beings, works toward a long-range future, and is accessible.

ACTIVITIES INVOLVING NURSES IN PARTICIPATORY MANAGEMENT

Some of the activities that can involve nurses in participatory management include job enrichment, personalization, gainsharing, participation, primary nursing, and response to identified factors causing job dissatisfaction.

Job Enrichment

Job enrichment satisfies the motivational force for higher-order need fulfillment. This includes variety within and among jobs and a strategy that challenges, with performance output stressed over job processes. Job enrichment creates jobs with greater responsibility and more flexibility and promotes personal development.

Personalization

Personalization is a strategy that focuses on people and knowledge, not numbers and politics. Its users stress empathy and involve professionals in critical decisions that affect them. Career development opportunities are facilitated by advertising jobs, allowing transfers, giving feedback to job applicants, allowing and providing liberal training and development opportunities, and promotions based on objective measures.[26]

Entrepreneurship

There is a great opportunity for professional nurses to be involved in entrepreneurship as decentralization and vertical integration strategies are implemented in health care organizations. Nurses can form small companies with the support of government agencies and private businesses. They require venture capital which can be obtained from government and the private health care industry. As an example, in the face of greater professional nurse shortages, hospitals could find it advantageous to contract with new small nurse companies through vertical integration that produces nurse staffing subsidiaries, durable medical goods subsidiaries, clinical nursing care subsidiaries, and others.

Entrepreneurship in nursing will be good for professional nurses and the health care industry, as it will create independent thinkers motivated to be productive, creative, and more competitive in the marketplace. They will become like other business people who have a strong desire to control their own careers.

Gainsharing

Gainsharing is a group incentive program in which employees share in the financial benefits of improved performance. It has many of the same advantages and disadvantages as other methods of participatory management. Top management is sensitive to employee's goals, and employees identify with the organization through greater involvement.

The results of gainsharing are measurable: savings, improved labor-management relations, fewer grievances, less absenteeism, and reduced turnover. Gainsharing adds money to intrinsic rewards. Stock ownership and profit sharing are economic rewards similar to gainsharing. Gainsharing, stock ownership, and profit sharing may not be legally possible in not-for-profit organizations. However, increased financial benefits can be made available through legal means such as merit pay, certification pay, and clinical promotions. Also, vertically integrated corporations have profit-making ventures under their corporate umbrellas.

Pay Equity

Pay equity between management and employees is an issue of participatory management. Employees resent announcements of huge salary increases, fringe benefits, and perquisites for top management. Incentive programs for employees are a part of participatory management programs. Although employees receive intrinsic satisfaction from public recognition and praise, they also obtain extrinsic rewards from financial bonuses, stock options, and profit sharing.[27]

SUMMARY

Decentralization disburses authority and power downward to the operational units of an organization. Japanese organizations practice decentralization by eliciting consensus of decision making in their management. Decentralization in nursing organizations facilitates communication and effectiveness of decisions, and clarifies roles.

Increased productivity, improved morale, increased favorable attitudes of people, and decreased absenteeism are the products of decentralized decision making. Decentralization supports participatory management, the characteristics of which are trust, commitment, involvement of employees in setting goals and objectives, autonomy, inclusion of employees in decision making, change and growth, originality, and creativity.

Decentralized and participatory organizations are usually flat or horizontal: employee centered and relationship centered. They are also vertically integrated to enhance revenue production by developing new markets for health care organizations.

Training is essential to the success of participatory management as managers are threatened by loss of authority. They have to be prepared for their new roles. Practicing nurses need to be able to perform as collaborators in the management of the nursing organization and the health care institution. With their new roles comes increased accountability for practicing nurses. Managers become facilitators.

Decentralization and participatory management are consistent with union participation. A memorandum of agreement is needed to keep grievance and contractual issues outside the employee involvement program. Some employers will opt to promote union decertification while bonding employees to the organization through participatory management.

Increased participation of nurses on organizational boards and committees will improve communication. Communication among units and departments becomes direct and hence faster and more accurate.

Although there are numerous benefits or advantages of participatory management, there are also some disadvantages. Among these disadvantages are occasional failures, occasional difficulty in fixing responsibilities, and difficulty in changing employee perceptions of previously authoritarian management.

Nurses can be involved in participatory management through such activities as job enrichment, personalization, primary nursing, case management, entrepreneurship, gainsharing, and pay equity.

EXPERIENTIAL EXERCISES

1. Using the reasons for decentralization of management and decision making in organizations given below, evaluate the organization in which you are a student.

Reasons for Decentralization:	Yes	No
1.1 Complex decisions are made and acted on at the lowest possible level. *Example:*		
1.2 Communication is facilitated at the lowest possible level. *Example:*		

1.3 Professional nurses indicate that they are making decisions at the lowest possible level.
  Example:

1.4 If your answer to any of the reasons for decentralization is "No," make a management plan for correcting the situation. If possible, do this with your colleagues.

MANAGEMENT PLAN

PROBLEM:

OBJECTIVE:

ACTIONS	TARGET DATES	ASSIGNED TO	ACCOMPLISHMENTS

2. *Scenario.* A newly employed nurse administrator finds that she is the chair of numerous committees and councils including the nursing directors' council and the division nursing council, the latter composed of all nurse managers of the institution. Bylaws for the division of nursing do not exist. Statements of mission, philosophy, and objectives exist but are unknown to most nursing personnel.

2.1 How can the characteristics of participatory management (trust, commitment, goals and objectives, autonomy, and inclusion) be developed by this newly employed nurse administrator?

3. Evaluate the structure of the organization in which you are a student.

Organization Structure	Yes	No
3.1 Flat?		
3.2 Democratic?		
3.3 Emphasizing all employees?		
3.4 Emphasizing manuals?		
3.5 Emphasizing job titles?		
3.6 Emphasizing management perks?		
3.7 Participatory?		
3.8 Assigning people by education and ability?		
3.9 Promoting teamwork?		
3.10 Enriching, enlarging, and rewarding jobs?		

4. What are the salable products of the organization in which you are a student?

5. Use the list under the heading, "Advantages of Participatory Management," to evaluate the division of nursing in the organization in which you are a student. Summarize your findings.

6. Six activities that can involve nurses in participatory management are:

   a. Job enrichment
   b. Personalization
   c. Gainsharing
   d. Participation
   e. Primary nursing
   f. Response to identified factors causing job dissatisfaction.

For each of the following anecdotes, place the letter of the activity being used to involve nurses in participatory management.

____ 6.1 Professional nurses have complained that record keeping takes too much time away from clinical patient care. The nurse manager has asked each nurse to look at one or more parts of the patient's record and suggest ways to streamline it. Two nurses are working together to develop problem-oriented patient-care records that will combine physician and nurses' histories, physicals, orders, and progress notes.

____ 6.2 The president of the organization has been marketing the notion that if one or more professional nurses designs a profitable outpatient case management product, the hospital will finance its startup as a joint venture. The nurses will be part owners and/or managers of the new enterprise. Several nurses are working on proposals.

____ 6.3 A nurse manager reduced overtime by giving her staff control over the work schedules. She provided legal and managerial guidelines. Absenteeism has been reduced 78 percent.

____ 6.4 As a reward for reducing absenteeism 78 percent and thereby increasing productivity, the president of the organization has increased the nurse manager's pay 5 percent.

____ 6.5 When a marked increase in patient census occurred, the nurse administrator called a meeting of the staff nurse councils to plan staffing. They decided to use overtime and expand the student cooperative education program.

____ 6.6 Even though the professional nurses are using techniques of case management, each patient has one professional nurse assigned to oversee care from admission through discharge.

7. *Group Exercise*

7.1 Form groups of six to eight persons each by random selection.

7.2 Select group leader and recorder.

7.3 List characteristics of decentralization and participatory management evident in your organization. (15 minutes)

7.4 List characteristics of centralized management evident in your organization. (15 minutes)

7.5 List changes you would like to see implemented to increase decentralization of decision making in your organization. (20 minutes)

7.6 Report. (20 minutes)

8. Fun is becoming part of the corporate culture with companies promoting "Hawaiian Shirt Day" for the Fourth of July, morning encounters with the company robot, hot-tub hours, entertainment breaks, masseuses to untie the stress knots, sampling edible products, and other special events to make work fun.[28]

8.1 Sample the attitudes of colleagues and managers in the organization in which you are a student. Is the corporate culture one in which holidays can be special fun days? If so, plan some appropriate activities for the next holiday. Use the management plan format following.

MANAGEMENT PLAN

PROBLEM:

OBJECTIVE:

ACTIONS	TARGET DATES	ASSIGNED TO	ACCOMPLISHMENTS

8.2 Form a group of peers or use an appropriately constituted committee of the nursing staff. Discuss the need for fun in your workplace. Summarize your conclusions.

8.3 Make a list of events that could be developed to promote fun in your workplace.

9. Read the following set of anecdotes from the perspective that nursing is a clinical practice discipline in which clinical nursing decision making is decentralized to the clinical practice level. Management solutions can be applied to remedy identified deficits.

The 61-year-old female patient was admitted to the medical center with a fractured neck of the left femur. The clinical nurse manager asked the patient's husband to complete the nursing history, which he did. The nursing history revealed that the patient had neurological deficit that included a paralyzed left arm for which the patient had a muscle stimulator applied 15 min. q.a.m. and passive/active exercises q.h.s. Also, when tired, the patient had slight drooping of the upper lip. This could be corrected by the patient when reminded to do so. Although the patient was in the hospital 16 days, neither nursing problem was ever addressed by the nursing personnel.

During the first 3 days of hospitalization the patient could not turn to either side due to Buck's extension and pain. Pain medication was administered as needed. The patient had IVs running during this time which caused her to void frequently and precipitously. By the time she called for nursing assistance, she had voided in the bed. Even when a "female" urinal was furnished, the patient had difficulty in placement and would get her bed wet.

Receiving a telephone call from her elderly and anxious mother, the patient could not talk to her because a portable phone was not handy. When the husband became angry and obnoxious the ward personnel insisted that the "phone was not a priority." Although the husband apologized for his behavior, he later noted that the ward clerk could use a call system to each patient's room to locate the telephone. The situation was resolved when the husband bought a conversion plug and brought a telephone from home.

Approximately 1 week postoperatively, the patient was ambulatory with a hemi-walker. At night she would fall soundly asleep and would awake early in the morning saturated with urine. This caused the patient to be very embarrassed.

During early hospitalization the patient had elastic support hose applied. When asked if these were released for 15 minutes q.8 hours, the head nurse replied such procedure was controversial. The patient was never measured for the support hose.

Other facts pertaining to the care of this patient:

- Except for A.M. care, there was little attention paid to the personal hygiene of this patient by the nursing staff.

- Meals were sometimes left at the bedside with plastic wrap tightly covering them which could not be removed by the patient.

- The room was seldom organized for the patient's protection: phone and urinal would be left on floor or chair which was out-of-reach.

- Mouth and bath cleaning utensils would be left dirty on the sink; dirty paper towels and debris from dead flowers would lay on stands for several days.

9.1 Assuming that decentralization of clinical nursing decisions is delegated to the clinical nurse staff, what are the management assets or deficits evident in the preceding scenario?

9.1.1 Assets

9.1.2 Deficits

9.2 What theory of management including that of decentralization would prevent or correct the deficits?

10. Delegation from nurse managers to clinical nurses is a part of the participatory management process. Mature nurse managers accept the principle of delegation which leads to a more productive and enjoyable relationship with clinical nurses. Use Figure 13–2 to audit your ability to delegate duties to licensed practical nurses, nursing assistants, and other professional registered nurses when appropriate.

10.1 Review your own delegation audit. Choose three areas you intend to refine, assign them priorities, and outline three steps to improve your performance in each area.

10.2 Narrate an experience in delegating that convinced you of the importance of exercising this basic responsibility and strengthened your confidence in your ability to delegate effectively.

How effective are you in

	Low				High	
1. Establishing work priorities for your subordinates?	1	2	3	4	5	6
2. Giving subordinates the necessary freedom and authority to work effectively?	1	2	3	4	5	6
3. Building confidence through guidance and direction?	1	2	3	4	5	6
4. Defining requirements clearly but not rigidly when you delegate work?	1	2	3	4	5	6
5. Relinquishing work you would like to do to others who can do it as well?	1	2	3	4	5	6
6. Spelling out the purpose and importance of a task, as well as other related duties?	1	2	3	4	5	6
7. Assigning someone to coordinate your activities when you are away?	1	2	3	4	5	6
8. Taking advantage of others' specialized skills when delegating?	1	2	3	4	5	6
9. Injecting challenge and motivation into tasks that you delegate?	1	2	3	4	5	6

TOTAL = _____

AVERAGE (total divided by 9) = _____

INTERPRETATION: Average Score of:
5–6 — Terrific; 3–4 — So-So; 1–2 — You're "Doing," not "Delegating"

SOURCE: E. C. Murphy, "Delegation—From Denial to Acceptance," *Nursing Management,* Jan. 1984, 56. Permission requested and granted.

Figure 13–2 • *Delegation Audit*

11. Read the following case study and summarize the characteristics of decentralization of decision making and participatory management evident in it.

CASE STUDY: Staff Nurses and Administration Team Up to Decrease Job Turnover Rate

By Sandra C. Kirkland, RN, BS, BSN, MSN, CETN

Director, Enterostomal Therapy/Wound Management
University of South Alabama Medical Center
Mobile, Alabama

Because nurses are the largest group of health care providers in the United States, their job turnover rate has a significant impact on the cost of health care delivery. "It has been reported that 64% to 75% of the turnover rate among nurses is voluntary and therefore could be reduced."[29]

When nursing administrators are seriously interested in reducing nurse turnover rates they must begin to seek out and find answers to questions like the following:

1. What affects a nurse's decision to accept a particular position?
2. What conditions contribute to job satisfaction for a nurse?
3. What changes will result in retention of nurses? Wandelt, Pierce, and Widdowson found that of 10 job conditions pertaining to nurse dissatisfaction, nurses ranked "support given by the administration of the facility" as #3 and "support given by nursing administration" as #6. Highly ranked but not included in the top 10 was "environment that does not provide a sense of worth as a member of the health care team."[30]

Additional studies show that nurses want "increased participation in decision making in the organizational structure" and the "right and responsibility to determine the nature and scope of their practice."[31]

Clearly, the communication between the nurse care provider and nursing administration is the key to solving many of the problems that result in nurses' job turnover.

A Direct Line of Communication

At the University of South Alabama Medical Center (USAMC), our primary nursing care provider is called the Registered Teaching Nurse I (RTN I). Considering recent literature and problems in our institution, our Nursing Administrator decided to establish a direct line of communication between the RTN Is and administration.

On August 24, 1981, he addressed a letter to a Nursing Service Supervisor expressing a desire for the establishment of an RTN I Committee. The purpose of the committee would be to facilitate communication between administration and practice (RTN Is). The objectives were:

1. Communicate viewpoints of clinical nurses to administration.
2. Advise on staff development and continuing education needs of the clinical nurse.
3. Consult on problems in nursing practice.
4. Assist in developing the nursing program within the medical center.

A supervisor consented to act as adviser to the committee. To establish beginning membership, each head nurse was asked to select an RTN I to represent his/her unit. At the first meeting, held on October 27, 1981, with 17 RTN Is in attendance, the adviser introduced the Assistant Administrator for Nursing and the Hospital Administrator. The purpose, objectives, and goals of the committee were discussed.

Organization: Officers, Goals and Bylaws

At the next committee meeting a temporary governing body was elected. The governing positions were chair, vice-chair, secretary, and parliamentarian. The people initially elected to these offices temporarily were reelected in January of 1982 by secret ballot for full 1-year terms. The committee immediately identified its prime objectives as:

1. Promoting quality patient care.
2. Promoting the problem-solving process by:

   a. Identifying problems.
   b. Recommending possible solutions to identified problems.
   c. Helping nurses cope with unresolved problems.
3. Promoting positive attitudes and morale among nurses.
4. Promoting cost effectiveness.
5. Promoting an environment that is conducive to the optimum practice of nursing.

One of the first orders of business was to establish a subcommittee to develop bylaws. This subcommittee consisted of the officers and six other RTN I committee members. Using guidelines from *Robert's Rules of Order* and Nursing Council Committee Bylaws, 10 articles were chosen around which to formulate the RTN I committee Bylaws. The articles were:

I. Name
II. Functions
III. Membership
IV. Officers
V. Meetings
VI. Quorum
VII. Standing Committees
VIII. Parliamentary Procedure
IX. Amendments
X. Standing Rules

The bylaws were drafted and accepted unanimously at the December meeting. They became effective immediately. The same individual remained as adviser to the committee.

Out of necessity during its formulation stage, the committee met weekly for several weeks, then biweekly, and in approximately 6 months, only monthly meetings were being held.

Accomplishments

From its inception on October 27, 1981, to date, the committee has been actively involved in pursuing the objectives it established. Its accomplishments have been numerous and obviously address some of the concerns expressed by nurses as indicated in the introduction.

One of the committee's most significant accomplishments has been the development of a career ladder for clinical advancement. The committee developed the entire ladder from the job descriptions to the performance appraisal summary. It was approved by administration and implemented May 1, 1985.

Other accomplishments include the formation of a Pharmacy Task Force. The group consists of RTN I committee members and pharmacy staff. Its purpose is to identify and solve problems between nursing and pharmacy that interfere with optimum patient care delivery. The meetings have resulted in many improvements a few of which are:

1. Expansion of the Pharmacy IV admixture program.
2. Regular, frequent pickup and delivery of orders and medications by paid and volunteer workers.
3. Institution of intensive care unit stock carts for medications that are frequently used and must be administered quickly.

The committee also has had a positive impact on the nursing orientation program. By meeting with the Director of Staff Development the committee members were made familiar with the then-current orientation schedule. Suggestions were made which resulted in an updated orientation program. The updated program stresses clinical time and provides a smoother transition from classroom to clinical setting. A yearly library update is conducted by the committee. Staff nurses are given this yearly opportunity to request that periodicals and books pertinent to their clinical practice be stocked in the library. This service may be found to be beneficial for continuing education.

Recently, many RTN Is were voicing great concern over the interpretation and enforcement of certain hospital policies regarding sick leave and vacation time. Disagreements were arising due to differing interpretations of these policies by head nurses and staff nurses. When the RTN I committee discussed these concerns with administration, it was obvious that some clarification was necessary. Nursing Service Administration handled the problem by holding several open forum meetings. In

Please circle the number that best correlates with your response.

    1—very well
    2—fair
    3—poor
    4—very poor

1. Has the RTN I Committee established a direct line of communication between staff nurses and administration?   1   2   3   4

2. Has the RTN I Committee's communication with Staff Development resulted in continuing education programs specific to your clinical practice?   1   2   3   4

3. Has the RTN I Committee consulted specifically on problems in nursing practice (such as problems with pharmacy, physical therapy, or physicians)?   1   2   3   4

4. Has the RTN I Committee assisted in developing the clinical nursing program within the Medical Center?   1   2   3   4

5. What one thing would you need to increase the effectiveness of the RTN I Committee?

6. Comments:

Evaluation Form Results

Question #	Ratings			
	1—very well	2—fair	3—poor	4—very poor
1	32	0	0	0
2	10	12	8	2
3	20	12	0	0
4	22	10	0	0
5	*	*	*	*
6	*	*	*	*

* Not included, as these questions were essay style.

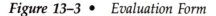

Figure 13–3 • *Evaluation Form*

these meetings, the RTN Is' rights and responsibilities were clarified. Both head nurses and staff nurses appreciated and benefitted from the way this problem was solved.

A current project under way is the evaluation of the staff need for hospital-affiliated day care. If a significant need is identified, the committee will proceed to evaluate methods and alternatives for hospital-affiliated day care, therein helping relieve a major concern among nurse parents.

In addition to specific accomplishments, the establishment of a direct line of communication between administration and practice has been most rewarding. It has enabled the staff nurse to receive direct administrative information about concerns that affect practice. Examples of this are:

1. Inclusion of the RTN I Chairperson in JCAHO rounds.
2. Detailed explanation given to the committee when the hospital retirement program added an IRA tax-sheltered retirement plan.
3. Encouragement of input into the discussions on the management information system purchased.
4. Active and ongoing relationship between personnel/nurse recruitment and the RTN I Committee to decrease nurse turnover rate.
5. Inclusion of the RTN I chairperson as a committee representative to attend all Nursing Council (Administration) meetings.

Self-Evaluation

An anonymous questionnaire was sent to former and present RTN I committee members. See Figure 13–3. Of the 32 questionnaires returned, 100 percent indicated that they indeed have direct and open communication with administration. See the table in Figure 13–3. Both question number five (5) and six (6) indicated an area the committee members wanted to see improved. This was the communication of information and activities in progress to the general staff nurse population, a problem they are now addressing.

The RTN I Committee demonstrates a continued cycle of nursing process in which assessment, planning, implementation, and evaluation are critical. Although not wholly attributable to the development of the RTN I Committee, we believe the committee's achievements have helped decrease our nurse attrition rate from 46.6 percent in August 1981 to the present 31 percent.

NOTES

1. L. C. Megginson, D. C. Moseley, and P. H. Pietri, Jr., *Management: Concepts and Applications*, 2d ed. (New York: Harper & Row, 1986), 266; H. Shoemaker and A. El-Ahraf, "Decentralization of Nursing Service Management and Its Impact on Job Satisfaction," *Nursing Administration Quarterly*, Winter 1983, 69–76.
2. C. W. Joiner, Jr., "SMR Forum: Making the 'Z' Concept Work," *Sloan Management Review*, Spring 1985, 57–63.

3. R. Edfelt, "A Look at American Management Styles," *Business*, Jan.-Mar. 1986, 51–54.

4. Ibid.

5. B. J. A. Simons, "Decentralizing Nursing Service—Six Months Later," *Supervisor Nurse*, Oct. 1980, 59–64; R. B. Fine, "Decentralization and Staffing," *Nursing Administration Quarterly*, Summer 1977, 59–67.

6. Shoemaker and El-Ahraf, op. cit.

7. Megginson, Moseley, and Pietri, op. cit., 266–267.

8. J. A. Raelin, C. Sholl, and D. Leonard, "Why Professionals Turn Sour and What to Do," *Personnel*, Oct. 1985, 28–41.

9. Fine, op. cit.; R. E. Walton, "From Control to Commitment in the Workplace," *Harvard Business Review*, Mar.-Apr. 1985, 77–84.

10. Raelin, Sholl, and Leonard, op. cit.

11. M. V. Batey and F. M. Lewis, "Clarifying Autonomy and Accountability in Nursing Services: Part I," *Journal of Nursing Administration*, Sept. 1982, 13–17.

12. F. M. Lewis and M. V. Batey, "Clarifying Autonomy and Accountability in Nursing Services: Part II," *Journal of Nursing Administration*, Oct. 1982, 10.

13. J. E. Bragg and I. R. Andrews, "Participative Decision Making: An Experimental Study in a Hospital," in B. Fuszard, *Self-Actualization for Nurses* (Rockville, MD: Aspen, 1984), 102–110.

14. G. Klaus, "Corporate Pyramids Will Tumble When Horizontal Organizations Become the New Global Standard," *Personnel Administrator*, Dec. 1983.

15. E. A. Elpern, P. M. White, and A. F. Donahue, "Staff Governance: The Experience of the Nursing Unit," *Journal of Nursing Administration*, June 1984, 9–15.

16. C. W. Clegg and T. D. Wall, "The Lateral Dimension to Employee Participation," *Journal of Management Studies*, Oct. 1984, 429–442.

17. Simons, op. cit.

18. Raelin, Sholl, and Leonard, op. cit.

19. Walton, op cit.

20. Ibid.; M. H. Schuster, and C. S. Miller, "Employee Involvement: Making Supervisors Believers," *Personnel*, Feb. 1985, 24–28.

21. C. L. Cox, "Decentralization: Uniting Authority and Responsibility," *Supervisor Nurse*, Mar. 1980, 28, 32; Shoemaker and El Ahraf, op. cit.; M. P. Lovrich, "The Dangers of Participative Management: A Test of Unexamined Assumptions Concerning Employee Involvement," *Review of Public Personnel Administration*, Summer 1985, 9–25; W. J. Bopp and W. P. Rosenthal, "Participatory Management," *American Journal of Nursing*, Apr. 1979, 671–672; J. A. Fanning and R. B. Lovett, "Decentralization Reduces Nursing Administration Budget," *Journal of Nursing Administration*, May 1985, 19–24; G. W. Poteet, "Delegation Strategies: A Must for the Nurse Executive," *Journal of Nursing Administration*, Sept. 1984, 18–27; Walton, op. cit.; S. R. Hinkley, Jr., "A Closer Look at Participation," *Organizational Dynamics*, Winter 1985, 57–67.

22. Bragg and Andrews, op. cit.

23. W. J. Weisz, "Employee Involvement: How It Works at Motorola," *Personnel*, Feb. 1985, 29–33.

24. Lovrich, op. cit.; Schuster and Miller, op. cit.

25. Shoemaker and El-Ahraf, op. cit.; Lovrich, op. cit.; Weisz, op. cit.; Cox, op. cit.

26. Raelin, Sholl, and Leonard, op. cit.

27. Walton, op. cit.

28. D. Gentile, "Fun Becoming Part of Corporate Culture," *Augusta Chronicle*, July 30, 1989, 7.

29. B. H. Munru, "Young Graduate Nurses: Who Are They and What Do They Want?", *Journal of Nursing Administration*, June 1983, 21.

30. M. A. Wandelt, P. M. Pierce, and R. R. Widdowson, "Why Nurses Leave Nursing and What Can Be Done about It," *American Journal of Nursing*, Jan. 1981, 73.

31. National Commission on Nursing, *Summary of the Public Hearings* (Chicago: Hospital Research and Educational Trust, 1981), 5.

FOR FURTHER REFERENCE

Dixon, N., "Participative Management: It's Not as Simple as It Seems," *Supervisory Management*, Dec. 1984, 2–8.

Ertl, N., "Choosing Successful Managers: Participative Selection Can Help," *Journal of Nursing Administration*, Apr. 1984, 27–33.

Hatcher, L. L., and Ross, T. L., "Organizational Development through Productivity Gainsharing," *Personnel*, Oct. 1985, 42, 44–50.

Levinson, R. E., "Why Decentralize?," *Management Review*, Oct. 1985, 50–53.

Malkin, S., and Lauteri, P., "A Community Hospital's Approach—Decentralized Patient Education," *Nursing Administration Quarterly*, Winter 1980, 101–106.

Muczyk, J. P., and Reimanu, B. C., "Has Participative Management Been Oversold?" *Personnel*, May 1987, 52–56.

Ondrack, D. A., and Evans, M. G., "Job Enrichment and Job Satisfaction in Quality of Working Life and Nonquality of Working Life Work Sites," *Human Relations*, Sept. 1986, 871–889.

O'Toole, J., "Employee Practices at the Best Managed Companies," *California Management Review*, Fall 1985, 35–65.

Probst, M. R., and Noga, J. M., "A Decentralized Nursing Care Delivery System," *Supervisor Nurse*, Jan. 1980, 57–60.

Sashkin, M., "Participative Management Remains an Ethical Imperative," *Organizational Dynamics*, Spring 1986, 62–75.

Vlcek, D. J., Jr., "Decentralization: What Works and What Doesn't," *Journal of Business Strategy*, Fall 1987, 71–74.

Wagel, W. H., "Working (and Managing) without Supervisors," *Personnel*, Sept. 1987, 8–11.

·14·

The Directing Process

INTRODUCTION AND BACKGROUND

In describing the functions of management, Fayol stated that managers must know how to handle people and must be able to defend their point of view with confidence and enthusiasm. Managers must learn continuously and must educate people at all levels for success in their assigned tasks.[1]

Fayol stated that command occurs when the manager gets "the optimum return from all employees of his [sic] unit in the interest of the whole concern."[2] To do this the manager must know the personnel, eliminate the incompetent, be well versed in binding agreements with employees, set a good example; conduct periodic audits; confer with chief assistants to focus on unity of direction, not become mired in detail, and have as a goal unity, energy, initiative, and loyalty among employees.[3] Fayol defined coordination as creating harmony among all activities to facilitate the working and success of the unit.[4] In modern management, command and coordination are labelled "directing."

According to Urwick, the purpose of command and the function of directing is to see that individual interests do not interfere with the general interest.[5] Command, (directing) protects the general interest and should ensure that each unit has a competent and energetic head. Command functions to promote esprit de corps and to carefully select a staff that can be of most service.[6] Urwick's premise is that bringing in new blood rather than promoting may excite resentment. He indicated the need for a grievance procedure, for common rules to be observed by all, and for regulation that allows for self-discipline. Managers should explain regulations and cut red tape. They should "decarbonize," clean out rules and regulations as needed.[7]

Rowland and Rowland stated that directing is "closely interrelated with leadership."[8] They suggested that a manager's choice of leadership style will be the major factor in exercising the directing function. Among the activities of directing are delegation, communication, training, and motivation.[9]

Kron used the term "implementing" as a synonym for "directing." The activities noted under this function include supervision, making assignments and giving directions, observation, evaluation, and leadership and interpersonal relationships with coworkers, dissemination, assignment of patient care, motivating workers, and maintaining morale.[10]

Douglass provided the following definition:

Directing is the issuance of assignments, orders, and instructions that permit the worker to understand what is expected of him or her, and the guidance and overseeing of the worker so that he or she can contribute effectively and efficiently to the attainment of organizational objectives.[11]

Douglass considered interpersonal relationships and communication to be directing functions, leadership and management taking effect through communication. According to Douglass, there are twelve technical activities or objectives related to the directing function at lower or first-level management. These activities are part of the directing function of the nurse manager and include:

1. Formulating objectives for care that are realistic for the health agency, patient, client, and nursing personnel.
2. Giving first priority to the needs of the patients/clients assigned to the nursing staff.
3. Providing for coordination and efficiency among departments that provide support services.
4. Identifying responsibility for all activities under the purview of the nursing staff.
5. Providing for safe, continuous care.
6. Considering the need for variety in task assignment and for development of personnel.
7. Providing for the leader's availability to staff members for assistance, teaching, counsel, and evaluation.
8. Trusting members to follow through with their assignments.
9. Interpreting protocol for responding to incidental requests.
10. Explaining procedure to be followed in emergencies.
11. Giving clear, concise, formal and informal directions.
12. Using a management control process that assesses the quality of care given and evaluates individual and group performance given by nursing personnel.[12]

Fulmer and Franklin defined a manager or supervisor as "someone who is responsible for directing the performance of one or more workers so that organizational goals are accomplished."[13] Rubin, Fry, and Plovnick wrote of directing in terms of theories of leadership effectiveness, group dynamics, values and value conflicts, effective interpersonal transactions, working with teams, and managing teams in organizations.[14] Barrett referred to development of personnel and supervision of work; Alexander to communication, assignments, and staffing.[15]

According to Donovan, standards are a basis for directing and controlling. They provide direction for performance. Other sources for direction are procedure and policy manuals. A nurse manager orients a new worker to the use of these manuals and thereby facilitates the following of standards in the performance of nursing work. Other sources of standards are job descriptions arrived at through job analysis. They subsequently form the basis for personnel evaluation. Donovan indicated that nursing care plans, nursing care conferences, and patient care conferences are the vehicles for directing nursing care. Directing is also influenced by the physical plant, how the facilities are organized, and by patient distribution according to degree of illness.[16]

DIRECTING AND NURSING MANAGEMENT

Directing is a physical act of nursing management, the interpersonal process by which nursing personnel accomplish the objectives of nursing. To understand fully what it entails, the nurse manager examines the conceptual functions of nursing management, that is, planning and organizing.[17] From the statement of mission or purpose, the statement of beliefs or philosophy, and the written objectives, the nurse manager develops management plans, the process by which methods and techniques are selected and used to accomplish the work of the nursing unit. Directing is the process of applying the management plans to accomplish nursing objectives. It is the process by which nursing personnel are inspired or motivated to accomplish work. Three of the major elements of directing are embodied in supervision of nursing personnel: motivation, leadership, and communication.[18] These elements are discussed in succeeding chapters.

Nurse managers will learn something of the nature of human beings. Subordinates are hired as total human beings and have to be managed as total human beings who respond to many institutions within society: church, school, government, family, service organizations, professional societies, and all of the other social groupings. There are similarities and differences between supervisors and subordinates. Both are complex human beings with known and conscious needs for food, safety, sex, and human associations. People react to the stresses and strains of a fast-paced society and may need some time for solitude if they are to function effectively and survive. Most individuals place their own concerns before those of others. They enjoy work from which the benefits exceed the costs, and they take a job that meets their established priorities for income and, maybe, social life.

People can be led and will accept leadership for various reasons, among them admiration, power, income, and safety. The zest with which they pursue achieving the objectives of the nursing division, department, service, or unit will correspond to the leader's ability to create an internal environment that inspires them to work at the levels of their capabilities. It is inherent in the acceptance of a management position that the person develop and use leadership abilities. These include:

1. Identification of personal training needs of individuals and establishment of programs to meet them.
2. Establishment of a system of performance appraisal to identify personal competencies and assignment and promotion based on competency.
3. Development of trust and subsequent delegation of responsibility and authority for decision making.

A good leader will contribute to creating a work environment that has the following properties:

1. Jobs that offer a living wage as well as adequate work.
2. Group identity and group purpose—the opportunity to work with others.
3. Pleasant surroundings and coworkers.
4. Interesting work.
5. Recognition that employee's work is valued and well done.
6. Opportunity for accomplishment and challenge.
7. Harmony between organizational and individual goals: equality of opportunity to be safe and secure, to achieve differently, to have choices

about shifts, to have job enlargement, and to be recognized as an individual.

Like other human beings, nurse leaders who are also nurse managers are in many ways different from subordinates. They persuade the group to work to achieve organizational objectives. Nurse leaders know more about organizational policies, goals, new programs, and plans for change. They are believed to have good judgment based on a breadth of experience. Nurse leaders are expected to behave in a socially acceptable manner, to exhibit personal qualities acceptable to subordinates, and to demonstrate skill in leadership, communication, and motivation techniques.

Effective directing increases subordinates' contributions to achievement of nursing management goals. Effective directing creates harmony between nursing management goals and nursing workers' goals. Effective directing operationalizes the principle of unity of command; a subordinate is answerable to one boss as completely as is possible.[19]

DELEGATING

Delegating is a major element of the directing function of nursing management. It is an effective management competency by which nurse managers get the work done through their employees. One of the criticisms of new nurse managers is that they emerge from clinical nurse roles and fail to develop identification with their management roles. They have been rewarded for their nursing, not for their skill in leading nurses. Delegation is a part of management that requires professional management training and development to accept the hierarchical responsibilities of delegation. Nurse managers need to be able to accept delegation of some of their own duties, tasks, and responsibilities as a solution to overwork leading to stress, anger, and aggression.

As nurse managers learn to accept the principle of delegation they become more productive and come to enjoy relationships with the staff. They learn to delegate by purposefully thinking about the delegation process, by doing careful planning for it, by gaining knowledge of clinical nurses' capabilities, by planning and implementing effective interpersonal communications, and by being willing to take risks. As they learn to delegate they become freed of daily pressures and time-consuming chores and have time to manage.

The following is a list of ways for nurse managers to delegate successfully:

1. Train and develop subordinates. It is an investment. Give them reasons for the task, authority, details, opportunity for growth, and written instructions if needed.
2. Plan ahead. It prevents problems.
3. Control and coordinate the work of subordinates. Do not peer over their shoulders. Develop ways of measuring the accomplishment of objectives with communication, standards, measurements, and feedback to prevent errors. Nursing employees want to know the nurse manager's expectations of them. They understand expectations when there are clear, consistent messages and behavior that prevents confusion. They understand expectations from clearly defined jobs, work relationships, and expected results.
4. Visit subordinates periodically. Spot potential problems of morale, disagreement, and grievance.
5. Coordinate to prevent duplication of effort.
6. Solve problems and think about new ideas. Emphasize employees solving their own problems.
7. Accept delegation as desirable.
8. Specify goals and objectives.
9. Know subordinates' capabilities and match the task or duty to the employee. Be sure the employee considers it important.
10. Agree on performance standards. Relate managerial references to employee performance.
11. Take an interest.
12. Assess results. Expect what is clearly and directly asked for as the deadline set for completing and reporting arrives. The nurse manager should accept the fact that employees will perform delegated tasks in their own style.
13. Give appropriate rewards.
14. Do not take back delegated tasks.[20]

Build professional nurses' self-esteem by delegating as much of the authority for nursing practice as possible. Professional nurses want authority over their practice and can be educated to perform management tasks related to it. Nurse managers will determine what authority to delegate through communication with clinical nurses. It will be commensurate with assigned responsibility. As professional nurses gain individual self-esteem, organizational self-esteem follows. Employees respond to participation in decision making and gain satisfaction with their jobs and the organization.

Reasons for Delegating

Five reasons for delegating include;

1. Assigning routine tasks
2. Assigning tasks for which the nurse manager does not have time
3. Problem solving
4. Changes in nurse manager's own job emphasis
5. Capability building[21]

The nurse manager should be careful not to misuse the clinical nurse by delegating tasks that can be done by nonnurses or nonlicensed personnel. This error can be avoided by consulting with clinical nurses to determine what authority they want.

Techniques for Delegating

Nurse managers at all levels can prepare lists of duties that can be delegated, from nurse executive to department head, from department head to unit head, and from unit head to clinical nurse. Delegation includes authority to approve, recommend, or implement. The list of duties should be ranked by time required to perform them and their importance to the institution. One duty should be delegated at a time.

When Not to Delegate

Do not delegate the power to discipline, responsibility for maintaining morale, overall control, a "hot potato," jobs that are too technical, or duties involving a trust or confidence.[22] These are complicated areas of nursing management requiring specialized knowledge and skills. Nurse managers who handle them should be well educated in the sciences of management and behavioral technology. Delegating these duties and responsibilities will cause clinical nurses to assume that managers are incompetent to handle these areas of nursing leadership and management.

MANAGEMENT BY OBJECTIVES

Management by objectives (MBO) as a directing element was first advocated by Peter Drucker and made famous by George Ordiorne who defined it as:

"a process whereby the superior and subordinate managers of an organization jointly identify its common goals, define each individual's major areas of responsibility in terms of the results expected of him (sic), and use these measures as guides for operating the unit and assessing the contribution of each of its members."[23]

Ordiorne further defines MBO as a system for making organizational structure work, to bring about vitality and personal involvement in the hierarchy by means of statements of what is expected from everyone involved and measurement of what is actually achieved. It stresses ability and achievement rather than personality.[24]

MBO allows the individual nurse to contribute to the common goal of the enterprise while nurse managers focus on the business goals. It promotes high standards, focusing on the job and not on the manager or the worker.

MBO spells out the results expected of the clinical nursing unit and of the unit in relation to other units. It emphasizes teamwork and team results. It will include short-range and long-range objectives, as well as tangible and intangible objectives. Intangible objectives include development of the individual, performance and attitude of workers, and public responsibilities. Objectives should include those that indicate the contributions to higher levels of the enterprise.

MBO allows people to control their own performance, to measure themselves, and to exercise self-control. Through MBO, clinical nurses make demands upon themselves. Nurse managers will assume that clinical nurses want to be responsible, want to contribute, want to achieve, and have the strength and desire to do so.

Procedure and Process

Training. Begin the training for the MBO process with the nurse managers of the enterprise. They will learn the characteristics of the process, the objectives of initiating an MBO program, the procedures to be used, and methods for evaluating its effectiveness. During this training program nurse managers can simulate the procedures to be used.

Once nurse managers are trained, all nursing employees are given similar training. Employees will be made aware of the necessity for writing and working toward their personal objectives as they seek to achieve those of the organization. They will be taught the value of synergism of personal and organizational objectives. They will bring their written lists of objectives to the first meeting with their superiors. See Figure 14–1.

First Meeting. The first MBO meeting should be held in quiet surroundings, with sufficient time for discussion. The nurse manager should set the employee at ease. As they present each personal objective the nurse manager relates it to an objective of the enterprise. Thus they create the conditions for them to fulfill these needs. This includes the removal of obstacles, encouragement of growth, and provision of guidance.

Nurses, like other workers, do not have their higher-level needs met by their employers. They meet these higher-level needs by using their capabilities, having responsibility, being active, having meaningful work, being self-controlled and self-directed, and being treated as mature adults. They want to participate by setting their own targets and evaluating themselves in obtaining them.[25] Nurse managers can facilitate these processes by establishing a climate and environment that supports achievement of the higher-level needs of clinical nurses.

Nurses are professionals and will not be controlled. Nurse managers and clinical nurse employees can explain their jobs to each other during the MBO process. The nurse manager may learn that the clinical nurse wants management to promote dignity and personal responsibility, peer status and acceptance, and recognition for achievement and creativity. The clinical nurse may learn that the nurse manager represents an organization that will create the conditions for them to achieve their own goals by directing their efforts toward the goals of the organization.[26]

During this first meeting nurse managers and clinical nurses set goals that are specific, promote teamwork, are measurable in terms of being quantified or described qualitatively, and are attainable. Goals should involve enough risk to challenge but not defeat. They should include objectives that are routine, problem solving, creative or innovative, and for personal development.[27]

At the end of the first meeting both nurse manager and clinical nurse should be satisfied with the written objectives. Each will have a copy. They will part with an understanding of how future meetings will progress and mutual expectations, including a time for the next meeting.

Phase	Key Activities	Participants
Planning	Identify and define key organizational goals.	Manager
	Identify and define key departmental goals that stem from overall goals.	
	Identify and define performance measures (operational goals) for employees.	
	Formulate and propose goals for specific job.	Subordinate
	Formulate and propose measures for specific jobs.	
	Participate in management conferences.	Manager and subordinates
	Achieve joint agreement on individual objectives and individual performance.	
	Set up timetable for periodic meetings for performance review.	
Performance review	Continue to participate in management conferences.	Manager and subordinates
	Adjust and refine objectives based on feedback, new constraints, and new inputs.	
	Eliminate inappropriate goals.	
	Readjust timetable as needed.	
	Maintain ongoing comparison of proposed timetable and actual performance through use of control monitoring devices, such as visible control charts.	
Feedback to new planning stage	Review overall organizational and departmental goals for the next planning period, such as the next fiscal year.	Manager

Reprinted from *Management Principles for Health Professionals* by J. G. Liebler, R. E. Levine, and H. L. Dervitz, p. 37, with permission of Aspen Publishers, Inc. © 1984.

Figure 14–1 • Summary of MBO Cycle

Actions. Between meetings employees perform work that meets their agreed-on objectives. They should periodically review these objectives and summarize their accomplishments.

Second Meeting. Conditions for the second MBO meeting will be as for the first meeting. It will be a time for evaluation of results, review, appraisal, and setting further goals.

Employees should be encouraged to spell out gratifying and exhilarating experiences, to do self-examination, and to relate their thoughts about work. Nurse managers should listen and make the employees feel safe while helping them to have a person-organization fit.

Superiors examine their own reactions without criticizing the subordinates. They build trust and confidence as well as an ethical relationship. In doing so they establish an organizational climate for personal and organizational achievement.[28]

MBO should include appraisal of managers by subordinates. The latter will appraise how well the manager helps employees do their jobs, supports them, assists with problems, and demonstrates proficiency and visibility.[29]

Both nurse manager and employee should exit this meeting with a sense of accomplishment. This does not mean they will not be made aware of deficiencies or shortcomings. It will be recognized in the form of needed additions or changes, increased progress, and even deletions. All will be tied to patient care and organizational development. The feedback process tells employees what is expected and when they make errors.

This process will be repeated at intervals, with dates and times agreed on at each meeting. At the end of an appraisal period, performance-results contracts will be signed off and sent to the personnel department for the employees' records. These performance appraisals can be used to identify promotion potential and determine merit pay increases.

Figure 14–1 illustrates the MBO process and Figure 14–2 is a list of standards for evaluating the directing function of nursing management.

A theory of nursing management explores the

1. Managers have established a medium by which nursing workers feel free to ask for advice, counsel, and consultation.

2. Needed written directions are available in the form of policies, procedures, standards of care, job analyses, job descriptions, job standards, and nursing care plans. They are clearly stated and current.

3. A training program is in effect that meets nursing employees' needs as they perceive them. They participate.

4. Supervisors are competent in needed knowledge and skills of administration and clinical specialization.

5. Nurse managers periodically work evening, night, weekend, and holiday shifts to keep abreast of clinical and administrative behaviors peculiar to these shifts.

6. The nurse administrator has operationalized ANA *Standards for Organized Nursing Services* and *Responsibilities of Nurse Administrators across All Settings.*

7. The nurse managers have operationalized the ANA *Standards of Nursing Practice.*

8. Nurse managers are knowledgeable about and apply the appropriate Standards of the Joint Commission on Accreditation of Healthcare Organizations, National League for Nursing, and Medicare and Medicaid.

9. The nurse administrator uses techniques of operations analysis. (This service is available at no charge to member hospitals of the American Hospital Association and its state affiliates.)

10. Nurse managers use a system of management by objectives.

11. The nurse administrator works with the consent and knowledge of patients, and solicits input from consumers regarding nursing services desired.

12. Nursing unit personnel are organized into and working as direct care personnel and clerical personnel.

13. Nurse managers use the physical plant to the best advantage for patients and personnel.

Figure 14–2 • *Standards for Evaluation of the Directing Function*

cause-effect relationship between clinical nurses and their performances. It has as object the removal of controls that create distrust, fear, and re-

sentment and the promotion of conditions (climate) that provide opportunities for clinical nurses to achieve their goals.

SUMMARY

Effective directing will result in greater harmony in the actions of supervisors and subordinates and in the achievement of the objectives of personnel as well as of the enterprise. Directing will be most effective when subordinates have a single superior with whom they have direct personal contact. Directing that encourages leadership, motivation, and communication techniques and that emphasizes the human aspects of managing individuals is most desirable. It can be fostered by nursing administrators who desire to improve their directing activities.

EXPERIENTIAL EXERCISES

1. Look at the statements of mission, philosophy, and objectives of a unit or division of nursing in which you work as a student.

1.1 What is the work of the unit or division?

1.2 What is the inference for the directing function of the unit or division?

2. Scenario: Jennie Lynd, RN, has been working in the newborn nursery for 1 year. Her performance in caring for babies, in teaching parents, and in supporting other unit personnel has been exemplary. She has been told this. Jennie Lynd tells her head nurse she is interested in a transfer to the Pediatric Intensive Care Unit.

With a group of your peers, decide how the head nurse should handle this request.

3. Scenario: As a nurse manager, Ms. Pressley, RN, has studied career development theory because she believes that clinical nurses do not really have careers. This is particularly true when a clinical ladder is nonexistent. Ms. Pressley plans to counsel her clinical nurses regularly and to push for a clinical promotion ladder that recognizes advanced competence, education, and certification. This activity falls within the directing category of management. Compare Ms. Pressley's actions with those of several other nurse managers you know or have known. Summarize your findings.

4. Scenario: Mr. Thompson, RN, is a director of emergency department nursing. His department is extremely busy and he is required to attend many meetings. As a policy, he is teaching members of his clinical RN staff to be his representative at selected meetings. He has one accompany him to each meeting so he can introduce the individual to other committee members and orient him or her to the committee's business. Each RN has one or more such assignments.

4.1 Which of the following directing activities is Mr. Thompson primarily performing?

____ *4.1.1* Delegating.

____ *4.1.2* Communicating.

____ *4.1.3* Training.

____ *4.1.1* Motivating.

4.2 Compare Mr. Thompson's performance with that of one or more equivalent nurse managers you know or have known. Do this specifically to identify delegating activities. Make a list of activities they delegate to their subordinate managers and clinical RN staff.

4.3 Make a list of activities that *could have been delegated* to their subordinate managers and clinical R.N. staff.

4.4 Summarize your assessment of this delegation observation.

5. Scenario: S. Baez, RN, is a nurse administrator who believes that to give professional clinical nurses autonomy, they can be delegated such activities as time schedules, policy and procedure development, quality assurance activities, authority to call other departments for service, and a host of other activities. As a reward for participation, these activities count toward clinical promotion, pay increases, and paid travel to professional meetings.

5.1 What activities are being delegated?

5.2 How are clinical nurses rewarded when they accept delegated activities?

6. Select one or more goals you would like to accomplish in the unit in which you work as a student. Make a management plan to accomplish the selected goal or goals. The process should:

6.1 Cover *your* individual objectives.

6.2 Be discussed and adjusted with your boss.

6.3 Have a plan for achieving each objective.

6.4 Set a time to evaluate accomplishment with your boss.

MANAGEMENT PLAN

PROBLEM:

OBJECTIVE:

ACTIONS	TARGET DATES	ASSIGNED TO	ACCOMPLISHMENTS

7. Use Figure 14–2, Standards for Evaluation of the Directing Function, to evaluate one of these entities in which you work as a student. Identify one concrete example for each. Summarize your results.

7.1 If the directing function does not meet the standards, use a problem-solving approach and implement a plan of improvement. Use the following format to make a management plan.

MANAGEMENT PLAN

PROBLEM:

OBJECTIVE:

ACTIONS	TARGET DATES	ASSIGNED TO	ACCOMPLISHMENTS

NOTES

1. H. Fayol, *General and Industrial Management*, trans. by C. Storrs (London: Sir Isaac Pitman & Sons, 1949), 82–96.
2. Ibid., 97.
3. Ibid., 97–98.
4. Ibid., 103.
5. L. Urwick, *The Elements of Administration* (New York: Harper & Row, 1944), 77.
6. Ibid., 81–82.
7. Ibid., 90–96.
8. H. S. Rowland and B. L. Rowland, eds., *Nursing Administration Handbook*, 2d ed. (Rockville, MD: Aspen, 1980), 7.
9. Ibid., 8.
10. T. Kron and A. Gray, *The Management of Patient Care: Putting Leadership Skills to Work*, 6th ed. (Philadelphia: W. B. Saunders, 1987), 155–176.
11. L. M. Douglass, *The Effective Nurse: Leader and Manager* 3d ed. (St. Louis: Mosby, 1988), 115.
12. Ibid., 117–118.
13. R. M. Fulmer and S. G. Franklin, *Supervision: Principles of Professional Management*, 2d ed. (New York: Macmillan, 1982), 6.
14. I. M. Rubin, R. E. Fry, and M. S. Plovnick, eds., *Managing Human Resources in Health Care Organizations* (Reston, VA: Reston Publishing, 1978), 128–129, 154–161, 182–189, 198, 236–243.
15. J. Barrett, *The Head Nurse: Her Changing Role* (New York: Appleton Century Crofts, 1968), 310–332; E. L. Alexander, *Nursing Administration in the Hospital Health Care System*, 2d ed. (St. Louis: Mosby, 1978), 198–246.
16. H. M. Donovan, *Nursing Service Administration: Managing the Enterprise* (St. Louis: Mosby, 1975), 128–154.
17. C. Arndt and L. M. D. Huckabay, *Nursing Administration: Theory for Practice with a Systems Approach*, 2d ed. (St. Louis: Mosby, 1980), 92–106.
18. H. Koontz, C. O'Donnell and H. Weihrich, *Essentials of Management*, 4th ed. (New York: McGraw-Hill, 1986), 392.
19. R. C. Swansburg, *The Directing Function of Nursing Service Administration* (Hattiesburg, MS: University of Southern Mississippi School of Nursing, 1977), 3–5.
20. B. B. Beegle, "Don't Do It—Delegate It!," *Supervisory Management*, Apr. 1970; J. K. Matejka and R. J. Dunsing, "Great Expectations," *Management World*, Jan. 1987, 16–17.
21. Rowland and Rowland, eds., op. cit., 54–57.
22. Ibid.
23. R. M. Hogdetts, *Management: Theory, Process and Practice*, 4th ed. (Orlando, FL: Academic Press, 1986), 575.
24. Ibid.
25. D. McGregor, *Leadership and Motivation* (Cambridge, MA: MIT Press, 1966).
26. Ibid.
27. M. L. Bell, "Management by Objectives," *Journal of Nursing Administration*, May 1980, 19–26.
28. H. Levinson, "Management by Whose Objectives?," *Harvard Business Review*, July–Aug. 1970, 125–134.
29. Ibid.

FOR FURTHER REFERENCE

Beck, A. C., Jr., and Hillman, E. D. "OD to MBO or MBO to OD: Does It Make a Difference?," in A. T. Hollingsworth and R. M. Hodgetts, *Readings in Basic Management* (Philadelphia: W. B. Saunders, 1975), 190–196.

Drucker, P. F., *Management: Tasks, Responsibilities, Practices* (New York: Harper & Row, 1973, 1974), 430–442.

Gibson, J. L., Ivancevich, J. W., and Donnelly, J. H., Jr., *Organizations: Behavior, Structure, Processes*, 6th ed. (Homewood, IL: Richard A. Irwin, 1988).

Holley, W. H., and Jennings, K. M., *Personnel Management: Functions and Issues* (New York: Dryden Press, 1983), 237–240.

Leadership

SHARON FARLEY, PhD, RN

Associate Professor
School of Nursing
Auburn University at Montgomery
Montgomery, Alabama

"Florence Nightingale, after leaving the Crimea, exercised extraordinary leadership in health care for decades with no organization under her command."[1]

"One of the purest examples of the leader as agenda-setter was Florence Nightingale. Her public image was and is that of the lady of mercy, but under her gentle, soft-spoken manner, she was a rugged spirit, a fighter, a tough-minded system changer. In mid-nineteenth Century England a woman had no place in public life, least of all in the fiercely masculine world of the military establishment. But she took on the establishment and revolutionized health care in the British military services. Yet she never made public appearances or speeches, and except for her two years in the Crimea, held no public position. She was a formidable authority on the evils to be remedied, she knew exactly what to do about them, and she used public opinion to goad top officials to adopt her agenda."[2]

Florence Nightingale was both leader and manager.

LEADERSHIP DEFINED

Researchers have studied leadership for decades, but experts still do not agree on exactly what it is. Many persons use the term leadership as if it were a magic quality, almost as if one must be born with it or as if one simply has a talent for it. However, like talent for music and art, leadership requires much knowledge and disciplined practice. Many definitions of leadership have been written, among them that of Stogdill, who defines it as " 'the process of influencing the activities of an organized group in its efforts toward goal setting and goal achievement.' "[3] There is a difference in responsibilities among group members, and each influences the groups' activities. A leader is one others follow willingly and voluntarily.[4]

Stogdill's definition of leadership can be applied to nursing. In nursing practice, goals of patient care are set. Each patient has a nursing care plan that lists the problems that interfere with achieving physical, emotional, and social needs. For each problem a goal is set and an approach or nursing prescription is written. An interdisciplinary team may identify problems, set goals, and write prescriptions. They are influenced by the most highly skilled nurse available, the registered nurse who coordinates the care. Each interdisciplinary team member assumes different responsibilities in performing the total team functions. This process holds true when the modality of team nursing is practiced or when there is a mixed staff of RNs, LPNs, and nursing assistants.

The same principles may be applied to the entire division of nursing. Usually the head of the division is titled assistant administrator, vice-president, chair, or director of nursing services. This person is responsible for influencing all nursing employees in achieving the stated purpose and objectives of the division of nursing. The nurse administrator is influenced by a stated philosophy or statement of beliefs about the kinds of services to be rendered by the personnel of the division of nursing. The total staff includes personnel in different job categories, including head nurses, clinical nurse managers of shifts, and clinical nursing personnel, each with differing nursing responsibilities.

Gardner defines leadership as "the process of persuasion and example by which an individual (or leadership team) induces a group to take action that is in accord with the leader's purposes or the shared purposes of all."[5] Numerous other definitions of leadership exist. Embodied in these definitions are the terms leader, follower or constituent, group, process, and goals. One would conclude that leadership is a process in which a person inspires a group of constituents to work together using appropriate means to achieve a common mission and common goals. They are influenced to do this willingly and cooperatively, with zeal and confidence and to their greatest potential.[6]

Merton described leadership as a social transaction in which one person influences others. He stated that persons in authority do not necessarily exert leadership. Rather, effective people in authoritative positions combine authority and leadership to assist an organization to achieve its goals. Merton described effective leadership as satisfying four primary conditions:

1. A person receiving a communication understands it.
2. This person has the resources to do what is being asked in the communication.
3. This person believes the behavior being asked is consistent with personal interests and values.
4. This person believes it is consistent with the purposes and values of the organization.[7]

According to McGregor, "there are at least four major variables now known to be involved in leadership: (1) the characteristics of the leader; (2) the attitudes, needs, and other personal characteristics of the followers; (3) the characteristics of the organization, such as its purpose, its structure, the nature of the task to be performed; and (4) the social, economic, and political milieu."[8] McGregor said that leadership is a highly complex relationship that changes with the times, such changes being brought about by management, unions, or outside forces. In nursing, changes in leadership are wrought by nursing management, nursing educators, nursing organizations, unions, and the expectations of the clientele—patients and their families.

Talbott said, "Leadership is the vital ingredient that transforms a crowd into a functioning, useful organization."[9] The theme seems always to be the same: "Leadership is the process of sustaining an initiated action. It is certainly not a matter of pointing in a direction and just letting things happen. Leadership is the conception of a goal and a method of achieving it; the mobilization of the means necessary for attainment; and the adjustment of values and environmental factors in the light of the desired end."[10]

In all of the definitions, leadership is viewed as a dynamic, interactive process that involves three dimensions—the leader, the followers, and the situation. Each of the dimensions influences the others. For instance, the accomplishment of goals depends not only on the personal attributes of the leader but also on follower needs and the type of situation.[11]

LEADERSHIP THEORIES

Trait Theories

Much of the early work on leadership focused on the leader. This research was directed toward identifying intellectual, emotional, physical, and other personal traits of effective leaders. The underlying assumption was that leaders are born, not made.

Intelligence	Personality	Abilities
Judgment	Adaptability	Ability to enlist cooperation
Decisiveness	Alertness	Popularity and prestige
Knowledge	Creativity	Sociability (interpersonal skills)
Fluency of speech	Cooperativeness	Social participation
	Personal integrity	Tact, diplomacy
	Self-confidence	
	Emotional balance and control	
	Independence (nonconformity)	

SOURCE: Adapted from B. M. Bass, *Stogdill's Handbook of Leadership* (New York: Free Press, 1982), in J. Gibson, J. Ivancevich, and J. Donnelly, *Organizations: Behavior, Structure, Processes*, 6th ed. (Homewood, IL: Richard D. Irwin, 1988), 375.

Figure 15–1 • *Traits Associated with Leadership Effectiveness*

After many years of research, no particular set of traits has been found that predict leadership potential. There are some possible reasons for this failure to find specific traits. According to McGregor, "research findings to date suggest that it is more fruitful to consider leadership as a relationship between the leader and the situation than as a universal pattern of characteristics possessed by certain people."[12] This statement implies that leadership is a human relations function and that different situations may require quite different characteristics or traits of a leader. Is it not to a large degree universally accepted in nursing that authoritarian power is effective in times of crisis but that it otherwise promotes instability?

Despite the shortcomings of the trait theory, some traits have been identified that are common to all good leaders. A summary of some of the most researched traits is shown in Figure 15–1.

Intelligence. Traits related to intelligence include knowledge, decisiveness, and fluency of speech. Perceived knowledge and competence in a specific job is one of the most important factors in a leader's effectiveness. A competent leader has expert power when it is used to inspire subordinates to excel in performance. Leaders who are competent and expert have greater latitude in their relationship with subordinates.

Personality. Personality traits such as adaptability, self-confidence, creativity, and personal integrity are associated with effective leadership. A leader is effective and knows how to motivate workers to achieve the goals of the organization.

Abilities

A leader has sufficient popularity, prestige, and interpersonal skills to symbolize, extend, and deepen collective unity among members of the system. In most nursing situations, the leader is appointed by the hospital or nursing administrator. Without losing authority and control, an appointed leader has to demonstrate understanding and achieve the worker's understanding of and motivation for achieving the goals of the organization. Too often the supervisor has been appointed because of technical and administrative talents rather than leadership abilities or acceptance by the group. This fact points up the relative emphasis given to leadership abilities and attitudes.

All of these traits and characteristics can be used by leaders either to inspire or to deflate morale and esprit de corps. Nurse managers need to develop those nurses who inspire high morale and esprit de corps.

Although it may be that leaders are made, not born, there are some persons who are natural leaders. They emerge from a group in which they have made known their talents for representing and articulating group values and goals. These natural leaders have plans for meeting the personal needs of the group, and thus the group willingly accepts their direction. *The group gives the person in the lead-*

ership role influence. According to Holloman, "Leadership results when the appointed head causes the members of his (*sic*) group to accept his directives without any apparent exertion of authority or force on his part."[13]

Behavioral Theories

Among the behavioral research and theories are those of Douglas McGregor's Theory X and Theory Y, Rensis Likert's Michigan Studies, Blake and Mouton's managerial Grid®, and Kurt Lewin's studies. Each of these is described in more detail following.

McGregor's Theory X and Theory Y. McGregor's Theory X and Theory Y are described elsewhere in this book. McGregor related his theories to the motivation theories of Maslow.

McGregor stated that each person is a whole individual living and interacting within a world of other individuals. What happens to this person happens as a result of the behavior of other people. The attitudes and emotions of others affect this person. The subordinate is dependent on the superior and desires to be treated fairly. A successful relationship is desired by both and depends on the action taken by the superior.

Security is a condition of leadership. Subordinates need security and will fight to protect themselves against real or imagined threats to these needs in the work situation. Superiors must act to give subordinates this security through avenues such as fair pay and fringe benefits. Unions act to solidify job security.

A superior provides a further condition for effective leadership by creating an atmosphere of approval for subordinates. This atmosphere is created through the leader's manner and attitude. Given the genuine approval of their superior, subordinates will be secure. Otherwise they will feel threatened, fearful, and insecure.

Knowledge is another condition of effective leadership espoused by McGregor. People have security when they know what is expected of them, including:

1. Knowledge of overall company policy and management philosophy
2. Knowledge of procedures, rules, and regulations
3. Knowledge of the requirements of the subordinate's own job—duties, responsibilities, and place in the organization
4. Knowledge of the personal peculiarities of the subordinate's immediate superior
5. Knowledge by subordinate of their superior's opinion of their performance
6. Advance knowledge of changes that may affect the subordinate[14]

Consistent discipline is another condition for effective leadership. People are met with approval when they do their jobs according to the rules. They should know what to expect in terms of disapproval when they break these rules. Superiors should be consistent in setting standards and expecting subordinates to meet them. Even discipline must occur in an atmosphere of approval.

Security encourages independence, another condition for effective leadership. Insecurity causes a reactive fight for freedom. Security that stimulates independence is desired. Subordinates need to be actively independent by becoming involved in contributing ideas and suggestions concerning activities that affect them. When workers are secure and are encouraged to participate in solving the problems of work, they provide new approaches to solutions of problems. They work to achieve the goals of the organization and feel they are a part of the organization.

With security and independence, subordinates develop a desire to accept responsibility. The level of responsibility can be increased at a pace commensurate with preservation of their security. It will give them pleasure and pride. Superiors need security before they can delegate responsibility to subordinates.

All subordinates need provision for appeal, for an adequate grievance procedure by which they take their differences with their superiors to a higher level in the organization. Superiors who do the jobs expected of them, who treat subordinates in ways to meet their needs and give them security, achieve self-realization and self-development.[15]

Likert's Michigan Studies. Likert and his associates at the Institute for Social Research at the University of Michigan did extensive leadership research. They identified four basic styles or systems of leadership: exploitive-authoritative, benevolent-authoritative, consultative-democratic, and participative-democratic. These systems are summarized in Figure 15–2.

It is generally conceded that leadership behav-

Authoritative		Participative	
System I: Exploitive-authoritative	System II: Benevolent-authoritative	System III: Consultative-democratic	System IV: Participative-democratic
Top management makes all decisions	Top management makes most decisions	Some delegated decisions made at lower levels	Decision making dispersed throughout organization
Motivation by coercion	Motivation by economic and ego motives	Motivation by economic, ego, and other motives such as desire for new experiences	Motivation by economic rewards established by group participation
Communication downward	Communication mostly downward	Communication down and up	Communication down, up, and with peers
Review and control functions concentrated in top management	Review and control functions primarily at top	Review and control functions primarily at the top, but ideas are solicited from lower levels	Review and control functions shared by superiors and subordinates

SOURCE: Adapted from R. Likert, *The Human Organization* (New York: McGraw-Hill, 1967), 4–10. Reprinted with permission of McGraw-Hill Book Co. © 1967.

***Figure 15–2* •** *Likert's Leadership Systems*

ior improves in effectiveness as it approaches System IV.

Blake and Mouton's Managerial Grid®. The Managerial Grid® (or, as it is labeled in its latest form, the Leadership Grid® [Blake & McCanse, 1991]) is a two-dimensional leadership model. Dimensions of this model are tasks or production and employee or people orientations of managers.

Grid® Synopsis. *Two key dimensions of managerial thinking are depicted on the Grid®:* Concern for Production *on the horizontal axis, and* Concern for People *on the vertical axis. They are shown as 9-point scales where 1 represents low concern, 5 represents an average amount of concern, and 9 is high concern.*

These two concerns are interdependent; that is, while concern for one or the other may be high or low, they are integrated in the manager's thinking. Thus, both concerns are present to some degree in any management style. Study of the Grid® enables one to sort out various possibilities and the attitudes, values, beliefs, and assumptions that underlie each approach. When one is able to objectively see personal behavior in contrast with the soundest approach, it provides motivation to change in order to more closely approximate the soundest management. When group

members come to share 9,9 values, beliefs, attitudes, and assumptions, they develop personal commitment to achieving group goals as well as their individual goals. In doing so, they develop standards of mutual trust and respect that cause them to elevate cooperation and communication.

Blake and Mouton contend that the 9,9 style is the one most likely to achieve highest quality results over an extended period of time. The 9,9 style, unlike the others, is based on the assumption that there is no inherent conflict between the needs of the organization for performance and the needs of people for job satisfaction.

Finally, as an orienting framework, the Grid® serves as a road map toward more effective ways of working with and through others. When group members have this common frame of reference for what constitutes an effective and or an ineffective approach to issues of mutual concern, they are able to take corrective action based on common understanding and agreement about the soundest approach and objectivity when actions taken are less than fully sound.[16]

Figure 15–3A illustrates general management application of the Grid®, and Figure 15–3B illustrates its application to the job of the nurse administrator.

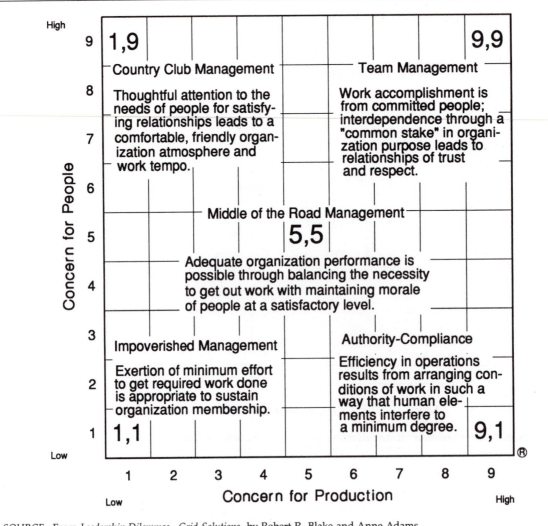

High

9 | **1,9**   **9,9**

Country Club Management   Team Management

Thoughtful attention to the needs of people for satisfying relationships leads to a comfortable, friendly organization atmosphere and work tempo.

Work accomplishment is from committed people; interdependence through a "common stake" in organization purpose leads to relationships of trust and respect.

Middle of the Road Management

5,5

Adequate organization performance is possible through balancing the necessity to get out work with maintaining morale of people at a satisfactory level.

Impoverished Management   Authority-Compliance

Exertion of minimum effort to get required work done is appropriate to sustain organization membership.

Efficiency in operations results from arranging conditions of work in such a way that human elements interfere to a minimum degree.

1,1   **9,1**

Concern for People (vertical axis, Low to High)

Concern for Production (horizontal axis, 1 2 3 4 5 6 7 8 9, Low to High)

SOURCE: From *Leadership Dilemmas—Grid Solutions*, by Robert R. Blake and Anne Adams McCanse. Houston: Gulf Publishing Company, p. 29. Copyright © 1991, by Scientific Methods, Inc.. Reproduced by permission of the owners.

Figure 15–3A • *The Leadership Grid®*

Kurt Lewin's Studies. Lewin's leadership studies were done in the 1930s. He examined three leadership styles related to forces within the leader, within the group members, and within the situation. These three leadership styles are summarized in Figure 15–4.

Other behavioral studies include the Ohio State studies using a quadrant structure that relates leadership effectiveness to initiating structure with emphasis on the task or production, and consideration, with emphasis on the employee. These studies identified four primary leadership styles as illustrated in Figure 15–5.

These researchers used the Leader Behavior Description Questionnaire. Items related to "initiating structure" and "consideration" describe how leaders carry out their activities. Both factors are considered simultaneously rather than on a continuum. As to which combination works best, the situation determines the style.[17]

LEADERSHIP STYLE

Other studies of leadership focus on style. These include contingency-situational leadership models that focus on a combination of factors such as the people, the task, the situation, the organization,

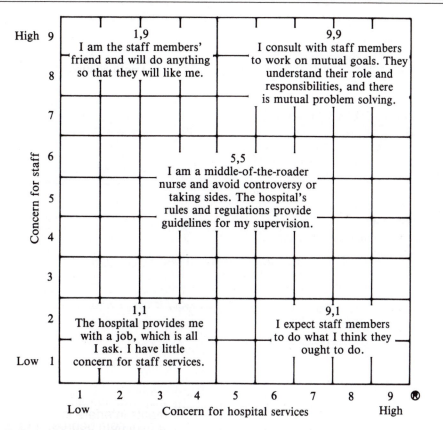

SOURCE: From *Grid Approaches for Managerial Leadership in Nursing*, by Robert R. Blake, Jane Srygley Mouton, and Mildred Tapper. St. Louis: C. V. Mosby Company. Copyright © 1981, page 2. Reproduced by permission.

Figure 15–3B • *The Nurse Administrator Grid®*

and a number of environmental factors. Such approaches combine theories of Fred F. Fiedler, William J. Reddin, Paul Hersey and Kenneth H. Blanchard, William Ouchi, and John W. Gardner whose contributions are discussed in the following sections.

Fiedler's Contingency Model of Leadership Effectiveness

There must be a group before there can be a leader. Fiedler indicates three classifications that measure the kind of power and influence the group gives its leader. The first and most important of these is the relationship between the leader and the group members. Personality is a factor but its influence depends on the group's perception of the leader. Second is the task structure, the degree to which details of the group's assignment are programmed.

If the assignment is highly structured, the leader will have less power. If it requires planning and thinking, the leader will be in a position to exert greater power. Third is the positional power of the leader; it should be noted that greater power does not yield better group performance. The best leader has been found to be one who has a task-oriented leadership style. This style works best when the leader has either great influence and power or when the leader has no influence or power over group members. When the leader has moderate influence over group members, a relationship-oriented style works best.

The organization shares responsibility for the leader's success or failure. Leaders can be trained to learn in which situations they do well and in which they fail. The job can be fitted to the leader. The appointee can be given a higher rank or can be assigned subordinates who are nearly equal in rank and status. Most appointees can be given sole

Autocratic. Leaders make decisions alone. They tend to be more concerned with task accomplishment than with concern for people. Autocratic leadership tends to promote hostility and aggression or apathy and to decrease initiative.

Democratic. Leaders involve their followers in the decision-making process. They are people-oriented and focus on human relations and teamwork. Democratic leadership leads to increased productivity and job satisfaction.

Laissez faire. Leaders are loose and permissive and abstain from leading their staff. They foster freedom for everyone and want everyone to feel good. Laissez-faire leadership results in low productivity and employee frustration.

SOURCE: Adapted from *Management: Concepts and Applications* by Leon Megginson et al. Copyright © 1986 by Harper & Row, Publishers, Inc. Reprinted by permission of HarperCollins Publishers.

Figure 15–4 • *Kurt Lewin's Studies of Leadership Styles*

authority or can be required to consult with the group. The appointee can be given detailed instructions or independence. Highly successful and effective leaders will avoid situations in which failure is likely. These leaders will seek out situations that fit their leadership style. Knowledge of strengths and weaknesses will help in choosing this style.[18]

Fiedler's theory is one of situations. Leadership style will be effective or ineffective depending on the situation.

The Life-Cycle Theory of Hersey and Blanchard

Blanchard and Hersey follow a situational approach to leadership. This theory predicts the most appropriate leadership style from the level of maturity or immaturity of the constituents.

With immaturity the leadership style will focus on the task, constituents being relatively passive and dependent. The leadership style will focus on relationship behaviors as the constituents become more mature, active, and independent.[19] This theory is illustrated in Figure 15–6.

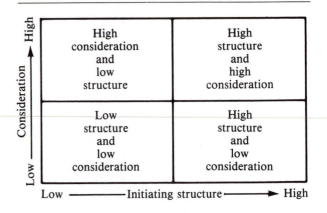
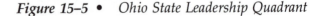

SOURCE: From *Management: Concepts and Applications* by Leon Megginson et al. Copyright © 1986 by Harper & Row, Publishers, Inc. Reprinted by permission of HarperCollins Publishers.

Figure 15–5 • *Ohio State Leadership Quadrant*

Reddin's Three-Dimensional Theory of Management

Reddin combined Blake and Mouton's managerial Grid® with Fiedler's contingency leadership style theory. The outcome was a three-dimensional theory of management, the dimensions being adapted from:

1. Managerial Grid® theory
2. Contingency leadership style theory
3. Effectiveness theory

The possible combinations result in four basic leadership styles (see Figure 15–7):

1. *Separated*, in which both task orientation and relationship orientation are minimal.
2. *Dedicated*, in which task orientation is high and relationship orientation low. Dedicated leaders are dedicated only to the job.
3. *Related*, in which relationship orientation is high and task orientation is low. Related leaders relate primarily to their subordinates.
4. *Integrated*, in which both task and relationship orientation are high. Integrated leaders focus on managerial behavior combining task orientation and relationship orientation.

These management styles are represented by the first two dimensions of Figure 15–7. The third dimension of effectiveness represents the degree of

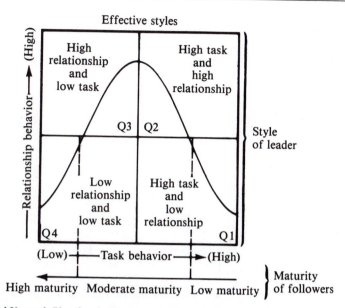

Effective styles

High relationship and low task — Q3

High task and high relationship — Q2

Low relationship and low task — Q4

High task and low relationship — Q1

Relationship behavior (High)

Task behavior — (Low) — (High)

Style of leader

High maturity Moderate maturity Low maturity

Maturity of followers

SOURCE: Paul Hersey and Kenneth Blanchard, *Management of Organizational Behavior: Utilizing Human Resources*, 3rd ed., © 1977, p. 164. Reprinted by permission of Prentice-Hall, Englewood Cliffs, New Jersey.

Figure 15–6 • *Life-Cycle Theory of Leadership*

the leader's achievement of position objectives and is situational:

- *Executive* leaders are integrated and more effective than *compromiser* leaders who are less effective integrated leaders.
- *Developer* leaders are related and more effective than *missionary* leaders who are less effective related leaders.
- *Bureaucrat* leaders are separated and more effective than *deserter* leaders who are less effective separated leaders.
- *Benevolent autocrat* leaders are dedicated and more effective than *autocrat* leaders who are less effective dedicated leaders.

The range of effectiveness is a continuum. As in other theories of leadership, the effective behavior of the leader is relative to the situation. Effective leaders apply leadership styles after assessing situations.[20]

Theory Z Organizations

Theory Z organizations focus on consensual decision making. Its democratic leadership style includes decentralization, participatory management, employee involvement, and quality of life. Leaders are managers who concentrate on developing and using their interpersonal skills. These theories have been attributed to William Ouchi.[21]

LEADERSHIP AND POWER

Gardner defines power as "the capacity to ensure the outcomes one wishes and to prevent those one does not wish."[22] Power is dispersed in a pluralistic society. The desirable social dimension of power brings about intended consequences and behavior that benefits people. The intended consequences and behavior can sometimes become malevolent even in a democratic society.

Power Bases

French and Raven suggested five interpersonal bases of power: legitimate, reward, coercive, expert, and referent.[23]

Legitimate Power. Legitimate power is a person's ability to influence because of that person's position. A person with a higher organizational position has power over people below. Legitimate

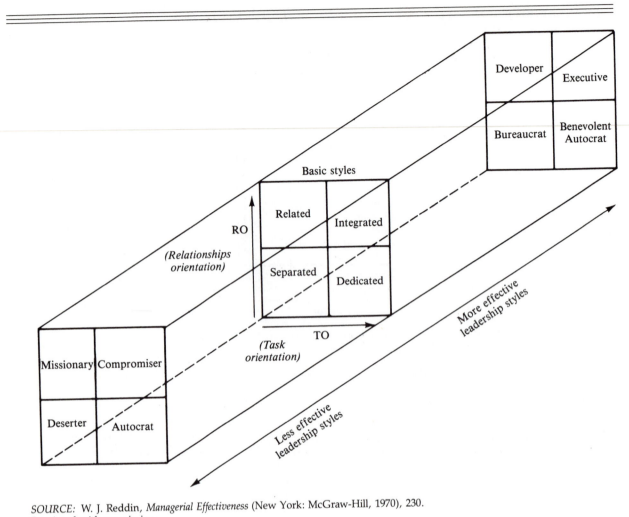

SOURCE: W. J. Reddin, *Managerial Effectiveness* (New York: McGraw-Hill, 1970), 230. Reprinted with permission.

Figure 15–7 • *Reddin's Three-Dimensional Management Styles*

power is dependent on subordinates. A supervisor who tries to coerce employees to contribute to a favorite political candidate may find that only some people comply.

Reward Power. A leader with legitimate power can use rewards to gain the cooperation of subordinates. Followers may respond to directions or requests if a leader can provide valued rewards such as raises, bonuses, or a choice job assignment. For example, a head nurse who can reward employees with requested time off or merit pay increases can exert reward power.

Coercive Power. Coercive power is the power to punish. Followers may comply because of fear. Managers may punish employees by blocking promotions or pay raises or by harassment. Even though coercive power may be used to correct nonproductive behavior in organizations, it often brings about the opposite effect. Those being punished may attempt to escape or avoid (through absenteeism or turnover) or show hostility toward management (through sabotage).

Referent Power. Charisma is the basis of referent power. A charismatic leader can influence people because of such a leader's personality or behavior style. Even though charisma is often used in reference to politicians, actors, or sports figures, some managers are regarded as charismatic by their employees.

Expert Power. A person with special expertise that is highly valued has expert power. Expert power is not tied to rank. A ward secretary can have high expert power if that secretary knows details of how the nursing unit functions. A staff nurse, because of years of employment, may have more information or job-specific expertise than a new head nurse and so may have more power.

The five types of interpersonal power are interdependent because they can be used in various combinations and each can affect the other.[24] For example, a nursing supervisor may lose referent power if that supervisor punishes staff by cancelling merit pay increases.

People use power to accomplish goals and to strengthen their positions in the organization. The use of power is legitimate when used in a fair and ethical way to achieve organizational, group, and individual objectives. Good managers desire power to influence the behavior of employees for the good of the organization, not for personal gain.

Preparation of Leaders as Managers

Young nurse managers need to be entered into a leadership-management development program. Such a program would teach them to recognize the worth and feelings of employees while having employees evaluate their personal goals in relation to those of the organization. This is one reason for agreement on a set of job standards and for the cooperative process of management by objectives. Principles that are applicable here include:

1. People need to know the standards expected of them. These standards should be flexible with details negotiated. If a person does not meet a standard, that person should be helped to plan a program to meet it.
2. People should know where they stand; they should be helped to improve when necessary.
3. People should be praised when they deserve it. A person should not be praised publicly unless it is important that others know the manager has a high opinion of the person.
4. Managers should show caring for people.
5. People should be made independent by helping them achieve their fullest potential.
6. Managers should be tactful, polite, and diplomatic.
7. Managers can learn from employees.
8. Managers should show confidence in themselves and in personnel.
9. People should be allowed freedom of expression.[25]

Organizational managers including nurse executives should teach managers the nature of leadership. They should train nurse managers in leadership skills. They should put managers in the proper environment to learn leadership. This will include "starting up an operation, turning around a troubled division, moving from staff to line, working under a wise mentor, serving on a high-level task force and getting promoted to a more senior level of the organization."[26]

Nurse executives and managers should be trained to coach their subordinates on leadership skills. Subordinates can be trained to help managers in leadership. Leaders can listen and articulate, can persuade and be persuaded, can use collective wisdom to make decisions, and they can teach subordinates to relate or communicate upward.

Persons who are only managers control. Managers who are leaders create commitment. They create a work unit that stands out, with culture and values that distinguish it from others. Forward-looking businesses are developing leadership at the lower levels. Most governments are not.[27]

LEADERSHIP AND NURSING

Nursing is usually conspicuous by its absence from lists of national leaders. National consumers do not perceive nurse leaders as having power. Cutler's perspective on nursing educators and nursing service personnel is that they have been the product of directive and authoritarian leadership.[28]

Historically, nurses have avoided opportunities to obtain power and political muscle. The profession now understands that power and political savvy will assist in achieving its goals, which are to improve health care and to increase nurses' autonomy. Milio believes that nurses have the capacity for power to influence public policy and recommends the following steps to prepare:

1. Organize.
2. Do the homework: learn to understand the political process, interest groups, specific people and events.
3. Frame arguments to suit the target audience by appealing to cost containment, political support, fairness and justice, and other data relevant to particular concerns.
4. Support and strengthen the position of converted policy makers.
5. Concentrate energies.
6. Stimulate public debate.
7. Make the position of nurses visible in the mass media.

8. Choose as the main strategy the most effective one.
9. Act in a timely fashion.
10. Maintain activity.
11. Keep the organizational format decentralized.
12. Obtain and develop the best research data to support each position.
13. Learn from experience.
14. Never give up without trying.

Nurses in leadership positions are most influential.[29]

SUMMARY

Theory of nursing leadership is a part of the theory of nursing management.

Leadership is a process of influencing a group to set and achieve goals. There are several major theories of leadership. One of the earliest theories of leadership is the trait theory. This theory infers that leaders have many intellectual, personality, and ability traits. Trait theory has been succeeded by other leadership theories indicating that managers, including nurse managers, can learn the knowledge and skills requisite to leadership competencies.

Behavioral theories of leadership include McGregor's Theory X and Theory Y, Likert's Michigan studies, Blake and Mouton's managerial Grid®, and Lewin's studies.

Other studies of leadership focus on contingency-situational leadership styles and factors such as people, tasks, situations, organizations, and environmental factors. Theorists include Fiedler, Reddin, Hersey, Blanchard, and Ouchi.

Nurse managers should learn to practice leadership behaviors that stimulate motivation within their constituents, practicing professional nurses and other nursing personnel. These behaviors will include promotion of autonomy, decision making, and participative management by professional nurses. It should be noted that these behaviors are facilitated by effective nurse manager-leaders.

EXPERIENTIAL EXERCISES

1. *Scenario:* Tom Kelly was the clinical nurse manager in the pediatric intensive care unit. His patients were well cared for physically and he and the staff nurses had the technological skills needed to work in the intensive care unit. After receiving letters of criticism from parents who stated Mr. Kelly and his staff were "cold and uncaring," the head nurse suggested that Mr. Kelly pay attention to the emotional needs of the children and parents and plan time for talking, explaining, and teaching. Mr. Kelly replied, "We don't have time for talking or teaching. That is the doctor's responsibility." Later he said to his nursing staff, "Ms. Barber wants us to plan time for emotional care. Do any of you have time for this? I certainly don't have time to just sit and talk. We do try to talk with the children and their parents while we are caring for them." The staff agreed with him, and no plans were made for teaching patients and their families.

1.1 How is each of the four essential components of leadership either present or lacking in the case of Mr. Kelly?

2. *Scenario:* A director of nursing, Ms. Carter, tells nurses on two medical units and two surgical units that their units have been chosen for a pilot project and that they will effect the case management model of nursing care by a specific date. She does not look at the organizational structure of the personnel or the staffing patterns on the units. She does not know what nursing personnel on the units are doing and has not taken time to find out. Contrast her approach to that of another director of nursing, Ms. Castro, who closely examines her unit organization. She staffs the units with adequate support personnel such as licensed practical nurses, nursing assistants, messengers, and transport personnel. The education coordinator arranges classes for the nurses to learn how to be case managers. Throughout this training, the departmental mission, philosophy, and goals are extolled. When training is completed, Ms. Castro asks the nurses to set a target date for complete implementation of case management. Within the 90 days set by themselves they are performing these functions.

2.1 Which director of nursing is meeting the conditions of leadership described by Merton and why?

3. The following questions pertain to your personal knowledge of a nurse leader.

3.1 Name a nurse you consider to be an outstanding leader.

3.2 State why you consider her or him to be outstanding.

4. Match each characteristic of leadership listed in Section I with an example from Section II by placing the correct letter in the space provided.

I

a. Does not blame others for failures; accepts role of scapegoat.

b. Helps personnel adapt to a changing environment.

c. Knows the goals of the organization and its employees; evaluates all the resources available for their use in achieving goals.

d. Arbitrates and mediates conflicts to give group members the feeling that justice has been accomplished.

II

____ 4.1 When a physician and a head nurse appeared bent on making a minor incident into a major labor relations problem, the clinical director assembled all parties including the union president. She presented the case to show that the head nurse had rights and feelings and the conflict was resolved to everyone's satisfaction.

____ 4.2 After trying an organizational pattern for many months, the head nurse admitted it would not work. She stated that the people involved had certainly been cooperative and industrious in their attempt to support her efforts.

____ 4.3 When head nurses were asked to become involved in preparing budgets, the director of nursing planned education programs to help them with the role change.

____ 4.4 The hospital administrator's objective was to increase productivity on the nursing units while maintaining quality care. The clinical nursing director decided to appoint unit managers and increase the number of nursing support personnel to meet the objective.

5. *Scenario:* Ms. Walsh, a director of nursing, had her scheduled counseling session with Ms. Walters, clinical nurse manager of the orthopedic unit. Ms. Walters appeared with her unit philosophy, objectives, and a written report of plans and accomplishments for each of the objectives. Ms. Walsh read the report and complimented Ms. Walters on the many achievements. She told Ms. Walters that the progress made on the unit had been the best in years and that she had seldom seen such enthusiasm and productivity on the part of a clinical nurse manager with only 6 months of experience in that position. Ms. Walsh commented on specific accomplishments that included a system for initiating the nursing history on admission of the patient by the shift personnel on duty at that time. Another area of progress had been the use of written assignment sheets that included a plan for achievement of unit objectives related to communication, organization, quality and quantity of care, teaching, and the team nursing concept.

During the conference, Ms. Walsh referred to the job performance standards for a clinical nurse manager, as did Ms. Walters, to whom she had given a copy. One area in which no plan was reported was for a planned counseling program for Ms. Walters' unit personnel. She stated that she counseled them when they needed it, but this was usually about something they did wrong.

In further discussion, Ms. Walters stated she felt the session so beneficial that she would make plans for doing the same with each of her people. She could use the job standards for each category and would begin as soon as she had the plan finalized. Her final remarks were that there had been many things she wanted to learn about her people, and she wanted to help them accomplish their personal goals and that she was anxious to get the program going. She agreed to report on this project at the end of 90 days.

5.1 What did Ms. Walsh do to tell Ms. Walters the standards expected of her?

5.2 What did she do to let Ms. Walters know where she stood and how to improve?

5.3 What did she do to praise Ms. Walters?

5.4 What did she do to show Ms. Walters she cared for her?

5.5 What did she do to help Ms. Walters achieve independence?

5.6 How was she tactful, polite, and diplomatic?

5.7 What evidence was there that both Ms. Walsh and Ms. Walters learned from others?

5.8 What evidence was there that either was confident?

5.9 What evidence was there of freedom of expression?

6. Brower describes the leader in politics as a person of stature who can rally the people, a person with outstanding ability and character. He says

there is an emotional bond between the leader and the led, a "bond which must exist between a leader and his people if either is to confront greatness." It is his thought that the abrasive strains of television may have irreparably damaged the bond between leader and led. Television shows leaders in their weaknesses because it constantly focuses on them. Formerly, it had been thought that such talent as Jefferson pictured in a natural aristocracy would freely rise to the top. American leaders would be people of ability and morality; they would be wise and virtuous. According to Brower,

Leadership, a relationship, depends very much on the basis of current enthusiasm or negation. Indeed it cannot exist at all in this country without the consent of the governed. We may very well be short on leadership because we are short on ourselves.[30]

6.1 Assuming that the characteristics of leadership are universally applicable to occupations, to government, to business, to industry, and certainly to service institutions and professions, list three characteristics described by Brower and make them applicable to nursing.

7. Kurt Lewin suggests that there are three leadership styles—autocratic, democratic, and laissez faire.

7.1 Which leadership style does your supervisor exhibit?

7.2 List three of his/her activities or decisions that illustrate that style.

7.3 How does your supervisor's leadership style affect your work and attitude?

8. Match the base of power listed in Section I with the descriptions in Section II by placing the correct letter in the space provided.

I

a. Legitimate power
b. Reward power
c. Coercive power
d. Referent power
e. Expert power

II

____ 8.1 Ms. Green, a staff nurse, was well liked by all staff. They listened and often agreed with her suggestions.

____ 8.2 Mr. Wilet, the director of a home health agency, blocked promotions if staff exceeded their budget by 2 percent.

____ 8.3 The vice-president of nursing has a right to set budget goals.

____ 8.4 The nursing assistant intimidated the new clinical nurse manager because she was more familiar with unit procedures.

____ 8.5 The head nurse gave staff nurses choice assignments when their quality assurance ratings improved significantly.

9. Place a check by each of the following statements that is true. Rewrite each false statement with changes that make the statement a true one.

____ 9.1 Perceptions of leaders by the followers are not relative to their power.

____ 9.2 A strong structural assignment gives more power to the leader.

____ 9.3 People should all be made as independent as possible.

____ 9.4 People should all be made as dependent as possible.

____ 9.5 A leader should tell people the standards expected of them and should help them improve.

____ 9.6 When the leader has great influence over group members, a relationship-oriented style works best.

____ 9.7 In Theory X organizations, the leadership style is an autocratic one that includes decisions only by top management.

____ 9.8 Coercive power improves productivity.

____ 9.9 Managers emphasize control, decision making, and results.

____ 9.10 Managers who are leaders create employee commitment.

NOTES

1. J. W. Gardner, *The Nature of Leadership: Introductory Considerations* (Washington, DC: Independent Sector, 1986), 8.

2. ———, *The Tasks of Leadership* (Washington, DC: Independent Sector, 1986), 15; E. Huxley, *Florence Nightingale* (New York: G. P. Putnam's Sons, 1975).

3. C. R. Holloman, "Leadership or Headship: There Is a Difference," *Notes & Quotes*, No. 365, 1969, 4; C. R. Holloman, " 'Headship' versus Leadership," *Business and Economic Review*, Jan.-Mar. 1986, 35–37.

4. L. B. Lundborg, "What Is Leadership?," *The Journal of Nursing Administration*, May 1982, 32–33.

5. Gardner, *The Nature of Leadership*, op.cit., 6.

6. Holloman, " 'Headship' versus Leadership," op. cit.; A. Levenstein, "So You Want to Be a Leader?" *Nursing Management*, Mar. 1985, 74–75; G. R. Jones, "Forms of Control and Leader Behavior," *Journal of Management*, Fall 1983, 159–172; D. McGregor, *Leadership and Motivation* (Cambridge, MA: MIT Press, 1966): 70–80.

7. R. K. Merton, "The Social Nature of Leadership," *American Journal of Nursing*, Dec. 1969, 2614–2618.

8. McGregor, op. cit., 73.

9. C. M. Talbott, "Leadership at the Man-to-Man Level," *Supplement to the Air Force Policy Letter for Commanders*, No. 8, Aug. 1971, 13.

10. D. G. Mitton, "Leadership—One More Time," *Industrial Management Review*, Fall 1969, 77–83.

11. J. Kilpatrick, "Conservative View," *Sun-Herald* (Biloxi, MS), Feb. 2, 1974, 4.

12. McGregor, op. cit., 75.

13. Holloman, "Leadership or Headship," op. cit.

14. McGregor, op. cit., 55–57.

15. Ibid, 49–65.

16. This Grid® synopsis was furnished courtesy of Scientific Methods, Inc., Box 195, Austin, TX 78767.

17. L. Megginson, D. Mosley, and P. Pietri, Jr., *Management: Concepts and Applications* (New York: Harper & Row, 1986), 397.

18. F. E. Fiedler, "Style or Circumstance: The Leadership Enigma," *Notes & Quotes*, No. 358, Mar. 1969, 3; Megginson, Mosley, and Pietri, op. cit., 419–422.

19. P. Hersey and K. H. Blanchard, *Management of Organizational Behavior*, 3d ed. (Englewood Cliffs, NJ: Prentice-Hall, 1977).

20. W. J. Reddin, *Managerial Effectiveness* (New York: McGraw-Hill, 1970), 230; R. M. Hodgetts, *Management: Theory, Process and Practice*, 4th ed. (Orlando, FL: Academic Press, 1986), 319–320.

21. W. G. Ouchi, *Theory Z* (Reading, MA: Addison-Wesley, 1981).

22. Gardner, *Leadership and Power*, op. cit., 3.

23. J. French and B. Raven, "The Basis of Social Power," in *Studies in Power*, D. Cartwright, ed. (Ann Arbor: Institute for Social Research, University of Michigan, 1959).

24. J. Gibson, J. Ivancevich, and J. Donnelly, Jr., *Organizations: Behavior, Structure, Processes*, 6th ed. (Homewood, IL: Richard D. Irwin, 1988), 335–337.

25. M. R. Feinberg, *Effective Psychology for Management* (Englewood Cliffs, NJ: Prentice-Hall, 1965), 133–141.

26. J. H. Zenger, "Leadership: Management's Better Half," *Training*, Dec. 1985, 44–53.

27. Ibid; J. W. Gardner, *The Nature of Leadership*, op. cit.

28. M. J. Cutler, "Nursing Leadership and Management: An Historical Perspective," *Nursing Administration Quarterly*, Fall 1976, 7–19.

29. N. Milio, "The Realities of Policymaking: Can Nurses Have an Impact?," *Journal of Nursing Administration*, Mar. 1984, 18–23.

30. B. Brower, "Where Have All the Leaders Gone?" *Life*, Oct. 8, 1971, 70B.

FOR FURTHER REFERENCE

Campbell, R. P., "Does Management Style Affect Burnout?," *Nursing Management*, Mar. 1986, 38A–38B, 38D, 38F, 38H.

Catton, J. J., "Applying Leadership to People Problems," *Supplement to the Air Force Policy Letter for Commanders*, No.9-1971, Sept. 1971, 30.

Davis, C. K., Oakley, D., and Sochalsk, J. A., "Leadership for Expanding Nursing Influence on Health Policy," *Journal of Nursing Administration*, Jan. 1982, 15–21.

Dunning, H. F., "Nobody Can Give You Leadership," *Notes & Quotes*, Sept. 1963, 3.

Gardner, J. W., *The Heart of the Matter: Leader-Constituent Interaction*; and *Leadership and Power* (Washington, DC: Independent Sector, 1986).

Glucksberg, S., "Some Ways to Turn on New Ideas," *Think* (IBM), Mar.-Apr. 1968.

Goldberg, D., "What Makes a Leader?," *Mississippi Press*, Nov. 23, 1978, 6D.

Jennings, E. E., "The Anatomy of Leadership," *Notes & Quotes*, No. 274, Mar. 1962, 1, 4.

Jones, G. R., "Forms of Control and Leader Behavior," *Journal of Management*, Fall 1983, 159–172.

Kaprowski, E. J., "Toward Innovative Leadership," *Notes & Quotes*, No. 351, Aug. 1968, 2.

Koontz, H., "Challenges for Intellectual Leadership or Management," *Notes & Quotes*, No. 315, Aug. 1965, 1, 4.

Levenstein, A., "Where Nurses Differ," *Nursing Management*, Mar. 1984, 64–65.

———, "Leadership Under the Microscope," *Nursing Management*, Nov. 1984, 68–69.

Likert, R., *The Human Organization* (New York: McGraw-Hill, 1967), 4–10.

Lundborg, "What Is Leadership?," *Journal of Nursing Administration*, May 1982, 32–33.

Mitchell, W. N., "What Makes a Business Leader?," *Notes & Quotes*, No. 350, July 1968, 2.

Phillips, J. S., and Lord, R. G., "Notes on the Practical and Theoretical Consequences of Implicit Leadership Theories for the Future of Leadership Measurement," *Journal of Management*, Spring 1986, 33.

Pike, O., "Rutan, Yeager Showed What Leadership Is About," *Mobile Press Register*, Jan. 1987, 4A.

Podsakoff, P. M., Todor, W. D., and Schuler, R. S., "Leader Expertise as a Moderator of the Effects of Instrumental and Supportive Leader Behaviors," *Journal of Management*, Fall 1983, 173–185.

Smith, H. L., and Mitry, N. W., "Nursing Leadership: A Buffering Perspective," *Nursing Administration Quarterly*, Spring 1984, 45–52.

Smith, H. L., Reinow, F. D., and Reid, R. A., "Japanese Management: Implications for Nursing Administration," *Journal of Nursing Administration*, Sept. 1984, 33–39.

Yanker, M., "Flexible Leadership Styles: One Supervisor's Story," *Supervisory Management*, Jan. 1986, 2–6.

Zaleznik, A., "Managers and Leaders: Are they Different?," *Harvard Business Review*, May-June 1977, 68.

·16·

Motivation

THEORIES OF MOTIVATION

Introduction

Motivation is a concept that describes both extrinsic conditions that stimulate certain behavior and intrinsic responses that demonstrate that behavior in human beings. The intrinsic response is sustained by sources of energy, termed "motives." They are often described as needs, wants, or drives. All living people have them. Motivation is measured by observable and recorded behaviors. Deficiencies in needs stimulate people to seek and achieve goals to satisfy their needs.

Why do some registered nurses pursue an area of nursing specialization to the extent of continuously acquiring new knowledge and skills that enable them to make rapid and accurate nursing diagnosis and prescription? Why does a pediatric nurse pursue development of a role in which professional practice is extended into such areas as teaching parents to enjoy their children, providing follow-up health observations of high-risk newborns, and health teaching of their parents after they have been discharged to their homes? Why does that nurse go a step further and teach others to extend themselves and then write articles to provide the information for all?

Why does a mental health nurse pursue a role as a co-therapist of a group even in off-duty time and in addition to rotating shifts as a staff nurse? Why does another work to sell the concept and then conduct a psychodrama therapy program, and to ask for the privilege of answering mental health consultations for medical and surgical patients? Why does a professional nurse work many hours as a committee member for a district nurses' association?

Why does a professional nurse contribute numerous hours of volunteer work to community organizations? Why does that nurse continuously pursue off-duty education courses for academic credit to update clinical practice?

Why does one professional nurse pursue any of these activities without watching the clock or setting limits to accepting responsibility for patient care?

Why do some nurses perform in a positive manner and others negatively?

Why do some people always act with truthfulness and integrity to support principles they believe in, whereas others remain silent and passive?

Why are some nurses goal oriented and others not? Why are some nurses actively dedicated to improving their quality of life, whereas others merely exert minimal effort to maintain it?

What makes some nurses come on duty on time, work hard and without error, maintain a pleasant demeanor, and meet all standards of performance, appearance, and behavior, whereas others do just the opposite? Some persons do not do well in an organization. This does not mean these persons are no good; the organization may be lacking the means of making them productive, useful, satisfied employees.

The answer to all these questions is motivation. Some nurses are motivated to excel and be creative, whereas others put forth just enough effort to do their jobs. Theories of motivation have been classified into content theories and process theories.[1]

Content Theories of Motivation

Content theories of motivation focus on factors or needs within a person that energize, direct, sustain, and stop behavior. The most widely recognized work in motivation theory is that of Maslow. Although not universally accepted because of its lack of scientific evidence or research base, it is universally known, and many managers attempt to use it as they turn to a human behavior approach to management.

Much has been said in support of Maslow's theories of motivation relative to human needs and goals. Like every science, nursing is a human creation stemming from human motives, having human goals, and being created, renewed, and maintained by human beings called nurses.

Nurses are motivated as are other scientists by physiological needs including that for food; by needs for safety, protection, and care; by social needs for gregariousness, affection, and love; by ego needs for respect, standing, and status leading to self-respect or self-esteem; and by a need for self-fulfillment or self-actualization of the idiosyncratic and species-wide potentialities of the individual human being. Many but not all are also motivated by cognitive needs for sheer knowledge and understanding, voraciously questioning others, reading textbooks, journals, and patients' charts and continuously pursuing courses in their specialty and in the liberal arts, particularly the humanities. Others are motivated by aesthetic needs for beauty, symmetry, simplicity, completion, and order, and by their need to express themselves. How many of these needs are related to a nurse's need for continuing to learn and to apply new knowledge and skills? What can the nurse manager do to spark the motive of curiosity in a nurse that sets in motion a desire to understand, explain, and systematize? These and many other human needs may serve as the primary motivations for pursuing a career in nursing and updating and expanding knowledge and skills. The need may be a feeling of identification and belongingness with people in general, a feeling of love for human beings, a desire to help people, the need to earn a living, a means of self-expression, or a combination of all these needs working at the same time. Certainly the diversity in needs is individualistic.[2]

Herzberg did research on a content theory, which he labelled a two-factor theory of motivation. One factor is labeled extrinsic conditions, hygiene factors, or dissatisfiers. These include salary, job security, working conditions, status, company procedures, quality of technical supervision, and quality of interpersonal relations among peers, with supervisors, and with subordinates. They must be maintained in quantity and quality to prevent dissatisfaction. They become dissatisfiers when not equitably administered, causing low performance and negative attitudes. The other set of factors is labeled intrinsic conditions, motivators, or satisfiers. They include achievement, recognition, responsibility, advancement, the work itself, and the possibility of growth. They create opportunities for high satisfaction, high motivation, and high performance. The individual must be free to attain them. Herzberg's research was criticized for its limited sample of accountants and engineers and for being simplistic.[3]

Many nursing personnel enjoy working together and are motivated by their affiliations. In some situations, such as nursing homes, they do not receive the recognition they need from clients, so they look for it from colleagues. Many nursing personnel want to talk to and socialize with each other on the job. They enjoy and prefer group-centered work activities, teamwork, interdependence, dependability, and predictability. The nurse manager works with them to maintain this affiliation need at a mutually acceptable level.[4]

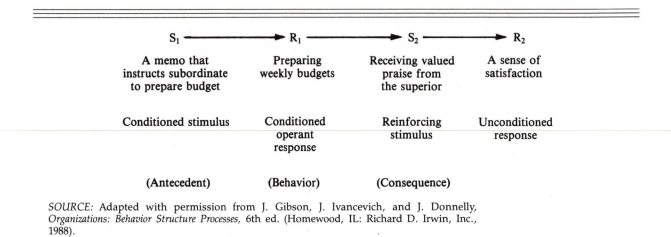

S_1 $\longrightarrow$	R_1 $\longrightarrow$	S_2 $\longrightarrow$	R_2
A memo that instructs subordinate to prepare budget	Preparing weekly budgets	Receiving valued praise from the superior	A sense of satisfaction
Conditioned stimulus	Conditioned operant response	Reinforcing stimulus	Unconditioned response
(Antecedent)	(Behavior)	(Consequence)	

SOURCE: Adapted with permission from J. Gibson, J. Ivancevich, and J. Donnelly, *Organizations: Behavior Structure Processes,* 6th ed. (Homewood, IL: Richard D. Irwin, Inc., 1988).

Figure 16–1 • *Reinforcement Theory*

Process Theories of Motivation

Four process theories of motivation are reinforcement theory, expectancy theory, equity theory, and goal setting. Most behavior within organizations is learned behavior: perceptions, attitudes, goals, emotional reactions, and skills. Practice that occurs during the learning process results in a relatively enduring change in behavior.

Skinner advanced a process theory of motivation called operant conditioning. Learning occurs as a consequence of behavior. This is also called behavior modification. Behaviors are the operants and are controlled by altering the consequences with reinforcers or punishments (reinforcement theory), as illustrated in Figure 16–1.

A second process theory of motivation is the expectancy theory of Vroom. This theory postulates that most behaviors are voluntarily controlled by a person and are therefore motivated. There is an effort-performance expectancy or belief by a person that a chance exists for a certain effort to lead to a particular level of performance. The performance-outcome expectancy or belief of this person will have certain outcomes. Given choices, the individual selects the choice with the best expected outcome. Research on expectancy theory is increasing although not systematic or refined. It is a complicated process in which unconscious motivation is avoided.[5]

Equity theory is a third process theory. People believe they are being treated with equity when the ratio of their efforts to rewards equals those of other persons. Equity can be achieved or restored by changing outputs, attitudes, the reference person, inputs or outputs of the reference person, or the situation. Research on equity theory has focused on pay.[6]

A fourth process theory of motivation is the goal-setting theory of Locke. This theory is based on goals as determinants of behavior. The more specific the goals the better the results produced. Research indicates goals are a powerful force. They must be achievable. The difficulty level of goals should be increased only to the ceiling to which the person will commit. Goal clarity and accurate feedback increase security.[7]

Maslow

Maslow's theory of motivation is a positive one and is based on a holistic-dynamic theory.

At the base of a needs system are physiological needs. These needs are based on homeostasis, which is a condition of constancy of body fluids, functions, and states; the constancy is maintained automatically by uniform interaction of counteracting processes. It should be noted that human beings do not just eat, they eat selectively to maintain homeostasis. The same is probably true of other physiological needs. Not all physiological needs are homeostatic, and they are relatively independent of each other while at the same time interdependent; for example, smoking may satisfy the hunger need in some persons. Some are in opposition, such as the tendency to be lazy at the same time one has a desire to be industrious.

Physiological needs are the most prepotent or strongest of human needs when unsatisfied. A starving person will steal food and perform other acts that threaten safety. Dominance of a physiological need changes the individual's philosophy for the future.

Human needs are organized in a hierarchy of prepotency: higher ones emerge as lower ones are satisfied. When the physiological needs are satisfied, the human being is no longer motivated by them. However, when deprived of a long-satisfied need, that person tolerates it better than one who has been long or previously deprived.

Safety needs are the second group in the hierarchy. Among these are security, protection, dependency, and stability; freedom from anxiety, chaos, and fear; need for order, limits, structure, and law; strength in the protector, and others. Their satisfaction influences a person's philosophy of life and of values. What threatens the safety of nursing? Are nurses threatened by increased consumer interest in their shortcomings, which may lead to consumer control of practice? What motivates people? Is it a fear of the high cost of extended illnesses and poor results of care? The average person likes law, order, predictability, and organization, and this may be one reason people resist change. Insurance programs, job tenure, and savings accounts are expressions of safety needs. People prefer familiar to unknown things. Today's managers are often threatened by the new generation of personnel who question regulations and use the law to achieve their goals.

Once the physiological and safety needs have been satisfied, the needs for love, affection, and belongingness emerge. Most individuals in nursing today have had their physiological and safety needs satisfied, although there are notable exceptions, the nonpromoted workers being among them. Now they want to be part of a group or family with love, acceptance, friendliness, and a feeling of belonging. Are these needs thwarted by frequent moves? How are the needs of the individual as well as those of the organization satisfied? A society that wants to survive and be healthy will work to satisfy these needs. Otherwise people will be maladjusted and will exhibit severe emotional and behavioral pathology.

Two categories emerge under the fourth set of needs—the esteem needs. All people share these needs. First they desire strength, achievement, adequacy, mastery and competence, confidence before the world, independence, and freedom. Second they desire reputation or prestige, status, fame and glory, dominance, recognition, attention, importance, dignity, or appreciation. A person whose self-esteem is satisfied has feelings of self-confidence, worth, strength, capability, adequacy,

usefulness, and being needed in society. For it to be stable and healthy, self-esteem must be based on known or deserved respect. The reason for it must be known and recognized within the recipient.

Finally, at the pinnacle of the hierarchy of needs is the emotional gold—the need for self-actualization, the effort of people to be what they can be. Nurses want to become everything that they are capable of becoming, to achieve their potential, to be effective nurses, to be creative, and to meet personal standards of performance.

Usefulness to Nurse Managers

Although there are many theories and much has been written about motivation, there is no easy way to motivate employees. Human motivation is diverse, subtle, and complex. To use the available information on motivation effectively, the nurse manager will read it and select and use those elements that appear to be practical and workable.

Some theories of motivation are contradictory. They provide useful knowledge when used selectively and carefully. Theories of motivation are really constructs and not theories, as motivation cannot be directly observed and measured.[8]

Knowledge of motivation theories is essential to improving job performance of employees. Individual employees have different needs and goals. Nurse managers will learn and use motivation theories selectively.

DISSATISFACTIONS

There are many dissatisfactions in nursing, and many have been enumerated in nursing studies. The following paragraphs relate to dissatisfaction among nurses. Dissatisfactions can be alleviated by learned approaches to change by nurse managers within nursing organizations.

Productivity

Nurses respond negatively and become dissatisfied when managers use force, control, threats, and repeated applications of institutional power. Productivity decreases or stagnates! The new breed of nurses questions authority and gives loyalty to those who earn it. An attitude of mutual respect between clinical nurses and managers is essential to productivity.

To promote mutual respect there must be free interaction and communication in which expectations are clarified, feedback on performance is given, and promises that cannot be delivered are avoided. There must be role modeling of expected and desired performance. In more than seven out of ten working relationships, employees do not know what is expected of them. Expectations must be clear. In a Productivity Attitude Test developed and administered to production workers by Pryor and Mondy over a 2-year period, 75 percent of respondents said that their supervisors did not keep promises they made. Broken promises anger employees and decrease productivity.[9]

Nurse managers are powerful models for staff. They are emulated, whether this example is good or bad. The obvious inference is that nurse managers should do self-assessment and modify their behavior to depict roles beneficial to both staff and organization.

Like other workers, all nurses work to survive and to meet their needs and aspirations. The complexity of the technological environment for patient care can lead to specialization and the depersonalization of jobs and work. This alienates nursing employees, and the quality of their work thus declines.

The Nurse as Knowledge Worker

Drucker indicates that knowledge workers are productive only with self-motivation, self-direction, and achievement. We have wasted over 200 years learning this. There is no one dominant dimension to working. People are motivated to work based on Maslow's hierarchy of needs. Even though satisfied, a human need remains important. Economic rewards that are not properly taken care of create dissatisfaction with work. They become deterrents.[10]

Nurses are knowledge workers. Their basic economic needs are related to other human needs or human values. Performing work of equal difficulty, they want economic rewards of equal value to those of other knowledge workers. Pay is part of the social or psychological dimension of nurses. They also want economic rewards to give them increased rank, power, and status, commensurate with other knowledge workers.

Education makes fear a demotivator. Educated people are mobile. Nurses can move laterally to jobs in other organizations. The role of discipline is to take care of marginal friction. If used to drive nurses, discipline causes resentment and resis-

tance; it demotivates. Direction and control are useless in meeting ego needs.

The nurse as knowledgeable worker is self-directed and takes responsibility. Rewarding and reaffirming self-direction and responsibility produce learning; fear produces resistance. Psychological manipulation is only a replacement for the carrot-and-stick approach to management. It does not work.

Thwarted needs or deficiencies lead to sick or negative behavior. Focus on already satisfied needs is ineffective, however, employees will demand more of what they already have unless attention is given to self-esteem and self-actualization. In such a situation money becomes the only means available of satisfying needs. Nurses want it to purchase material goods and services. Inflation increases the demand as it takes more money to satisfy other desires. However, this increased demand for money and material rewards destroys their usefulness as incentives and managerial tools.

Nurses are adults and as such have outgrown dependence. They want to be independent. They want to be treated as adults and partners, with dignity and respect. It is the practicing clinical nurses who achieve health care productivity gains, not capital spending and automation.

Nursing personnel retreat from association and identification with organizations in which they cannot meet their perceived care requirements. Even though more nurses believe themselves competent and able to do good work, they are dissatisfied because they cannot live up to the standard of care they want to provide. They care, and because they care they are dissatisfied.

SATISFACTIONS

The Science of Human Behavior

How do we apply the knowledge of the social sciences so that our human organizations will be truly effective? We have the knowledge, just as we have the knowledge of physical sciences to develop alternative sources of energy such as solar, tidal, atomic, and geothermal energy. Application of vast knowledge in both physical and social sciences is expensive and time-consuming.

Theory X and Theory Y

Although Douglas McGregor died in 1964, his theories of leadership and motivation live on. Unfortunately, his Theory X has not been replaced by his Theory Y. He summarized Theory X in terms of the world of business as follows:

1. *Management is responsible for organizing the elements of productive enterprise—money, materials, equipment, people—in the interest of economic ends.*

2. *With respect to people, this is a process of directing their efforts, motivating them, controlling their actions, modifying their behavior to fit the needs of the organization.*

3. *Without this active intervention by management, people would be passive—even resistant—to organizational needs. They must therefore be persuaded, rewarded, punished, controlled—their activities must be directed. This is management's task—in managing subordinate managers or workers. We often sum it up by saying that management consists of getting things done through other people.*

Behind this conventional theory there are several additional beliefs—less explicit, but widespread:

4. *The average man (sic) is by nature indolent—he works as little as possible.*

5. *He lacks ambition, dislikes responsibility, prefers to be led.*

6. *He is inherently self-centered, indifferent to organizational needs.*

7. *He is by nature resistant to change.*

8. *He is gullible, not very bright, the ready dupe of the charlatan and the demagogue.*[11]

How many nurse managers demotivate practicing nurses by falling into the trap of voicing the very statements embodied in Theory X? How may nurse managers motivate practicing nurses by following the contrasting precepts of Theory Y?

1. *Management is responsible for organizing the elements of productive enterprise—money, materials, equipment, people—in the interest of economic ends.*

2. *People are not by nature passive or resistant to organizational needs. They have become so as a result of experience in organizations.*

3. *The motivation, the potential for development, the capacity for assuming responsibility, the readiness to direct behavior toward organizational goals are all present in people. Management does not put them there. It is the responsibility of management to make it possible for people to recognize and develop these human characteristics for themselves.*

4. *The essential task of management is to arrange organizational conditions and methods of operation so that people can achieve their own goals best by directing their own efforts toward organizational objectives.*[12]

Nurse Managers and Motivation

Motivation is an emotional process, being psychological rather than logical. Learn how a nurse wants to feel and help this nurse use the tools that will permit achievement of those feelings. Such feelings may relate to associations with people on the job that make the nurse feel accepted, performance of those acts for which the nurse is highly skilled, and recognition for a satisfactory performance, among others.

As previously stated, motivation is basically an unconscious process. When asked why a nurse did a certain thing, that nurse may not be able to give the answer. Even though people's basic motives are hidden and intangible, their actions or behavior makes sense to them.

Each person is unique, the key to behavior lying within the self. A supervisor must use judgment to figure out why each person reacts in a given way to any situation.

Within each unique individual, motivating needs differ from time to time. The key lies in figuring out which need is currently prepotent.

People shape a nurse's needs and actions, making the nurse a social being and motivation a social success. People help satisfy these needs.

The motivational patterns are learned early and followed for years. There is no conscious selection, judgment, or decision involved in 95 percent of what people do.

Perhaps with hard work nurse managers may be able to influence the motivational processes that cause practicing nurses to do things that will benefit the organization. In evaluating nurses, the supervisor will observe how well each one defines and solves problems on the job. They will be tested on their capacities to generalize—to tie facts together and predict the outcome; to see degrees of difference—what make one solution better than another; and ability to abstract—to weed out the unessential. They will be tested on their abilities to depart from orderliness and demonstrate creative and imaginative solutions to problems. They will be tested for their feelings, emotions, and attitudes to determine the stability of their individual personalities. All nurses will be tested for their social skills. They will be tested for their insight as well as their insight into others. Can they look objectively and thoughtfully at the actions of both? They will be tested for their ability to use good work habits and to discriminate among tasks. They will be tested on their individual philosophy of life and the code of standards they set and follow for themselves.

Can you as a nurse manager influence all the aspects of individual nurses so as to meet their inner drives or needs? Perhaps a question would be, Can you provide those things from the outside world that will satisfy the inner drives or needs of the individual? Such actions will earn respect, self-satisfaction, and love. Money usually cannot buy loyalty, creativity, or morale. Positive motivation and consistent fairness are the marks of good leadership. Satisfied employees will be happy and as productive as their capacities allow. The secret of success, then, is to enable them to achieve an exciting and satisfying life by doing the things that you need to have done. Successful people usually are well motivated.[13]

Human beings, including nurses, motivate themselves. The nurse manager will provide practicing nurses the opportunity for satisfaction of their needs, or deprive them of it.

The motivational theory under discussion asserts that man (sic)—if he is freed to some extent, by his presence in an affluent society, from the necessity to use most of his energy to obtain the necessities of life and a degree of security from the major vicissitudes—will by nature begin to pursue goals associated with his higher-level needs. These include needs for a degree of control over his own fate, for self-respect, for using and increasing his talents, for responsibility, for achievement both in the sense of status and recognition and in the sense of personal development and effective problem solving. Thus freed, he will also seek in many ways to satisfy more fully his physical needs for recreation, relaxation, and play. Management has been well aware of the latter tendency; it has not often recognized the former, or at least it has not taken into account its implication for managerial strategy.[14]

Hard versus Soft Approach to Nursing Management. What are the effects of a hard approach to personnel management such as coercion and disguised threats, close supervision, and tight controls over behavior? Experience has shown that such an approach causes counterforces, including the restriction of output, militant unionism, and subtle but effective sabotage of the objectives of management.

Nurses turn to labor organizations when they fail to achieve results with their supervisors. They do this when authoritarian managers manage from the top down with job descriptions, performance standards and evaluations, rules, pay incentives, promotions, management objectives, and dismissal threats. They are not consulted on any of these management tools and activities.

The soft approach to personnel management, such as permissiveness, satisfying people's demands, and achievement of harmony, has been proven to cause indifferent performance, with expectations of receiving more and giving less. As a consequence, people try to take the middle-of-the-road approach.

Observation and evidence of the social sciences indicate that employees' behavior shapes itself to management perceptions. This behavior does not result from inherent human nature but from the nature of organizations, management philosophy, policy, and practice.

The nursing leader looks for simple, practical, immediate ideas to solve personnel problems. There are no magic wands, but that does not mean there are no solutions.

Solutions

Career Planning. Career planning is a continuous process of self-assessment and goal setting. It is a cooperative venture between the organization and the employee, the career counselor (who could also be a mentor or sponsor) and the individual nurse. Career planning is an organized system with short-term and long-term career goals fitted to those of the organization.

To build a career development program requires major effort. The following outline stresses the major activities:

1. Assess the future goals and labor power needs of the nursing organization relative to recruitment, promotion, hiring, placement, retention, and turnover.
2. Develop job structures with career paths and qualifications including career opportunities within the nursing organization.
3. Recruit qualified applicants, including those already employed within the nursing organization.
4. Assess each applicant for personal expectations.

    4.1 Why are they making this career choice?
    4.2 What are their needs, motivators, and job satisfiers?
    4.3 What stressors make them frustrated and dissatisfied?

4.4 What stressors excite them?

4.5 What are their career goals?

4.6 How does their present performance relate to their career goals?

4.7 What are their competencies and interests?

4.8 What potential performance will be needed to achieve their career goals?

5. Develop an individual career development plan for the individual nurse.

6. Provide developmental opportunities for the individual nurse to achieve career goals.

There can be a career development program advisory committee. Staff development personnel can be career counselors. The real goal is self-development of a career plan for every nurse fostered by the nursing organization. For this reason the individual nurse is best involved in the entire career development program from its inception. Most nurses will benefit from participation in a career development program, even if it only improves the quality of their working lives.[15]

Communication. To produce quality nursing products and services requires highly motivated practicing nurses. Nurse managers can motivate nurses by sharing information about the organization. Consultative managers consult with nurses on problems, solutions, and decisions, and share information about results.

Communication involves giving feedback as information and as reinforcement. It avoids surprising nurses by keeping them informed of changes. Communication media are used to recognize nurses, thereby improving their self-esteem and to clarify expected behavior and job performance. They can be part of an effective open door policy and a complaint system, and they can be used to inform nurses about a workable career ladder and educational opportunities to upgrade their knowledge and skills. Communication media implement uniform grievance procedures.

Effective communication by nurse managers, along with other motivators, boosts morale and keeps practicing nurses from turning to labor organizations for need satisfaction that includes security.[16] Communication is discussed more fully in Chapter 17.

Teamwork. Nurse managers can motivate practicing nurses by encouraging teamwork. Teams can be built from work groups for discussion and resolution of work-related issues. Teams should have identifiable output, inclusive membership, leaders with carefully circumscribed authority, agreement on purpose, rules of procedure, and measurable goals, resources, and feedback.

Allender suggests the following ways to enhance productivity through teamwork:

1. Form teams by common activity and include all people associated with each activity from top management to lowest level.

2. Manager chooses a results-oriented leader who is a motivator, compassionate, respected, and organized. This leader keeps the team on schedule as its chair and summarizes and distributes the minutes. The leader ensures that decisions are reached by consensus.

3. The team develops a written statement of team purpose with which numbers totally agree. This agreement is reached through discussion.

4. Meeting times are set to accommodate all members, usually about an hour every 1 to 2 weeks.

5. The team develops measurement criteria for team performance, uses them, and records the results on charts.

6. The team gathers data on past and present performance and sets goals. It displays the performance data of graphs at each meeting.

7. The team identifies indirect issues of the work environment and attends to them. Completion addresses concerns of team members as items are never left hanging.

Through using teams, Hewlett-Packard has cut labor costs, reduced defects, solved vendor problems, eliminated jobs, decreased inspections, cut scrap production, and reached targets ahead of schedule. Teamwork achieves personal recognition, raising self-esteem, motivation, and commitment. It is stimulated by trust, support, completion, acknowledgement, communication, and agreement.[17]

Cornett-Cooke and Dias describe the use of teamwork to raise the spirits of nurses during a time of economic recession, cutbacks, and curtailment of capital expenditures. They showed that teamwork could be used to clarify the purpose or mission of a department or unit, to define a vision of the process and product of team effort, to identify blocks and barriers to their vision, to look at ways the work group members support each other, to make requests and agreements about how each can better work together with others on the team, and to plan the team's work goals and activities and commit each member to accomplishing them. The result would be an effective team with personally satisfied members.

1. Head nurses have strength when they know that other employers want to hire them because of their demonstrated influence with nurses, physicians, and others. They have self-esteem when this gives them satisfaction.

2. Nurse administrators have strength when chosen by the top management to expand their spheres of responsibility to direct other departments and when recognized by other administrators for skills and knowledge—being consulted by legislators, or leaders in nursing and health care. They have self-esteem when this gives them satisfaction.

Figure 16–2 • *Examples of Self-Esteem Based on Strength*

This strategy was used to build a team. They made a schedule of their sessions to include one on team building. They planned for input from representatives of all shifts. Their kickoff included posters, including one of each nurse team member's graduation picture and school on a U.S. map.

They had a productive session in which they agreed on ground rules including what the manager would do and what the manager would ask the staff to do. They explored such vision areas as patient care, staffing, interpersonal communication, and professional relationships. They analyzed problems and set about solving them with action plans. Each month they recognized each other with "warm fluffy days," giving each team member a compliment and a cotton ball on a pin. They even had an intrashift team session to share experiences when they became curious about each other. They developed spirit through teamwork.[18]

Teamwork recognizes people as worthy. It provides support and commitment of goals leading to productivity. It motivates practicing nurses. Nurse managers can develop it.

Self-Esteem. Self-esteem is having a stable, firmly based, usually high evaluation of oneself, having self-respect, and being self-confident from being able to act independently, from achieving one's personal and professional goals, and from competence in personal and professional skills and knowledge. Being held in esteem by others by reason of one's personal accomplishments and reputation gives a person status and recognition. It makes one feel appreciated and respected and increases one's self-esteem. It satisfies the desire for

1. A professional nurse satisfies the desire for self-esteem by running for and winning a government office or an office in some service or professional organization.

2. A professional nurse satisfies the desire for self-esteem by achieving credentials such as certification, an advanced degree, or the skill of using a computer.

3. A professional nurse manager satisfies the desire for self-esteem by lowering the absenteeism and turnover rates of personnel in the nursing division.

Figure 16–3 • *Examples of Self-Esteem through Achievement of Goals*

having strength among family, friends, colleagues, supervisors, patients, visitors, and others.[19] See Figure 16–2 for examples of self-esteem based on strength.

Self-esteem is also satisfaction of the desire for achievement of personal, professional, and organizational goals, as illustrated in Figure 16–3.

Self-esteem comes from satisfaction of the desire for adequacy, feeling worthwhile as a person in society and as a worker, as illustrated in Figure 16–4.

Self-esteem involves satisfying the desire for mastery and competence in the knowledge and skills needed to perform a role in clinical practice, management, education or research, as a member of a family, and as a citizen, as shown in Figure 16–5.

Self-esteem comes from acquiring a feeling of confidence in the face of the world, as in Figure 16–6.

Self-esteem involves satisfying the desire for independence and freedom. To satisfy the need for self-esteem, a person must be free to speak, free to act without hurting others, free to express oneself, free to investigate and seek information, and free to defend oneself. Each person must be treated with justice, fairness, honesty, and orderliness in the group. See Figure 16–7.

Other terms can be used to describe self-esteem. These include valuing oneself or estimating one's worth. Our goal is to value ourselves highly, to consider ourselves favorably, to appreciate and think well of ourselves. We also want others to have a high regard for us, to honor and admire us.

In terms of Maslow's hierarchy of needs, self-

1. A professional nurse feels that she is a good wife and mother because she can work a schedule compatible with her husband's, be involved in the activities of her family, and save money for a future college education for her children.

2. A staff nurse in the recovery room feels that she has time to assess, plan, and give good care and attend to good documentation of care. She even has opportunity to obtain reading references she needs to keep her knowledge and skills updated.

Figure 16–4 • *Examples of Self-Esteem through Adequacy*

esteem is a higher level need in the ego category. It emerges after physiological, safety, belonging, and love needs are fairly well gratified. Although self-actualization needs are higher in the hierarchy, this hierarchy of needs does not follow the same order in everyone. The self-esteem needs are rarely fully satisfied.

People want a good reputation and to have prestige (respect or esteem from others). They want to be recognized, to have attention, to be important, and to be appreciated.

People meet their esteem needs in different ways. They are influenced by culture, including the culture of the organization in which they work. The ends or results are more important than the roads taken to achieve those ends. All human be-

1. A nurse manager involves clinical nurses in preparing strategic objectives for a unit. The plan is approved by the organization's administrators.

2. A clinical nurse is selected to implement a theory of nursing about which she is considered an authority.

Figure 16–5 • *Examples of Self-Esteem through Mastery*

ings want esteem unless they are pathological. Persons lacking self-esteem feel inferior, weak, helpless, and discouraged. They become indolent, passive, resistant to change, lacking in responsibility, and unwilling to follow a dialogue. They focus on salary and fringe benefits by making unreasonable demands for economic benefits. They can become neurotic or emotionally sick when they have a deficiency in self-esteem.[20]

Meeting the self-esteem needs of employees is of great significance to management—in nursing as everywhere. Most nurses work in bureaucratic organizations such as hospitals, home health care agencies, nursing homes, clinics, and the like. In these bureaucratic organizations work is organized to meet many concerns including those of the organization and physicians, and the routines and personnel of other departments. The lower levels of the hierarchy have few opportunities to meet their ego needs. Nurses must schedule care of their pa-

1. A professional nurse goes to work confident that she can perform as well as any other nurse, and better than some; that she can learn anything she needs to learn to do a job well; that other people recognize her abilities and give her credit for them; that she will earn full merit pay; and that she will do this while meeting standards of her employers, the ANA, the JCAHO and other internal and external agencies.

2. A professional nurse decides that she has the capacity to win support for her candidacy and wages a successful campaign.

Figure 16–6 • *Examples of Self-Esteem through Confidence*

1. A supervisor decides she would like to know something about joint practice as a modality of nursing. She obtains information and writes a position paper on it. Her administrator tells her to go ahead with making a plan to practice it. She sets a specific schedule to orient and gain approval of the clinical nurses and then the physicians who use the unit.

2. Clinical nurses are given complete freedom to manage the care of their patients including coordination with personnel of x-ray, medical laboratory, nutrition and food service, physicians, and others.

Figure 16–7 • *Examples of Self-Esteem through Independence*

tients around everyone else. They are often the servants of the organization.

Direction and control are useless methods of motivating professional nurses where social, ego, and self-fulfillment needs are predominant. Intellectual creativity is a characteristic of professional nurses. They do not get ego satisfaction from wages, pensions, vacations, or other benefits of work. The job itself must be satisfying and fun if professional nurses are to satisfy their self-esteem needs. They get their ego needs met by having a voice in decision making. Professional nurses will commit to organizational objectives when allowed to determine the steps to take to achieve them. They want to collaborate with other professionals, both internal and external to the environment in which they work.

Full utilization of their talent and training is another desire of professional nurses. They want critical attention paid to the nature of nursing as a clinical practice discipline, to the organization of nursing functions and job challenges. They do *not* want close and detailed supervision. One reason for the success of primary nursing has been the control professional nurses have over the nursing process of patients who are their primary nursing responsibility. This success will not continue unless management gives attention to a career development plan. Such a plan is the logical evolution into joint practice in which physicians and nurses collaborate to give total care to patients. Professional nurses want opportunities to develop within their professional careers *as clinical nurses.* Career ladder progression must relate to clinical practice.

Professional nurses want status, internally and externally. This includes publication, with clerical support services from employers. It includes participation in the affairs of professional societies to which employers pay annual dues and expenses of attending meetings for at least representative groups.[21]

What can management do? Management can set the conditions under which professional nurses become committed to organizational goals and exercise self-control and self-direction. This leads to creativity.

Strategic planning by top management can involve professional clinical nurse participation. Is not the end result accomplished through professional nursing? The strategic plan can then be submitted to the department level for input by clinical nurses and other professionals. They will contribute to it by critiquing it, strengthening it, and making it a plan to which they can commit. This management process will be a difficult task, the accomplishment of which gives professional nurses new knowledge and skills, opportunity for creativity, and recognition and prestige in other peoples' eyes, meeting their ego needs for self-esteem. In the area of performance evaluation, nurse managers can again set the stage for meeting the self-esteem needs of professional nurses who want to be evaluated, promoted, rotated, and transferred in terms of their clinical or other personal career motivations. Self-evaluation in which individuals plan and appraise their contributions to organizational objectives promotes self-esteem. Conventional performance appraisal attacks self-esteem.[22]

It is obvious that management can create the conditions in which professional nurses can meet their esteem needs. They can make nurses feel good about themselves by providing adequate staffing to give good nursing care, by correct placement and orientation to achieve mastery, independence, and freedom, by respecting them for a job well done, and by promoting deserved respect from coworkers and employees.[23]

What do managers get from their jobs? Freedom? Social satisfaction? Opportunities for achievement? Knowledge? Ability to create? Who gets the reward and for what? Who must provide the opportunities for increased dignity, achievement, prestige, and social satisfaction?

Self-esteem involves the personhood of all professional nurses, be they managers, clinical nurses, researchers, or teachers. Each should enrich the esteem of the other person, should be the peer pal, mentor, sponsor, and guardian of the person within the profession. Esteem results in leading and influencing. One can listen to other people, treat them as individuals, show earnest exhilaration in responding to their creativity, offer ideas for improvement, and share the excitement of their success with victories and wins. Success gives a good self-image. It builds self-esteem. It avoids the pain of failure.[24]

Self-Actualization

Self-actualization was defined by Maslow as an ego need at the top of the needs hierarchy. It does not exist by itself and in some persons may be no stronger than the love and belonging need or the self-esteem need.

Self-actualized people are better able to distinguish the real world, seeing reality more clearly. Comfortable with the unknown, self-actualized people are attracted to it. All are creative in whatever they do and perceive.

Accepting and adjusting to their own shortcomings, self-actualized people are less defensive and less artificial. They feel guilty if they are not doing something about improvable shortcomings, prejudice, jealousy, envy, and the other shortcomings of humanity. They have autonomous codes of ethics, yet are the most ethical of people. They conform when no great issues are involved.

In the area of values, self-actualized people accept their own nature, human nature, the realities of social life, and the constraints of physical reality. Self-actualized people are problem centered, not ego centered. Their values are broad, universal, and transcend their time. Being deeply democratic as opposed to authoritarian by nature, they respect people and have a strong sense of right and wrong, of good and evil. Self-actualized people are not interested in hostile humor. Their humor is of a philosophical bent, stated only to produce a laugh.

Self-actualized people like solitude and privacy. They are detached and objective under conditions of turmoil. They are self-movers with more free will. Although they generally want to help the human race and can sometimes feel like strangers in a strange land, their relationships with people are more profound and their circle of friends small. They love children and humanity but can be briefly hostile to others when it is deserved or for the others' good. In social terms, self-actualized people are godly but not religious.

Even though they are not conventional, they conform to social graces with toleration. They can be radical.

Maslow indicates that living at the higher need level is good for growth and health, both physically and psychologically. Self-actualized persons live longer, have less disease, sleep and eat better, and enjoy their sexual lives without unnecessary inhibitions. For them life continues to be fresh, thrilling, exciting, and ecstatic. They count their blessings.

Self-actualized people have mystic or peak experiences. These are natural experiences. Happiness can cause tears. It comes from appreciation of the transcendence of poetry, music, philosophy, religion, interpersonal relationships, beauty, or politics. They can have the peak experience from doing or sensing.

Self-actualized people merge or unify dichotomies such as selfishness, considering every act to be both selfish and unselfish. They perceive work as play, duty as pleasure, and so on. The purpose of higher needs is a "healthward" trend—when people experience them they place a higher value on them.

Self-actualized people are "metamotivated." Their motivations are for character growth, character expression, maturation, and development. They place more dependence on self-development and inner growth than the prestige and status of others' honors.

Self-actualizing people are not perfect. They can be (or can be perceived to be) joyless; mundane; silly, wasteful, or thoughtless in habits; boring, stubborn, or irritating; superficially vain or proud; partial to their own productions, family, friends, or children; temperamental; ruthless; strong and independent of others' opinions; shocking in language and behavior; concentrated to the point of absent-mindedness or humorlessness; mistaken; needing improvement. They can feel guilt, anxiety, sadness, self-castigation, internal strife, and conflict.

Self-actualized people develop detachment from the culture. They become autonomous and accepting.

Higher needs require more preconditions such as more people, larger scenes, longer runs, more means and partial goals, and more subordinate or preliminary steps. To achieve the higher needs requires better environmental conditions.

Pursuit and gratification of higher needs have desirable civic and social consequences: loyalty, friendliness, civic consciousness. People who are living at this level make better parents, spouses, teachers, public servants, and so on. They also create greater, stronger, and true individualism. They are synergistic.

A conclusion could be that the self-actualized person achieves a highly satisfactory quality of life, and that this quality of life extends from the gratified self-actualized person into society. Gratification or satisfaction of the higher level needs can be positively influenced by the social environment of work, family, community, government, and the like.

Applying these insights to nursing, the nurse manager would selectively apply knowledge and skills of the social and behavioral sciences to creating an environment or climate in which practicing nurses could become self-actualized. In so doing, nurse managers become self-actualized, and the products and services of nursing increase in quantity and quality.

Although critics of Maslow's work say it is based on too narrow a population, it is widely accepted and used. He analyzed the profiles of sixty subjects including Lincoln, Jefferson, Einstein, and Frederick Douglass. Maslow suggested that our population may be limited to being between 5 to 30 percent self-determined, another forecast criticized by other scientists.[25]

SUMMARY

To summarize:

1. A person is motivated.
2. A person has goals.
3. Management has goals.
4. An environment needs to be established in which a person can achieve personal goals by achieving management's goals (or vice versa).
5. The person will be rewarded by work achievements that are successful. Management will have provided the setting for success through managerial practices, perhaps by removing restraints or giving other intrinsic rewards. High level ego needs are met on the job.
6. There will be a cooperative interaction between manager and employees, because the latter will be participating in decisions that affect them.
7. Motivation occurs.
8. Personal and motivational goals are met as the nurse is motivated to be ambitious, and responsible, to show initiative, to be proud of fellow nurses and the employing institution, to welcome change, and to demonstrate individual abilities.

This law will apply to successful leadership in nursing: find out where nurses want to go and what they want to accomplish and bring these wants into line with those of the organization. Then nurses will accomplish organizational goals as their own.

EXPERIENTIAL EXERCISES

1. Match each approach to personnel management listed in Section I with an example in Section II by placing the correct letter in the space provided.

I

a. The hard approach to personnel management

b. The soft approach to personnel management

c. The social sciences approach to personnel management

II

____ 1.1 Ms. Gompertz says she has a regulation to cover everything. When nurses ask if they can abandon caps, she says "No" but the only reason she gives is, "They'll always wear them while I'm director of nursing."

____ 1.2 Ms. Phillips tells her nursing staff to write a policy for the wearing of uniforms and for personal appearance. She gives them guidelines from management. When they are completed, she meets with the group, and the policy is modified, ratified, and put into effect.

____ 1.3 When a nurse complains that she does not agree with her performance rating by her clinical nurse manager, the director of nursing tells her that she will have the nurse manager change it to suit the employee.

____ 1.4 When a technician complains that a nurse will not allow his girl friend to visit him during duty hours, the director of nursing agrees to the technician's demands and advises the nurse to let the girl friend visit.

____ 1.5 When a patient's visitor complains that a nurse is too rough in handling her patients, the director of nursing tells the visitor she will look into the matter. She then proceeds to develop an interviewing technique to determine how patients view this nurse. The result is an opposite finding, and she makes an appointment with the visitor to discuss the results of her observations. Before doing this she discusses the entire matter with the nurse and assures her that she is satisfied with her performance.

____ 1.6 When a nurse complains about the amount of clerical work she is required to do on night duty, the director of nursing tells her this is the least busy shift and she is being paid a good salary to work it.

2. *Scenario:* In a large medical center a newly employed director of nursing was faced with making decisions about staffing. She did not know whether she had enough registered nurses. Her theory was that she might have enough registered nurses, but they were not performing primary nursing care functions. She employed a qualified nurse to do a staffing study. After making a survey of the literature on the subject, this nurse designed the instruments by which she intended to collect

data. These included an instrument for rating patients based on the amount and kinds of care needed; an instrument for measuring satisfaction with nursing care by nursing personnel, physicians, and patients, and an instrument to measure the types and numbers of activities that consumed the greatest amount of nursing care. Some of the data collected indicated the following:

1. Equipment such as suction apparatus was not centrally stored and maintained but was located on patient units where nursing personnel cleaned and maintained them.

2. Unit clerk positions were practically nonexistent, making a large clerical workload for nursing personnel. On one unit, twenty-seven resident physicians visited patients and wrote orders on an 8-hour shift.

3. Nurses mixed, poured, and administered as many as 160 doses of medication per 8-hour shift. This consumed 2 hours per shift per unit sampled.

4. Nursing personnel performed ECGs and IPPB treatments on some shifts. A sampling of one unit showed them performing ten IPPB procedures on one 8-hour night shift.

5. Laboratory rounds were made once daily at approximately 6 A.M. Monday through Friday. After that, most venipunctures for blood specimens were performed by nursing personnel. This amounted to approximately eight to twelve per day per acute care nursing unit.

6. All surgical preparations, including those for cardiac catheterization, were done by unit nursing personnel.

7. Many inpatient units did not have central piped-in oxygen or compressed air. IPPB machines were not fitted with compressors. Consequently, nursing personnel transported eight to ten tanks of compressed gases throughout the medical center each day.

8. There were six separate intensive care units, all separately staffed for maximum workload but uncoordinated so that maximum-care patients were frequently left on the units.

9. Nursing care planning was poor to nonexistent, and nurses complained they were too busy doing nonnursing duties to perform the basic components of nursing care that would meet physical, emotional, and other needs. Volunteer RNs were used to assist with data collection.

Once she had gathered all the needed information, the director of nursing made plans that included the following.

1. A detailed plan for placement of patients according to their degree of illness or ability to help themselves. This included coordinating intensive care units and took into consideration the availability of facilities. It covered the entire medical center on a phase-in basis with estimated costs for changes in physical plant.

2. Assignment of nonnursing tasks to nonnursing departments, with accompanying reductions in nursing personnel. This included supply, laboratory, inhalation therapy, and pharmacy functions, as well as increased clerical coverage on all shifts.

3. Identification of duties that would be performed by RNs, LPNs and nursing assistants according to types of patients and procedures being performed during specific hours. Her goal was maximum use of each category of personnel. Job classification for differentiated practice was initiated.

4. Experimentation with new systems of care. As one example, she proposed three types of offerings to patients: at the highest rate they would receive total care by staff; at the next rate they would do everything they could for themselves; and at the lowest rate they would be assisted by their families who would be given care plans and access to staff by telephone or other form of communication.

5. Maximum patient teaching programs to enable patients to take over their own care as soon as possible.

The director of nursing presented the plan to her nursing staff and received their suggestions, incorporating many of them into her original plan. When she was satisfied that the plan was as perfect as she could make it, she presented it to the hospital administrator.

2.1 What evidence was there that the director of nursing performed a problem-seeking, question-asking, hunch-encouraging, hypotheses-producing function?

2.2 What did she do to satisfy the fact-gathering and verifying function?

2.3 How did she search for larger generalities?

2.4 How did she perform a history-collecting, scholarly function?

2.5 What scientific instruments, methods, or techniques were used by this director of nursing?

2.6 How did she accomplish the administrative, executive, and organizational side of the study?

2.7 How did she accomplish the publicizing and educational functions?

2.8 How did she apply the study to human uses?

2.9 How did she accomplish its appreciation?

3. Place a check in the blank beside the statement that represents the best course of action by a nurse manager.

____ 3.1 Ms. Hauk, a director of nursing, listens for complaints and remarks that indicate dissatisfaction among her employees. She records them in their personnel records so that they will be available should any employee make a formal complaint.

____ 3.2 One of the activities of Ms. Goldberg, a director of nursing, is to discuss the goals and plans for their accomplishment with all employees so as to find out their satisfactions and dissatisfactions. She uses the information to modify both goals and plans so that the employees are able to accomplish many of their desires.

4. *Scenario:* Ms. Sanchez has been director of nursing of a 250-bed hospital for 8 years. Although her management operation has followed traditional patterns, she has read extensively on the subject and has been taking business administration courses in the evenings at the state university. Ms. Sanchez has decided to make some management changes in her institution.

Although meetings with members of the nursing staff had been held on a scheduled basis, they were never productive and served mainly as a medium for information to flow from management downward. She carefully planned an agenda for her next clinical nurse manager meeting and distributed it a week in advance. An item of new business on the agenda was to write specific objectives for these meetings that would benefit the clinical nurse managers and ultimately the nursing employees working for them. At the same time she would present a working draft of an operational plan for accomplishing the objectives of the department of nursing. The nurse manager group would be asked to discuss the mission, philosophy, objectives, and operational plan from the point of view of supporting it so as to achieve the objectives.

At the clinical nurse manager meeting, Ms. Sanchez was pleased with the active participation by the members. They had many suggestions for changes and for additional activities that would be helpful in achieving the objectives. During the discussion she learned many major dissatisfactions of these personnel. As an example, they did not understand the personnel rating system and wanted to know how she arrived at decisions for promotions. One of the suggested activities for accomplishment of objectives was that job standards be written and that they use the ANA Standards for Nursing Practice as a basis for them. They appointed an ad hoc committee to do this without the prodding of Ms. Sanchez, and they set a target date for completion. It was their intent to help Ms. Sanchez strengthen the objectivity of the rating system, thereby giving them input into the promotion process.

Next, Ms. Sanchez asked if the department's mission, philosophy, objectives, and operational plan should be presented to all the nursing staff, and a large majority of members agreed that it should. They also recommended that she do this, since the staff would be impressed with being able to discuss it with the boss. A suggestion was made that she meet with the staff of each unit, and they wrote a schedule acceptable to her. They then decided to develop statements of mission, philosophy, objectives, and operational plans for each of the units and to have them done by a specific date.

Ms. Sanchez discussed means of encouraging the nursing staff to be more productive and better satisfied with their working conditions. Several suggestions were made by the nurse manager group. These included modifications in policies related to wearing of the uniform and to staffing and time schedules. They also stated that many nursing personnel had expressed the desire to become more involved in unit in-service education and other nursing activities but had not been encouraged to do so. Ms. Sanchez said she would welcome all suggestions for change but that she could not guarantee that all would take place immediately. Some would have to be approved by the hospital administrator, and if Ms. Sanchez did not agree with some recommendations she would tell the people involved the reasons why. They agreed that this was acceptable to them, and the meeting was adjourned.

4.1 List a fact that encourages or discourages freedom to speak—communication.

4.2 List a fact that encourages or discourages freedom to do what one wishes to do without harming others—choice of jobs, friends, or entertainment.

4.3 List a fact that encourages or discourages freedom to express oneself—creativity.

4.4 List a fact that encourages or discourages freedom to investigate and seek information.

4.5 List a fact that encourages or discourages freedom to defend oneself, justice, fairness, honesty, or orderliness in the group.

5. *Scenario:* Ms. Rather is clinical nurse manager of a pediatric unit and encourages her employees to discuss their families and their off-duty activities. They tell her of their hopes and dreams and even of confidential personal happenings. Mr. Pottinger is clinical nurse manager of an intensive care unit. He gives his personnel needed supervision and training and supports them well while on duty. He lets it be known that he does not want to know anything about their personal lives unless it relates to their work.

5.1 Which clinical nurse manager exhibits the best understanding of motivational theory?

5.2 What knowledge of motivational theory has been exhibited by the clinical nurse manager you selected?

6. *Small Group Session*

6.1 Write a statement that provides a "vision" of what you want to accomplish in stimulating the motivation of your peers or employees. (20 minutes)

6.2 Outline a process for accomplishing this "vision." (20 minutes)

6.3 Report. (20 minutes)

7. *Exercise*

7.1 Place a large spike in a bulletin board that is read by many employees.

7.2 Hang a sign "SPIKE THAT RUMOR" above the bulletin board.

7.3 Provide a method for employees to write down rumors they have heard and hang them on the bulletin board.

7.4 Management hangs a reply within 24 hours.[26]

8. An "Investment Model of Motivation" involves the employees as *investor* and the manager as *the broker or investment adviser* for the employee.

8.1 The broker (manager) has the investors (employees) identify their investment objectives. These will include short-range and long-range objectives such as career goals and promotions. They will include those to be achieved inside the organization and outside the organization.

8.2 Broker and investors specify the components of the investment portfolio. How or what are the investors going to invest in the organization to achieve their objectives? (Long hours? Development of requisite skills? High level of involvement with, and commitment to, the organization?)

8.3 The broker actively helps the investors set realistic objectives and select the investments to be made to acquire the objectives. The broker also helps the investors analyze outcomes, assess objectives, and even seek employment elsewhere. There must be harmony between investors and organization.

8.4 Broker and investors periodically review the portfolio and modify it.

8.5 Make a management plan for implementing an Investment Model of Motivation.[27]

MANAGEMENT PLAN

OBJECTIVE:

ACTIONS	TARGET DATES	ASSIGNED TO	ACCOMPLISHMENTS

Place a Y (yes), N (no), or I (insufficient) before each statement:

In my current job I am

___ Happy with being able to help others.

___ Intellectually stimulated and challenged.

___ Given opportunity to progress educationally.

___ Learning new skills.

___ Sharpening old skills.

___ Learning a new discipline.

___ Qualifying for more responsibility.

___ Qualifying for more respect.

___ Given opportunities to attend staff meetings, patient care conferences, and staff development programs.

___ Rewarded for doing my job well.

___ Adequately paid.

___ Given opportunity for advancement.

___ Given opportunity to innovate and be creative.

___ Given opportunity to choose shifts and hours of work.

___ Given opportunity to be a leader.

___ Given opportunity to grow as a bedside nurse.

___ Able to trust my supervisors and peers.

___ Supported by administration.

___ Communicated with by administration.

___ Being paid for my total knowledge and experience.

___ Confident of job security.

___ Working with adequate staffing.

___ Feeling satisfied with my accomplishments.

___ Supported by nursing management in resolving physician-nurse conflict.

___ Able to resolve peer conflict.

___ Adequately paid for overtime.

___ Given opportunity to schedule extra time off above and beyond holidays and vacation.

___ Given opportunity to schedule my working hours.

___ Prepared to function as a team leader or clinical nurse manager.

___ Supported by competent professional nurses who assist and teach me.

My job satisfaction could be increased by:

Identify specific steps to gather the information or make the changes that will help you reach your goal.

One of my job satisfaction goals is:

As a step toward reaching this goal, I will talk to:

about:

and I will undertake the following activities myself:

Figure 16–8 • *Checklist for Assessing Job Satisfaction*

9. Read and prepare an abstract on two articles on motivation. You may select from the following or locate two published at a later date than 1986.

J. Fanslaw, "Motivating Groups," *Nursing Management,* Sept. 1986, 51–52.

M. Sinetar, "SMR Forum: Entrepreneurs, Chaos, and Creativity—Can Creative People Really Survive Large Company Structure?," *Sloan Management Review,* Winter 1985, 51–62.

T. Kempner, "Motivation and Behavior—A Personal View," *Journal of General Management,* Fall 1983, 51–57.

10. Complete the following exercise.

Complete Figure 16–8, Checklist for Assessing Job Satisfaction, and use it to develop goals that

you can achieve. Don't forget that all responsibility for personal satisfaction in life is ultimately your own. We have to take action to help ourselves, to be informed, to become better educated, to improve our interpersonal relationships, and to make our lives meaningful.

Setting personal goals is a person's way of planning ahead. It gives them momentum because it means they have made a decision to pursue what they want and have decided to obtain the qualifications to do it. It is important they recognize their personal limitations and abilities and use that awareness to initiate the changes necessary to achieve future goals. They must look at positive attitudes, too. Social and leadership goals gained

You will want to set goals in at least three areas:

1. **Personal Goals.** What would you really like to do with your life? Write down the personal goals you want to accomplish. Examples are, "Become a role model of the profession," "Achieve as a writer in the field of clinical nursing" or "Serve people who need, but lack, the means to buy health care."

_____

_____

2. **Family Goals.** Do you want to save money to travel? To put you and your family through school? To supplement a primary income? To buy something special? You may want to discuss these with your spouse and children, but write down your family goals.

_____

_____

3. **Professional goals.** Do you want to become a professor? A director of nursing? A consultant in nursing care of cancer patients? A clinical researcher? Something outside of nursing altogether? Write down your professional goals.

Figure 16–9 • *Future Goals Worksheet*

Standards for Evaluating Goals	Yes	No
1. I have reviewed my short-range goals within the last 3 months.		
2. I have reviewed my long-range goals within the last year.		
3. My goals reflect my personal philosophy or beliefs and the purpose or reason I want to achieve them.		
4. My goals can be measured or verified as being achieved.		
5. I have set my goals in the priority or sequence in which I want to accomplish them.		
6. My goals are clear to me. They are specific and indicate actions to take to achieve them.		
7. My goals are flexible and realistic so that I will have as many opportunities as possible.		
8. I have the resources to accomplish my goals.		
9. My goals are stated for a specific job.		

Figure 16–10 • *Goal Evaluation Checklist*

from family, community, church, and other aspects of living are often overlooked credentials to achieving self-improvement and self-fulfilment. Use the Figure 16–9, Future Goals Worksheet, to develop a list of goals. Once you have them written down, they can be evaluated, using Figure 16–10, Goal Evaluation Checklist.

11. Using Herzberg's two-factor theory of motivation, which of the items in Figure 16–8, Checklist for Assessing Job Satisfaction

11.1 Summarize the results of the extrinsic conditions, hygiene factors, or dissatisfiers related to *yourself and your job?*

11.2 Summarize the results of the intrinsic conditions, motivators, or satisfiers related to *yourself and your job?*

12. *Self-Esteem Exercises*

12.1 List the strengths or abilities to influence others that you have and that give you self-esteem.
How can you improve them?

12.2 List those personal, professional, and organizational goals of achievement that will make you think well of yourself.
What would improve them?

12.3 List those things that make you feel adequate in your personal life and your job.
What would improve them?

12.4 List two or more major areas in which you have achieved mastery and competence.
List one or more in which you desire to achieve mastery and competence.

12.5 List those qualities that give you confidence in the face of the world.
How can they be enlarged or improved?

12.6 List those areas in which your desire for independence and freedom are limited.
How can your independence and freedom be expanded?

12.7 List those activities that tell you you have a good reputation and prestige. Indicate whether

A	B
Vivacious	Languid
Intelligent	Stupid
Bright	Dull
Clever	Clumsy
Funny	Solemn
Courteous	Rude
Prompt	Late
Tolerant	Prejudiced
Gracious	Surly
Unpretentious	Complacent
Sincere	Devious
Friendly	Antagonistic
Humble	Arrogant
Honest	Dishonest
Truthful	False
Accurate	Deceptive
Confident	Pessimistic
Respectful	Rude
Pleasant	Obnoxious
Candid	Deceitful
Courageous	Fearful
Decent	Gross
Unselfish	Egotistic
Integrity	Fraudulent
Sincere	Sly

SOURCE: Russell C. Swansburg and Philip W. Swansburg, *Strategic Career Planning and Development for Nurses* (Rockville, MD: Aspen, 1984), p. 76.

Figure 16–11 • *Personal Characteristics*

they come from patients, visitors, supervisors, physicians, personnel, or others.

12.8 List those activities that give you feelings of self-confidence, value, strength, or being useful and needed in the world.

12.9 List those activities that make you feel inferior, weak, helpless, and discouraged.

13. Figure 16–11 is a list of matched pairs of personal characteristics. Complete the list and write a statement summarizing your personal characteristics.

Make a plan to change any personal characteristics you believe should be changed to improve your self-esteem.

13. Figure 16–12 is one approach to developing standards for the motivation aspects of the directing aspects of nursing management.

Standards:
There is evidence to show that the nurse administrator demonstrates a knowledge of:

1. Maslow's hierarchy of needs: The manager demonstrates ability to identify employees' physiological, safety, social, esteem, and self-actualization needs, and to create work situations that help meet their needs.

2. Modern motivational theory that relates needs to behavior.

   2.1 Argyris' immaturity-maturity theory: The manager attempts to make jobs challenging and subordinates as independent as they are capable of being.

   2.2 Herzberg's two-factor theory of motivation: The manager attempts to prevent dissatisfaction through providing hygiene factors and prompt satisfaction through motivators.

   2.3 Expectancy theory and learned behavior: The manager promotes an environment in which subordinates see a high probability of achieving objectives that are desirable and reinforces satisfactory performance with recognition.

      2.3.1 Vroom's theory: The manager recognizes productivity of subordinates and recommends promotions accordingly, causing them to expect such outcomes.

      2.3.2 Porter and Lawler's theory: The manager acts so that subordinates expect reward based on performance.

   2.4 Equity or social comparison theory: The manager recognizes that subordinates adapt. They weigh what they give to the enterprise against rewards or benefits.

Figure 16–12 • *Standards for the Evaluation of the Motivational Aspects of Directing Nursing Personnel*

13.1 Apply the standards for evaluation of the motivation aspects of directing nursing personnel and determine whether there is adequate evidence to show that nurse managers are using modern motivational theory at division, department, service, or unit levels. Summarize your findings.

13.2 If the nurse managers are not meeting the standards, discuss with them how they can devise and implement programs to identify and meet needs of personnel. Summarize your results.

NOTES

1. R. M. Hodgetts and D. F. Kuratko, *Management* 2d ed. (New York: Harcourt Brace Jovanovich, 1988), 285, 294.

2. A. H. Maslow, *Motivation and Personality,* 2d ed. (New York: Harper & Row, 1970).

3. Hodgetts and Karatko, op. cit., 287–289; D. McGregor, *Leadership and Motivation,* (Cambridge, MA: MIT Press, 1966).

4. E. C. Murphy, "What Motivates People to Work?," *Nursing Management,* Feb. 1984, 58, 61–62; G. K. Gordon, "Developing a Motivating Environment," *Journal of Nursing Administration,* Dec. 1982, 11–16.

5. J. L. Gibson, J. M. Ivancevich, and J. M. Donnelly, *Organizations: Behavior, Structure, Processes,* 6th ed. (Homewood, IL: Richard D. Irwin, 1988), 381–384.

6. Ibid.

7. Ibid.

8. Gordon, op. cit.

9. K. L. Roach, "Production Builds on Mutual Respect," *Nursing Management,* Feb. 1984, 54–56; M. G. Pryor and W. Mondy, "Mutual Respect Key to Productivity," *Supervisory Management,* July 1978, 10–17.

10. P. F. Drucker, *Management: Tasks, Responsibilities, Practices,* (New York: Harper & Row, 1973–1974), 176, 195–196.

11. McGregor, op. cit., 5–6.

12. Ibid., 15.

13. M. Miller, "Understanding Human Behavior and Employee Motivation," *Notes & Quotes,* 1968; McGregor, op. cit., 211–212.

14. Ibid.

15. M. K. Kleinknecht and E. A. Hefferin, "Assisting Nurses Toward Professional Growth: A Career Development Model," *Journal of Nursing Administration,* July-Aug. 1982, 30–36; J. C. Crout, "Care Plan for Retaining the New Nurse," *Nursing Management,* Dec. 1984, 30–33; R. C. Swansburg and P. W. Swansburg, *Strategic Career Planning and Development for Nurses* (Rockville, MD: Aspen, 1984).

16. B. Conway-Rutkowski, "Labor Relations: How Do You Rate?," *Nursing Management,* Feb. 1984, 13–16; W. L. Ginnodo, "Consultative Management: A Fresh Look at Employee Motivation," *National Productivity Review,* Winter 1985–1986, 78–80.

17. M. C. Allender, "Productivity Enhancement: A New Teamwork Approach," *National Productivity Review,* Spring 1984, 181–189.

18. P. Cornett-Cooke and K. Dias, "Teambuilding: Getting It All Together," *Nursing Management,* May 1984, 16–17.

19. Maslow, op. cit.

20. B. Fuszard, ed., *Self-Actualization for Nurses: Issues, Trends, and Strategies for Job Enrichment* (Rockville, MD: Aspen, 1984), 140.

21. McGregor, op. cit.

22. Fuszard, op. cit.

23. Ibid., 40.

24. Ibid., 207.

25. Maslow, op. cit.

26. D. L. Niehouse, "Job Satisfaction: How to Motivate Today's Workers," *Supervisory Management,* Feb. 1956, 8–11. 37.

27. L. Ackerman and J. P. Gruenwald, "Help Employees Motivate Themselves," *Personnel Journal,* July 1984, 55–57.

FOR FURTHER REFERENCE

Ackerman, L., Let's Put Motivation Where It Belongs—Within the Individual," *Personnel Journal,* July 1970.

Battalia, O. W., "Style Changes in the Way Men Lead Men," *Psi Phi Quarterly,* Fall 1971, 4–7.

Campbell, L. R., "What Satisfies . . . and Doesn't?," *Nursing Management,* Aug. 1986, 78.

Donovan, L., "What Nurses Want (and What They're Getting)," *RN,* Apr. 1980, 23–30.

Godfrey, M. A., "Job Satisfaction—or Should That Be Dissatisfaction?," *Nursing,* June 1978, 82.

Holt-Ashley, M., "Motivation: Getting the Medical Units Going Again," *Nursing Management,* June 1985, 28–30.

Jenkins, R. L., and Henderson, R. L., "Motivating the Staff: What Nurses Expect from Their Supervisors," *Nursing Management,* Feb. 1984, 13–14.

Joiner, C., Johnson, V., Chapman, J. B., and Corkrean, M., "The Motivating Potential in Nursing Specialties," *Journal of Nursing Administration,* Feb. 1982, 26–30.

Lancaster, J., "Creating a Climate for Excellence," *Journal of Nursing Administration,* Jan. 1985, 16–19.

Maslow, A. H., "A Theory of Human Motivation," in R. A. Sutermeister, *People and Productivity,* 2d. ed. (New York: McGraw-Hill, 1969), 91–95.

Swansburg, R. C., and Swansburg, P. W., *Strategic Career Planning and Development for Nurses* (Rockville, MD: Aspen Publishers, 1984), 1–41.

Youker, R. B., "Ten Benefits of Participant Action Planning," *Training,* June 1985, 52, 54–56.

Communications

Between two beings there is always the barrier of words. Man has so many ears and speaks so many languages. Should it nevertheless be possible to understand one another? Is real communication possible if word and language betray us every time? Shall, in the end, only the language of guns and tanks prevail and not human reason and understanding?

Joost A. M. Meerloo[1]

COMPONENTS OF COMMUNICATION

In answering the question of who is involved in communication, one could simply answer, everyone! However, there are several aspects to be considered. The first of these is that the person who wants to be heard is involved in communication. For example, the Bantam fried chicken facility wants to sell chicken and wants people to know that it has chicken to sell. Its manager will therefore advertise in an effort to communicate this desire to sell an appetizing product. The manager will do this through such media as newspapers, billboards, radio, and television. All kinds of tempting pictures will fill these advertisements. If the manager is successful, if people buy lots of Bantam fried chicken as a result of these advertisements, then they have received the message and the manager has communicated to them.

A second type of communication occurs when a person seeks out desired information. Suppose a working wife is just plain tired of cooking and wants Bantam fried chicken to serve her family for Sunday dinner. She knows where the nearest location is, because she has heard it advertised on TV or seen it on a billboard. She may have driven by the facility and seen the sign and markings that identify the product. She may have been reminded of it in the Sunday paper as she sipped her cup of coffee that morning. And even if she can't remember the address, she can always refer to the Yellow Pages for an address and phone number or call directory assistance. When she wants the information, she has many sources from which to obtain it. All these sources are media of communication.

Elements of Communication

At least two people are involved in communication, a sender or provider and a receiver. Senders usually have something they want to communicate, although they could conceivably have to provide information of a nature distasteful to themselves. Receivers usually have need of some information, good or bad. Regardless of the medium, information is transmitted from senders to receivers and communication occurs.

Regardless of whether money is involved, there is always a buyer or seller involved in a communication. The buying or selling is based on a need. Sometimes the receiver's need to hear is not as acute as the sender wants it to be. An example of this is the communication between a parent and a child. The parent can tell the child to be in by midnight on Saturday but has said the same thing before, and when the child did not return by midnight, nothing happened. Now the child does not even hear the parent, because he has no reason for listening. When he returns after midnight and is told he will not be allowed out after 8:00 P.M. for 4 weeks, he has a reason to listen. Communication now takes place, since he finds there is sufficient reason for listening.

Communication is a human process involving interpersonal relationships—and therein lies the problem. Some managers view their knowledge of events as power; they see sharing knowledge through communication as sharing power and they do not want to share power. Other managers do not realize the importance of communication in an information age because they are not up to date on the advantages of decentralization and participatory management. They frequently fall into crisis management, treating the symptoms of poor communication and never identifying the root causes. A third group of managers recognize that communication is like the central nervous system. It directs and controls the management process.

More than 80 percent of a higher-level manager's time is spent on communication: 16 percent reading; 9 percent writing; 30 percent speaking; and 45 percent listening. Is there any question that communication skills are absolutely essential to career advancement in nursing?[2]

There are three basic principles for successful communication:

1. Successful communication involves a sender, a receiver, and a medium.
2. Successful communication occurs when the message sent is received.
3. Successful nurse managers achieve successful communication.

Climate for Communication

Organizational climate and culture are discussed in Chapter 11, "Organizing Nursing Services." The communication climate should be in harmony with the corporate culture and should be used to encourage positive values among nursing employees. These include values of quality, independence, objectivity, and client service. Communication is used to support the mission (purpose or business) and vision of the nursing organization. It is used to tell the consumers or clients that nursing is of high quality. The media used will include performance, nursing records, and marketing. It will be objective when it is accurately portrayed with descriptions of factual outcomes judged on the basis of objective outcome criteria.

Nursing literature abounds with evidence of nurses' desire for autonomy. Nurse managers will use this knowledge to communicate their support of autonomy. They will also provide a climate in which the nursing business remains as free of political constraints as possible. When political considerations are imperative, the imperative will be communicated to employees. Employees make decisions based on the institution's values and beliefs.

Although organizational culture is more difficult to change than organizational climate, both can be modified with managerial effort and skill. The first step for nurse managers is to sample employees' attitudes or ideas of how they receive information and effect communication. Managers and employees know the formal structure, including roles and modes of operation used to inform and communicate. What is the informal structure? It involves people who are heroes or role models who can be involved in communication if they are positive and enthusiastic. Otherwise they may have to be replaced, particularly if they are destructive.

Cultural Agendas. Cultural agendas publicize the mission or business of the organization. They tell what the organization stands for. They will tell what the nursing division, department, or individual unit places value on.

Cultural agendas are used to communicate promotions, new hires, marriages, deaths, and other personal news about personnel. Heroes are highlighted with features that illustrate support of desired values and beliefs: the nurse who presents a paper, authors a book, achieves prominence in the profession or in the community; the nurse who is a champion bowler, an elected officer in an organization, an appointed official in the health care system; the nurse who is a volunteer in community activities. The cultural agendas are used to publicize nursing units and special achievements such as ongoing research in burn care or rehabilitation.

Various media are used to publicize cultural agendas including newsletters, memoranda, awards ceremonies, and external communications via publications, radio, television, and organizational meetings. Such communication will be most effective when they depict the people who are directly involved in the publicized events.

Cultural agendas can be effectively used to change the organizational climate and culture.[3] The nurse manager has to establish the climate for effective communication. Wlody recommends:

Step I: Review your own communication technique.

Step II: Concentrate the staff's attention on communication as a needed skill which everyone can develop.

Step III: Lead the staff into more positive interaction within the unit.

Step IV: Make daily rounds with the whole team.

Step V: Form a group to reduce stress.[4]

Nature of Communication Climate. Important communication occurs between supervisor and employees at the work level where climate is set. A supportive climate encourages employees to ask questions and give solutions to problems. Figure 17–1 summarizes characteristics of supportive and defensive communication climates. Nurse managers would strive for a supportive climate. There is a strong relationship between good communication skills and good leadership.

Open Door Policy. Communication climate influences the success of an open door policy. An open door policy of a nurse manager implies that an employee can walk into that person's office at any time. Usually, the one who does will find the manager has a schedule and it is more convenient for both for the employee to make an appointment.

The communication climate associated with some organizations has made employees wary of the open door policy. Line managers are threat-

ened when they see their employees in the boss's office. They find out the reason for the visit by any means possible. Some punish employees by telling them to use the chain of command. Some adjust performance evaluations, ostracize, adjust pay increases, or work to fire the employee. This climate quickly teaches the employee not to use the open door policy.

A nurse manager who believes in the open door policy will clearly state the rules, including whether the employee needs anyone's permission to make an appointment with the manager. A democratic manager who believes in setting a climate for open communication will encourage visits. Such a manager knows how to deal with confidential communication to protect employees and their supervisors.

COMMUNICATION AS PERCEPTION

In nursing as in other disciplines, communication is perception. Sound is created by the sensory perceptions people have associated with it. The noise aspect of communication is voice. There is communication only if the receiver hears, and people hear or perceive only what they are capable of hearing. It is important that the communication be uttered in the receiver's language, and the sender must have knowledge of the receiver's experience or perception capacity.

Conceptualization conditions perception: a person must be able to conceive to perceive. In writing a communication, writers must work out their own concepts first and ask whether the recipients can receive it. The range of perception is physiological, because perception is a product of the senses. However, the limitations to perception are cultural and emotional. Fanatics cannot receive a communication beyond their range of emotions.

Different people seldom see the same thing in a communication, because they have different perceptual dimensions. Drucker has said that to communicate, the sender must know what the recipient, the true communicator, can see and hear, and why. Perhaps if we focus on the recipient as the true communicator, we will improve communications. The unexpected is not usually received at all or is ignored or misunderstood. The human mind perceives what it expects to perceive. To communicate, the sender must also know what the recipient expects to see and hear. Otherwise the recipient has to be shocked to receive the intended message.[5]

People have selective retention by emotional

Supportive Climate	Defensive Climate	Supportive Climate	Defensive Climate
1. The individual is free to talk to managers at any level of the organization without fear of retribution of any kind. Opportunities for this are planned and made known to the entire staff.	1. The individual works within traditional management principles of chain of command, line of authority, and span of control.	information at specific intervals and when indicated.	
		4. Spontaneity.	4. Strategy is kept at managerial planning level.
2. Equality: management by objectives (MBO) supports equality by encouraging two-way communication in which both supervisor and employee evaluate progress and make future plans.	2. Superiority: pyramids, hierarchies, and chains of command support superiority.	5. Problem orientation emphasizes joint view, bringing employee into the process.	5. Control emphasizes supervisor's view.
		6. Provisionalism encourages adaptation and experimentation.	6. Certainty is dogmatic; it squelches.
3. Descriptive evaluation with management analysis and employee input. The employee gets	3. Traditional evaluation with one-way communication done on an annual basis.	7. Empathy indicates concern and respect. Use to counteract neutrality by using nontraditional management techniques.	7. Neutrality indicates nonconcern. It is fostered by orientation to numbers as in outcomes, profits, and even standardization of orientation procedures.

SOURCE: C. E. Beck and E. A. Beck, "The Manager's Open Door and the Communication Climate." Adapted from *Business Horizons*, Jan.–Feb. 1986, pp. 15–19. Copyright 1986 by the Foundation for the School of Business at Indiana University. Used with permission.

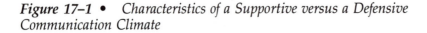

Figure 17–1 • *Characteristics of a Supportive versus a Defensive Communication Climate*

association and receive or reject based on good or bad experiences or associations. Communications make demands on people. It is often propaganda and so creates cynics. It demands that the recipient become somebody, do something, or believe something. It is powerful if it fits aspirations, values, and goals. It is most powerful if it converts, because conversion demands surrender.

Leveling with Employees

Leveling is being honest with employees. It makes all information known to them, both the good and the bad. It gives them a chance to improve. Managers can control the content of negative information, not by concealing it but by sharing ideas, feelings, and information with affected employees. Nurse managers address issues as they arise. They focus on employee needs, offering help as indicated. Communication is a major factor in performance evaluation. See Chapter 22 on "performance appraisal."[6]

COMMUNICATION DIRECTION

For effective communication the place to start is with the perceptions of the recipients. Listeners do not receive the communication if they do not understand the message. Know what they can perceive, what they expect to perceive, and what they want to do. Then formulate the message. Many nurse managers focus on what they want to say and then cannot understand why it is not understood by the recipients.

The information load should be kept down. This will help to increase communication. Management by objectives focuses on perceptions of both recipients and senders. Recipients have access to the experience of the manager. The communicative process focuses on aspirations, values, motivations: the needs of the subordinates. Performance evaluation or appraisal should focus on the recipient's concerns, perceptions, and expectations. Communication then becomes a tool of the recipient and a mode of organization, because it is used by the employee.

Feedback

Feedback completes or continues communication, making it two-way. Today's workers are better managed under a climate that promotes Theory Y and participation or involvement. Most are more affluent, better educated, have increased leisure, and retire earlier, all indications of their changed values.

Feedback is one of the most important factors influencing behavior. People want to know what they have accomplished and where they stand. Feedback works best when specific goals are set to specify the improvements sought, with measurable targets, specific deadlines, and specific methods of attaining goals.

Effective communication includes giving and receiving suggestions, opinions, and information. If this two-way interaction does not occur, there is little or no communication. Communication requires mutual respect and confidence.

One-way communication prevents input or feedback and interaction. It causes nurses to depersonalize their relationships with patients and families. It serves as a barrier between nurses and physicians. It causes distorted communications that result in distorted and inaccurate feedback; scapegoating of peers, patients, and families; and emotional blowups, skepticism concerning all messages, frustration, stress, delay of therapeutic intervention, and negative socioeconomic consequences.[7]

INFORMATION

Although they are interdependent, communication and information are different. Communication is perception; information is logic. Information is formal and has no meaning. It is impersonal and not altered by emotions, values, expectations, and perceptions.

Computers allow us to handle information devoid of communication content, an example being personnel information. Information is specific and economical. It is based on need by a person and for a purpose. Information in large amounts beyond that which meets a person's needs is an overload. Communication may not be dependent on information; it may be shared experience. Information should be passed to the person who needs to know it, and that person must be able to receive it and act on it. Perception and communication are primary to information, and as the latter increases the communicator or receiver must be able to perceive its meaning.[8] In the interest of time management nurse managers need skills that sort information according to its import, skills that require clear communication and acute perception.

LISTENING

Communications take place between employer and employee, and herein lies the crux of the situation. An employer must hear what employees are saying as well as what they are *not* saying. That employer must do so to have satisfied, productive employees. To hear them requires concentration because most people speak at 125 to 150 words per minute. It is just like church on Sunday. While the preacher talks, the congregation hears only by concentrating. Otherwise they are planning next week's work. Many managers do not listen effectively to what people are saying to them. They shut off the person who wants to say something about a problem but knows that it either will not be heard or will have no effect.

Because a person can listen four times as fast as words are spoken is one reason personnel have a problem listening to the change-of-shift report. As a consequence they forget to give a person a message about an appointment or to do something for a patient. It is usually more efficient to read change-of-shift reports or to listen to tape-recorded reports.

According to Haakenson, working persons are engaged in some form of verbal communication 70 percent of their waking day, or approximately 11 hours and 20 minutes out of 16 hours. Of that time, 45 percent is spent listening to what is 50 percent forgotten within 24 hours. Another 25 percent is forgotten in the next 2 weeks.[9] If this is true of nursing personnel, you will forget 75 percent of what you hear today within the next 2 weeks.

Others claim we remember only 50 percent of what we hear immediately after a 10 minute speech. Twenty-five percent is considered a good retention level.[10]

Causes of Poor Listening Habits

Remember that it is a bad habit to call a subject uninteresting or boring. Listen for useful information from what is considered a dull subject. Sift and screen, separate wheat from chaff, and look for something useful. Be an interested person and make the subject interesting. Good listeners attempt to hear what is said.

It is a bad habit to criticize the delivery. Concentrate on finding out what the speaker has to say that is interesting or useful. Keep from being overstimulated by the subject. Otherwise you mentally prepare an argument or rebuttal and miss what the speaker says. Hear the speaker out before making judgments. Listen for the main idea rather than the facts and identify principles, concepts, and generalizations. Facts merely support the generalizations. Accept the face value of the message rather than evaluate it.

Avoiding the speaker's eye contact is a bad habit as it decreases trust. Remember that 60 percent of a message is nonverbal.

Defensive listening occurs when the speaker's message threatens the listener with blame or punishment for something. It is a bad habit as it prevents accurate listening and perceptions. Defensive listening is stimulated when a person's speech implies a listener's behavior is being evaluated. Defensive response is reduced when the speaker describes behavior objectively.

Speech that indicates the sender is trying to control the receiver evokes defense. People don't want their values and viewpoints controlled and will shut them out. They want to have freedom to choose. When the sender solicits the collaboration of the receiver in solving mutual problems, the receiver responds positively.

Receivers defend themselves against perceived strategies to change their behaviors or control them, which they regard as deceitful. They respond to spontaneity and honesty that they perceive as free of deceit.

Speech perceived as unconcerned about a group's welfare evokes defense. Speech perceived as empathetic evokes acceptance. People want to hear speech that indicates they are valued. Gestures communicate neutrality or empathy.

Speech, verbal or nonverbal, that indicates superiority evokes defense, while speech indicating equality is accepted and supported. Certainty indicates dogmatism and evokes defense. Defensiveness is reduced by professionalism in speech. It indicates the sender wants help, information, data, or input from the listener.[11]

Other reasons supervisors give for not listening include:

1. Thinking employees do not expect supervisors to listen.
2. Thinking employees have nothing of value to say.
3. Thinking listening is not part of supervisors' jobs.
4. Thinking employees should listen to them.
5. Thinking employees will change supervisors' minds and they will have to reevaluate employees.[12]

Techniques to Improve Listening

There are many ways of improving listening ability.

Summarize what is being said for better understanding and retention. Give empathetic attention to the speaker and try to understand the substance of what is being said. Seek to be objective and to apply creativity. Go beyond the speaker's dialect, stance, gestures, and attire to understand the meaning of the speaker's words. Try to counter your own emotionality or prejudice even though you may have opposite convictions.

It is important to discriminate among those to whom you listen. Listen to people who keep you informed and lighten your workload or save time. Listen to those who argue constructively and force you to sharpen your judgment. Know the kind of people who want to listen to you and the situation in which they will try to make you hear. Learn to recognize when you are prone to listen and when not. Some people give good information and one should listen to them. They are trusted troubleshooters, line managers in charge of the bread-and-butter functions of primary patient care, staff specialists delegated tasks such as the staff development specialist, and those who need the decisions only you can make. Graciously avoid exaggerators, opportunists, office politicians, gossips, and chronic complainers.[13]

Things said by the speaker, appearance, facial expression, posture, accent, skin color, or mannerisms can all turn off the listener. So if a person wants to hear, that person must put aside all preconceived ideas or prejudices and give the speaker full attention so that the speaker will be motivated to do a better job of attempting to communicate. While the person is talking, the listener analyzes what is being said for ideas and facts. The receiver must also listen for feelings, which appear in what a person says in relation to background and performance, tone of voice, gestures, and facial expressions.

The literature abounds with examples of practical suggestions for encouraging people to listen. Listening shows respect and value for employees. It encourages their cooperation and their acceptance of change. It helps to relieve stress and prevent burnout. A manager who talks and listens to an employee helps that person to figure out how to do the job.

Listening elicits suggestions that lead to profitability. It prevents operating deficiencies and cuts costs. Listening saves disciplinary actions and jobs when it reveals the real cause of an error. It promotes loyalty.[14] Poor listening can cost millions of dollars.

Practical suggestions for encouraging people to listen if you are the speaker include:

1. Be prepared; answer the questions, Who? and What?
2. Identify and evaluate the purpose of your remarks.
3. Organize and outline the report or speech to convey the facts.
4. Make efficient notes and use them. Outline.
5. Remember that you are part of the package.
6. Make your voice work for you with proper breathing and pitch.
7. Communicate with your eyes.

Results

The results of effective listening are that (1) two people hear each other, (2) beneficial information is furnished on which to base right decisions, (3) a better relationship between people is established, and (4) it is easier to find solutions to problems.[15]

MEDIA OF COMMUNICATIONS

Meetings

Meetings of all kinds are a media for communication, often for purposes of dissemination of information as well as true communication. Refer to Chapter 12 on committees.

Supervisors

Supervisors or managers at all levels are also a media for communication.

Questions

Questions are an important part of communications. They are asked to obtain information; the goal is mutual understanding. The tone of voice must encourage confidence and trust from the person questioned. Facial expression is important, as is the physical conduct of the questioner. Always go beyond the answer to a primary question; do not flatly agree or disagree with the answer.

Successful questioning consists of creating and maintaining a climate for communication, asking the right questions in the right way and listening to the responses.

Oral Communication

Oral communication is the most common form used by executives, who spend 50 percent to 70 percent of their time listening and talking and as much as 80 percent communicating. Since oral communication takes so much of a nurse manager's time, one should use the most effective words. Verbal messages are said to be 7 percent verbal (word choice), 38 percent vocal (oral presentation), and 55 percent facial expression.[16]

An advantage of face-to-face communication is that each person can respond directly to another or to others. The larger the group, the less effective is face-to-face communication. An effective message requires a knowledge of words and their various meanings as well as the contexts within which they can be used. In short, effective communication may depend on use of the dictionary for effective vocabulary formation. Many people cannot adequately read or write the English language. They can improve their ability by reading books and articles on techniques of effective speaking and writing, by using dictionaries and grammars books, and by taking courses that teach the skills of speaking and writing. The communicator of messages should learn to transmit them so they will be understood by the recipients, who are the true communicators. The sender should know their backgrounds, interests, and motives so that the message will give the desired meaning and motivate the recipients. Courtesy, tact, and finesse are more effective than giving orders. The listener must listen for understanding of the meaning of the message being conveyed by the speaker. The listener must keep the mind from straying and must grasp the main ideas, organize them, and translate them into order for future action.

Figure 17–2 summarizes other techniques to use in preparing and giving an oral presentation.

1. Prepare carefully. What is the goal of your presentation? Is it to inform? Persuade? Entertain? It can be a combination of these and to be effective should probably combine at least two, such as entertainment with information or persuasion.

2. Prepare the presentation carefully. Make an outline and develop the content to fit the outline. Start well in advance so that you can read and adjust the material for a smooth flow of ideas.

   2.1 What is the purpose of the presentation? Did you select the topic or was it given to you? In both instances clarify the purpose with the organizers of the event or whoever has engaged you to do the presentation.

   2.2 Prepare an introduction that will gain the attention of the audience. Spark their interest. Humor often helps but be careful of using cynicism or making derogatory remarks. References to religion, sex, and other controversial subjects should be carefully selected, if used at all. They are better avoided if you wish to persuade or inform, unless they are a part of your topic. Remember, words convey feelings, attitudes, opinions, and facts. Use them to turn the audience on, not off.

   2.3 Make the main points in the body of the presentation. Support them with appropriate and specific examples.

   2.4 Prepare or select and use visual aids to support the key points of the presentation effectively. They are an extension of your presentation designed to appeal to the senses and increase reception.

   2.5 Know who the audience will be and tailor the message to it. Provide useful material.

   2.6 Plan for audience participation with questions or appropriate exercises to involve listeners.

   2.7 Tie the message together with interval summaries and an effective conclusion. How do you want to leave the audience?

   2.8 If you plan to speak extemporaneously, make notes on cards or put outlines on a visual aid such as a poster, a chalkboard, an overhead transparency, or a slide projection screen.

3. Prepare the environment beforehand. Surroundings are important and should be as attractive as possible. Bear this in mind when you have input into selection.

   3.1 If you want to speak from a podium, make sure it is in place. If you want to sit, have a table and chair in place.

   3.2 Check lighting and sound equipment.

   3.3 Check audiovisual equipment.

   3.4 Remove unneeded barriers such as screens, furniture, and other movable objects. If pillars are in the way, rearrange your position or the audience seating if this is possible. Arrange your proximity to the group to facilitate a feeling of closeness.

   3.5 Prepare your person for the presentation. Wear clothes that present you best. Conventional clothes are best as the audience will then focus on your words rather than on your appearance. Be well groomed.

   3.6 Good preparation will help you to be relaxed. Get a good night's sleep the night before the presentation. Plan your schedule so as not to be excited beforehand. Eat and drink moderately. Sit and do deep breathing exercises immediately before.

4. Be on time and use time effectively.

5. Speak to be heard.

   5.1 Use your voice, varying pitch, volume, rate, and tone for planned effect.

   5.2 Practice pronouncing words with which you have trouble.

   5.3 Pause to enhance your delivery. Short silences emphasize points and allow the audience to think about them.

   5.4 Make your presentation sound natural even if you read it.

SOURCE: Adapted from J. Lancaster, "Public Speaking Can Be Improved," *Journal of Nursing Administration*, Mar. 1985, 31–35; D. Caruth, "Words: A Supervisor's Guide to Communications," *Management Solutions*, June 1986, 34–35; W. D. St. John, "You Are What You Communicate," *Personnel Journal*, Oct. 1985, 40–43.

Figure 17–2 • *Techniques for Effective Public Speaking*

6. Use body language effectively.

   6.1 Develop the audience's awareness of your nonverbal behavior slowly. Be aware of it yourself.

   6.2 Maintain eye contact.

   6.3 Plan your movement: walking, standing. Your posture should convey energy, interest, approval, confidence, warmth, and openness.

   6.4 Keep the space between you and the audience open.

   6.5 Use positive gestures. They are positive in themselves.

   6.6 Use head movements for effect.

   6.7 Use facial expression for effect.

   6.8 Know where your hands and feet are at all times.

   6.9 Be genuine! An audience can quickly identify a fake.

7. Adapt to audience feedback, being sensitive to listeners' interests and moods.

   7.1 Listen for unrest, shifting in seats, whispering, muttering.

   7.2 Watch for nonverbal responses. Pay attention to body language, facial expressions, gestures, body movements. Leaning backward or away is perceived as a negative response.

   7.3 Be prepared to answer questions if there are breaks in the presentation. You may want to plan for them. Repeat them before answering, whether they are oral or written. You are giving additional information.

   7.4 Treat your audience with respect in every way and they will view you as genuine.

Figure 17–2 *(Continued)*

Written Communication

Writing is one of the most common media of communication, not only in nursing but in society in general. It comes in massive proportions; publications and memos to be read and passed on even if they go into the wastebasket; letters that need to be answered. How should one go about handling all this material? First make a mental decision: It must be dealt with, so organize yourself and attend to it. A system must be established for assigning priorities to the mass of written communications. Go through them by scanning, and then answer or delegate what can be handled immediately. Lay aside whatever can be taken care of at a future date, but do not put things where you will forget them. You can put them in a folder in priority sequence until you can attend to them.

You are writing to the receiver; a reader, viewer, listener, observer, or member of an audience. They are not interested in you as the author, only the message you are sending. Write everything to the reader or listener, the receiver. Use good marketing techniques and sell your product.[17]

Figure 17–3 lists nine principles or rules to follow when writing.

Words are an important part of written communication. Put the reader's interest first. Begin with a provocative question or striking statement to jar them. Go right to the point: the purpose of the letter and the request for action. A personal letter is always better than a form letter. People like personal letters. Use a personal friendly tone, with first names and personal pronouns. You are expressing interest in the reader. Contractions such as "aren't" should, however, be used with discretion.

Use active voice verbs for strength. About 10 percent of total words should be verbs. Use strong nouns. Use the subject and main verb early in the sentence. Avoid overuse of adjectives and adverbs and be specific when using adjectives. State the specific amount such as "100" instead of "much," "any" or "a lot."

Be as brief as possible. Use short rather than long words. Use sentences that contain one idea and are no longer than sixteen to twenty words. Vary the sentence length. Write naturally using friendly, conversational language.

Reread and revise written communication. Look at the nouns and verbs; the simplicity or wordiness of your sentences. Have you stated what you intended? Do you mean what you say? Eliminate unneeded words. You may want to add a personal handwritten note to the bottom.[18]

Evaluate your written communication using the Gunning Mueller Fog Index presented in Figure 17–4.

Interviews

Interviewing is a basic tool of communication. A prospective employee is interviewed. If good counseling and guidance techniques are practiced, in-

1. Empathize—be sensitive to the needs and desires of those who will read what you are writing. Arouse and maintain the reader's interest by appealing to the mind and emotions. For example, compose a message that will transmit respect for the nurse while offering a credible and unique inspiration to take nursing histories or prepare nursing care plans. When you give orders, tell the person why you are having her do something. You-centered rather than I-centered communications are interesting to the reader or listener. Give people honest and deserved praise, the kind of flattery that makes them feel they are worth flattering. If you are addressing a particular person, a unique human personality, put that person's name in the salutation as well as in the body of the letter or memo. Make an effort to please the receiver by using tact, respect, good manners, and courtesy.

2. Attempt to avoid the COIK fallacy ("clear only if known" to the reader or listener already). Think of the misunderstanding that could occur in a written message using abstract terms. Your aim should be to create mental pictures using language that is suitable to the experience and knowledge level of the receiver.

3. Do not repeat anecdotes frequently or the reader will be insulted. Avoid overcommunication, overdetailing, and redundancy. Necessary repetition can be achieved by using pleasant and meaningful examples, illustrations, paraphrasing, and summaries. Repetition is essential to the mastery of a skill.

4. Express yourself in clear, simple language. Lincoln's Gettysburg Address contains 265 words, three-fourths of them of one syllable. Abstract, technical-sounding jargon, cliches, and trite platitudes may cover up insecurity in writers afraid of committing themselves in writing. Avoid archaic commercial expressions, specialized in-house jargon, and fading journalese by writing clearly and concisely.

5. Make yourself accessible to the reader by positively and courteously requesting a response. You can ask a direct question and expect a reply by a certain date. You can also encourage response by giving a special return address, a private box or phone number, writing instructions, a postcard, or a return envelope. Make it easy, desirable, and pleasant for the reader to reply.

6. Use the format of the newspaper story: accuracy, brevity, clarity, digestibility, and empathy. Arouse the reader with a headline opener. Follow it with a summary that tells significant highlights in the opening paragraph. Then tell the details. Here is an example of a memo form that has worked for others.

Date _____ Time _____

To: _____ Subject: _____

From: _____

Objective: _____

1. _____

_____

2. _____

_____

3. _____

_____

7. Break up a solid page of print with a variety of forms: underline, space, italicize, capitalize, enumerate, indent, box, summarize, and illustrate. Make your reading attractive and digestible.

8. Back up what you write by what you do; build a reputation for integrity.

9. Organize your material.
    9.1 Outline key points.
    9.2 Compile data into groups according to commonality.
    9.3 Arrange materials in a logical sequential order.
        9.3.1 Chronological
        9.3.2 Cause-effect relationship
        9.3.3 Increasing complexity
    9.4 Tie the groups together using transitional devices.
        9.4.1 Time-order words (first, later, finally)
        9.4.2 Guide words (as a result, therefore, on the other hand)
    9.5 Link the communication with the previous message by referring to:
        9.5.1 Date
        9.5.2 Subject
        9.5.3 Sender of correspondence
    9.6 Furnish appropriate excerpts from past correspondence.

Figure 17–3 • *Nine Principles or Rules to Follow When Writing*

The Gunning Mueller Fog Index presents a way to measure the reading ease of a piece of writing. It produces a number that approximates the grade level at which a person must read to comprehend the material. Here is how to use it.

Take a 100-word sample of your writing and:

1. Find the average number of words per sentence. (If the final sentence in the sample runs beyond the hundredth word, use more than 100 words for this step.)

2. In the first 100 words, count the number of words that contain three or more syllables. Do not count proper nouns, combinations of short words like "bookkeeper" or "manpower," or verbs made into three syllables by adding "-ed" or "-es."

3. Add the average number of words per sentence and the number of words containing three or more syllables. Multiply the sum by 0.4.

The result tells you the grade level of the writing sample. Remember, the average person reads at about a ninth grade level, and anything above a seventeenth grade level is difficult for college graduates.

Caution: Do not let the formula restrict your writing. Use it only to spot-check your writing periodically. Slavish devotion to the formula could result in choppy writing.

SOURCE: Reprinted with permission from *Communication Briefings,* "How to Write to Be Understood," 700 Black Horse Pike, Suite 110, Blackwood, NJ 08012.

Figure 17–4 • *The Fog Index*

terviews are used to apprise the employee of performance. An interview is essential to practicing management by objectives. In disciplining an employee, it is necessary to interview the individual. When an employee leaves, an exit interview is desirable to learn why the person is leaving and gain suggestions for strengthening the human relations management program. Questions for these interviews should be worded to obtain the most beneficial information. For effective interviewing:

1. Use plain and direct language rather than technical, professional, or slang terms.
2. Keep questions short.
3. Use familiar illustrations.
4. Don't assume the interviewee knows something. Check the extent of interviewee's knowledge beforehand.

5. Avoid improper emphasis so as not to indicate the answer you hope to elicit.
6. Be sure the interviewee gives words the same meaning as you do.
7. Be precise in picking words. Use accurate synonyms.
8. Use words with one pronunciation.

Refer to Chapter 5 on personnel management for more discussion of interviewing.

Organizational Publications

Barnard stated that the first function of an executive was to develop and maintain a system of communication.[19] The bigger the organization, the more difficult it is for the director of nursing to communicate to the employees who give direct care to patients. This problem is further complicated by the requirement for 24-hour-a-day, 7 day-a-week services. One medium for communication between nurse executives and employees is an organizational publication. This does not have to be confined to nursing but can be supported and used by nursing. Certainly the nurse executive will have input into the development and evaluation of an organizational publication.

OBTAINING INFORMATION

Receivers have a responsibility for obtaining information. Every professional employee feels some conflict between personal needs and the demands of the organization. Communication, the giving and receiving of information, helps the employee to control or tolerate this conflict. Assume that management controls information that will be given to employees. A conservative manager will give employees as little information as possible, because that manager considers the information will be distorted or misunderstood.

A director of nursing stated that although the registered nurse in the recovery room was totally competent, she would not give her the title of clinical nurse manager and bring her to nurse manager meetings because she would misinterpret the statements made there. The enlightened manager will be direct and honest, believing that employees need all the information they can get to do their jobs. Bad news usually leaks, and trying to keep it covered up only creates distrust and anxiety.

Poor communication is caused by caution and preoccupation with running the department. Some middle managers tend to treat information as private property. Organization geography and size effect communication. People tend to protect their egos and their prejudices, and employees have to seek out information.

Communication of information is a joint responsibility of employer and employee. So if you need to know something, go find out—ask. Gather intelligence. Find out how your organization is developing and what its future prospects are. Will its requirements continue to be compatible with your personal goals?

THE FUTURE

The success pattern of the industrial age is a liability to the information age; thus, corporations will have to reshape their policies and structure to recruit employees in the information age of the 1990s. We are not on the threshold but have entered the information age and will be in it for the next 50 years.

During this time the following changes have started and will continue to occur:

1. Agriculture will be reduced in people and productivity.
2. Only 10 percent of the population will be employed in manufacturing.
3. Sixty-five to 70 percent of the work force will be employed in the service industries.
4. The information/electronic industry is creating 4 to 4.5 million jobs a year.
5. Education will be a dominant industry because services are education-intensive.
6. Total training budgets will be $10 trillion per year.
7. There will be 350 million people in the United States.
8. Income will be $40,000 per capita at a 2 percent per year compound model of growth in gross national product.
9. A new accounting system will evolve to depreciate people. Education will become the capital to replace losses.
10. There will be more organizations with fewer employees per organization.[20]

People as Capital

Specialization, division of labor, and economics of scale do not work in a service organization. People are the capital resource and the return on people is the measurable outcome, not capital in building and machines. The cost basis of service organizations will continue to be in people.

What will the organization be like?

- Those that foster personal growth will attract the best and brightest people. Work enlargement yields greater productivity from such people. They want health and fitness and education programs from their employers. They want work integrated into their lives. They want to work in environments that are democratic and allow them to network and to work in small teams. They want work to be fun.
- Good employees want ownership. They want to own stock in the company. They also want psychic ownership in the company. They believe they are entrepreneurs. Within the corporation, "intrapreneurship" is already creating new products and new markets, revitalizing companies from the inside out.
- The service economy produces to meet unique human needs. Ideas come from employees with a rich mix of cultures. Customer demands and needs spur intuition and creativity leading to new products and services. Medical problems including nursing are not neatly packaged. They are organic and interdependent, requiring workers who will integrate the specialists to meet the needs of the people.
- Capital has to be compounded through education and software. Training and education will reduce general and administrative costs to maintain and increase competition. Information should be bought as direct cost because a productive employee must be up to date and have information to be competent and productive.

Organizations

To grow and profit organizations will have to eliminate their hierarchical orientation and become team oriented. They will have to emulate the positive and productive qualities of small business. The infrastructure of the organization will give way to networking and people orientation.

Many businesses are striving for monopoly through mergers, acquisitions, and coalitions to control their environments. Although success evolves from market feedback, market forces demand change from people and are brutally destructive when they fail. The market will become the arbiter of power, obliterating layers of bureaucracy unless seized by political means.[21]

Technology

Technology will be linked to the service orientation of surviving, adaptive, customer-oriented organizations. It will shift the cost curve, with labor continuing to have high income because of technology-increased productivity outcomes.

Quality will be paramount, requiring that the organization design and the technology be brought together as enablers for human resources. Computers can supplement, not replace, the human capital.

Technology will become overhead. Information technology will be used to solve problems where there is little intelligence and very little collective knowledge. When available the information technology should be bought, not generated directly, to decrease both overhead costs and the hierarchy. Otherwise managers have to establish entire teams of experts to develop and implement a system that may already be available. It will be cheaper to pay the experts by the minute, as many will be available electronically. Thus contract or consultative labor will replace hired labor, especially in the technological sphere.

Artificial intelligence will be a key enabler that will create generalists. It replaces experts and encapsulates and capitalizes knowledge. Knowledge is added to machines to become an extension of the user. There will be a symbiotic relationship between the manager and the expert machine.

Survival in the information age will depend on a combination of technology and strategic insights. Service organizations will have to find people who need services and deliver them. During the past 6,000 years information has belonged to the power structure. They did not trade it, market it, or give it away. The service industries of the information age will market services that are heavily information-based.

Technology is always in arrears as both people and systems quickly become obsolete in developing databases. Managers should go after strategic, not technical gains. They should not computerize what does not work nor maintain obsolete technology in hiring people. The people have to be developed and updated, adjusted to the system. They will career hop within and without the organization. Turnover is expensive as it throws away assets. Human resource assets generate more value added when they are managed, enriched, and involved in the enterprise.[22]

SUMMARY

Communications occur between government and governed, between governments, between buyers and sellers, between manufacturers and consumers, between pupils and teachers, between parents and children, and between neighbors, but most important communication occurs between people *only if they want it to.* The products of lack of communication are too costly to accept: misinformation, misunderstanding, waste, fear, suspicion, insecurity, and low morale.

People have difficulty accepting the fact that communication is not the answer to all problems of human relations and personnel management. There is a gap between senders and receivers that must be recognized before it can be bridged—a gap in background, experience, and motivations.

Good communication is frequently an illusion. It is not achieved with open doors, geniality, or jokes. It is helped by listening to what people are really saying and perceiving what they are projecting through their words, their facial expressions, their tones of voice, and their actions. They may be worrying about what is on the boss's mind. To induce greater numbers of people to accept direction and not undermine it, they must participate. They will listen for genuineness in the words of the boss as demonstrated by actions.

EXPERIENTIAL EXERCISES

1. *Scenario:* Communication in nursing to a large extent depends on reports. Change-of-shift reports are given on most wards and units and between managers or supervisors. A clinical nurse manager decided that her change-of-shift reports were not being listened to by the employees. They were tape-recorded reports, and the team members were always returning to ask questions, the answers to which were given in the reports. They also referred to patient's records to get information given in the reports. She asked the staff to write objectives for the reports. They decided that the purpose of the report was to give them needed information to do their day's work but that it did not need to repeat physicians' or nurses' orders. They preferred to get these from the original plans. They also decided that all oncoming team members would listen to report but offgoing ones would not. This eventually led to a change of hours, because no overlapping was needed for anyone except the clinical nurse manager and team leader who could work while report was listened to by others. The team members also decided on an outline of information that would be reported. It was also their decision that listeners would critique the recorders so

that they could improve the quality of their voice recordings.

Answer the following questions.

1.1 What was decided about who the listeners would be and what they would listen to?

1.2 How was the purpose identified and evaluated?

1.3 How was the report outlined and organized?

1.4 How were efficient notes made and used by the recorder?

1.5 How was the recorder a part of the communication package?

1.6 How did the recorder communicate with her eyes?

2. Match each of the principles or rules to follow in writing in Section I with the correct example in Section II by placing the letter in the blank. Choices may be used more than once.

I

a. Empathize—be sensitive to the needs and desires of those who will read it.
b. Attempt to avoid the COIK (**C**lear **O**nly **I**f **K**nown) fallacy.
c. Do not repeat anecdotes frequently. The reader will be insulted.
d. Express yourself in clear, simple language.
e. Make yourself accessible to the reader by positively and courteously requesting a response.

II

____ 2.1 "If you are interested in the project, please tell me by November 10."
____ 2.2 "If you do not do the nursing care planning, the patient will not receive the care he deserves, and the hospital will have its accreditation compromised."
____ 2.3 As a young student was registering for class at a southern university, the clerk, noting that she was from Iowa, asked, "How did you get away down here?" The confident reply of "I flew!" did not answer the implication of the question. A listener thought the student was being sarcastic, but neither tone of voice nor facial expression verified this. The clerk was interested in the process or reasons that had brought the student to the university, but the student did not know this.

Standards:

1. An information system exists for the nursing division, department, service, or unit.
2. The nurse manager makes a concerted attempt to communicate with nursing workers according to their abilities to perceive and to hear in terms of their own experience.
3. The nurse manager knows what nursing workers expect to hear and see.
4. The nurse manager attempts to tune communication into nursing workers' values, thereby making demands on them.
5. The nurse manager attempts to find out what nursing workers want to know and what they are interested in.
6. The communication system focuses on the values, beliefs, and aspirations of nursing workers.
7. The communication system encourages feedback (is two-way) vertically and horizontally.

Figure 17–5 •   Standards for Evaluation of the Communication System of a Nursing Division, Department, Service, or Unit

____ 2.4 A writer often repeated the same story but used different words or more words.
____ 2.5 When the grateful patient wrote a laudatory letter to the hospital administrator about Ms. O'Rourke, he endorsed it to Ms. Kathleen O'Rourke, Team Leader, Unit 4N, and said, "Thank you, Ms. O'Rourke, for the great job you are doing in providing high quality care to our patients, and thank you also for the personalized efforts you make in helping us achieve our objectives."
____ 2.6 Instead of writing, "Enclosed please find a check for the sum of ten dollars to cover the purchase of a book entitled *A Bird in the Bush*," write, "Here is ten dollars. Please send me the book *A Bird in the Bush*."

3. *Scenario:* The objective of the department of nursing is "to provide individualized care in a safe environment to meet the total therapeutic needs of each patient—physical, emotional, spiritual, environmental, social, economic, and rehabilitative." The 24-hour nursing report to the director of nursing states the following:

Criscraft, Pauline Age 40, Dx Ca with metast
HD No.:___
Prob: Hydration; in acceptance phase.
Sol: IVs as ordered; try to give her realistic goals.

Previous reports have indicated that Ms. Criscraft is obstructed and that she is going through the stages of grief over her terminal illness. The hospital day number was omitted, and the report of continuity of progress was not continued by the evening and night nurses.

3.1 How does the report on Ms. Criscraft meet the stated objectives of the department of nursing?

3.2 What indication is there that the information on Ms. Criscraft is or is not provided in a manner that is simple, functional, qualitative, and indicative of the workload of the unit?

4. Use the Gunning Mueller Fog Index in Figure 17–4 on a piece of your own writing or on an assigned one.

5. Use Figure 17–5 to evaluate the communication system of a nursing division, department, service, or unit in which you are practicing as a student.

Summarize your findings. If the standards are not being met, use a problem solving approach to build and implement a communication system model. Use the management plan format.

MANAGEMENT PLAN

PROBLEM:

OBJECTIVE:

ACTIONS	TARGET DATES	ASSIGNED TO	ACCOMPLISHMENTS

6. Group Exercise: Communication

Goal: To find out how well we communicate

Exercise One

1. Use two groups of five to seven persons each.

2. Arrange chairs and members of one group in a center circle.

3. Arrange chairs and members of other group in an outer circle.

4. The center group will discuss a controversial topic until told to stop. (about 5 minutes)

5. Have group change places and the center group discusses another controversial topic until told to stop. (about 5 minutes)

6. Have each group summarize exactly what the other group said in their discussion. (about 5 minutes)

7. How close did each listening group come to hearing exactly what the inner group was talking about? Which principle of communication was demonstrated?

Suggested topics:

Marijuana use should be legalized.

Certain information should be kept from employees.

Exercise Two

1. Use a group of five to seven persons.

2. Select a person to *describe* a drawing. Do not *tell* the group what the drawing is. Each person will draw the item as the one person describes it. The person will not answer questions nor use any gestures. Take 3 to 5 minutes.

3. Select a second person to describe the same drawing. Now tell each person to ask any questions they want to about the diagram as they redraw it. Use any gestures to help describe the diagram. Take 3 to 5 minutes.

Reassemble and answer the following questions:

1. How much does a person control receiving or getting information?

2. What things help a person to get correct information?

Exercise Three

1. Identify five to ten areas of concern in interpersonal relationships with people: *peers* (co-workers), *colleagues* (physicians, dietary personnel, etc.), and *management*. (15 minutes)

2. How can these areas of concern be improved through improved communication by us? (10 minutes)

3. How can these areas of concern be improved through improved communication by them? (10 minutes)

4. Present summary. (15 minutes)

NOTES

1. J. Anderson, "What's Blocking Upward Communication?," *Personnel Administration*, Jan.-Feb. 1968, 5ff.
2. P. Morgan and H. K. Baker, "Building a Professional Image: Improving Listening Behavior," *Supervisory Management*, Nov. 1985, 34–36; J. A. Griver, "Communication Skills for Getting Ahead," *AORN Journal*, Aug. 1979, 242–249.
3. W. J. Corbett, "The Communication Tools Inherent in Corporate Culture," *Personnel Journal*, Apr. 1986, 71–72, 74.
4. G. S. Wlody, "Communicating in the ICU: Do You Read Me Loud and Clear?," *Nursing Management*, Sept. 1984, 24–27.
5. P. F. Drucker, *Management: Tasks, Responsibilities, Practices* (New York: Harper & Row, 1973), 483.
6. W. D. St. John, "Leveling with Employees," *Personnel Journal*, Aug. 1984, 52–57.
7. Wlody, op. cit.
8. Drucker, op. cit., 487–489.
9. R. Haakenson, "How to Be a Better Listener," *Notes & Quotes*, No. 297, Feb. 1964, 3.
10. H. K. Baker and P. Morgan, "Building a Professional Image: Using 'Feeling-Level' Communication," *Supervisory Management*, Jan. 1986, 20–25.
11. J. R. Gibb, "Defensive Communication," *Journal of Nursing Administration*, Apr. 1982, 14–17.
12. D. E. Shields, "Listening: A Small Investment, A Big Payoff," *Supervisory Management*, July 1984, 18–22.
13. N. Stewart, "Listen to the Right People," *Nation's Business*, Jan. 1963, 60–63.
14. Shields, op. cit.
15. N. B. Sigband, "Listen to What You Can't Hear?," *Nation's Business*, June 1969, 70–72.
16. W. D. St. John, "You Are What You Communicate," *Personnel Journal*, Oct. 1985, 40–43; D. Caruth, "Words: A Supervisor's Guide to Communication," *Management Solutions*, June 1986, 34–35.
17. R. Wilkinson, "Communication: Listening from the Market," *Nursing Management*, Apr. 1986, 42J, 42L.
18. R. Dulik, "Making Personal Letters Personal," *Supervisory Management*, May 1984, 37–40.
19. C. I. Barnard, *The Functions of the Executive* (Cambridge, MA: Harvard University Press, 1938), 226.

20. P. A. Strassman and S. Zuboff, "Conversation with Paul A. Strassman," *Organizational Dynamics,* Fall 1985, 19–34; A. J. Rutigliano, "Naisbitt & Aburdene On 'Re-Inventing' the Workplace," *Management Review,* Oct. 1985, 33–35.
21. Ibid.
22. Ibid.

FOR FURTHER REFERENCE

Auger, B.Y. "How to Run an Effective Meeting," *Commerce,* October, 1967.

Finsher, S., "Rework, Revise, Rewrite," *Business,* Jul.-Sept. 1985, 54–55.

Gelfand, L. I., "Communicate through Your Supervisors," *Harvard Business Review,* Nov.-Dec. 1970, 101–104.

Guncheon, J., "To Make People Listen," *Nation's Business,* Oct. 1967, 96–102.

"Is Anybody Listening?," *Fortune,* Sept. 1950, 77ff.

Joblin, F. M., "Formal Structural Characteristics of Organizations and Superior-Subordinate Communication," *Human Communication Research,* Summer 1982, 338–347.

Levenstein, A., "Feedback Improves Performance," *Nursing Management,* Feb. 1984, 64, 66.

———, "Back to Feedback," *Nursing Management,* Oct. 1984, 60–61.

Lynch, E. M., "So You're Going to Run a Meeting," *Personnel Journal,* Jan. 1966, 22ff.

Nathan, E. D., "The Art of Asking Questions," *Personnel,* July-Aug. 1966, 63–71.

O'Sullivan, P. S., "Detecting Communication Problems," *Nursing Management,* Nov. 1985, 27–30. Research report.

Tingey, S., "Six Requirements for a Successful Company Publication," *Personnel Journal,* Nov. 1967, 638–642.

Zelko, H. P., "How to Be a Better Speaker," *Notes & Quotes,* No. 311, Apr. 1965, 3.

Nursing Management Information Systems

RICHARD J. SWANSBURG, BSN, MS, RN

Health Systems Coordinator
University of South Alabama Medical Center,
Mobile, Alabama

INTRODUCTION

Communication is important in a health care institution because many departments are involved in patient care. Hospitals spend $7 to $10 billion a year on communication.[1] Because hospitals are only one part of the health care industry, the total price for communication in the industry could be in the vicinity of $25 billion.

Nursing services and nurse managers have entered the information age, an age that is here to stay. Already the computer is absolutely essential to the management of:

1. An increasingly complex financial environment
2. Reporting requirements of numerous agencies
3. Communication needs of a diverse health care team
4. Knowledge related to all areas of patient care[2]

Computers are affecting practice, administration, education, and research, and their impact will continue to spread. The information age is the biggest social and technological change in recent history, and it will continue to shape how people live and work for decades. This chapter gives a brief overview of computers, focusing on aspects that relate to nursing management.

HISTORICAL PERSPECTIVE

The electronic computer was introduced about fifty years ago. The first computers of the 1940s and 1950s were bulky machines that used vacuum tubes for calculation and control. In the late 1950s the transistor replaced the vacuum tube, making computers smaller, more reliable, and more efficient.

A big break came in the early 1960s with the introduction of integrated circuits. The first integrated circuits combined hundreds of transistors on a single silicon chip as small as a fingertip. Then in the 1970s large-scale integrated circuits containing thousands or tens of thousands of transistors were introduced. These large-scale integrated circuits started the microcomputer revolution.

Hospitals were slow to catch on to the computer revolution. In a 1962 survey only 39 hospitals reported using computer services. By 1974 this figure had grown to almost 6,000 hospitals using some type of computer services.[3] Today almost every hospital uses computer resources, at least for financial management.

Nursing has been even slower to experience the benefits of computerization. Early attempts at nursing computerization in the late 1960s and 1970s included:

1. Automation of nurses' notes to describe the patient's status and care.[4]
2. Storage of census and nursing staff figures to analyze for future staffing trends.[5]

In the middle 1970s, the idea of hospital information systems (HISs) caught on and nursing began to experience the benefits of management information systems. Finally the 1980s brought extremely powerful microcomputers and specialized software for nursing known as nursing management information systems (NMISs).

THE STATE OF THE ART IN NMIS

"State of the art" is a phrase commonly used by salesmen and consultants. It means that something is as advanced as is technologically possible. More often than not, what is state of the art today is old technology tomorrow.

HARDWARE

Computers are the hardware of NMISs. These devices accept numbers or alphabetical characters, otherwise known as data, process these data in some way, and then record the processed data. Data that have been processed or manipulated are called information. Information can be viewed on a screen and/or printed. See Figure 18–1. Information is stored temporarily in the computer's memory. For permanent storage it is put on magnetic tapes or disks. The computer is like a factory with a work area, storage area, tool crib, and administration.[6]

The stored information is the database, which is used as a source for decision making by nurse managers. The data are processed by the computer at the request of users. Computers organize and communicate data quickly. Because nurse managers will facilitate the use of NMISs, they need knowledge and skills in computer use. With computers involved in more than 75 percent of all jobs, nurse managers need to take the initiative in making computer applications to nursing.[7]

Hardware is extremely diverse. Large mainframe computers are being used as system controllers. They run the hospital information systems and may be connected to, or interfaced with, smaller minicomputers and microcomputers. Minicomputers run the smaller departmental subsystems such as central supply, laboratory, and pharmacy. For example, if a hospital has over 300 beds, a mainframe computer may not be able to handle its total information needs. Only the information useful to all areas of the hospital will be located on the mainframe, such as admissions, medical records, business office records, and order management applications. These applications are basic to all HISs. Areas such as central supply, pharmacy, nursing, and the laboratory have complex additional needs not shared by all other areas of the hospital. Therefore applications in these areas may run on their own dedicated computer, with information that needs to be shared passing from one computer to another via an interface.

In smaller hospitals the entire system may be run by a mainframe or, in some situations, by a minicomputer. For example, in hospitals with 100 to 300 beds a mainframe computer is capable of handling all the information needs of all areas. In a hospital of 100 beds or less a minicomputer may be all that is needed. The two factors determining the size of computer needed are:

1. The amount of information that needs to be managed and stored.
2. The number of users that will be working with the computer.

The more people that use the system and the more information that needs to be managed, then the larger the computer needs to be.

Microcomputers are capable of running departmental subsystems by themselves. Currently there are systems on the market for pharmacy,

NS	Total Type				Total C/NC	Total Census	Avg Acuity	Hrs Per Pat Day	Wkld Indx	Hrs Per Wkld Indx	Required Staffing	Reg Staff 7–3	Reg Staff 3–11
	1	2	3	4									
BURN	00	00	02	03	05 01	06	4.0	13.0	20.0	3.2	8.5	2.9	2.8
CCU	00	00	04	02	06 01	07	3.3	10.3	20.0	3.1	8.2	2.8	2.7
CRU	00	00	02	01	03 01	04	3.3	10.3	10.0	3.1	4.1	1.4	1.4
ICN1	00	00	07	05	12 01	13	3.5	11.1	42.5	3.1	17.5	6.0	5.8
ICN2	00	00	09	00	09 00	09	2.5	7.0	22.5	2.8	8.4	2.9	2.8
L&D	00	00	00	00	00 04	04	.0	.0	.0	.0	.0	.0	.0
MICU	00	00	00	05	05 00	05	5.0	17.0	25.0	3.4	11.3	3.8	3.7
MINU	00	00	00	00	00 02	02	.0	.0	.0	.0	.0	.0	.0
NBN	00	00	00	00	00 23	23	.0	.0	.0	.0	.0	.0	.0
NTIC	00	00	00	03	03 00	03	5.0	17.0	15.0	3.4	6.8	2.3	2.2
PICU	00	00	00	00	00 00	00	.0	.0	.0	.0	.0	.0	.0
PN	00	00	13	00	13 00	13	2.5	7.0	32.5	2.8	12.1	4.8	3.6
SICU	00	00	00	04	04 00	04	5.0	17.0	20.0	3.4	9.0	3.1	3.0
SINU	00	00	03	00	03 00	03	2.5	7.0	7.5	2.8	2.8	1.0	.9
3	02	00	00	00	02 21	23	.5	1.0	1.0	2.0	.2	.1	.1
4	00	00	00	00	00 19	19	.0	.0	.0	.0	.0	.0	.0
5N	00	03	10	00	13 02	15	2.1	6.0	28.0	2.8	10.4	4.7	3.1
5S	05	03	12	00	20 02	22	1.7	4.9	35.5	2.7	12.7	5.7	3.8
6	00	00	00	00	00 26	26	.0	.0	.0	.0	.0	.0	.0
7	00	08	24	00	32 01	33	2.1	6.0	68.0	2.8	25.3	12.7	8.9
8N	00	00	00	00	00 12	12	.0	.0	.0	.0	.0	.0	.0
8S	00	00	00	00	00 10	10	.0	.0	.0	.0	.0	.0	.0
9N	00	02	13	00	15 02	17	2.3	6.4	34.5	2.8	12.8	5.1	4.5
9S	01	06	07	00	14 02	16	1.7	4.8	24.0	2.8	8.9	3.6	3.1

SOURCE: University of South Alabama Medical Center, Mobile, Alabama. Reprinted with permission.

Figure 18–1 • *University of South Alabama Medical Center Patient Classification Summary*

(Continued)

Nursing Station MICU

PROBE CONTINUE FOR STAFFING

Number of Patients Classified as Type 1 = 00
Number of Patients Classified as Type 2 = 00
Number of Patients Classified as Type 3 = 00
Number of Patients Classified as Type 4 = 00

Total Number of Patients Classified   = 05
Total Number of Patients Not Classified = 00

Total Number of Patients   = 05

SNC1CSUM	CONTINUE	RE-INQUIRE	MASTER
NURSING STATION STAFFING SUMMARY	06/05/89		2450

Nursing Station MICU

Average Acuity	= 5.0	Required Staffing (7–3)	= 3.8
Hours per Patient Day	= 17.0	Required Staffing (3–11)	= 3.7
Workload Index	= 25.0	Required Staffing (11–7)	= 3.7
Hours per Workload Index	= 3.4	Required Staffing (24 hrs)	= 11.3

Actual Staffing:	RN	LPN	NA	NU FTE	WC	TOT FTE
11–7	00.0	00.0	00.0	00.0	00.0	00.0
7–3	00.0	00.0	00.0	00.0	00.0	00.0
3–11	00.0	00.0	00.0	00.0	00.0	00.0
24 Hours	00.0	00.0	00.0	00.0	00.0	00.0

	PAGE BWD	RE-INQUIRE CENSUS	MASTER
SNI1CSTF			

Figure 18–1 (Continued)

nursing, radiology, medical records, and central supply that run on microcomputers. These microcomputer subsystems are intended to meet special departmental needs and to provide a degree of independence from the mainframe HIS. Often some information must be shared between these systems. Today much attention is being focused on this information sharing and the micro-to-mainframe link. Actually, microcomputers are still predominantly used to do word processing, spread-sheets, and file/database management. Even so, microcomputers are fast becoming the machines of choice for running nursing management information systems.

Personal computers or microcomputers are the computers of the 1990s and beyond. These computers are extremely powerful and are becoming more so every year. Today some microcomputers are capable of doing the same work as minicomputers and smaller mainframe computers. The only thing holding them back is the lack of adequate operating system software.

Microcomputers can run software applications for personal productivity, and they can interface to the NMIS and to the HIS. For approximately two to three times the price of a single mainframe terminal, a nurse manager can have a microcomputer with a hundred times the capability and functionality.

SOFTWARE

There are many areas in which microcomputers are better suited than mainframes to assist nursing functions. Such applications include scheduling, report writing, unit budget planning, unit policy and procedure documentation, research, unit-specific personnel records, continuing and in-service education records, programmed instruction, and clinical support.[8]

Although more are appearing, there are still relatively few specialized nursing application programs for microcomputers. Most nursing applications are incorporated into NMISs.

Nurse managers should not let the lack of a specialized program prevent them from reaping the benefits of a microcomputer, especially if they have easy access to one. There are many general-purpose software programs available that can meet nursing needs,[9] such as word processing programs, spreadsheet programs, file/database management programs, and graphics programs.

Spreadsheets

A spreadsheet is a tool used to record and manipulate numbers. Originally spreadsheets were paper ledgers used for business accounting such as the recording of debits and credits. With the coming of the microcomputer revolution, electronic spreadsheets were developed.

An electronic spreadsheet is a software package that turns a microcomputer into a highly sophisticated calculator. Huge quantities of numbers can be recorded, manipulated, and stored quite simply and easily. Nurse managers could use spreadsheets to maintain statistics, create graphics, plan budgets, and evaluate quality assurance. See Figures 18–2 through 18–5 for examples.

A spreadsheet is made up of columns and rows of memory cells. These cells can be variable in size to allow for small or very large numbers. Besides numbers, cells can store text and formulas. Text is used in a spreadsheet to allow for titles, column and row headers, comments, and instructions. Formulas are used to perform the actual mathematical manipulation of memory cells and their numbers, such as addition, subtraction, multiplication, and division.

Formulas really make a spreadsheet a powerful number-crunching tool. For example, a formula can be inserted in the last cell of a column to add all the numbers in that column and display the total (see Figure 18–6). The formula could just as easily have added the cells, divided that number by the number of cells in the column, and given an average. Formulas can also be inserted to subtract one cell from another or multiply one cell by another.

Spreadsheets also have functions for copying, moving, inserting, and deleting cells. One of the most important spreadsheet functions is graphing, which allows numbers to be displayed in the form of a line graph, a bar graph, or a pie graph (see Figure 18–7).

Although electronic spreadsheets are a relatively new tool for nurse managers, they are the best tool to use in situations that require the management of a lot of numbers. For this reason they are particularly pertinent to financial management when they speed up the processes of budgeting, forecasting, developing tables and schedules, and so on.

Middleton recommends teaching employees to use spreadsheets before word processing and database management programs, although word processing is often used more. He suggests the

	Oct	Nov	Dec	Jan	Feb	Mar	Apr	May	Jun	Jul	Aug	Sep
Triage Out	482	428	524	515	510	412	356	353	358	346	301	342
Treated & Released	1862	1761	1637	1599	1553	1853	1766	2043	1962	2064	1868	1983
Admitted	503	510	548	499	523	584	514	540	482	566	549	546
DOA	8	10	3	10	7	8	2	0	4	4	2	2
ED DEATH	8	8	10	6	7	2	7	12	9	8	7	6
OB	360	362	338	342	269	300	303	329	351	358	425	381
Total	3223	3079	3060	2971	2869	3159	2948	3277	3166	3346	3152	3260
Year to Date:	3223	6302	9362	12333	15202	18361	21309	24586	27752	31098	34250	37510
TO%	14.96	13.90	17.12	17.33	17.79	13.04	12.08	10.77	11.31	10.34	9.55	10.49
TR%	57.77	57.19	53.50	53.82	54.13	58.66	59.91	62.34	61.97	61.69	59.26	60.83
A%	15.51	16.56	17.91	16.90	18.23	18.49	17.44	16.48	15.22	16.92	17.42	16.75
DOA%	0.25	0.32	0.10	0.34	0.24	0.25	0.07	0.00	0.13	0.12	0.06	0.06
DEATH%	0.25	0.26	0.33	0.20	0.24	0.06	0.24	0.37	0.28	0.24	0.22	0.18
OB%	11.17	11.76	11.05	11.51	9.38	9.50	10.28	10.04	11.09	10.70	13.48	11.69
	Oct	Nov	Dec	Jan	Feb	Mar	Apr	May	Jun	Jul	Aug	Sep
Triage Out	300	346	365	435	409	328	312	276	223	237	279	255
Treated & Released	2098	1840	1887	2016	1972	1957	2205	2318	2218	2392	2397	2125
Admitted	551	547	612	706	607	589	577	562	592	576	558	613
DOA	4	4	5	8	0	1	2	1	3	3	3	4
ED DEATH	13	13	13	13	12	8	10	16	12	15	15	8
OB	370	353	423	388	364	318	340	382	376	396	393	419
Total	3336	3103	3305	3566	3364	3201	3446	3555	3424	3619	3645	3424

SOURCE: University of South Alabama Medical Center, Mobile, Alabama. Reprinted with permission.

Figure 18–2 • *Report of Emergency Department Statistics*

	Oct	Nov	Dec	Jan	Feb	Mar	Apr	May	Jun	Jul	Aug	Sep
Year to Date:	3336	6439	9744	13310	16674	19875	23321	26876	30300	33919	37564	40988
TO%	8.99	11.15	11.04	12.20	12.16	10.25	9.05	7.76	6.51	6.55	7.65	7.45
TR%	62.89	59.30	57.10	56.53	58.62	61.14	63.99	65.20	64.78	66.10	65.76	62.06
A%	16.52	17.63	18.52	19.80	18.04	18.40	16.74	15.81	17.29	15.92	15.31	17.90
DOA%	0.12	0.13	0.15	0.22	0.00	0.03	0.06	0.03	0.09	0.08	0.08	0.12
DEATH%	0.39	0.42	0.39	0.36	0.36	0.25	0.29	0.45	0.35	0.41	0.41	0.23
OB%	11.09	11.38	12.80	10.88	10.82	9.93	9.87	10.75	10.98	10.94	10.78	12.24

	Oct	Nov	Dec	Jan	Feb	Mar	Apr	May	Jun	Jul	Aug	Sep
Triage Out	161	152	128	223	220	211	160	242	229	0	0	0
Treated & Released	2390	2182	2252	2238	2287	2444	2378	2497	2512	0	0	0
Admitted	662	570	551	559	567	626	580	577	600	0	0	0
DOA	1	5	2	4	6	2	7	5	2	0	0	0
ED DEATH	11	9	17	14	15	16	10	14	16	0	0	0
OB	331	374	331	377	316	313	248	293	326	0	0	0
Total	3556	3292	3291	3415	3411	3612	3383	3628	3685	0	0	0

	Oct	Nov	Dec	Jan	Feb	Mar	Apr	May	Jun	Jul	Aug	Sep
Year to Date:	3556	6848	10129	13544	16955	20567	23950	27578	31263	0	0	0
TO%	4.53	4.62	3.90	6.53	6.45	5.84	4.73	6.67	6.21	0	0	0
TR%	67.21	66.28	68.64	65.53	67.05	67.66	70.29	68.83	68.17	0	0	0
A%	18.62	17.31	16.79	16.37	16.62	17.33	17.14	15.90	16.28	0	0	0
DOA%	0.03	0.15	0.06	0.12	0.18	0.06	0.21	0.14	0.05	0	0	0
DEATH%	0.31	0.27	0.52	0.42	0.44	0.44	0.30	0.39	0.43	0	0	0
OB%	3.31	11.36	10.09	11.04	9.26	8.67	7.33	3.08	3.35	0	0	0

Figure 18–2 • *(Continued)*

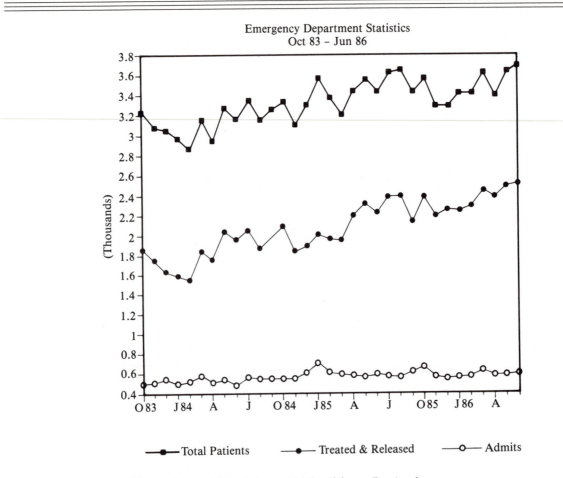

Emergency Department Statistics
Oct 83 – Jun 86

──■── Total Patients   ──●── Treated & Released   ──○── Admits

SOURCE: University of South Alabama Medical Center, Mobile, Alabama. Reprinted with permission.

Figure 18–3 • *Computer-Generated Graphic Display*

following tips for learning spreadsheet software use:

1. Use the package immediately.
2. Apply it to something practical such as mortgage payments or personal budgets.
3. Take a course even if it is self-training.
4. Find the learning method best liked: manual, audiocassette, interactive video.
5. Decide whether to take the course or do self-study.
6. Set a schedule and keep it.
7. Share the results with a friend or colleague.
8. Keep up to date and include reviews.
9. Avoid plateaus.
10. Enjoy it![10]

Word Processing

Word processing is the manipulation of words and special characters to produce a printed document. Examples are memorandums, letters, policies/procedures, forms, labels, instruction sheets, manuals, signs, books, and others. See Figures 18–8 through 18–11 for examples.

A word processing program is a specialized software package that allows a computer and a printer to do word processing. In a sense, a word processing program makes a computer and a printer act like a super deluxe typewriter. Some advantages of word processing are:

1. A document can be displayed on a computer screen exactly as it will look when printed.

Patient Name _____   Date of Audit _____

Account # _____   Audit Firm _____

Surgical Record
_____   Auditor _____

Admission Date ____/____/____

Discharge Date ____/____/____

Department	Amount Billed	Undocumented		Unbilled		Adjusted	
		Amount	Percent	Amount	Percent	Amount	Percent
Anesthesia							
Blood Bank							
Burn Center							
Cath Lab							
Central Supply							
Circulation Tech							
Dialysis							
EEG							
EKG							
Emergency Department							
Enterostomal Therapy							
Fiber Optic Lab							
GI Lab							
Guest Charges							
L & D Charges							
Laboratory							
Operating Room							
Orthopedics							
Pharmacy							
Physical Therapy							
Pulmonary Function							
Radiology							
Radiology—US/NM/MAM							

SOURCE: University of South Alabama Medical Center, Mobile, Alabama. Reprinted with permission.

Figure 18–4 • *University of South Alabama Medical Center Report of Patient Account Audit*

Department	Amount Billed	Undocumented		Unbilled		Adjusted	
		Amount	Percent	Amount	Percent	Amount	Percent
Recovery Room							
Respiratory Therapy							
Room Charges							
Transport							
Vascular Lab							
Total							

Comments _____

_____

Figure 18–4 (Continued)

Total Number of Records Audited — 17
AUDIT FIRM AUDITS — 8
PATIENT AUDITS — 9
NUMBER OF INCORRECT BILLS — 17

Department	Amount Billed	Undocumented		Unbilled		Adjusted	
		Amount	Percent	Amount	Percent	Amount	Percent
Anesthesia	$4,957.00	$299.75	6.05%	$72.25	1.46%	($227.50)	−4.59%
Blood Bank	$4,733.50	$0.00	0.00%	$0.00	0.00%	$0.00	0.00%
Burn Center	$0.00	$0.00	0.00%	$0.00	0.00%	$0.00	0.00%
Cath Lab	$0.00	$0.00	0.00%	$0.00	0.00%	$0.00	0.00%
Central Supply	$25,737.25	$652.50	2.54%	$500.25	1.94%	($152.25)	−0.59%
Circulation Tech	$1,021.62	$0.00	0.00%	$0.00	0.00%	$0.00	0.00%
Dialysis	$0.00	$0.00	0.00%	$0.00	0.00%	$0.00	0.00%
EEG	$833.75	$0.00	0.00%	$0.00	0.00%	$0.00	0.00%
EKG	$286.00	$0.00	0.00%	$31.25	10.93%	$31.25	10.93%
Emergency Department	$1,705.25	$390.50	22.90%	$0.00	0.00%	($390.50)	−22.90%
Enterostomal Therapy	$0.00	$0.00	0.00%	$0.00	0.00%	$0.00	0.00%
Fiber Optic Lab	$0.00	$0.00	0.00%	$0.00	0.00%	$0.00	0.00%
GI Lab	$0.00	$0.00	0.00%	$0.00	0.00%	$0.00	0.00%
Guest Charges	$15.00	$0.00	0.00%	$0.00	0.00%	$0.00	0.00%
L & D Charges	$1,497.18	$0.00	0.00%	$0.00	0.00%	$0.00	0.00%

SOURCE: University of South Alabama Medical Center, Mobile, Alabma. Reprinted with permission.

Figure 18–5 • *University of South Alabama Medical Center Audit Summary Report, June*

(Continued)

Department	Amount Billed	Undocumented		Unbilled		Adjusted	
		Amount	Percent	Amount	Percent	Amount	Percent
Laboratory	$19,200.50	$46.75	0.24%	$169.25	0.88%	$122.50	0.64%
Operating Room	$10,580.63	$148.50	1.40%	$0.00	0.00%	($148.50)	−1.40%
Orthopedics	$0.00	$0.00	0.00%	$0.00	0.00%	$0.00	0.00%
Pharmacy	$27,058.73	$4,782.78	17.68%	$7,322.60	27.06%	$2,539.82	9.39%
Physical Therapy	$2,451.95	$261.25	10.65%	$117.50	4.79%	($143.75)	−5.86%
Pulmonary Function	$13,955.75	$0.00	0.00%	$110.50	0.79%	$110.50	0.79%
Radiology	$12,920.50	$295.00	2.28%	$57.25	0.44%	($237.75)	−1.84%
Radiology—US/NM/MAM	$373.75	$0.00	0.00%	$0.00	0.00%	$0.00	0.00%
Recovery Room	$1,302.50	$415.00	31.86%	$0.00	0.00%	($415.00)	−31.86%
Repiratory Therapy	$39,046.25	$1,764.00	4.52%	$2,152.75	5.51%	$388.75	1.00%
Room Charges	$55,470.75	$140.00	0.25%	$115.75	0.21%	($24.25)	−0.04%
Transport	$218.95	$0.00	0.00%	$0.00	0.00%	$0.00	0.00%
Vascular Lab	$0.00	$0.00	0.00%	$0.00	0.00%	$0.00	0.00%
	$41.75	$0.00	0.00%	$0.00	0.00%	$0.00	0.00%
Total	$223,408.56	$9,196.03	4.12%	$10,649.35	4.77%	$1,453.32	0.65%
Total—Ancillary Only	$167,937.81	$9,056.03	5.39%	$10,533.60	6.27%	$1,477.57	0.88%

Figure 18–5 (Continued)

ED Admits
Jan to Jun

Jan	559
Feb	567
Mar	626
Apr	580
May	577
Jun	600
Total	3509

ED Admits
Jan to Jun

Jan	559
Feb	567
Mar	626
Apr	580
May	577
Jun	600
Total	3509
Average	585

SOURCE: University of South Alabama Medical Center, Mobile, Alabama. Reprinted with permission.

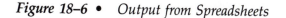

Figure 18–6 • *Output from Spreadsheets*

2. A document can be modified or changed very quickly and easily without having to redo it.
3. A document can be printed numerous times with the same material in different formats.
4. Special graphics can be used to enhance or highlight the content of a document.
5. Multiple documents (up to 350 typed pages) can be stored as compressed electronic files with a removable and transportable magnetic disk as small as $3\frac{1}{2}$ inches square by 2 millimeters deep. See Figure 18–12 as an example of an electronic file listing.

Some word processing programs have facilities for multiple document profiles. The document's profile establishes:

1. Line spacing, such as single, double, or triple
2. Character pitch, such as pica, elite, or compressed (number of characters per inch)
3. Font or type style such as script, italics, or standard
4. Number of lines per inch, such as 6 or 8 lines per inch
5. Margins and tabs
6. Page headers or footers
7. Footnote or outline formats
8. Printer types, such as letter quality or graphics
9. Paper size and type
10. Different keyboard types

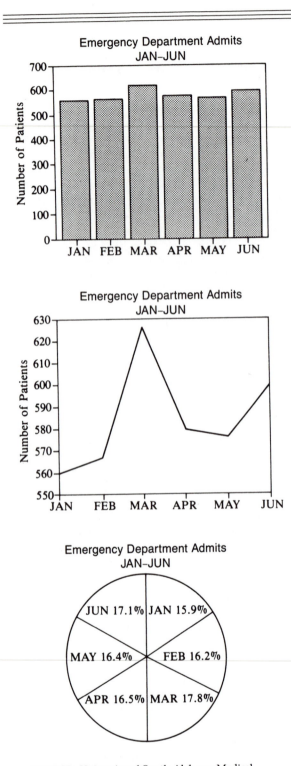

Emergency Department Admits
JAN–JUN

Emergency Department Admits
JAN–JUN

Emergency Department Admits
JAN–JUN

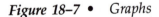

SOURCE: University of South Alabama Medical Center, Mobile, Alabama. Reprinted with permission.

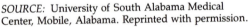

Figure 18–7 • *Graphs*

May 7

TO: Assistant Administrator, Finance

FROM: Health Systems Coordinator
           Data Processing

SUBJECT: HIS Orientation and Training for New
           Employees

I would like to recommend that all new hospital employees, who are issued an ID to use the HIS, be required to attend an orientation class in use of the computer and the HIS. An ID would not be issued until the employee had attended this class and had been instructed in areas of HIS security, user signon, information confidentiality, terminal operation, and HIS overview. Also, I would like for you to consider additional training which is departmental specific. Objectives for this training would be developed jointly between the department heads and myself. Records of all employee training should also be maintained.

RJS:djm

SOURCE: University of South Alabama Medical Center, Mobile, Alabama. Reprinted with permission.

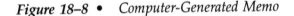

Figure 18–8 • *Computer-Generated Memo*

Different profiles can be set up and used when different documents are to be produced.

Most word processing programs have utilities for checking spelling within a document. These utilities usually contain a standard dictionary to which the text in a document can be compared. Often words can be added to the dictionary. When the dictionary is called, words that are misspelled can be highlighted for correction. If the word is not recognized, then a list of words that are similar can be generated and the user can choose the correct word.

Utilities for performing block functions are also standard in most word processing programs. It is easy to insert, move, copy, or delete words, sentences, paragraphs, or pages of text within a document. Simple insertion or deletion of characters can be accomplished with a few keystrokes. A particular word or sentence can be searched for and found anywhere within a document by a simple request.

A document can be paginated after it is completely typed. This function can justify the text within set margins; hyphenate words that are too long for a line; establish a set number of lines per

University of South Alabama Medical Center
Personal Computer Inventory Form

Date: _____

Department: _____ Contact: _____ Phone: _____

Location: _____ Use: _____

PC Model: _____ SN: _____ Date Purchased: _____

System Board Memory: _____ Expanded Memory: _____ Total Memory: _____

System Board Slots: _____ Slots Used: _____ Slots Available: _____

Display Type: _____ SN: _____ Date Purchased: _____

Keyboard Type: _____

Floppy Disk Drives:

Type	Disk Size	Memory Capacity	Drive Height
_____	_____	_____	_____
_____	_____	_____	_____
_____	_____	_____	_____

Hard Disk Drives:

Type	Memory Capacity	Drive Height
_____	_____	_____
_____	_____	_____

Tape Backup: _____ Expansion Unit: _____

Expansion Unit Board Slots: _____ Slots Used: _____ Slots Available: _____

Attached Printers:

Type	Model	Graphics	Letter Quality
_____	_____	_____	_____
_____	_____	_____	_____

Add-On Circuit Boards:

	Type	Use	SN	Date Purchased	Main/ Expansion Unit	Slot
1.	_____	_____	_____	_____	_____	___
2.	_____	_____	_____	_____	_____	___

SOURCE: University of South Alabama Medical Center, Mobile, Alabama. Reprinted with permission.

Figure 18–9 • *Computer-Generated Form*

(Continued)

3. _____ _____ _____ _____ _____ _____

4. _____ _____ _____ _____ _____ _____

5. _____ _____ _____ _____ _____ _____

6. _____ _____ _____ _____ _____ _____

7. _____ _____ _____ _____ _____ _____

8. _____ _____ _____ _____ _____ _____

Additional Accessories:

Type	Use	SN	Date Purchased	Main/Expansion Unit	Slot
1. _____	_____	_____	_____	_____	_____
2. _____	_____	_____	_____	_____	_____
3. _____	_____	_____	_____	_____	_____

Comments: _____

_____

_____

Figure 18–9 (Continued)

page; and establish page numbers for the document's pages.

Shell documents can be created where the main content of a document never changes, but some areas are reserved for text that will change each time the document is printed. The best examples of this are memorandums and letters, when the same memo or letter goes to many different people. The document and the list of variable information can actually be created separately and then merged at printing time.

In a division such as nursing where there are many different typing tasks, changing to a word processing program could greatly improve document-handling efficiency.

File/Database Management

Electronic files and databases are the computer counterparts to the standard file cabinet and its contents. They store data and are manipulated for information much like paper files. Nurse managers could use a computer and a database software package instead of a manual filing system to handle many of their information and record-keeping needs. Examples might include personnel records, education records, and equipment inventory.

A microcomputer database program allows for databases to be created by defining their record layouts and data fields. When a data field is defined, its maximum length is set and the type of data that can be stored in it established. Data types can be character (allowing letters, numbers, and special symbols), numeric (allowing only numbers), logical (allowing only yes or no; true or false), or date (allowing only numbers in a date format). See Figure 18–13 for an example of data fields and Figure 18–14 for an example of actual data entry.

Once a database is created, procedures can be established to:

1. Add information
2. Update information
3. Display information
4. Delete information
5. Generate printed reports

A menu can also be created to allow easy access to and execution of the procedures; see Figure 18–15 for an example. Most database tools have ap-

Edward, Pat	7344	Data Entry	7982
Jean	7345	Terry, Clint	7983
Richard, Rose	7679	Jim	7984
Darlene	7979	Susan	7985
Sangeeta	7980	Lisa	7986
Gloria	7981		

SOURCE: University of South Alabama Medical Center, Mobile, Alabama. Reprinted with permission.

Figure 18–10 • *Computer-Generated Form Labels*

plication generators that will lead the user through a series of steps to define a database and its procedures and menus.

The greatest advantage to electronic database management is the ease in maintaining information and the timely retrieval of this information in report format as illustrated in Figure 18–16.

Today some software companies have actually integrated all three types of programs into one package. This allows a person the ability to perform word processing, number crunching, and database management all with the same information. Once a person begins using one of these programs, that person will begin to develop ideas for other ways to use the program. The big problems a person faces are getting started and ensuring that a particular company's software will accomplish the work and function on the microcomputer available.

USING NMISs

Nursing management information systems (NMISs) are software packages developed specifically for nursing services divisions. These software packages have multiple programs or modules that can perform various nursing management functions. Most NMISs have modules to do patient classification, staffing, scheduling, personnel records, and report generation. Other modules may be included such as budget development, resource allocation and cost control, diagnostic-related group (DRG) analysis, quality control monitoring, staff development records, modeling and simulation for decision making, strategic planning, short-term demands forecasting and work planning, and program evaluation.

NMIS modules for patient classification, staff-

Scheduling of Personal Computer and Training Room *NOTE:* The PC and the training room will be scheduled in the same manner, using the wall calendar to the right of this memo. If the training room is scheduled for a particular day and time, then that means the PC will be unavailable during that period.

Guidelines

1. To schedule yourself for use of the PC, write the time, PC, and your name or department in the top-most available slot for the day desired on the calendar (i.e., 8:00 A.M.–9:00 A.M., PC, Richard Swansburg). To schedule the training room, confirm availability of the room with the Health Systems Department, and indicate that it is reserved by writing the time, ROOM, and your name or department where desired (i.e., 8:00 A.M.–5:00 P.M., ROOM, Data Processing).

2. Schedule use of the room or PC at least a day ahead of time, but try not to schedule more than a week in advance.

3. Limit your PC sessions to 2 hours. If the PC is available, then this time limit may be extended.

4. Do not schedule the PC for more than 5 working days in a row. This may be negotiated according to need.

5. Please notify the Information Center of cancellation of reserved time at least 30 minutes prior to that time. If you are 15 minutes late for your reserved time and someone else wishes to use the PC, then your time will be forfeited.

SOURCE: University of South Alabama Medical Center, Mobile, Alabama. Reprinted with permission.

Figure 18–11 • *Computer-Generated Procedure*

ing, scheduling, personnel records, and report generation are often closely interrelated. Patients are classified according to established acuity criteria. The patient classification information is entered into the staffing module, and needed staffing is then calculated according to various workload formulas. Also, actual staffing is entered and a comparison of census, patient acuity, needed staffing, and actual staffing can be made. Schedules are then prepared using the information from the staffing and personnel records modules.

```
The IBM Personal Computer DOS
Version 3.20 (C) Copyright International Business Machines Corp 1981, 1986
              (C) Copyright Microsoft Corp 1981, 1986


DisplayWrite 3 DOS Command Task
Type EXIT to Return to Task Selection
<D> Type Command: dir/w

  Volume in drive D has no label
  Director of D: \

CHARGES    TXT    SCHEDULE   TXT    CAUSES    TXT    PPSEX      TXT    HIST    TXT
PROGRESS   TXT    FORM       TXT    PTCLSCH   TXT    RESPONSE   TXT    DAY1    TXT
RESPDAYS   TXT    TERMMOVE   TXT    STUSCH    TXT    STUSCHSH   TXT    ROUNDS  TXT
MISCLST    TXT    RECOMEND   TXT    ORIENT    TXT    RJS        UPR
          19 File(s)        483328 bytes free


DisplayWrite 3 DOS Command Task
Type EXIT to Return to Task Selection
<D> Type Command:
```

SOURCE: University of South Alabama Medical Center, Mobile, Alabama. Reprinted with permission.

Figure 18–12 • *List of Documents Stored as Compressed Electronic Files*

DRG analysis and quality control monitoring are done to associate patient acuity, quality of care, and DRG. This is helpful for establishing future guidelines and care needs for patients according to their DRGs. Budget development is also supported by the census, patient acuity, and needed staffing patterns. This information is invaluable to support requests for additional full-time or part-time help. Finally, the report generation module allows all of the stored information to be retrieved and generated in a timely and presentable manner.

Clinical Uses

NMISs and computers can make patient care more effective and economical. Clinical nurses use them for patient care management. Clinical components include patient history, nursing care plans, direct and remote physiological monitoring, physician's order entry and results reporting, nursing progress notes and charting, and discharge planning. This can all be done in the nurses' station or, with the most advanced systems, from individual rooms.

Clinical nurses can use the NMIS to replace manual systems of data recording. This may reduce costs while permitting improved quality of care as well as quality of work life. Those who work in remote locations have access to the clinical components of NMIS to increase effectiveness and quality of care. All clinical nurses can collect and input clinical data and use the computer to analyze it to formulate treatment plans. They can use quantitative decision analysis to support clinical judgments. Automated consultation can be applied to screen for adverse drug reactions, interactions, and preparation of correct dosages. Computers can be programmed to reject orders that could cause problems in these and other areas, thus preventing medication errors.[11]

Curtin reminds nurses to provide "high touch" in this inhuman "high-tech" world. Technology, computers, and information systems provide the knowledge to save lives or prolong them. Nurses can return control over their lives to patients and families who have lost freedom of action or become unable to understand. Nurses can keep control of cybernetics through the exercise of human compassion.[12]

"High tech" includes the new scientific knowledge of microelectronics, computers, information,

Num	Field Name	Type	Width	Dec
1	NAME	Character	24	
2	STR_ADDR	Character	24	
3	CITY	Character	14	
4	STATE	Character	2	
5	ZIP_CODE	Numeric	9	0
6	PHONE	Numeric	10	0
7	SEX	Character	1	
8	EMP_TYPE	Character	5	
9	LICENSED	Character	1	
10	LICENSE_NO	Character	14	
11	LIC_REN_NO	Character	14	
12	LIC_DATE	Date	6	
13	EXP_DATE	Date	6	
14	LIA_INS	Character	1	
15	INS_AMOUNT	Numeric	8	0
16	PRIM_AREA	Character	24	
17	UNIT_ASSG	Character	24	
18	PRIM_SHIFT	Character	5	

MODIFY STRUCTURE: >A:\NUPER   Field: 1/18
Enter the field name.
Field names begin with a letter and may contain letters, digits, and underscores.

SOURCE: University of South Alabama Medical Center, Mobile, Alabama. Reprinted with permission.

Figure 18–13 • Data Fields and Types

sensors, processors, displays, and education. It has as object the solution of society's total problems, not just those of health care, including nursing.[13]

The Patient Care Profile

Hinson and others describe the use of a total clinical nursing system that includes one computerized form for treatment, Kardex, nursing care plan, and nursing notes, as illustrated in Figures 18–17 and 18–18.

The PCP can be updated by the nurse and/or the unit secretary. It becomes a part of the patient's medical record. Clinical nurses can use it to individualize patient care while nurse managers use it as a source of nursing cost data. It is practical and efficient.

The PCP system includes:

1. A Patient Care Profile: activities of daily living, identification data, active orders, treatments, nursing goals, nursing interventions, and nursing notes.

2. Use of nursing diagnoses.

3. Provision of space for handwritten nursing notes.

4. Provision for each nurse to have PCPs of assigned patients on a clipboard.

5. A copy of the PCP for nursing assistant assignments to provide information and make notes and reports.

6. Updating with each shift when a new PCP is printed.

7. A Master Reference Care Plan file from which to select "inappropriate defining characteristics, nursing diagnosis, discharge goals, day-to-day goals, and interventions."

8. A Team Leader worksheet listing patients, diagnoses, and active orders.

9. Patient classifications and staffing requirements.

10. Costing out of nursing care per patient.

11. Completed orders on demand.

In the development of this PCP a vendor was to develop a software package for the HIS. A task force worked with the vendor to develop the care

Num	Field Name	Entry
1	NAME	Swansburg, Richard
2	STR_ADDR	31 Country Lane
3	CITY	Mobile
4	STATE	AL
5	ZIP_CODE	36608
6	PHONE	2053432361
7	SEX	M
8	EMP_TYPE	RN
9	LICENSED	Y
10	LICENSE_NO.	02861
11	LIC_REN_NO	1-35855
12	LIC_DATE	123188
13	EXP_DATE	123190
14	LIA_INS	Y
15	INS_AMOUNT	1000000
16	PRIM_AREA	Medicine
17	UNIT_ASSG	MICU
18	PRIM_SHFT	7-3

EDIT: >A:\NUPER   Rec: 1/18

SOURCE: University of South Alabama Medical
Center, Mobile, Alabama. Reprinted with permission.

Figure 18–14 •   *Data Entry*

Nursing Personnel   **10:21:31 PM**
Master Menu

1. Add Nursing Personnel Record
2. Update Nursing Personnel Record
3. Display Nursing Personnel Record
4. Delete Nursing Personnel Record
5. Report Generation Menu
6. Exit

Key selection number and press enter: 6

SOURCE: University of South Alabama Medical
Center, Mobile, Alabama. Reprinted with permission.

Figure 18–15 •   *Menu of Procedures*

nurses. The number of forms was reduced. It required top management commitment.[14]

Almost all NMISs have been developed by various management, accounting, and software firms to operate on microcomputers or PCs. These developers sell the hardware, software, documentation, training, and maintenance for their NMISs. Prices will vary according to the hardware bought, how complex and extensive the software is, whether on-site training is wanted, and how much continued support is desired. Nurse administrators can expect a complete system to cost $50,000 to $250,000.

program which was pilot tested. Training of the staff included tutoring.

This system resulted in better documentation and information. It promoted accountability of

Registered Nurses
with Licenses Expiring December

Name	License No.	Unit	Shift
Abbott, Patricia M.	1-42345	5S	11–7
Daniels, Mark J.	1-55476	ED	3–11
Meyers, Mary Beth	1-23111	NBN	7–3
Munroe, Jane H.	1-65432	6	7–3
Parker, Harold T.	1-34567	SICU	11–7
Swansburg, Richard J.	1-35855	MICU	11–7
Zieman, Margaret A.	1-43298	3	3–11

Total: 7

SOURCE: University of South Alabama Medical Center, Mobile, Alabama. Reprinted with permission.

Figure 18–16 •   *A Computer-Generated Report*

PATIENT CARE PROFILE

| PIEDMONT HOSPITAL | 5/16/84 | 11:45AM | PAGE 1 | SHIFT: 1 |

ACTIVITIES OF DAILY LIVING
VITAL SIGNS   RT
OOB   W/ASSIST MJ
BATH   W/ASSIST MJ
FLUIDS   FORCE
TRANSPORT BY W/C MJ

ALL   REGULAR
CRANBERRY JUICE AT BEDSIDE
NPO AFTER MIDNIGHT

PRC: HARD OF HEARING

ACTIVE ORDERS
CBC W DIFF (PLATEL 5/16 7:30AM JD
SMA 18 BIOCHEM PRO 5/16 7:30AM JD
PYELOGRAM INTRAVEN 5/16 AM JD
1:MAY HAVE LIQUIDS ON THE DAY OF EXAM
   UNLESS UPPER G.I. SERIES, GALLBLADDER
   SERIES OR SONOGRAM IS ORDERED

TREATMENTS
1:ANESTHESIA TO SEE PT.
2:SHAVE AND PREP:MID NIPPLE TO MID
   BACK AND FROM MID AXILLA TO HIP ON
   RIGHT SIDE
3:PRE OP ON CALL.   DATE:5/17
4:STRAIN ALL URINE. D/E/N: MJ
5:INTAKE & OUTPUT Q SHIFT. D/E/N: MJ

TRN–09   000187023   2555555   TRN
   TESTPAT JACK   SEX:M
   ADM: 5/15/84   SRV:URO   SMK:N
   DOB:10/06/21   62   COND:G   LEVEL:1
   HT :5/11   F/I   WT:180/000   P/O
   10000 INTERNIST OTHER
   ALG:PENICILLIN
   DX :NEPHROLITHIASIS

NURSING GOALS
GL :PT. WILL RECEIVE PRE-OP TEACHING AS
      PER PROTOCOL
GL :PT. WILL UNDERSTAND WHAT TO EXPECT
      PRE-OP AND IMMEDIATELY POST-OP

NURSING INTERVENTIONS
1:REVIEW INFORMATION IN PRE-OP BOOKLET
   W PT. INCLUDING PRE-OP PROGRAMS ON
   CHANNEL 13. JD
2:REVIEW EXERCISES & EXPECTED
   LIMITATIONS POST-OP WITH PT. (TCDB,
   LOG ROLL, ETC)
3:EXPLAIN WHAT PT. SHOULD EXPECT PRE-OP
   (PREPS, MEDS, DRESSING, ETC) JD
4:REVIEW SEQUENCE OF EVENTS ON DAY OF
   SURGERY (PRE-OP MEDS, STRETCHER TO
   OR, TIME IN RR, RETURN TO ROOM)

DATE: NURSING NOTES   SIGNATURE

8am Clear yellow urine. No evidence of stones or ® flank pain. Pt. prepared
     for IVP this a.m. Dr. Jones visited ————
                                        Jane Doe RN

10³⁰/A Returned from x-ray. Demerol 100mg. IM RUD for ® flank pain. Sally Smith RN

11³⁰/am Pain subsided. Pt. verbalized understanding of information in pre-op
     booklet and able to give return demonstration of TCDB ——— Jane Doe RN

1³⁰/pm Urine remains clear yellow. No evidence of stones or ® flank pain— Jane Doe RN

| INT | SIGNATURE | INT | SIGNATURE | INT | SIGNATURE |
| JD | Jane Doe RN | MJ | Mary Jones NA | SS | Sally Smith RN |

SOURCE: I. Hinson, N. Silva and P. Clapp, "An Automated Kardex and Care Plan,"
Nursing Management, July 1984, p. 36. Reprinted with permission.

Figure 18–17 •   Patient Care Profile

Piedmont Hospital	5/16/89 11:41 A.M.	Page 1

TRN-09   000187023   2555555   TRN
TESTPAT JACK   SEX: M
ADM: 5/15/89   SRV: URO   SMK:N
DOB: 10/06/21   62   COND: G   LEVEL:1
HT : 5/11   F/1   WT : 180/000P/0
10000 Internist other
ALG: Penicillin
DX : Nephrolithiasis

Knowledge Deficit Pre-op
Comfort Alteration Physical
Urinary Elimination Alt Incontinence

Discharge goal	:Pt. verbalizes understanding of significant S&S to report to MD after discharge	Active
Discharge goal	:Pt. verbalizes understanding of type pain to report to MD after discharge	Active
Goal	:Pt. will receive pre-op teaching as per protocol	Active
Goal	:Pt. will understand what to expect pre-op and immediately post-op	Active
Goal	:Pt. will have increased physical comfort	Active
Intervention	1:Review information in pre-op booklet w pt. including pre-op programs on Channel 13.	5/16/84 JD
Intervention	2:Review exercises & expected limitations post-op with pt. (TCDB, log roll, etc.)	Active
Intervention	3:Explain what pt. should expect pre-op (preps, meds, dressing, etc.)	5/16/84 JD
Intervention	4:Review sequence of events on day of surgery (pre-op meds, stretcher to OR, time in RR, return to room)	Active
Intervention	5:Explain what to expect immediately post-op (IV, tubes, dressings, etc.)	Active
Intervention	6:Change dressing PRN	
Intervention	7:Teach pt. to request pain med before pain becomes acute	5/16/84 SS
Intervention	8:Encourage rest (quiet room, limit visitors)	Active
Intervention	9:Change position gradually D/E/N: ____	
Intervention	10:Assist pt. to dangle D/E: ____	
Intervention	11:Assist pt. to ambulate progressively D/E/: ____	
Intervention	12:Teach pt. S&S to report to doctor after D/C (cloudy urine, itching, burning, etc.)	Active

SOURCE: I. Hinson, N. Silva, C. P. Clapp, "An Automated Kardex and Care Plan," *Nursing Management*, July 1984, p. 40. Reprinted with permission.

Figure 18–18 • *Patient Care Plan*

HOSPITAL INFORMATION SYSTEMS

Hospital information systems (HISs) are large, complex computer systems designed to help communicate and manage the information needs of a hospital. An HIS will have applications for admissions, medical records, accounting, business office, nursing, laboratory, radiology, pharmacy, central supply, nutrition/dietary services, personnel, and payroll. Numerous other applications can exist for any department and for practically any purpose. See Figures 18–19A through 18–19E.

Admissions applications include patient scheduling, preadmissions, admissions, discharges,

```
Jun 2                        Univ. of So. Alabama Med Ctr—NINplus              1:42 PM
ID: PMED010A/881118            A. Demographic Information          User ID:      JYE
```

```
Name:                                                    Employee ID:
Home Unit: PICU    Job Title: WC                             Status: Full Time


_____ ADDRESS _____

  1550 Main St

                                                _____ GENERAL _____
  City: Mobile              St: AL 36617-        Telephone : (   )   -
                                                Soc. Sec.:     -   -
_____ TRAVEL INFO _____     Birth Date:   /  /
                                                Maiden:
  Drivers License Number:                       Special Sort Code: 1863
  Drivers License Status:
  Distance From Hospital:  0.0 Miles
  Travel Time to Hospital:  0 Hrs   0 Mins
  Means of Transportation:


  Comments: WC POSITION
```

```
CMNDS: A(dd C(hg R(em B(rowse F(ind N(xt P(rv <F1> = Help S(el Q(uit M(ore [   ]
Record Status: AVAILABLE
```

Figure 18–19A • *Personnel Management System: Demographic Information*

transfers, and census procedures. Some medical records applications include master patient index maintenance, DRG/diagnosis/procedure coding, physician incompletion of medical records, and medical record locator procedures. Business and accounting procedures include patient insurance verification, billing, billing follow-up, billing inquiry, accounts payable, accounts receivable, and cash processing.

Nursing applications are many. Some applications include order entry, results reporting, nursing care plans, patient classification, staffing, scheduling, nurse's notes, discharge planning, and patient assessments.[15] Other applications include nursing histories, medication profiles, nursing education, nursing research, patient education, quality monitoring, and nursing worksheets or checklists.[16] Still other nursing applications exist.

Applications in other areas such as the laboratory, radiology, pharmacy, and central supply may be so voluminous and complex that they have their own subsystems. These subsystems can stand alone and run independently of the HIS but are usually interfaced to the HIS for information transfer.

Hospital information systems are developed specifically for large mainframe computers and minicomputers. Often several computers are networked together to handle the information needs of large hospitals.

Selection, development, and installation of an HIS can easily take 2 to 5 years. The initial cost can be millions of dollars for the hardware and software. Continued yearly maintenance is required and can cost hundreds of thousands or even millions of dollars.

JOBS AND THE FUTURE

Nurse managers need to be computer literate, which includes being familiar with commonly used

```
Jun 2                        Univ. of So. Alabama Med Ctr—NINplus                    1:43 PM
   ID: PMED010A/881118                 B.  Job Information              User ID:      JYE
```

```
┌─────────────────────────────────────────────────────────────────────────────┐
│                                                                               │
│   Name:                                              Employee ID:             │
│   Home Unit: PICU    Job Title: WC                       Status: Full Time    │
│                                                                               │
│ _____ JOB INFO _____        _____ TERMINATION INFO _____│
│                                                                               │
│   Job Title: WC                               Term. Date:   /  /              │
│   Job—Grade                                   Reason:                          │
│   Hours per Week: 0.0    Status: Full Time    Len. of Service    Yr    Mo      │
│   Hire Date: 11/19/64    Pay Status: FT-Perm  Rehire Consideration:            │
│                          Time on Job: 24 Yr 7 Mo                               │
│                                                                               │
│ ═══════════════════════════ TRANSFER HISTORY ═══════════════════════════════ │
│      No          From           To         Date          Reason               │
│                                                                               │
│                                                                               │
│                                                                               │
│                                                                               │
│                                                                               │
└─────────────────────────────────────────────────────────────────────────────┘
```

```
CMNDS: A(dd C(hg R(em B(rowse F(ind N(xt P(rv <F1> = Help S(el Q(uit M(ore [   ]
Record Status: AVAILABLE
```

Figure 18–19B • *Personnel Management System: Job Information*

computer terms. See Figure 18–20. All nurses need to know how to interact with a computer; typing will become a necessary technical skill. Computer literacy is beginning to be included in nursing school curriculums.

This means that teaching jobs will change and new positions will open for instructors with computer backgrounds. This will also be true in the work environment. Special positions are already opening in hospitals. Nurses are considered the personnel of choice to fill computer user liaison positions.

These liaison personnel are often referred to as user coordinators. User coordinators promote and improve communication between the data processing or information systems department and the other hospital departments. They assist and provide input into the systems analysis and design of new computer applications. They help with computer information and training. Finally, they are an invaluable resource for helping the end user with computer-related problems.

In the future one can expect that all nursing jobs will be affected by the computer, and many more new positions will be developed for nurses in the computer area.

Among the jobs generated by computer and information technologies are training, education, technical support, coaching, information analyst, macro design, fourth generation language programmer, librarian, product specialist, using computer manager, and systems development auditing.[17] It has even been suggested that computers will lead to an electronic cottage industry.[18]

With entry into the information age nurse managers should do career planning for themselves and their clinical nurses. New careers in NMIS may be one of the answers to nurse burnout.

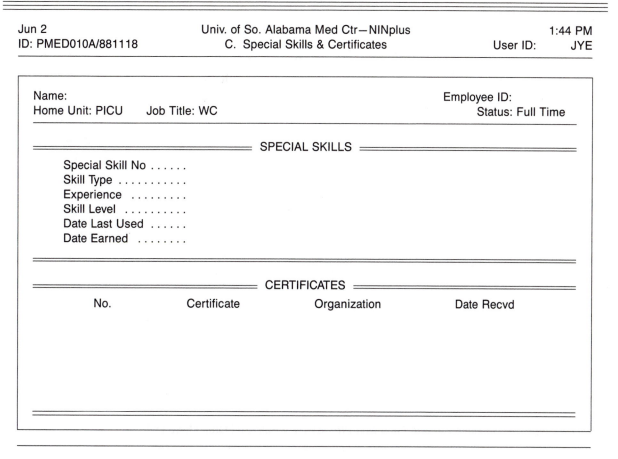

| Jun 2 | Univ. of So. Alabama Med Ctr—NINplus | 1:44 PM |
| ID: PMED010A/881118 | C. Special Skills & Certificates | User ID: JYE |

Name: Employee ID:
Home Unit: PICU   Job Title: WC   Status: Full Time

═══════════════════════ SPECIAL SKILLS ═══════════════════════

Special Skill No . . . . . .
Skill Type . . . .
Experience . . . .
Skill Level . . . .
Date Last Used . . . . . .
Date Earned . . . .

═══════════════════════ CERTIFICATES ═══════════════════════

No.   Certificate   Organization   Date Recvd

CMNDS: A(dd C(hg R(em B(rowse F(ind N(xt P(rv <F1> = Help S(el Q(uit M(ore [   ]
Record Status: AVAILABLE

Figure 18–19C • Personnel Management System: Special Skills and Certificates

TRENDS FOR THE FUTURE

There is little doubt that computers will continue to grow smaller with yet greater capacities. In all likelihood microcomputers will replace minicomputers and maybe even mainframes. Other areas in which we can expect change include robotics, voice communication, optical disks, and expert systems and artificial intelligence.

Robotics

Robots will assist nurses in performing numerous tasks. The most practical use of robotics is in electronic carts, which are used to store and transport drugs, linens, and other supplies. These carts can be remote-controlled and can actually follow predefined routes along the floor. Another example is robotic arms which can be used to do heavy lifting. Possible future applications include procedures humans are unable to perform such as delicate microscopic eye, brain, or spinal surgeries; or procedures for which direct contact is contraindicated due to health hazards, such as a patient with no immune system or exposure to toxic chemicals or radioactive elements.

Voice Communication and Optical Disks

Voice communication will allow nurses to talk to their computers. Keyboards and bar code readers will not be needed to enter or retrieve information.

```
Jun 2                          Univ. of So. Alabama Med Ctr—NINplus              1:45 PM
ID: PMED010A/881118              D.  Recruitment/LOA Information         User ID:    JYE
```

```
Name:                                                    Employee ID:
Home Unit: PICU    Job Title: WC                            Status: Full Time


_____ EDUCATION IN PROGRESS _____     ____ PREVIOUS EMPLOYER ____
                                                 Employer No.:

    School:                                      Previous Job:
    Address:                                     Prev. Employer:
    Course:                                      City:
    Degree Program:                              State:
    Expected Finish:   /  /                      Time On Prev. Job.:  Yrs.   Mnths


================ LEAVE OF ABSENCE ================
        No              LOA Type          LOA Start          LOA Return
```

CMNDS: A(dd C(hg R(em B(rowse F(ind N(xt P(rv <F1> = Help S(el Q(uit M(ore [   ]
Record Status: AVAILABLE

Figure 18–19D • *Personnel Management System:*
Recruitment/LOA Information

The computer will be requested to retrieve information or to record it by voice command. Optical disks will revolutionize information storage with their ability to store many times the information in the same space. Microcomputers today use removable floppy diskettes for limited information storage and nonremovable hard disks for volume information storage. New optical laser disks will be removable and the same size as floppy diskettes, but will store up to fifty times as much information as a hard disk.

Conversant computers are widely used in industry. They tell airline baggage handlers which conveyor to put bags on and bank customers their account balances. Conversant computers can identify product deficiencies during manufacturing. They can maintain supply inventories, recording the voice print and processing a spoken reply. They are used to move cameras on spacecraft and to turn on lights and roll up windows of cars. With use of conversant computers, productivity on assembly lines has increased by 25 to 40 percent. Complete

units are available at a cost of about $40,000. Such machines are about 85 percent accurate at present.

Speaker-dependent machines use voice prints so they must be programmed with the user's voice. Speaker-independent machines can understand any speaker. All IBM PCs and Apple Macintoshes have standard built-in speakers but little software is available. Users have not responded well to computer-synthesized voices.[19]

Software today has become much more user friendly. Almost all software today has help screens and is menu driven. This means users only have to elect what they want to do from a list of items on the screen, and if a problem is encountered help is only a keystroke away. Some computer languages today are almost like English. What used to take weeks and months to program can now be done in days or weeks. Users are becoming more involved in designing applications on mainframes and handling most things themselves on microcomputers.

Continued or expanded user involvement is a

```
Jun 2                    Univ. of So. Alabama Med Ctr—NINplus              1:46 PM
ID: PMED010A/881118         E.  Continuing Ed.—Optional        User ID:     JYE
```

```
 Name:                                              Employee ID:
 Home Unit: PICU    Job Title: WC                     Status: Full Time

 ════════════════════════ OPTIONAL CONTIN. ED. ════════════════════════
       Program Rec. No  ....
       Program Name  ......
       Internal Program  ...?
       Start Date  .........
       End Date  ...........
       Involvement  ........
       Sponsor ............
       CEUs/Cont. Hrs ......
       Hospital Cost  ...... $
       Employee Cost  ..... $
```

```
CMNDS: A(dd C(hg R(em B(rowse F(ind N(xt P(rv <F1> = Help S(el Q(uit M(ore [   ]
Record Status: AVAILABLE
```

SOURCE: University of South Alabama Medical Center, Mobile, Alabama. Reprinted with permission. System by MDAX.

Figure 18–19E • Personnel Management System: Continuing Ed.—Optional

trend of the future. This will occur as users become more knowledgeable about computer hardware and software. Software will continue to become easier for users to manipulate, and software vendors will provide greater support. The best examples are already evident in laboratory, pharmacy, central supply, and nursing management systems, where very little help is involved from data processing personnel.

Expert Systems and Artificial Intelligence

Other future trends in software are expert systems and artificial intelligence. Expert systems are possible today. Nurse managers have access to a huge quantity of information that is capable of assisting them in making everyday decisions. With expert systems the nurse manager identifies the management situation, the criteria defining the problem,

and objectives for handling the situation. The expert system evaluates the information and provides a listing of alternative ways to manage the situation. The nurse manager then evaluates the alternatives and makes decisions.

Expert systems encode the relevant knowledge and experience of experts to make it available to less knowledgeable and experienced persons. An example would be to take the total knowledge and experience of clinical nurse specialists in neuroscience nursing, encode it in a computer program, and make it available to clinical nurses working in the neuroscience area. They would consult it to solve nursing care problems.

Expert systems encode specialized knowledge including rules and product descriptions to solve difficult problems by supporting human reasoning. They use symbolic reasoning and perform above the level of competence of nonexpert humans. They use heuristic techniques rather than al-

ABEND: abnormal end of task.

Algorithm: a prescribed set of rules for the solution of a problem in a finite number of steps.

Artificial Intelligence: the capability of a machine that can proceed or perform functions that are normally concerned with human intelligence such as learning, adapting, reasoning, self-correction, automatic improvement.

Bar Code Reader: an optical scanning unit that can read documents encoded in a special bar code. A laser scanner.

Batch Processing: a system approach to processing where similar input items are grouped for processing during the same machine run.

Binary: (1) the number system based on the number 2; and (2) pertaining to a choice or condition where there are two possibilities.

Bit: the smallest unit of data, a binary digit of 0 or 1.

Buffer: intermediate storage, used in input/output operations to hold information temporarily.

Bug: a mistake or error in a computer program.

Byte: a set of eight adjoining bits thought of as a unit.

Central Processing Unit (CPU): the part of the computer that contains the circuits that calculate and perform logic decisions based on a set of instructions.

Compact Disk: a type of disk storage that uses magnetic optical recording and lasers.

CRT (Cathode Ray Tube): cathode ray terminal. The typewriter keyboard or input station.

Data: representation of information in a form suitable for processing.

Database: an electronic storage structure similar to a file.

Disk Storage: a storage device that uses magnetic recording on flat rotating disks.

DOS: disk operating system.

Downtime: the elapsed time when a computer is not operating, may be scheduled for maintenance or unscheduled because of machine or program problems.

Expert Systems: systems that rely on large amounts of information to provide assistance in decision making.

Field: a unit of information within a record.

File: an electronic storage structure for related records.

Forecasting: describing the possible future, anticipating the impact of present decisions or actions on future activities of nursing. Forecasting uses simple techniques such as graphs and hand calculators, and complicated mathematical models that can be developed using desk top computer software packages.

Hard Copy: printed computer output: reports, listings, documents.

Hardware: the physical computer equipment.

Hospital Information System (HIS): a system designed to facilitate the day-to-day needs of a hospital; a system that stores and manipulates information for interhospital communication and decision support.

Input/Output (I/O): the transfer of data between an external source and internal storage.

Interface: the point at which independent systems or computers interact.

Keyfield: a field within a record that makes that record unique with respect to other records in a file.

Kilobyte: 1,024 bytes of characters.

Laser Scanner: a type of device that uses a laser to recognize and receive input.

Mainframe Computer: a large computer capable of being used and interacted with by hundreds of users seemingly simultaneously.

Management Information System (MIS): a system designed to manipulate information to assist in management decision making.

Microcomputer: a small desktop computer built around a microprocessor.

Minicomputer: a medium-size computer smaller than a mainframe but larger than a microcomputer.

Modeling: development of mathematical equations that can be used to fit and balance relationships between or among variables. Forecasting uses models. Managers decide which variables to include and the form of

SOURCE: Reprinted from *The Nurse Manager's Guide to Financial Management* by R. C. Swansburg, P. W. Swansburg, and R. J. Swansburg, pp. 330–332, with permission of Aspen Publishers, Inc., © 1988.

Figure 18–20 • Glossary of Commonly Used Computer Terms

(Continued)

models. In management there are budget models, inventory models, production process models, cash-flow models, models for work-force planning, models of distribution systems, linear programming resource allocation models, and many others.

Modem: a device that converts computer signals into signals for transmission over a telephone line, or vice versa.

Number Crunching: a process of taking huge quantities of numbers and performing mathematical functions on them.

Nursing Management Information System (NMIS): a type of information system geared toward assisting nurse managers in performing their management functions.

On-Line Processing: a form of input processing where information is input and updated at that time.

Operating System: an organized collection of techniques and procedures combined into programs that direct a computer's operation.

Optical Disk: same as a compact disk.

Printer: a terminal that produces hard copy or printed output.

Program: a set of computer instructions directing the computer to perform some operation.

Random Access: a storage technique whereby a record can be addressed and accessed directly at its location in the file.

Record: a group of related fields of information treated as a unit.

Robotics: machines that work automatically and perform physical movements.

Scenario Projection: use of a scenario or set of planning assumptions to describe and plan for the possible future state of the environment at a point in time and considering the economic, political, social, technological, and natural effects. Scenario projections use trends and trend analysis.

Sequential Access: a storage technique

whereby a record can only be addressed and accessed after all those before it have been.

Simulation Forecasting: risk analysis, a procedure that mimics possible or probable business conditions to describe the possible future of each. Simulations stress model structure.

Software: a program or set of programs written to tell the computer hardware how to do something.

Spreadsheet: a specialized type of software for manipulation of numbers.

Table: a collection of data in a form suitable for ready reference.

Trend: systematic pattern of change (increase or decrease) over time based on history or a particular theory. *Example:* an increase in the acuity level of patients over a 1-year period.

Trend Impact Analysis: analysis of the impact or consequences of the pattern of change (increase or decrease) over time. *Example:* How will the increased acuity level of patients over a 1-year period affect operational costs, use of resources, cash flow, etc?

Trend Line: a straight line fitted to a graph plotting trends in a time series. It shows the pattern of change (increase or decrease) over time.

Trends Extrapolation Forecasting: describing the possible future by projecting the systematic pattern of change (increase or decrease) using the prevailing tendencies of a time series.

User Friendly (software): easier to use because of menus and help facilities.

Voice Communication: interaction with a computer by voice recognition.

Word Processing: the manipulation of words within documents by a computer.

Word Processing Program: a specialized type of software for manipulation of printed material.

Figure 18–20 (*Continued*)

gorithms to provide good answers, but they do not always reach the optimum ones. Heuristic programs use rules of thumb to search through alternative solutions to problems.[20]

Expert systems are software products combining sophisticated representational and computing techniques with expert knowledge. Eventually they will support nursing decision making. Although they are not widely used, their use will increase as regional computer systems are established with extensive nursing and medical databases to link clinical nurse specialists.

SUMMARY

This chapter provides an overview of nursing and computers. The computer is a necessary information-handling tool, and most people feel the impact of it on their daily lives. In fact, the computer is now a necessity to manage the complex financial structure of today's health care.

Large mainframe computers are used to support and run highly complex hospital information systems. These HISs have tremendous capabilities for manipulation and storage of information. Almost any nursing application can be implemented through an HIS. With the introduction of the microcomputer, nursing management information systems have developed. These MISs assist nursing in doing patient classification, analyzing staffing needs and trends, billing patients for nursing care, and developing the nursing budget.

Other general-purpose microcomputer software is also available to assist nursing in doing word processing, number crunching, and record keeping.

Financial areas where nurses need to be particularly adept are in budgeting, tracking of charges and supplies, and patient classification. The budget is the prime tool for managing nursing revenue and expenses. Keeping up with charges and supplies can be simplified with computers; this is often a neglected area where much revenue is lost. Classification of patients is the way in which nurse staffing needs and patterns are determined.

In the future more and more will be accomplished through computers. All nurses will have to be able to interact with these machines. Nursing schools are already incorporating the use of the computer into the nursing curriculum. New positions are being developed for nurses in computer education and support.

The computer has come of age. These machines are tools that already assist nurse managers in performing numerous tasks. They are excellent for the management of all types of information.

EXPERIENTIAL EXERCISES

1. Compile a list of the general functions for which nursing personnel currently use a computer in the nursing management environment of a unit in which you are a student.

   1.1 Assess whether these functions are performed as part of personal, departmental, or organizational responsibilities.

   1.2 List the different computers used to perform different responsibilities?

2. Determine the dollar amounts that a nursing unit spends on computers and information management for 1 year.

   2.1 What percentage of the budgets do these amounts represent?

3. Do any regulations, guidelines, or laws require computerized information management in your current place of work?

   3.1 What are they?

   3.2 What organizations administer them?

   3.3 How do they apply?

4. Does the organization have an organizational information system?

   4.1 What applications are common to the entire organization?

   4.2 What applications are unique to the nursing department?

   4.3 What applications are unique to the unit to which you are assigned?

   4.4 What departments have their own computer information systems?

5. Identify instances in which microcomputers are used to manage specialized functions in a health care organization.

6. Identify instances where laser scanners are used to manage information.

7. Identify applications for which you feel you could use a microcomputer to manage personal information.

8. Identify applications of a spreadsheet that would be useful to you.

9. Create a document such as a memorandum or letter and print it.

   9.1 Revise the document and change the margins, line spacing, type style, and character pitch. Print it again.

10. Create a return address label for your mailings. Print it multiple times.

11. Identify whether the word processing program you use has a spelling function.

11.1 Does it have a supplement for storing words that are not in the dictionary?

11.2 Identify different aspects of the spell function.

12. What is meant by a block function?

12.1 What is the smallest workable block? What is the largest?

12.2 List the different block functions you can perform.

13. What type of searching tasks can you perform?

14. Identify a number of manual paper files that you feel could be converted to the computer and a database management package.

15. Identify and list computerized applications that clinical nurses may use for patient care management.

16. What two quality benefits may the clinical nurse receive from using these computerized applications?

17. Explain how the clinical nurse can use the computer to assist in performing analyses and making decisions.

18. Assess and list the possible components of a patient care profile (nursing care system or patient care system).

18.1 Discuss the purpose of each component.

18.2 Assess and list the benefits of a patient care profile.

19. Identify and explain how supplies are requisitioned in your area.

19.1 Are there differences in how patient-chargeable items and departmental-chargeable items are obtained?

19.2 Identify and explain how patient charges are captured in your area.

19.3 What kinds of reports are available to show supplies used and procedures performed?

20. Identify nursing personnel associated with the computer and information environment in your organization.

20.1 What are their job functions? Do any of them perform a liaison function?

NOTES

1. C. R. Carpenter, "Computer Use in Nursing Management," *Journal of Nursing Administration*, Nov. 1983, 17–20.
2. R. D. Zielstorff, "Cost Effectiveness in Computerization in Nursing Practice and Administration," *Journal of Nursing Administration*, Feb. 1985, 22–26.
3. D. E. Gagnon, "Use of Automation in Improving Nursing Efficiency and Operations," *World Hospitals*, Nov. 1983, 23–25.
4. R. F. Stein, "An Exploratory Study in the Development and Use of Automated Nursing Reports," *Nursing Research*, Jan.-Feb. 1969, 14–21.
5. B. Moores and I. Wood, "Nursing Allocation Using a Time-Shared Computer," *Nursing Times*, Aug. 18, 1977, 109–112.
6. E. B. Borner, "What Every Manager Should Know about Computers," *Supervisory Management*, May 1984, 16–23.
7. L. J. McCarthy, "Taking Charge of Computerization," *Nursing Management*, July 1985, 35–36, 38, 40.
8. K. Bellinger and J. Laden, "Nurse Use of General Purpose Microcomputer Software," *Nursing Outlook*, Jan.-Feb. 1985, 22–25.
9. S. A. Finkler, "Microcomputers in Nursing Administration: A Software Overview," *Journal of Nursing Administration*, Apr. 1985, 18–23.
10. B. Middleton, "Getting Up to Speed on Spreadsheet Software," *Supervisory Management*, Apr. 1986, 12–14.
11. H. W. Gottinger, "Computers in Hospital Care: A Qualitative Assessment," *Human Systems Management*, Fall 1984, 324–345.
12. L. Curtin, "Nursing: High Touch in a High-Tech World," *Nursing Management*, July 1984, 7–8.
13. P. McKenzie-Sanders, "The Central Focus of the Information Age," *Business Quarterly*, Winter 1983, 87–91.
14. I. Hinson, N. Silva, and P. Clapp, "An Automated Kardex and Care Plan," *Nursing Management*, July 1984, 35–36, 38–40, 42–43.
15. "What Nurses Think of Computers," *Nursing Life*, May-June 1985, 28–30.
16. R. D. Zielstorff, ed., *Computers in Nursing* (Rockville: Aspen, 1980); G. Clark, "Computers and the Nurse," *Australian Nurses' Journal*, Apr. 1984, 45–47; K. J. Sofaly, "The Nurse and Electronic Data Processing," *Medical Instrumentation*, May-June 1981, 169–170.
17. T. Guimaraes, "Human Resources Needs to Support and Manage User Computing Activities in Large Organizations," *Human Resource Planning*, Feb. 1986, 69–80.

18. McKenzie-Sanders, op. cit.
19. N. Madlin, "Conversant Computers," *Management Review*, Apr. 1986, 59–60.
20. F. L. Luconi, T. W. Malone, and M. S. Scott Morton, "Expert Systems: The Next Challenge for Managers," *Sloan Management Review*, Summer 1986, 3–14.

FOR FURTHER REFERENCE

Adams, R., and Duchene, P., "Computerization of Patient Acuity and Nursing Care Planning," *Journal of Nursing Administration*, Apr. 1985, 11–17.

American Hospital Association, *Strategies: Nursing Management Information Systems* (Chicago: American Hospital Association, 1985), 1–8.

Bagby, P. R., "Orienting Nurses to Computers," *Nursing Management*, July 1985, 30–33.

Chang, B. L., "Adoption of Innovations," *Computers in Nursing*, Nov./Dec. 1984, 229–235.

Charalambides, L. C., "Systematic Organizational Communications," *Human Systems Management*, Apr. 1985, 309–321.

Ernst, C. J., "A Relational Expert System for Nursing Management Control," *Human Systems Management*, Fall 1984, 286–293.

Gilliam, R., "The Use of Computers in Nursing," *International Nursing Review*, Oct. 1968, 308–328.

Graham, N., *The Mind Tool, Computers and Their Impact upon Society*, 4th ed. (St. Paul, MN: West Publishing Company, 1976), 27–28.

Grazman, T. E., "Managing Unit Human Resources: A Microcomputer Model," *Nursing Management*, July 1983, 16, 19–22.

Happ, B., "Should Computers Be Used in the Nursing Care of Patients?," *Nursing Management*, July 1983, 31–34.

Henney, C. R., and Bosworth, R. N., "A Computer-Based System for the Automatic Production of Nursing Workload Data," *Nursing Times*, July 10, 1980, 1212–1217.

Jecmen, C., and Stuerke, N. M., "Computerization Helps Solve Staff Scheduling Problems," *Nursing Economics*, Nov.-Dec. 1983, 209–211.

Jelinek, R. C., Zinn, T. K., and Brya, J. R., "Tell the Computer How Sick the Patients Are and It Will Tell You How Many Nurses They Need," *Modern Hospital*, Dec. 1973, 81–85.

Krampf, S., and Robinson, S., "Managing Nurses' Attitudes toward Computers," *Nursing Management*, July 1984, 29, 32–34.

Marks, F. E., "Computer Graphics for Nursing Managers," *Nursing Management*, July 1984, 19–20, 22–23, 25–26.

Minetti, R. C., "Computerized Nurse Staffing," *Hospitals*, July 16, 1983, 90, 92.

Nyberg, J., and Wolff, N., "DRG Panic," *Journal of Nursing Administration*, Apr. 1984, 17–21.

Quinn, S. J., "Computerizing Services in the Nursing Department," *Nursing Management*, July 1984, 16–18.

Rockart, J. F., and Crescenzi, A. D., "Engaging Top Management in Information Technology," *Sloan Management Review*, Summer 1984, 3–16.

Romano, C. A., "Computer Technology and Emerging Roles," *Computers in Nursing*, May/June 1984, 229–235.

Conflict Management

INTRODUCTION

Any organization in which people interact has a potential for conflict. Health care institutions include many interacting groups: staff with staff, staff with patients, staff with families and visitors, staff with physicians, and so on. These interactions frequently lead to conflicts.

Conflict relates to feelings including feelings of neglect, of being viewed as taken for granted, of being treated like a servant, of not being appreciated, of being ignored, and of being overloaded. It relates to a lack of self-esteem and not being treated as worthy. The individual's feelings build into anger to the point of rage. This results in overt behaviors like brooding, arguing, or fighting. The individual can let feelings and behavior get in the way of work. Productivity declines, sometimes purposefully, and mistakes are made.

CAUSES OF CONFLICT

Defiant Behavior

Defiant behavior can create conflict. It produces guilt feelings in the person to whom it is directed. The nurse manager should take the position that the person expressing defiance is responsible for the conflict. Defiance is a threat to rational dialogue; it violates the acceptable protocols for adult interaction.

The defiant person challenges the authority of the nurse manager through obstinate and intransigent behavior. This behavior may be both verbal or nonverbal.

Murphy describes three versions of the defier. The first of these is the Competitive Bomber who simply refuses to work. Such persons mutter statements that translate into "go to the devil." They scowl and will even walk away from the nurse manager or off the job.[1] Competitive defiers can be aggressive underminers who plan deliberate assaults. They comment about unfair and terrible working conditions, manipulation, and lousy schedules. These behaviors are done to provoke managerial response. If they do elicit a response, they sulk and pout to win the pity of peers or even higher management.

The second defier is the Martyred Accommodator, who uses malicious obedience. They work and cooperate but do so mockingly and contemptuously. They complain and criticize to enlist the support of others.

A third category of defier is the Avoider. These defiers avoid commitment and participation. They do not respond to the nurse manager. When conditions change they avoid participating.[2]

Stress

Conflict leads to stress, fear, anxiety, and disruption in professional relationships. These conditions can, in turn, increase the potential for conflict. Stressors include "having too little responsibility, lack of participation in decision making, lack of managerial support, having to keep up with increasing standards of performance, and coping with rapid technological change."[3] Stress costs in 1973 were estimated at 1 to 3 percent of the gross national product. If anything they have risen since then.

Burnout is a result of stress. Nurse managers burn out from trying to maintain a support system for the care givers. Clinical nurses burn out from trying to give high-quality nursing care.

Confrontation, disagreements, and anger are evidence of stress and of conflict. Stress and conflict are caused by poorly expressed relationships among people, including unfulfilled expectations.

Stress in patients leads to iatrogenic ailments, complications, and delayed recovery. It may be created by depression and anxiety. Stressed staff cannot cope with stressed patients, and this leads to inefficiency, job dissatisfaction, and insensitive care. Ultimately the staff are provoked into conflict. They too can develop iatrogenic ailments, just like their patients. Families of patients can add to stress if they are not managed appropriately. Increased stress for patients and staff decreases effective use of time. Such problems increase patient care costs, as they increase the length of the illness and decrease nursing efficiency and effectiveness. The next time the patients may go somewhere else for care, whether at their own initiative or on the recommendations of physicians, relatives, friends, or acquaintances.[4]

Space

When nurses have to work in crowded spaces they must interact constantly with other staff members, visitors, and physicians. This is particularly true of crowded critical care units. Such conditions cause stress that leads to burnout and turnover.

Physician Authority

Physicians are trained to be in authority over nurses. Today's nurses want to be more independent, to have professional responsibility and accountability for patient care. They spend more time with patients than physicians do and often have valid proposals for altering therapeutic measures. Physicians sometimes ignore their suggestions, indicating they do not want feedback. Nurses become angry as their self-worth diminishes. Communication fails, particularly two-way communication.[5]

Beliefs, Values, and Goals

Incompatible perceptions or activities create conflict. This is particularly evident when nurses hold beliefs, values, and goals different from those of nurse managers, physicians, patients, visitors, families, administrators, and so on. Nurses' values may boil over into conflicts related to ethical issues that include "do not resuscitate" orders, callous statements that belittle human worth, abortion, abuse, AIDS, and other problems. Personal goals frequently conflict with organizational goals, particularly with regard to staffing, scheduling, and the climate within which nurses work.

Nurses who have to violate their personal standards will lash out at the system. This is demeaning to them and causes loss of self-esteem and emotional stress. They must know that they are valued, that their beliefs, values, and personal goals are respected. Like other people, nurses act to protect their personal or public images when confronted or invaded. They respond in terms of other people's expectations of them, as they want approval. They will defend their rights and their professional judgments. The ego is easily bruised and becomes a big problem in conflict. Defense becomes more heated when one or both parties to the conflict are uninformed or manipulated. When nurses are not recognized or respected they feel helpless, and they feel hopeless when they are unable to control the situation.[6]

Other Causes[7]

Change creates conflict that in turn impedes change. People who are not prepared for change will fight it or fail to support it. They are threatened.

Organization climates and leadership style can create conflict if different managers set conflicting rules. Disciplinary problems can result from inadequate orientation and training and poor communication.

Off-the-job problems affect work performance, leading to disciplinary problems and conflict. These include marital discord, drug use, alcoholism, mental stress, and financial problems.

Age can create stress and conflict. As employees age, they resent increased scrutiny of their work. Clinical nurses cannot keep up with physical demands of work as they grow older. They become fearful of being able to compete with younger nurses and build up resentment that can lead to conflict.

Nurse managers are professional managers and directors of clinical nursing practice. They must cope with forces internal and external to the nursing organization. Pressures include cost containment, effectiveness of patient care, collective bargaining, consumer awareness and involvement, regulatory agencies, entry-level qualifications, scope of practice, and mandated continuing education.

Computers are replacing many activities of middle managers in business and industry. Centrally controlled departments are being replaced by ad hoc forces, project teams, and small, autonomous business units. This results in downsizing within the organization, with decentralization and fewer levels of management, thus increasing pressures to increase output without increasing the number of managers. Managers face increased accountability and more demanding performance evaluations. The remaining managers become anxious, insecure, and doubtful about the future, resulting in malaise and conflict. As hospitals implement nursing management information systems this situation can affect nurse managers.

People who have been discriminated against, such as racial minorities, may have "chips on their shoulders" and resent real or imagined slights. They may respond with confrontation, defensiveness, anger, and other conflict-producing behaviors. Persistent racial prejudice and discrimination are also an important source of workplace conflict.

CONFLICT MANAGEMENT

Discipline

In using discipline to manage or prevent conflict, the nurse manager must know and understand the organization's rules and regulations. If they are not clear, the nurse manager should seek help to clarify them. Discipline is the last resort in correcting undesirable employee behavior. Rules and regulations must be reasonable and work related. Rules that are unreasonable or reflect personal biases invite infractions.

The following rules will help in managing discipline:

1. Discipline should be progressive.
2. The punishment should fit the offense, be reasonable, and increase in severity for violation of the *same* rule.
3. Assistance should be offered to resolve on-the-job problems.
4. Tact should be used in administering discipline.
5. The best approach for each employee should be determined. Managers should be consistent and should not show favoritism.
6. The individual should be confronted and not the group. Disciplining a group for a member's violation of rules and regulations makes them angry and defensive, increasing conflict.
7. Discipline should be clear and specific.
8. It should be objective, sticking to facts.
9. It should be firm sticking to the decision.
10. Discipline produces varied reactions. If emotions are running too high, a second meeting should be scheduled.
11. The nurse manager performing the discipline should consult with her supervisor. One should expect to be overruled sometimes. Knowing the boundaries of authority and the supervisor will avoid most overrules.
12. A nurse manager should build respect, trust, and confidence in her ability to handle discipline.[8]

Considering Life Stages

Most organizations will include nurses at all life stages. Conflict can be managed by supporting individual nurses in achieving goals that pertain to their life stage. Three developmental stages are:

1. The young adult stage. This is the stage during which the nurse is establishing a career. People at this stage pursue knowledge, skills, and upward mobility. Conflict may be prevented or managed by facilitating career advancement.
2. Middle age, during which the nurse becomes reconciled with achievement of life's goals. This nurse helps to develop careers of younger nurses.

3. After age 55, adults integrate their own ego ideals with their accomplishments. At this stage the nurse is thinking in terms of completing her work and retiring.[9]

Communication

Communication is an art essential to maintaining a therapeutic environment. It is necessary to accomplishing work and resolving social and emotional issues. Supervisors prevent conflict with effective communication and should make it a way of life. To promote communication that prevents conflict:

1. Teach nursing staff effective communication and their role in it.
2. Provide factual information to everyone—be inclusive, not exclusive.
3. Consider all aspects of a situation—emotions, environmental considerations, verbal and nonverbal messages.
4. Develop basic skills of:
   4.1 Reality orientation, by direct involvement and acceptance of responsibility in resolving conflict.
   4.2 Physical and emotional composure.
   4.3 Having positive expectations that generate positive responses.
   4.4 Active listening.
   4.5 Giving and receiving information.[10]

Active Listening. Active or assertive listening is essential to managing conflict. To be sure the perceptions of nurse managers are correct, they can paraphrase what the angry or defiant employee is saying. Paraphrasing clarifies the message for both. It can help to cool off the situation as it gives the employee time and opportunity to hear the supervisor's perception of the emotions expressed.

Active or assertive listening is sometimes called stress listening. Powell suggests these techniques for stress listening:

1. Do not share anger; it adds to the problem. Remain calm and matter-of-fact.
2. Respond constructively in both verbal and nonverbal language. Be cheerful but sober. Maintain eye contact. Prevent interruptions. Get the problem into the open. Make the employee comfortable. Act serious. Always be courteous and respectful.
3. Ask questions and listen to the answers. Determine the reasons for the anger.

4. Separate fact from opinion, including your own.
5. Do not respond hastily. Plan a response.
6. Consider the employee's perspective first.
7. Help the employee find the solution. Ask questions and listen to responses. Do not be paternalistic.[11]

Solving problems of angry confrontation requires stress listening. The nurse manager guides the process to a joint solution.

Quality Circles

Quality circles have been used to reduce stress by increasing employee motivation. They have been used with participatory management, membership in standing committees, leadership development programs, exercise classes, career ladders, job enrichment, and nursing grand rounds. These programs reduced turnover from 37.6 percent in 1980 to 20 percent in 1982 at one hospital.[12]

Assertiveness Training

Assertive nurses, including managers, will stand up for their rights while recognizing those of others. They are straightforward, being free to be themselves. Assertive nurses know they are responsible only for their own thoughts, feelings, and actions. They can help others deal with their anger and thus prevent conflict. They know their strengths and limitations. Rather than attack or defend assertive nurses, the nurse manager should assess, collaborate, and support, remaining neutral and nonthreatening. They can then accept challenges.

Assertiveness can be taught through staff development programs. In these programs nurses are taught to make learned, thoughtful responses. They learn to accept responsibility rather than blame others. They learn when to say no, even to the boss. They learn to hold people to a standard. When they are dissatisfied they do something to increase their satisfaction. Most of these assertive behaviors can be learned with case studies, role playing, and group discussion.

When they finish their training, assertive nurses will reinforce their expectation that others will do their job by positive comments. Praise and consideration promote wellness and positive individual behavior, which are linked to effective management and communication. Nurse managers learn that direct communication of support to the staff increases their job satisfaction.

Assertive nurses focus on data and issues when offering constructive criticism to the boss or constructive feedback to the staff. This encourages dialogue and produces solutions to problems rather than conflict. They ask for assistance or for delay when it is needed.

People usually respond positively to assertion and negatively to aggression. Some people respond negatively to assertion.[13]

TECHNIQUES OR SKILLS FOR MANAGING CONFLICT

Aims

When involved in managing conflict, the nurse manager must aim for broadening of understanding about problems. Help the parties to see the big picture rather than the limited perspectives of each party. Aim to increase the possible number of alternatives in resolving the conflict. If possible, encourage conflicting parties to voice several possibilities acceptable to each. Then work on a compromise. This stimulates their interaction and involvement, another aim of conflict management. Other aims include better decisions and commitment to decisions that have been made.

Strategies[14]

Avoidance. Avoidance is a strategy that allows conflicting parties to cool down. The nurse manager involved in a conflict can sidestep the issue by saying, "Let's both take time to think about this and set a date for a future talk." This approach allows both parties to cool down and gather information. Avoidance can be used when the issue is not critical or when the potential damage of immediate confrontation outweighs the benefits. In the latter case a third party may have to be involved. Certainly the nurse manager as third party can tell the parties to a conflict: "I want you both to go on with your work while I take time to determine the facts and analyze them." Then set a not-too-distant date for the future meeting.

Accommodation. The nurse manager who is party to a conflict can accommodate the other party by yielding and placing the other's needs first. This is particularly good strategy when the issue is more important to the other person. It maintains cooperation and harmony and develops subordinates by allowing them to make decisions.

Competition. A nurse manager as supervisor can exert position power at a subordinate's expense. This enforces the rule of discipline. It is an assertive position that does not foster commitment to conflict resolution on the part of the subordinate.

Compromise. Taking a middle ground may resolve a conflict. It should be a temporary strategy when time is needed to work out a permanent satisfactory position. A compromise that leaves both parties dissatisfied is not a good one.

Collaboration. When both parties collaborate to resolve conflict, they will both be satisfied. This is especially true of important issues. There should be integration of insights. This takes time and energy. A consensual solution wins full commitment.

Collaboration leads to satisfaction among nurses. Collaboration can be better achieved through managerial factors and organizational factors than through personal factors.[15]

Specific Skills

The following is a list of skills to use in managing conflict. Many are preventive.

1. Establish clear rules or guidelines and make them known to all.
2. Create a supportive climate with a variety of options. This makes people feel comfortable to make suggestions. It energizes them, promoting creative thinking and leading to better solutions. It strengthens relationships.
3. Tell people they are appreciated. Praise and confirmation of worth are important to everyone for job satisfaction.
4. Stress peaceful resolution rather than confrontation. Build a bridge of understanding.
5. Confront when necessary to preserve peace. Do so by educating people about their behavior. Tell them the behavior you perceive, what is wrong with it, and how it needs to be corrected.
6. Play a role that does not create stress or conflict. Do not play an ambiguous and fluctuating role that creates confusion among employees.
7. Judge timing that is best for all. Do not postpone indefinitely.
8. Keep the focus on issues and off personalities.
9. Keep communication two-way. Tune into the message, to correct interpretation, and to the feeling level of the employee. Reassure people

by listening to them unload and dump. What is the real problem?

10. Emphasize shared interests.

11. Separate issues and confront those that are important to both parties.

12. Examine all solutions and accept the one most acceptable to both parties.

13. Avoid overriding your better judgment, becoming defensive, reprimanding the individual, cutting off further expression of feelings, and monopolizing the conversation. These responses increase frustration and are ineffective management techniques.

14. If conflict is evident at decision-making or implementation stages, work to reach an agreement. Commit to a course of action serving some interests of all parties. Seek agreement rather than power.

15. Understand barriers to cooperation or resolution and focus on the dynamics of conflict to resolve it.

16. Distinguish between defiant behavior and normal on-the-job mistakes. Defiance is usually an individual behavior. Determine who the defier is and prepare for the confrontation emotionally and intellectually. Deal with one defiant person at a time. Establish authority and competence. Interview privately; teach, evaluate, resolve, guide, and deal with the defier. Do this immediately and follow-up in 2 days. Discuss behavior and consequences including possible termination, keeping calm and steely. Assume adults have a sense of courtesy and cooperation. When challenged, respond on the spot and stand your ground. Then move to a private area or remove yourself from the scene.

17. Be a sponge to a charge by an angry person.

18. Determine who owns the problem. Take responsibility for it as if you own it and say thanks.

19. Determine needs that are being ignored or frustrated and need recognition and nurturing.

20. Help distinguish demands from dreams.

21. Build trust by listening, clarifying, and allowing the challenges to unwind completely. Give feedback to make sure you understand. Let people know you care and that you trust them. Indicate recognition of other viewpoints and willingness to work to improve the relationship. Be factual. Ask for feedback. Work out a common bridge of "must" items. If a staff nurse or other employee has a valid point, recognize it, apologize if need be, and be genuine.

22. Renegotiate problem-solving procedure to fore-

stall further anger, distrust, and defensiveness.[16]

RESULTS OF CONFLICT MANAGEMENT

If attention is given to the role of the nurse manager in creating a climate for productive work by nurses, many of the causes of conflict will be eliminated. Knowledge of and skill in managing conflict when it occurs is an active role of nurse managers.

Zemke indicates that stress and work pressure in themselves are stimulating. They make managers more positive, more upbeat, and more concerned about their employees. In his survey he found that downsizing motivates good performance, improves output, and eliminates nonproductive jobs that can cause morale problems and conflict. With changes in the reimbursement system for hospitals, nurse managers will be confronted with stress, work pressure, and downsizing.[17]

Conflict can be a positive source of energy and creativity; it can be constructive when properly managed. Otherwise conflict can become dysfunctional and destructive, draining energy and reducing both personal and organizational effectiveness.

Conflict can destroy initiative or creativity and cause hostile and disruptive behavior, loss of team spirit, and loss of the desire to work toward common goals, resulting in deadlocks and stalemates. Managed conflicts do not escalate.[18]

SUMMARY

The interrelationships among nurses and other personnel, patients, and families offer many potentials for conflict. For this reason nurse managers should know how to manage conflict.

Causes of conflict include defiant behavior, stress, crowded space, physician authority, and incompatibility of values and goals.

Conflict can be prevented or managed by discipline, consideration of people's life stages, communication including active listening, use of quality circles, and provision of assertiveness training for nurse managers.

Aims of conflict management include broadening understanding about problems, increasing alternative resolutions, and achieving a workable consensus on decisions and genuine commitment to decisions made. Specific strategies include avoidance, accommodation, competition, compromise, and collaboration. In addition nurse managers can learn and use specific skills to prevent and manage conflict.

Conflict management keeps conflict from escalating, makes work productive, and can make conflict a positive or constructive force.

EXPERIENTIAL EXERCISES

1. For each of the following statements place a + in the blank if the statement is true and a − if it is false.

____ 1.1 A nurse manager is the cause of conflict when an employee defies all suggsetions for patient care, thereby creating arguments with patients and visitors.

____ 1.2 There is potential for conflict when many personnel work in a crowded emergency room.

____ 1.3 A nurse stated she would not care for patients with AIDS. She told other nurses they should not do so either. When assigned to care for an AIDS patient in the postoperative recovery room, she walked off the job. This is an example of the defier who is a Martyred Accommodator.

____ 1.4 A clinical nurse was told by the resident physician that the patient was a "bum" and that treating him was a waste of time and effort. The nurse exploded, berating the physician for his lack of human compassion. She called her supervisor and stated she wanted an apology from the physician for herself and for the patient. The cause of this conflict is the nurse's beliefs, values, and goals.

2. Place a check mark in the space beside each statement that is a potential cause of conflict.

____ 2.1 The nurse manager announced that a new time-scheduling option for shift rotation would be implemented. All rotations would be voluntary and the clinical nurse personnel would all participate in developing the policy and procedure.

____ 2.2 A clinical nurse receives numerous calls from her husband while she is on duty. He accuses her of unfaithfulness and calls to check up on her. His calls are verbally abusive.

____ 2.3 Although Mrs. Casey, RN, is over 60 years of age, the younger nurses value

and seek her advice. They assist her with her assignments whenever they sense she needs it. They are very tactful as they regard her as an experienced resource.

____ 2.4 Although they do outstanding work and are well qualified for promotions, minority nurses who apply for promotions have never been selected.

The following questions can be done in groups. Form groups of five to eight persons. Select a leader to keep the group moving and a recorder to write the plan or report. Refer to the chapter for techniques or skills in assessing and managing conflict.

3. *Case Study:* You are called to a unit to resolve a conflict between an RN and an LPN. They are shouting at each other in the hallway. The RN is the supervisor of the LPN. As you approach them you hear the following dialogue:

RN: I asked you to get Mr. W. ready to go to x-ray and you ignored me. The transport person was here and left because you would not help him.

LPN: I was busy with Mrs. L. and could not leave. Why didn't you get Mr. W. ready? You apparently knew about it.

RN: It was your job. I assigned Mr. W. to you.

LPN: I do my own work and part of yours. You are the RN. You are supposed to be the leader in this hall.

RN: Don't get sarcastic with me. I don't have to put up with it. I'm going to call the supervisor and report you for your insolence.

LPN: My insolence! Go ahead and report me! I'll tell the supervisor what a lazy bitch you are!

Outline a plan to deal with this conflict. You may use the following format.

3.1 What is (are) the cause(s) of the conflict?

3.2 Decide on aims, strategies, and specific skills for resolving the conflict. List them.

4. *Case Study:* During P.M. change-of-shift report, an RN calls in ill and the staffing office says she cannot be replaced. This leaves only one RN, Mrs. K., for 26 patients. Mrs. K. says, "If you do not get another RN for this unit, I am going to quit this job. I will do it this shift but I will not put up with this constant shortage of help. I don't care if it is an RN, but I should have people with some skills to get the patients cared for. The reason everyone

quits around here is because they are overworked, underpaid, and the hospital management does not give a damn. The place needs to be investigated."

Outline a plan to deal with this conflict. You may use the following format.

4.1 What is (are) the cause(s) of the conflict?

4.2 Decide on aims, strategies, and specific skills for resolving the conflict. List them.

5. *Case Study:* A surgeon and a scrub nurse get in an argument during an operation. The surgeon tells the scrub nurse she is stupid and he does not want her to ever scrub for him again. The scrub nurse says that she is totally competent but that he expects her to read his mind. She says, "If you don't quit badgering me, I'm going to sue you and this hospital!" This comment leads to escalation of the dialogue into a shouting match.

Outline a plan to deal with this conflict. You may use the following format:

5.1 What is (are) the cause(s) of the conflict?

5.2 Decide on aims, strategies, and specific skills for resolving the conflict. List them.

6. Describe a recent instance of a conflict in which you were involved. Was it resolved satisfactorily? Can the gorup help in finding a better solution? Discuss.

7. Do a library computer search on conflict management. Look at indices of nursing, business, and management periodicals. Prepare an abstract of two recent publications. The abstract should describe the value of the publication to the performance of the nurse manager.

NOTES

1. E. C. Murphy, "Managing Defiance," *Nursing Management,* May 1984, 67–69.
2. Ibid.
3. D. R. Faulconer and V. B. Goldman, "Managerial Stress," *Nursing Administration Quarterly,* Winter 1983, 32.
4. E. C. Murphy, "Communication and Wellness: Managing Patient/Staff Relationships," *Nursing Management,* Oct. 1984, 64–68.
5. G. S. Wlody, "Communicating in the ICU: Do You Read Me Loud and Clear?," *Nursing Management,* Sept. 1984, 24–27.
6. M. B. Silber, "Managing Confrontations: Once More into the Breach," *Nursing Management,* Apr. 1984, 54, 56–58.
7. E. C. Murphy, "Practical Management Course," *Nursing Management,* Mar. 1987, 76–77; American Hospital Association, *Role, Functions, and Qualifications of the Nursing Service Administrator in a Health Care Institution* (Chicago: AHA, 1978); R. Zemke, "The Case of the Missing Managerial Malaise," *Training,* Nov. 1985, 30–33; M. A. Palich, "What Supervisors Should Know about Discipline," *Supervisory Management,* Oct. 1983, 21–24; and L. Greenhalgh, "SMR Forum: Managing Conflict," *Sloan Management Review,* Summer 1986, 45–51.
8. Palich, op. cit.
9. Murphy, "Practical Management Course," op. cit.
10. Murphy, "Communication and Wellness," op. cit.
11. J. T. Powell, "Stress Listening: Coping with Angry Confrontations," *Personnel Journal,* May 1986, 27–29.
12. Faulconer and Goldman, op. cit.
13. C. C. Clark, "Assertiveness Issues for Nursing Administrators and Managers," *Journal of Nursing Administration,* July 1979, 20–24.
14. H. K. Baker and P. I. Morgan, "Building a Professional Image: Handling Conflict," *Supervisory Management,* Feb. 1986, 24–29.
15. A. C. Alt-White, M. Charns, and R. Strayer, "Personal Organizational and Managerial Factors Related to Nurse-Physician Collaboration," *Nursing Administration Quarterly,* Fall 1983, 8–18.
16. Baker and Morgan, op. cit.; Murphy, "Practical Management Course," op. cit.; R. Lamkin, "Communicating Effectively," *B&E Review,* July 1984, 16; H. K. Baker and P. Morgan, "Building a Professional Image: Using 'Feeling Level' Communication," *Supervisory Management,* Jan. 1986, 20–25; Murphy, "Managing Defiance," op. cit.; L. Greenhalgh, op. cit.; and Silber, op. cit.
17. Zemke, op. cit.
18. Baker and Morgan, "Building a Professional Image: Handling Conflict," op. cit.

FOR FURTHER REFERENCE

Filmer, D., "Improving Communications in Large Organizations," *Work and People,* Feb. 1985, 12–14.

Levenstein, A., "Negotiation versus Confrontation," *Nursing Management,* Jan. 1984, 52–53.

Swansburg, R. C., and Swansburg, P. W., *Strategic Career Planning and Development for Nurses* (Rockville, MD: Aspen, 1984).

Templeton, J., "For Corporate Vigor, Plan a Fight Today," *Sales Management, The Marketing Magazine,* June 15, 1969, 32–36.

·20·

Controlling or Evaluating

INTRODUCTION

The final element of management discussed by Fayol was control. He defined control as:

> *verifying whether everything occurs in conformity with the plan adopted, the instructions issued, and principles established. It has for its object to point out weaknesses and error in order to rectify them and prevent recurrence.*[1]

Controlling or evaluating was defined by Urwick as "seeing that everything is being carried out in accordance with the plan which has been adopted, the orders which have been given, and the principles which have been laid down."[2] Urwick referred to three principles:

1. The principle of uniformity ensures that controls are related to the organizational structure.
2. The principle of comparison ensures that controls are stated in terms of the standards of performance required, including past performance. In this sense controlling means setting a mark and examining and explaining the results in terms of the mark.
3. The principle of exception provides summaries that identify exceptions to the standards.[3]

It is important that controlling be done on a factual basis. When issues arise people should be made to meet each other and settle them through direct contact. To stimulate cooperation, they need to participate from the beginning. Nurse managers can teach people to cooperate across departmental lines and to let reason and common sense prevail.[4] Management authors, including nurses, have described the controlling process as follows:

1. Establish standards for all elements of management in terms of expected and measurable outcomes. These are the yardsticks by which achievement of objectives are measured.
2. Apply the standards by collecting data and measuring the activities of nursing management, comparing standards with actual care.

3. Make any improvements deemed necessary from the feedback.
4. Keep the process continuous for all areas including:
   4.1 Management of the nursing division and each subunit.
   4.2 Performance of personnel.
   4.3 Nursing process/product.[5]

This may be expressed as a formula:

$$Ss + Sa + F + C \rightarrow I$$

Standards set plus Standards applied plus Feedback plus Correction will yield Improvement.

CONTROLLING AS A FUNCTION OF NURSING MANAGEMENT

Dovovan is one of the few nurse authorities who has written of controlling as a major function of nursing management. Other authors have expended considerable space devoted to quality assurance and performance evaluation. Dovovan stated that control is "the sum of the findings of the means in use to determine whether the goal is being achieved."[6] Control includes coordination of numerous activities, decision making related to planning and organizing activities, and information from directing and evaluating of each worker's performance. Control is also viewed as being concerned with records, reports, organizational progress toward aims, and effective use of resources. Kron and Gray indicated that control uses evaluation and regulation, whereas other authors have suggested that controlling is identical to evaluating.[7]

Koontz and Weihrich defined controlling as "the measurement and correction of the performance in order to make sure that enterprise objectives and the plans devised to attain them are accomplished.[8]

Controls as Management Tools

In the process of measuring the degree to which predetermined goals are achieved and applying necessary corrective actions to improve performance, policies and procedures are used as standards. Also, observations, questions, patient charts, patients, and health care team members serve as sources of data. Corrective actions can be corroborative, disciplinary, or educational.[9] In the process of feedback, a positive experience will stimulate motivation and contribute to the growth of employees.[10]

Controls are management tools for improving performance. Among the controls are rules needed to let people know what is expected of them and how functions can be coordinated. Communication as information is essential to control. Self-control is essential to managerial control as it is the highest form of control. Self-control includes being up to date in knowledge, giving clear orders, being flexible, understanding reasons for behavior, helping others improve, increasing skills of problem solving, standing calm under pressure, and planning ahead. People should be told the facts in language that they understand and words that have the intended meaning. Effective nursing managers set limits and make them known to their employees. Then when the line is crossed the appropriate disciplinary action should be taken. The latter is achieved by corrective action that is consistently applied after checking the facts.[11]

Ten characteristics of a good control system are:

1. Controls must reflect the nature of the activity.
2. Controls should report errors promptly.
3. Controls should be forward-looking.
4. Controls should point out exceptions at critical points.
5. Controls should be objective.
6. Controls should be flexible.
7. Controls should reflect the organizational pattern.
8. Controls should be economical.
9. Controls should be understandable.
10. Controls should indicate corrective action.[12]

Nurse managers will realize that the best way of ensuring the quality of nursing service provided in the patient units is to establish philosophy, standards of care, and objectives. At least two of these, philosophy and objectives, involve planning, further evidence that the major functions of management take place simultaneously.[13] Controlling mechanisms also include accreditation procedures, consultants, evaluation devices, rounds, reports, inspections, and nursing audits.[14]

Nurses activate the processes of control. This function involves the use of power and should be used by nurse managers to promote openness, honesty, trust, competence, and even confrontation. It involves value systems, ethical decision making, self-control, professional self-regulation, and control by an aggregate of professionals. It is emerging as a system of quality control programs. The dimensions of quality assurance programs are quality of care including accessibility and beliefs and attitudes of patients about health care, structure of health care, processes of care, professional competence, outcomes of care, and self-regulation. Audits and budgets are the major techniques of control.[15]

Control functions can be differentiated among levels of managers. For example, the head nurse manager of a unit is concerned with short-range operational activities including daily and weekly schedules, assignments, and effective use of resources. This nurse manager also keeps records of absences and incidents and prepares personnel appraisals: control activities subject to quick changes.

Two methods of measurement are used to assess achievement of nursing goals: task analysis and quality control. In task analysis, the head nurse inspects the motions, actions, and procedures laid out in written guides, schedules, rules, records, and budgets. It is a study of the process of giving nursing care. It measures physical support only, and relatively few tools have been used to do task analysis in nursing. In quality control the head nurse is concerned with measurement of the quality and effects of nursing care. Mechanisms or models for doing this have been developed by the American Nurses' Association (ANA), the Joint Commission on Accreditation of Healthcare Organizations (JCAHO), and others. Many quality assurance techniques are referred to as audits.[16]

STANDARDS

A prime element of the management of nursing services is a system for evaluation of the total effort. This includes a system for evaluation of the management process as well as of the practice of nursing and all nursing care services. Evaluation requires standards that can be used as the yardsticks for gauging the quality and quantity of services. The key sources for these standards, which are available in both management and practice, is the ANA, whose publications include *Standards for Organized Nursing Services and Responsibilities of Nurse Administrators across All Settings* and *Standards of Clinical Nursing Practice*. Several functional yardsticks can be developed using these source documents. They can assist in developing the objectives of the division of nursing and of each ward, unit, and clinic. Objectives are developed into operational or management plans, and systematic and periodic review of accomplishments of these objectives will be part of the evaluation system. In addition, a management evaluation system can be developed with a similar format. Further evaluation can be effected through development of criteria for nursing rounds by the nurse executive and other nurse managers.

Performance standards can be used for individual performance, and criteria can be developed for collective evaluation of patient care. The latter may include the standards for use during nursing rounds as well as criteria for the quality assurance program.

Performance evaluation and quality assurance are dealt with in succeeding chapters. Standards are established criteria of performance, planning goals, strategic plans, physical or quantitative measurements of products, units of service, personnel hours, speed, cost, capital, revenue, program, and intangible standards.[17] They have also been defined as "an acknowledged measure of comparison for quantitative or qualitative value, criterion, or norm," and as "a standard rule or test on which a judgment or decision can be based." Nurse managers develop, in collaboration with clinical nurses, the "clinical nursing criteria against which to measure patient outcomes and the nursing process."[18] These standards are stated as patient outcomes and as nursing care processes.

Figure 20–1 shows an example of an evaluation plan for nursing services.

CONTROLLING TECHNIQUES

Although evaluation operational plans are controlling techniques, other specific controlling techniques can be developed including planned nursing rounds by nurse managers from all levels, checklists from ANA *Standards for Organized Nursing Service and Responsibilities of Nurse Administrators Across All Settings*, ANA *Standards of Nursing Practice*, JCAHO *Accreditation Manual for Hospitals*, and other published standards of third-party payers such as Medicare and Medicaid.

Mission Statement to Which Objective Applies. The division of nursing has a stated philosophy and has objectives. Personnel of each department or unit within the division will have their own philosophy and will set up their own objectives. The objectives will be continuously evaluated, and a written statement as to progress will be sent to the chair office each August and February.

Philosophy Statement to Which Objective Applies. We believe that a continuous evaluation of the activities of the division of nursing is necessary to assess how effectively the needs of the patients are being met and to take action to improve nursing service when indicated. Research must be performed, and the results must be analyzed, adapted, and implemented to modify nursing procedures and practices for the attainment of more effective patient care.

Objective 6. The patient benefits from close nursing supervision to all nonprofessional personnel who give patient care, and the patient benefits from continuous evaluation of the nursing care given and of performances of all nursing service personnel based on professional standards.

Plans for Achieving Objective	Action and Accountability	Target Dates	Accomplishments
1. Plan and execute a system of continuous evaluation and appraisal of nursing services.	1. Make complete rounds throughout the hospital at least once a day from nursing office. Establish a system of formal nursing rounds by chair, assistants, and clinical nursing coordinators monthly.	Apr 23, 1992	Doing.
	2. Do a monthly nursing audit. Have committee chair brief the chair of the division of nursing afterward.	Dec. 1, 1992	Criteria for 45 conditions completed; 10 more under development. Committee combined with other disciplines. Criteria applied to four conditions with retrieval by medical records personnel and corrective actions taken.
	3. Develop standards for patient care. Obtain ANA *Standards of Nursing Practice* for evaluating patient care. Obtain copies for all clinical nurse managers.	Jan. 1, 1992	Obtained. Being developed into checklist by committee of staff nurses. Will cross-check with job performance standards.
	4. Develop standards for personnel performance.	Dec 31, 1992	Completed for clinical nurses I, II, and III, clinical nurse manager, in-service education coordinator, clinical coordinator, chair and assistants, operating room supervisor and staff nurses, public health nurse, and rehabilitation nurse.

Figure 20–1 • Operational Plan

Plans for Achieving Objective	Action and Accountability	Target Dates	Accomplishments
	5. Set up a system whereby supervisors attend: a. Change-of-shift reports b. Unit conferences c. Unit in-service programs	Jul 1, 1992	Receiving reports and need to plan for their use. Will discuss with supervisors.
	6. Review and use ANA *Standards for Organized Nursing Services* to develop an evaluation and inspection checklist.	Dec 1, 1992	
2. Study organization	1. Reorganize as needed. Have organizational chart printed.	Jul 1, 1992	Done as hospital policy.
	2. Write policy on unit policies and procedures.	Jul 1, 1992	Done as nursing operating instruction 160-2-4.
3. Establish a counseling program for all nursing pesonnel.	1. Program counseling sessions for all head nurses. Have them do the same for those they supervise.	Jan 1, 1992	All done once by Jan 1, 1992. Next sessions appointed.
	2. Use the job performance standards.		

Figure 20-1 (*Continued*)

Nursing Rounds

An effective controlling technique for nursing managers is planned nursing rounds. They can be placed on a schedule and can include all nursing personnel. Rounds cover such issues as patient care, nursing practice, and unit management. To be effective, the results should be discussed with appropriate nursing personnel in a follow-up conference. Part of the evaluation process takes place as a result of the communication occurring during the rounds. Figure 20-2 shows a protocol for planned monthly nursing rounds.

Nursing Operating Instructions

Nursing operating instructions or policies become standards for evaluation as well as controlling techniques. See Figure 20-3.

The ANA *Standards for Organized Nursing Services and Responsibilities of Nurse Administrators across All Settings* can be developed into a checklist for evaluating the management processes of nursing services. See Figure 20-4 for an excerpt from these standards.

The ANA *Standards of Clinical Nursing Practice* can be implemented in several ways. One way is to

1. The chair, assistant chair, and other appropriate nursing personnel will make nursing rounds monthly.
2. Time: 10:00 to 11:00 A.M. unless otherwise indicated
3. Schedule

Unit	Day
1F	1st Tuesday
2A	1st Wednesday
2B	1st Thursday
2F	2nd Tuesday
ICU	2nd Wednesday
4A	2nd Thursday
3A	2nd Friday
3-OB	3rd Tuesday 10:30 A.M. to 11:30 A.M.
3F	3rd Wednesday
4B	3rd Thursday 11:00 A.M. to 12:00 noon
5A, CCU	4th Tuesday
5B	4th Wednesday

4. All unit nursing personnel are welcome to attend these rounds with their head nurse and as patient care needs allow. The following areas will be covered as rounds are made to each patient's bedside:
   a. Nursing histories
   b. Nursing care plans
   c. Nursing diagnoses
   d. Nursing notes
   e. Nurse signatures on necessary documents
5. Other management areas of note will be discussed after bedside rounds:
   a. Equipment and supplies
   b. Staffing and assignments
   c. Controlled substance registers

Figure 20–2 • *Protocol for Planned Monthly Nursing Rounds*

convert these into a checklist and evaluate their use, as in Figure 20–5. The entire set of standards can be developed into a checklist along these lines.

Written protocols should be developed to effect a program for the evaluation process. Another way

1. Special care units will maintain policies and procedures relative to their mission. These procedures will be reviewed, updated, and signed at least annually.
   a. Intensive care unit
   b. Critical care unit
   c. Newborn/intensive care unit nursery
   d. Renal dialysis
2. Special care units will maintain a list of equipment needed to achieve their mission.
3. Supplies and equipment
   a. Blount resuscitator will have percent-adaptor to increase oxygen concentration.
   b. Ambu resuscitator will have tail on to increase oxygen concentration.
   c. Humidification will not be used with oxygen with Ambu resuscitator.
   d. Trays from Central Sterile Supply will be returned as soon as used so that instruments will not be lost or misplaced.

Figure 20–3 • *Operating Instructions*

they may be implemented is by using them to develop the evaluation standards as in Figure 20–6.

Gantt Charts

Early in this century, Henry L. Gantt developed the Gantt chart as a means of controlling production. It depicted a series of events essential to the completion of a project or program. It is usually used for production activities.

Figure 20–7 shows a modified Gantt chart that could be applied to a major nursing administration program or project. The five major activities that the nurse administrator has identified are segments of a total program or project. It could be applied to a project such as implementing a modality of primary nursing. These are possible nursing actions for such a project:

1. Gathering of data
2. Analysis of data
3. Development of a plan
4. Implementation of the plan
5. Evaluation, feedback, and modification

Figure 20–7 is only an example. Application of this controlling process by nurse managers would

Standard 1: Organized nursing services have a philosophy and structure that ensures the delivery of effective nursing care.

Criteria	Yes	No

1. The philosophy and structure are compatible with established professional standards, *Nursing: A Social Policy Statement* and *Code for Nurses with Interpretative Statements*, standards of regulatory agencies, and the mission of the organization within which nursing services are provided.

2. The philosophy of organized nursing services provides to individual nurses the authority and accountability for the clinical management of nursing practice.

3. The philosophy provides for a structure that facilitates participative management.

4. A written organizational plan specifies lines of authority, accountability, and responsibility for all nursing personnel.

5. The philosophy supports the representation and participation of nurses in professional organizations and community and governmental activities related to health care.

SOURCE: From *Standards for Organized Nursing Services and Responsibilities of Nurse Administrators across All Settings*, © 1988, American Nurses Association, Washington, D.C. Reprinted with permission.

Figure 20–4 • *Checklist: Standards for Organized Nursing Services and Responsibilities of Nurse Administrators across All Settings, Standard 1*

be specific to the project or program, the time elements for the various activities varying with each. Also, these five major activities could be modified by using subcategories of activities with estimated completion times. The nurse manager's goal is to complete each activity or phase *on or before* the projected date.

Future controlling or evaluating will focus on process evaluation in which the workforce prevents or corrects errors as they occur. Rigid inspection that creates fear is nonproductive. Total quality management (TQM), decentralization, and participatory management include their own evaluating process.

MASTER CONTROL PLAN

A master controlling or evaluating plan can be used by nurse managers to fulfill this important management function. It can be a general plan for all with each manager adding specific items for their management area. A sample basic master control plan is depicted in Figure 20–8.

SUMMARY

Controlling or evaluating is an ongoing function of nursing management occurring during planning, organizing, and directing activities. Through this process standards are established and then applied; followed by feedback that leads to improvements. The process is kept continuous.

Each nurse manager should have a master plan of control that incorporates all standards related to these actions. This plan can be applied to obtain immediate feedback and meet the objectives of control established for the unit, department, or division. The plan will verify results, provide instructions, and apply principles of uniformity, comparison, and exception.

Controls include policies, rules, procedures, self-control or self-regulation, discipline, rounds, reports, audits, evaluation devices, task analysis, and quality control. They should reflect the nature of the activity and be forward looking, objective, flexible, economical, and understandable. They should lead to continuous action.

Standards are the yardsticks for evaluation and include ANA *Standards for Organized Nursing Services and Responsibilities of Nurse Administrators across All Settings* and *Standards of Clinical Nursing Practice*. Other standards include management plans, goals, programs, costs, revenues, and capital. Physical standards use Gantt charts.

Each nurse manager should have a master evaluation plan that should involve input from all workers.

Section: 3C
Date: Oct. 15, 1992
Evaluator: F. Jules, RN

Standard 1: Assessment   Yes   No   Example
THE NURSE COLLECTS CLIENT HEALTH DATA

Measurement Criteria

1. The priority of data collection is determined by the client's immediate condition or needs.

2. Pertinent data are collected using appropriate assessment techniques.

3. Data collections involves the client, significant others, and health care providers when appropriate.

4. The data collection process is systematic and ongoing.

5. Referent data are documented in a retrievable form.

SOURCE: Reprinted with permission from *Standards of Clinical Nursing Practice,* © 1991, American Nurses Association, Washington, D.C.

Figure 20–5 • *Evaluation of Implementation of ANA Standards of Clinical Nursing Practice*

1. An evaluation plan exists and is used for each nursing department, service, or unit.

2. Each evaluation plan is specific to the needs and activities of the individual department, service, or unit.

3. Evaluation findings are given in immediate feedback to subordinate nursing personnel.

4. Standards are accurate, suitable, and objective.

5. Standards are flexible and work when changes are made in plans and when unforeseen events and failures occur.

6. Standards mirror the organizational pattern of the nursing division, service, or unit.

7. Standards are economical to apply and do not produce unexpected results or effects.

8. Nursing personnel know and understand the standards.

9. Application of the standards results in correction of deficiencies.

Figure 20–6 • *Standards for Evaluation of the Controlling (Evaluating) Function of Nursing Administration of a Division, Service, or Unit*

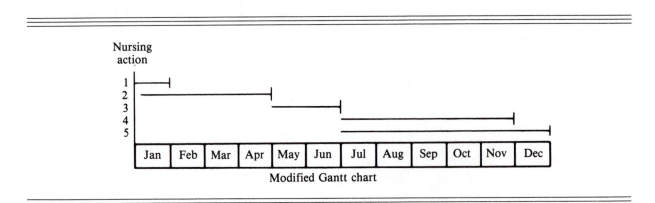

Figure 20–7 • *Modified Gantt Chart*

Objective 1. Inspect for and identify the presence of written, current, and practical statements of mission, philosophy, and objectives for the division of nursing and each of its component units. They should reflect the purposes of the health care organization and give direction to the nursing care program.

Actions

1. The written statements of mission, philosophy, and objectives were current (reviewed or revised within past year).
2. They existed for the division of nursing and for each department, unit, and clinic.
3. They were written by appropriate nursing personnel, representative of people who will accomplish them.
4. The philosophy reflected the meaning of clinical practice.
5. The philosophy was developed in collaboration with consumers, employees, and other health care workers.
6. The objectives were specified, written in behavioral terms, and achievable.
7. They guided the process of implementing the philosophy.
8. They were used for orientation of newly assigned personnel and were otherwise widely distributed and interpreted.
9. They supported the mission, philosophy, and objectives of the institution.
10. Nursing personnel knew the rights of individuals and served as advocates for those rights.

Objective 2. Inspect for and identify the presence of written operational or management plans for accomplishment of the objectives of the division of nursing and each of its component units.

Actions

1. The written operational or management plans were current (entries within past 30 days).
2. They existed for the division of nursing and for each department, unit, and clinic.
3. They included specific actions to be taken to achieve objectives, target dates, and names of personnel assigned responsibility for each action.
4. They were used to evaluate progress; accomplishments were listed.

Objective 3. Inspect for and identify the presence of an organizational plan for the division of nursing and each of its component units.

Actions

1. The organizational plan was current; it agreed with actual organization when checked.
2. It existed for the division of nursing and for each department, unit, and clinic.
3. It showed the relationships between component parts, spelling out the major functions of each, and it showed relationships with other services.
4. The organizational plan supported the mission assigned to personnel.
5. All nursing functions were managed by the nurse administrator.

Objective 4. Inspect for and identify the presence of adequate policies and procedures for guidance of personnel of the division of nursing and each of its component units.

Actions

1. Policies and procedures of the division of nursing and of each department, unit, and clinic were current (reviewed within past year).
2. Policies and procedures did not duplicate those of higher echelons.
3. Policies and procedures were not obsolete, restrictive, or inappropriate in context.
4. Content of location of policies and procedures was known by people who needed this information.
5. Policies and procedures for special care units included:
   a. Function and authority of unit director.
   b. Admission and discharge criteria.
   c. Criteria for performance of special procedures, including cardiopulmonary resuscitation, tracheostomy, ordering of medications, administration of parenteral fluids and other medications, and the obtaining of blood and other laboratory specimens.
   d. The use, location, and maintenance of equipment and supplies.
   e. Respiratory care.
   f. Infection control.
   g. Priorities for orders for laboratory tests.
   h. Standing orders, if any.
   i. Regulations for visitors and traffic control.

Figure 20–8 • *Master Controlling Plan*

(Continued)

6. The nursing annex to the disaster plan was current and included:
   a. Recall procedures.
   b. Assignment procedures.
   c. Training plan.

Objective 5. Inspect for and identify the presence of job descriptions and job standards for all personnel throughout the division of nursing.

Actions

1. Job descriptions and job standards existed and were current throughout the division of nursing (reviewed within past year).
2. Nursing personnel participated in formulating them.
3. Nursing personnel were classified according to competence, and salaries were commensurate with qualifications and positions of comparable responsibility within the agency and the community.
4. Job descriptions were used for purposes of counseling and for helping employees to be productive.
5. They were used for orientation of newly assigned personnel.
6. They described the functions, qualifications, and authority of each position identified in the organizational plan.
7. They were readily available and known to each employee.
8. There was a designated nurse leader for the division of nursing who was a registered nurse with educational and experiential qualifications in nursing practice and the administration of nursing services.

Objective 6. Inspect for and identify the presence of a master staffing plan for the division of nursing and each of its component units.

Actions

1. A master staffing plan existed and was current for the division of nursing and each department, unit, or clinic. It showed authorized versus assigned personnel and was reviewed at least monthly.
2. Adequate personnel policies existed to give guidance to nursing personnel in the planning of time schedules and to allow for mobility so that personnel could be matched to jobs.

3. Avenues of communication existed to give input from nursing personnel to the nurse administrator regarding staffing problems.
4. An active plan existed for sponsoring newly assigned personnel and for identifying their special training and experience and their desired assignments.

Objective 7. Inspect for and identify the presence of a planned counseling program for all personnel of the division of nursing.

Actions

1. The nurse executive had a planned program for counseling with managers, including clinical nurse managers.
2. Counseling occurred at least every 6 months on a scheduled basis.
3. Clinical nurse managers counseled with individual staff members on a scheduled basis at least once every 6 months.
4. The counseling process included discussion of progress toward personal objectives and revisions resulted from the sessions. Job standards were reviewed and special educational and experience goals were discussed and acted on.
5. Records of counseling sessions were available and were reviewed.
6. A career progression plan was operational.

Objective 8. Inspect for and identify the presence of a system of evaluation of nursing activities in the division of nursing and each of its component units.

Actions

1. A system for evaluation of the division of nursing and each of its departments, units, and clinics was in operation.
2. Change-of-shift reports and unit conferences were being periodically evaluated (at least once every 6 months).
3. Management plans indicated current evaluation of accomplishment of objectives (within past 30 days).
4. Management personnel, including the nurse executive, made planned unit rounds at least monthly and checked all aspects of department, unit, or clinic management including:

Figure 20–8 (Continued)

(Continued)

a. Controlled substance registers.
b. Nursing histories.
c. Nursing diagnosis.
d. Nursing care plans.
e. Nursing notes.
f. Drug levels and security.
g. Supplies and equipment.
h. Assignment procedures.
i. Patient records.

5. The quality assurance program was in effect, and at least one problem per month had been evaluated since June 1, 1991.

6. There was provision for inclusion of other health care disciplines and consumers in evaluating the nursing care programs.

7. Results of evaluation were used to assess planning for change.

Objective 9. Inspect for and identify the representation of division of nursing personnel on institutionwide and departmental boards, committees, and councils.

Actions

1. The division of nursing was represented on institutionwide boards, committees, and councils whose activities affected nursing personnel directly.
   a. Social actions.
   b. Personnel boards such as awards and benefits.

2. Nursing service committees had specific objectives.

3. Membership was current and representative of all appropriate segments of the nursing staff.

4. Minutes of meetings reflected progress toward objectives and follow-up of problems.

Objective 10. Inspect for and identify the existence of a working public relations program that serves as a means of communication between personnel of the division of nursing and the community they serve.

Actions

1. Evaluation programs existed to tell consumers of the nursing services available to them and to receive feedback from consumers on the types of services they needed.

2. There was a planned program to publicize nursing activities and recognize contributions and accomplishments of nursing personnel.

Objective 11. Inspect for and identify the existence of a planned program for training and continuing education for all division of nursing personnel.

Actions

1. Written statements of mission, philosophy, and objectives existed and were current (reviewed within past year).

2. An operational or management plan for the accomplishment of objectives was current (entries made within past 30 days).

3. The plan listed activities, set priorities and target dates, assigned responsibility, and provided for continuous evaluation.

4. The plan provided for identification of training and continuing education needs, including input from participants, translation of needs into objectives, and the accomplishment of objectives.

5. An orientation program existed and included philosophy and objectives of organization and nursing service, personnel policies, job descriptions, work environment, clinical practice policies and procedures, and operational policies and procedures.

6. Supplemental classes were taught to meet on-the-job training needs.

7. Training programs were documented.

8. The program supported career advancement.

Objective 12. Inspect for and identify the existence of procedures and policies for providing needed primary nursing care to patients.

Actions

1. Collection of data on each patient was sufficient to permit identification and assessment of the patient's needs and to institute an individual plan of care. Included were admission data and patient's nursing history.

2. The nursing care plans included the nursing diagnoses, prescriptions for care, and patients' teaching needs.

3. The plan was used to provide care to the patient, and there was an ongoing reassessment of the patient's needs with appropriate changes made in the plan of care.

4. There was evidence that nursing actions required by physicians' orders, plans of nursing care, and hospital policies were

Figure 20–8 (Continued)

(Continued)

accomplished appropriately. Observations of patient's progress and response to actions were made and recorded.

5. There was evidence of interpretation and implementation of the ANA *Standards of Nursing Practice.*

6. Nursing administration had a plan for reviewing the requirements for giving credentials to individuals and health-care organizations and for participating in their implementation.

7. Guidelines existed for assignment of personnel based on level of competence.

8. There were policies to use unit managers and unit clerks to perform clerical, managerial, and indirect service roles.

9. Nursing administration provided resources to accomplish primary nursing care to patients: facilities, equipment, supplies, and personnel. *Note:* Under TQM most of ths plan would be delegated to unit personnel.

Figure 20–8   (Continued)

EXPERIENTIAL EXERCISES

1. Obtain a copy of *Standards for Organized Nursing Services and Responsibilities of Nurse Administrators across All Settings.* Convert it to a checklist similar to Figure 20–4. Use the checklist to inspect a nursing unit or department in which you are a student.

1.1 List the deficiencies:

1.2 Make a management plan for correcting the deficiencies.

MANAGEMENT PLAN

DEFICIENCY:

OBJECTIVE:

ACTIONS	ASSIGNED TO	TARGET DATES	ACCOMPLISHMENTS

2. Obtain a copy of one of the ANA *Standards of Clinical Nursing Practice.* Convert it to a checklist similar to Figure 20–5. Use the checklist to audit a patient's chart in a nursing unit in which you are a student.

2.1 List the deficiencies:

2.2 Make a management plan for correcting the deficiencies.

MANAGEMENT PLAN

DEFICIENCY:

OBJECTIVE:

ACTIONS	ASSIGNED TO	TARGET DATES	ACCOMPLISHMENTS

3. Apply the standards for evaluation of the controlling (evaluating) function of nursing administration of a division, service, or unit from Figure 20–6 to the nursing unit, service (department), or division in which you are a student.

3.1 List the deficiencies:

3.2 Make a management plan for correcting the deficiencies.

MANAGEMENT PLAN

DEFICIENCY:

OBJECTIVE:

ACTIONS	ASSIGNED TO	TARGET DATES	ACCOMPLISHMENTS

4. Use Figure 20–8, Master Controlling Plan, to inspect the management functions of the nursing division in which you work as a student.

4.1 Summarize your findings:

4.2 Make management plans to correct deficiencies.

MANAGEMENT PLAN

DEFICIENCY:

OBJECTIVE:

ACTIONS	ASSIGNED TO	TARGET DATES	ACCOMPLISHMENTS

5. *Group Exercise*

5.1 Form groups of five to eight persons.

5.2 Elect a leader to keep the group progressing to project completion.

5.3 Elect a recorder to keep a written record of the work.

5.4 Examine the mission, philosophy, and objectives statements of a nursing unit in which you work as a student. Which statements relate specifically to controlling or evaluating a unit?

5.5 If the statements related to controlling or evaluating a unit do not exist or are inadequate, draft appropriate ones.

6. Do a library computer search on "controlling" or "evaluating." Look at indices of nursing, business, and management periodicals. Prepare abstracts of two recent publications. The abstracts should describe the value of the publication to the performance of the nurse manager.

NOTES

1. H. Fayol, *General and Industrial Management*, trans. by C. Storrs (London: Sir Isaac Pitman & Sons, 1949), 107.
2. L. Urwick, *The Elements of Administration* (New York: Harper & Row, 1944), 105.
3. Ibid., 107–110.
4. Ibid., 113–117.
5. H. Koontz and H. Weihrich, *Management* (New York: McGraw-Hill, 1988), 490–492; R. M. Hodgetts and D. F. Kurato, *Management: Theory, Process, and Practice* 2d ed. (New York: Harcourt Brace Jovanovich, 1988), 376; R. M. Fulmer and S. G. Franklin, *Supervision: Principles of Professional Management* 2d ed. (New York: Macmillan, 1982), 214–216; H. S. Rowland and B. L. Rowland, *Nursing Administration Handbook* 3d ed. (Germantown, MD: Aspen, 1992), 35–39; P. F. Drucker, *Management: Tasks, Responsibilities, Practices* (New York: Harper & Row, 1973), 495–505; and T. Kron and A. Gray, *The Management of Patient Care: Putting Leadership Skills to Work* 6th ed. (Philadelphia: W. B. Saunders, 1987), 179–180.
6. H. M. Donovan, *Nursing Service Administration: Managing the Enterprise* (St. Louis: C. V. Mosby, 1975), 155.
7. Kron and Gray, op. cit., 100.
8. Koontz and Weihrich, op. cit., 490.
9. P. Franck and M. Price, *Nursing Management*, 2d ed. (New York: Springer Publishing, 1980), 135.
10. M. L. Holle and M. E. Blatchly, *Introduction to Leadership and Management in Nursing* (Monterey, CA: Wadsworth Health Services Division, 1982), 178–185.
11. A. Levenstein, in *The Nurse as Manager*, edited by M. J. F. Smith (Chicago: S-N Publications, 1981), 17–33.
12. Fulmer and Franklin, op cit., 216–217.
13. I. G. Ramey, "Setting Standards and Evaluating Care," in Stone et al., eds., *Management for Nurses* (St. Louis: C. V. Mosby, 1976), 79.
14. Donovan, op. cit., 160–169.
15. M. Beyers and C. Phillips, *Nursing Management for Patient Care*, 2d ed. (Boston: Little, Brown, 1979), 109–141.
16. L. M. Douglass, *The Effective Nurse: Leader and Manager*, 3d ed. (St. Louis: C. V. Mosby, 1988), 180–184.
17. Koontz and Weihrich, op. cit., 490, 492–494.
18. J. M. Ganong and W. L. Ganong, *Nursing Management*, 2d ed. (Rockville, MD: Aspen, 1980), 191.

FOR FURTHER REFERENCE

Lemin, B., *First Line Nursing Management* (New York: Springer, 1977), 47–51.

Swansburg, R. C., *Management of Patient Care Services*, (St. Louis: Mosby, 1976).

Quality Assurance

OVERVIEW

As discussed in the preceding chapter, a master evaluation or controlling plan is needed to evaluate the whole program of any nursing department, service, or unit. One of the major elements of such a plan will be a quality assurance program. As the costs of hospital and all aspects of health care keep increasing, quality assurance programs are essential to assuring that the quality of care is maintained, and indeed, that quality care is delivered. The assumption is that nursing must be accountable to its clients for the care rendered by its practitioners.

Quality assurance programs began in hospitals in the 1960s with voluntary implementation of nursing audits. The term has emerged in the health care field as a synonym for evaluation or as a major evaluation activity. Quality assurance has been defined as "estimation of the degree of excellence in patient health outcomes and in activity and other resource outcomes."[1]

Part of evaluation involves determination of management effectiveness or how well objectives, outcomes, or results have been achieved. Another part involves efficiency, the cost of achieving objectives. Quality assurance not only involves evaluation, it involves its use to secure improvement.

COMPONENTS OF A QUALITY ASSURANCE PROGRAM

A quality assurance program or plan has the following components:

1. Clear and concise written statements of purpose, philosophy, and objectives.
2. Standards or indicators for measuring the quality of care.
3. Policies and procedures for using such standards for gathering data. These policies define the organizational structure for the quality assurance program.
4. Analysis and reporting of the data gathered, with isolation of problems.
5. Use of the results to prioritize problems.

Mission. The mission of the Quality Assurance Plan of the University of South Alabama Medical Center is directly reflective of the mission of the University of South Alabama Medical Center. As stated in the policy, "Functional Plan of Organization of the University of South Alabama Medical Center" (from Mission Statements), the Department of Quality Assurance "ensures that the quality of patient care at the University of South Alabama Medical Center is optimal through a unified program for patient care evaluation activities."

Purpose. The purpose of the Quality Assurance Plan of the University of South Alabama Medical Center is to ensure that all patients receive the optimal quality of care.

SOURCE: Courtesy of the University of South Alabama Medical Center, Mobile, Alabama.

Figure 21–1 • *Mission and Purpose Statements*

6. Monitoring of clinical and managerial performance and ongoing feedback to ensure problems stay solved.
7. Evaluation of the quality assurance system.

Statements of Purpose, Philosophy, and Objectives

The first element of a planned quality assurance (QA) program will be development of clear and concise statements of purpose, philosophy, and objectives. A group developing a tool to evaluate QA programs indicated that only 50 percent of studies done during a 7-year period in a 700-bed medical center stated their individual purposes.[2] Every program needs objectives and every study a purpose. See Figure 21-1 for an example of mission and purpose statements.

Standards for Measuring the Quality of Care

Standards define nursing care outcomes as well as nursing activities and structural resources needed. They are used for planning nursing care as well as for evaluating it. Outcomes include positive and negative indexes.

Various organizations issue indexes. The Health Care Financing Administration (HCFA) discloses projected and actual hospital mortality rates by diagnosis-related group (DRG) annually. HCFA is preparing to disclose physician quality indexes. The Joint Commission on Accreditation of Healthcare Organizations issued clinical and organizational performance measures and outcomes in 1991. Indicators include severity of illness or risk adjustment mechanisms. Providers doing an excellent job as well as those doing a poor job are being identified.

Other organizations collecting data to do quality measurement are the American Hospital Association, Voluntary Hospitals of America, National Committee for Quality Healthcare, and the National Association of Health Data Organizations. They will gather, analyze, and publish data on quality of health care for consumers, employers, and the government. These standards will include performance standards for providers. The objectives are to achieve improvement in the health status of patients, to reduce unnecessary use of health care services, and to meet specifications of patients and purchasers. The standards will address social, psychological, financial, clinical, and management concerns.[3]

Outcomes or indexes serve as an estimate or judge of the value, rank, or degree of excellence. See Figure 21-2.

Policies and Procedures

The third element of a quality assurance program is to develop policies and procedures for using standards or indicators for gathering data to measure the quality of care. They will define the organizational structure for the QA program and will prescribe the tools for gathering data.

TOOLS OR INSTRUMENTS FOR COLLECTING QA DATA

Standards are not evaluation instruments. Tools or instruments will be selected to collect evidence that indicates standards are being met. Various standardized instruments are available. If the QA committee decides to develop new tools it will need to determine reliability and at least content validity.

There are three basic forms for nursing audits: structure audits, process audits, and outcome audits.

The following standards are directed toward nursing care that is provided for all patients regardless of social, economic, or religious status.

Standard 1. When admitted to the Sixth Floor, the patient and family will be oriented to hospital and room by a nursing employee who will explain hospital policies, including visiting hours, smoking, etc., in an unhurried, warm manner.

Standard 2. A registered nurse will interview the patient, or family responsible for the patient, to obtain a complete health history. This information will be written on the admission data profile and will become a part of the medical record, accessible to all medical personnel.

Standard 3. An RN will make an assessment of the patient with regard to the reason for admission and chief complaint. The individualized nursing care plan will be developed from this assessment.

Standard 4. The nursing staff will evaluate and revise the nursing care plan as necessary. The care plan will be discussed with other patient care disciplines by means of report, patient care conferences, etc.

Standard 5. Patient care will include the following on a daily basis:

1. A.M. care:
   a. Daily bath—self, given, or with assistance
   b. Mouth care—self, given, or with assistance
   c. Hair grooming—self, given, or with assistance
   d. Skin care—special attention to be given to areas of potential breakdown
   e. Change linens on the bed, clean linens for bath
2. P.M. care:
   a. Skin care
   b. Mouth care

c. Freshen patient's linens and straighten room

3. HYGIENE
   a. Handwashing before and after meals
   b. Handwashing after use of bedpan and/or urinal

4. ACTIVITY
   a. As ordered—proper positioning in bed or chair
   b. Active or passive physical therapy

5. Assessment of nutritional needs and diet instruction

6. Assistance with meeting needs of bowel and bladder elimination

7. Ensurance of necessary rest and sleep

8. Administration of medication and treatments according to correct procedures

9. Ensure a safe environment

Standard 6. The nursing staff will give the patient and family support by:

1. Attentive listening
2. Reassurance
3. Observance of unusual behavior
4. Therapeutic intervention
5. Assistance with spiritual needs

Standard 7. An RN will provide the patient and/or family with appropriate patient teaching and discharge planning that include:

1. Explanation of all procedures and nursing measures used
2. Teaching of self-care
3. Discussion and presentation of discharge plan with other patient care disciplines

SOURCE: Courtesy of the University of South Alabama Medical Center, Mobile, Alabama.

Figure 21–2 • Standards of Nursing Care for Sixth Floor

Structure Audits

Structure audits focus on the setting in which care takes place. They include physical facilities, equipment, caregivers, organization, policies, proce-dures, and medical records. Standards or indicators will be measured by a checklist that focuses on these categories.

Structure can include such content as staff knowledge and expertise, in addition to policies and procedures. Content related to specific nursing care to meet established standards will be included in nursing process audits.

Process Audits

Process audits implement criteria for measuring nursing care to determine if nursing standards of practice are being met. They are task oriented. Process audits were first used by Maria Phaneuf in 1964 and were based on the seven functions of nursing established by Lesnick and Anderson. The Phaneuf audit is retrospective, being applied to measure the quality of nursing care received by the patient after a cycle of care has been completed and the patient is discharged. The seven subsections of the Phaneuf audit are:

1. Application and execution of physicians' legal orders
2. Observation of symptoms and reactions
3. Supervision of the patient
4. Supervision of those participating in care (except the physician)
5. Reporting and recording
6. Application and execution of nursing procedures and techniques
7. Promotion of physical and emotional health by direction and teaching

The Phaneuf model uses a Likert scoring system. It does not evaluate care not recorded.[4]

The *Quality Patient Care Scale (Qual PacS)* is a process audit that measures the quality of nursing care concurrently. Its six subsections are:

1. Psychosocial—individual
2. Psychosocial—groups
3. Physical
4. General
5. Communication
6. Professional implications

The nurse is evaluated by direct observation in a nurse-patient interaction. A 15 percent sample of nurses on a unit is considered adequate. Both of these process audits use the performance of the first-level staff nurse as a standard for safe, adequate, therapeutic, and supportive care.[5]

The Qual PacS audit was developed from the *Slater Nursing Competencies Rating Scale*. The Slater model references five staff nurses from best to poorest, contains eighty-four questions, and takes

$2\frac{1}{2}$ to 3 hours per nurse-patient interaction. Qual PacS reduced it to sixty-eight items.[6]

Other open-system audits include Commission on Administrative Service in Hospital (CASH) Scale and the Medicus Corporation Nurses Audit. They also measure or monitor action, assessment, and clinical skills.

Outcome Audits

Outcome audits are also either concurrent or retrospective. They evaluate nursing performance in terms of established patient outcome criteria. The National Center for Health Services developed an outcome audit based on Orem's description of nine categories of self-care requirements:

1. Air
2. Water/fluid intake
3. Food
4. Elimination
5. Rest/activity/sleep
6. Social interaction and productive work
7. Protection from hazards
8. Normality
9. Health deviation

These categories are evaluated in terms of:

1. Evidence that the requirement is met
2. Evidence that the patient has the necessary knowledge to meet the requirement
3. Evidence that the patient has the necessary skill and performance abilities to meet the requirement
4. Evidence that the patient has the necessary motivation to meet the requirement[7]

Outcome criteria are set for selected topics. They can evaluate specific aspects of nursing care for particular groups such as cancer patients, perioperative patients, intensive care patients, and others. Patients are grouped for efficiency: DRGs, like treatments, like needs, geography, life stages, illness stages, and like standards. A determination is made as to whether the outcomes are met. If not, deficiencies are corrected and followed up.

Triad Models

Some nursing quality assurance models use a triad of structure, process, and outcome. Measurement criteria are referenced by code to specific structure, process, or outcome standards. A modular approach has been used in which patient conditions were related to five areas: patient rights, developmental stage of patient, social groups, therapy-associated needs, and medical diagnoses. Standards for each patient group were developed and used to construct the evaluation instrument.

A modular design for QA provides discrete components that can be used independently or in different combinations. This design has three modules:

1. Patient care standards
2. Outcome, process, structure trail
3. The standard with derived measurement criteria[8]

Outcome indicators also include mortality rates and infection rates.

PROBLEM IDENTIFICATION

Analysis and reporting of the data gathered from the evaluation process leads to problem identification and isolation. Evidence comes from primary sources such as the patient and personnel and from secondary sources including the patient's chart and family. Evidence is gathered through rounds, observations, and records. There should be active patient and family participation. QA addresses current problems. Nurse managers look for patterns or trends of deviation from normal. They also identify deficiencies relating to other departments that affect nursing care.

PROBLEM RESOLUTION

Once problems have been defined and isolated, plans are made to solve them on a priority basis. Those that are critical are addressed first, and plans are immediately made and implemented to resolve them. Those involving the safety and welfare of the patient take first priority. Other factors used in determining priority will include severity, frequency, benefit, cost effectiveness, elimination, reduction, association with professional liability, and impact on accreditation. The first consideration is always based on the impact on patient care.[9]

Solutions and corrective action for problems will be assigned to appropriate nursing departments, services, and units. The need is to resolve problems, not just evaluate them.

MONITORING AND FEEDBACK

The QA process is a cyclic one that requires monitoring of clinical and managerial performance and feedback to ensure that problems stay solved. Follow-up can be expensive and difficult. Its breadth should determine what should be covered. Problems of a multidisciplinary nature such as those involving occupational therapy, physical therapy, speech pathology, and nursing can be one consideration.

The cyclic process will continue to set standards of care, take measurements according to those standards, evaluate data from multiple sources, recommend improvements, and above all, ensure that improvements are carried out.

SYSTEM EVALUATION

Although nurses defend their right to define and regulate good quality care, they often do not pursue QA activities. In a study of nurse managers, staff development nurses, and clinical nurses in ten metropolitan hospitals, it was found that most nurses believed QA involved all levels of nursing personnel but not as part of their daily work. Twenty-five percent viewed it as an accreditation requirement. Peer review and patient care audits ranked low against direct patient care activities. Less than 50 percent of respondents wanted to participate in these activities.[10]

Nurses with formal QA experience were more likely to want to write standards for their specialty, to participate in peer review, and to want to be on QA committees. They were more interested in QA associated with direct patient care.[11]

Many QA programs are developed without thorough assessment of the needs of those to be served or of the resources available. Many programs are continued without evaluation and evidence of their positive contributions to health care. These include hospice and cardiac rehabilitation programs.[12]

Several models for QA program evaluation have been developed. These include the James model and the Renzulli key features model.

The nurse manager will view QA as part of the total evaluating function of nursing management rather than as a distinct entity. A model for evalua-

Directions: Read the report of the study in its entirety. Respond yes to items below when you can find a specific statement to support your answer. Otherwise, respond no.

Study title _____ Type: Retrospective _____ Concurrent _____

Year _____ Dept. _____ Total # pts. studied _____

	% Yes	No			% Yes	No
1. Problem statement				b. Findings are reported in relation to total population at risk (e.g., # of UTI over # of catheterized patients)	___	___
a. Reason for study is stated	___	___				
b. Reason is based on an identified problem	___	___		c. A plan of action supported by study results is formulated	___	___
c. Study is related to nursing practice (versus activities of medical pharmacy or others)	___	___		d. Action plan aims at solving the problem defined	___	___
d. Reason is described as a nursing problem or diagnosis	___	___		e. Outcomes of action plan are measurable	___	___
e. Evidence that costs/risks of problem were considered (i.e., risks of problem identified are greater than costs of the study)	___	___		**4. Follow-up**		
				a. Person(s) or group(s) responsible for implementation of action plan are named	___	___
2. Methods				b. There is a specified time frame for implementation of action plan	___	___
a. Subject selection criteria are stated	___	___				
b. Rationale for sample size is described	___	___		c. Mechanisms for follow-up are described	___	___
c. Individuals collecting data are identified	___	___		d. There is evidence that follow-up occurred (e.g., dates of action, names of people contacted)	___	___
d. A description of how study tools and/or methods were developed is included	___	___				
e. Tools or forms used are included	___	___		e. There is evidence that the stated problem is either resolved or further action is planned	___	___
3. Findings/plan of action						
a. Findings are summarized	___	___		Total Score (add yes answers)	___	

SOURCE: Reprinted from "Quality Assurance: Evaluate Thyself," by L. F. Maciorowski, E. Larson and A. Keane, with permission of *Journal of Nursing Administration*, June 1985, 38–42.

Figure 21–3 • *Assessment of Quality Assurance Studies*

tion of all nursing services, including clinical practice, managerial, teaching, and research should be selected in consultation with representative nurses working in these areas. The model should produce results in a timely and economical manner.

MANAGEMENT PROCESSES INVOLVED IN QUALITY ASSURANCE

Quality assurance is important to accountability of nurses who want to control their practice areas.

Many groups are seeking evidence that outcomes of nursing care are of good quality and represent a cost-effective use of resources. Accountability for nursing practice is still diffused by the employment environment, and this fact must be corrected by nurse managers.

Involvement of Practicing Nurses

Practicing nurses can be stimulated to increase their positive attitudes about QA by direct behavioral experience. Nurse managers will find out reasons these nurses view QA unfavorably. They will correct and change this viewpoint by various strategies that include:

1. Having practicing nurses choose QA topics.
2. Providing release time for practicing nurses to participate in QA activities including attendance at committee meetings and time for QA audits.
3. Providing rewards such as performance results achievement records that can lead to pay raises, promotions, educational opportunities, or special assignments.
4. Targeting QA to patient care outcomes, the very essence of nursing practice.
5. Involving clinical nurses in management through such techniques as quality circles, employee involvement programs, participatory management, decentralization, "adhocracy," quality of work life, and TQM.

Resources

QA programs are labor intensive, requiring efficient and effective use of resources that include personnel, physical plant, supplies, equipment, policies, and procedures. Nurse managers should be selective in determining areas to be evaluated, considering time and difficulty as well as safety and urgency. They should sample the standards rather than dogmatically evaluating every one. This will require placing priority on standards and even making a decision whether to eliminate some that are not critical.

Efficiency

Efficiency is related to two questions: Was the care accomplished in a way that conserved resources? and Did it meet practice standards?[13] The computer is a labor-saving device for developing and con-

ducting a QA program. Nurse managers will use it and teach other practicing nurses to use it. It can help track the QA process.

Standards will be kept up to date and accessible to all units. A loose-leaf notebook or the computer memory are efficient for easy access. Standards should be cross-indexed.

Charts can be labelled so as to be easily retrieved for nursing QA evaluation. They can be coded by nursing diagnosis or nursing care standards.[14]

Consumer Involvement

Consumers will be involved in all aspects of a QA program including discharge planning. They know what they want and are demanding quality with economy. Nurses can teach patients to do pricing of health care that includes calling providers of all health services and establishing prices. Then consumers can negotiate with providers to accept their insurance as payment in full. Consumers can be taught to negotiate discounts for making prompt payments and billing their insurers themselves.

Training and Communication

Training and communication are important elements of a total QA program. Training includes interpersonal skills, stress management, and conflict management. Learning is a cyclic or continuous process. Nurse managers who play educator roles develop self-awareness by applying learning principles to their own behaviors. Patient education requires an interdisciplinary team approach.

Communication of QA findings including problems, resolution of problems, and results must be clear. Both physicians and employees need to be kept up to date. Quality must be provided and communicated to be successful. This means that providers as well as consumers will know the status of the quality of care being rendered.

Quality in the marketplace is defined by employers, employee benefit consultants, physicians, and consumers—not by providers (even though physicians are providers, as are hospitals, nurses, and other caregivers). The reason physicians determine quality is they have control over all orders for diagnosis and treatment procedures. Only one-half of consumers, employers, and employee benefit consultants ever differentiate between high and low quality hospitals. Two-thirds of physicians do.[15]

Good employee relations and consumer relations programs are necessary for success in the marketplace, and their good quality must be communicated. Consumers want quality factors in this order:

1. Warmth, caring, concern
2. Expert medical staff who are concerned, thorough, and successful
3. Up-to-date technology/equipment
4. Specialization/scope of services available
5. Outcome[16]

Nurses sometimes tend to emphasize technology and specialization rather than warmth, caring, and concern.

RISK MANAGEMENT

Risk management has an altogether different connotation today than it did in the 1960s. It was then touted by business and industry as the venture approach to new business, to taking a chance on the unknown. The risk manager was an entrepreneur who purposefully formed small new companies to develop new products that would create new sales and more profit dollars. This manager was responsible for the success or failure of the new venture, of patent protection, technical know-how and marketing methods.[17] Although venture management is still alive and well in U.S. business and industry, risk management has evolved into a defense against the spiraling costs of institutional liability premiums generated by successful and costly malpractice suits.

Goal of Risk Management

The goal of risk management is to have a program that will identify and correct deficient patterns of care, thereby preventing malpractice suits. Some liability insurers require that a risk management program be in place before insuring. Some states require a risk management program for licensure.[18] In its high-visibility context, a risk management program is designed to reduce system and personnel failures.

Since the 1960s, emphasis on civil and consumer rights has generated increased legal challenges to all health care providers, including nurses. The possibility that accidents or negative outcomes will occur in health care is a reality. The consumer knows this and frequently agrees to the possibility in writing. However, when a negative outcome occurs, the same consumers expect compensation for the loss. According to the National Association of Insurance Commissioners Closed Claims Study, 85 percent of all loss dollars paid by insurance companies are for claims originating in the hospital setting.[19]

Health care, including nursing, is big business and costly. The consumer views hospitals, physicians, and nurses as being in business to make money. Injuries and deaths occur in health care institutions and at the hands of professional personnel. Many can be prevented, a fact recognized by the general public that results in increased malpractice litigation even when care meets established standards of practice.

The objectives of a hospital risk management program are:

1. Protection of hospital assets and earning power from large awards that will cause financial instability. This frequently includes liability insurance for employees while they are working for the institution.
2. Injury control or elimination.
3. An effective and economical program.[20]

Activities

Risk management activities include internal audits of hospital procedures and educational activities, effective claims management by investigating and managing claims, an effective patient representative program, and effective insurance management.[21]

The risk management process consists of:

1. Identification of pure risks
2. Analysis of risks for possible loss frequency and severity
3. Development of risk control and risk financing techniques
4. Implementation techniques
5. Maintenance of program for effectiveness and modification as needed[22]

Audits

Audits of hospital procedures are a quality assurance technique and part of an evaluating function of nursing management. From initiatives of the risk management program, personnel must be educated in the process. This will include knowledge of the reasons for the program, its goals, their roles in the risk management program, and frequent feedback concerning their own status and that of the organization with regard to the risk management program. Audits and incident reports are usual sources of identification of pure risks.

The educational program should be coordinated through the staff development or education department. Specific classes can be given by the risk manager, who may act as a consultant for risk management content of other classes. Classes will be given over shifts and often enough to allow all employees to attend. They should be related to job factors for various classes of employees. Professional hands-on personnel will have different interests from technical and support personnel.

Claims Management

Claims management includes analysis of risks for possible loss frequency and severity—the assessment of potential claims based on data analysis. It also includes development of risk control and risk-financing techniques as well as implementation techniques. To accomplish this the risk manager uses written and verbal reports to investigate potentially compensable events and losses and their causes, thereby determining liability and settlement value. Recommendations are made to administrators that include write-offs of specific charges or entire bills. Also, many claims can be settled out of court for small sums.

It is important that the risk manager be able to determine where the institution and personnel are *not* at fault. Some claims should go to litigation with jury trials.

The risk manager's job is further described in Figure 21–4.

The Patient Representative. Many large health care institutions employ patient representatives. These individuals may be nurses or other professionally educated individuals with strong interpersonal skills. They see that patients and families are attended to and satisfied with all aspects of their care and treatment.

Among the services provided by patient representatives are orientation of patients and their families to hospital policies and procedures and to services provided, resolution of complaints, making phone calls, mailing letters, notarizing documents, making transportation arrangements, and daily follow-up survey samples of patients following discharge. Patient representatives can be assisted by volunteers.[23]

1. Keep and up-to-date manual including policies, lines of authority, safety roles, disaster plans, safety training, procedures, incident and claims reporting, procedures, and schedule and description of retention/insurance program.
2. Update programs with changes in properties, operations, or activities.
3. Review plans for new construction, alterations, and equipment installation.
4. Review contracts to avoid unnecessary assumptions of liability and transfer to others where possible.
5. Keep up-to-date property appraisal.
6. Maintain records of insurance policy renewal dates.
7. Review and monitor all premiums and other billings and approve payments.
8. Negotiate insurance coverage, premiums, and services.
9. Prepare specifications for competitive bids on property and liability insurance.
10. Review and make recommendation for coverage, services, and costs.
11. Maintain records and verify compliance for independent physicians, vendors, contractors, and subcontractors.
12. Maintain records of losses, claims, and all risk management expenses.
13. Supervise claim-reporting procedures.
14. Assist in adjusting losses.
15. Cooperate with director of safety and risk management committee to minimize all future losses involving employees, patients, visitors, other third parties, property, and earnings.
16. Keep risk management skills updated.
17. Prepare annual report covering status, changes, new problems and solutions, summary of existing insurance and retention aspects of the program, summary of losses, costs, major claims, and future goals and objectives.
18. Prepare an annual budget.

Figure 21–4 • Risk Manager Competencies

INCIDENT REPORTING

Incident reporting is an effective technique of a good risk management program. The tool itself should be constructed to collect complete and accurate information. This will include the name, address, age, and condition of the individual involved; exact location, time, and date of the incident; description of the occurrence; physician's examination data; bedrail status; reason for hospitalization; witnesses; and extent of out-of-bed privileges.

Use of Incident Reports

Incident reports are used to collect and analyze future data for the purpose of determining risk control strategies. They are prepared for any unusual occurrence involving people or property, whether or not injury or damage occurs.

The incident report is discoverable by the plaintiff's attorney. For this reason it should be prepared in a timely manner to ensure accuracy and objectivity of reporting. It must be complete and factual. The incident report is corrected as any other medical record and should not be altered or rewritten. It should contain no comments criticizing or blaming others. To keep the incident report from being discoverable it must be sent from preparer to attorney to assure confidentiality. Nurse managers frequently insist on reviewing them. They can obtain accurate information from the patient's chart and from conversation with the preparer. The incident report should be prepared in a single copy and should never be placed on the patient's chart.

Attorneys can prepare abstracts of data from collective incident reports. Thus they identify the number of occurrences of particular incidents. The information will be used by risk managers to do their job, including trend analysis to establish patterns and education and training of personnel.[24] See Figure 21-5.

Although it may be institutional policy to send the incident report to the risk manager, an alternative method of notification is better. The preparer can call the risk manager and the nurse manager and give them verbal information to investigate and evaluate deviations from the standard of care and for making corrections. To accomplish this managers will have to establish a climate of trust that supports incident reporting by nurses. The JCAHO requires incident reporting.

According to Poteet, the majority of successful suits against nurses fall into nine risk categories. These are:

1. Administration of medication
2. Assisting in the surgical suite
3. Falls
4. Burns
5. Electric shocks
6. Injuries due to faulty equipment
7. Nosocomial infection
8. Mistaken identity
9. Misinterpretation of signs and symptoms[25]

These would be included in a planned staff development program as would fire safety, disaster procedures, work hazards, radiological and laser safety, sanitation, and infection control. Specific staff development programs would focus on malpractice and legal liability, including standards of care, informed consent, documentation, professional competence, and relevant laws. Other programs would focus on these fundamental concepts in nursing care:

1. Sensitivity to patients
2. Identification of patients
3. Environment
4. Mental competence of patients
5. Moving and lifting
6. Transport of patients[26]

ACCIDENT REPORTING

Incidents involving employees are frequently referred to as accidents. Follow the same principles as for incident reporting. These will usually be covered by institutional policy and procedure. Perceptions vary too much to require personnel to discriminate between incident and accident. An accident is an incident and many incidents are accidents.

INFECTION CONTROL

A major area for quality control and risk management is infection control. Infections acquired in hospitals are termed *nosocomial* infections. Many hospitals will have full-time infection control nurses. They investigate all reported nosocomial infections. A source of data is the medical laboratory. It is good policy to have all laboratory reports positive for infectious diseases routed to the infection control nurse. They will be investigated and procedures implemented to prevent their spread and future development.

Staff development is a major function of infection control. Standards followed are those of the Centers for Disease Control.

DOs	DON'Ts
• For any event involving patient mishap or serious expression of dissatisfaction with care. • For any event involving visitor mishap or property. • Be complete. • Follow established policy and procedure. • Be prompt. • Act to reduce fear by the nursing staff. • Correct as any medical record. • Include names and identities of witnesses; record their statements on separate pages. • Report equipment malfunctions including control numbers. Remove them from service for testing. • Keep the report confidential. • Report to nurse manager. • Confer with risk manager. • Work to provide nursing care to meet established standards. • Attend all staff development programs. • Confirm all telephone orders in writing.	• Place blame on anyone • Place on the patient's chart. • Make entry about an incident report on the patient's chart. • Alter or rewrite. • Report hearsay or opinion. • Be afraid to consult, ask questions, or complete incident reports. They can be part of your best defense and protection. • Prescribe in the MDs domain. • Be cold and impersonal to patients, families, or visitors.

Figure 21–5 • *DOs and DON'Ts of Incident Reporting*

SUMMARY

Quality assurance programs make certain that patient care is delivered that meets established standards. QA programs have as their objective the determination of whether the actual service provided matches predetermined criteria of excellence. Quality assurance also involves continuous action to improve deficiencies.

QA is a management process that provides a sound basis for decision making and problem solving. Management of care by competent clinical nurses and nurse managers ensures the quality of that care.

EXPERIENTIAL EXERCISES

1. Figure 21-6 represents the standards for quality assurance measurement of patient care processes and outcomes. Select 10 charts of medical patients in the institution in which you work as a student,

five charts of current patients and five charts of discharged patients. Apply the standards to determine the percentage of compliance for each.

2. Summarize your results using Figure 21–7. Include your conclusions, actions to be taken, and follow-up to be done.

3. Group Exercise: Form groups of five to eight persons. Read the following case study.

Case Study: Ms. Alice Logan, a 91-year-old widow, was admitted to a nursing home by ambulance from the community hospital on February 1, 1984. She was assessed by a Registered Nurse as able to walk short distances with assistance and holding on to furniture, being blind, needing assistance with ADL, having adequate hearing and speaking ability, mucous membranes being pink and moist, skin cool and dry to touch with skin turgor being fair, heart rate regular and strong, respirations rapid at times and complaining of SOB, lung fields clear bilaterally and breath sounds de-

Standard I	% Compliance
1. The patient had a complete system assessment by a registered nurse on admission.	(100% compliance)
1.1 The initial assessment was completed within 30 minutes of arrival to the unit.	(100% compliance)
1.2 The complete assessment was done during the shift or as the condition changed.	(95% compliance)
2. The nursing diagnosis was made.	(100% compliance)
3. Nursing prescriptions (orders) were made.	(100% compliance)
4. Nurse and physician orders were carried out.	(100% compliance)
5. Outcomes were evaluated.	(100% compliance)
5.1 Daily effects of nursing prescriptions (orders) were done.	(100% compliance)
5.2 Outcomes of nursing prescriptions (orders) were evaluated for discharge.	(100% compliance)
6. Specific nursing diagnoses and prescriptions were accomplished.	(100% compliance)
6.1 IV fluids and medication were documented as to start date and time.	(100% compliance)
6.2 IV site evaluation was done and documented each shift.	(100% compliance)
6.3 IV fluid changes were done and documented each shift.	(100% compliance)
6.4 IV tubing was changed, dated, timed, and documented each 48 hours.	(100% compliance)
6.5 IV site was changed and documented each 72 hours	(100% compliance)

Standard II	% Compliance
1. The patient with a nursing diagnosis of *comfort, alteration in* was provided with appropriate nursing prescription during hospitalization and at discharge.	(100% compliance)
1.1 The nursing diagnosis of *comfort, alteration in* was documented when appropriate.	(100% compliance)
1.2 Nursing prescription for pain and/or discomfort was done and documented.	(100% compliance)
1.3 The patient and/or family were involved in nursing prescription for pain and/or discomfort.	(100% compliance)
1.4 Physician prescriptions for pain and/or discomfort were appropriately done and documented.	(100% compliance)
1.5 The patient was prepared to manage pain and/or discomfort following discharge (if appropriate).	(100% compliance)

Figure 21–6 • *Process and Outcome Indicators*

creased posteriorly, hand grip good in both hands, abdomen soft without tenderness and with active bowel sounds, and no broken skin areas noted.

Ms. Logan had lived in the community with anyone who would care for her. She was socially deprived. Her admitting diagnosis included:

1. Possible cerebral vascular accident with right-sided weakness; inability to walk.
2. Mild hypertension.
3. Abdominal pain; left renal cyst.
4. Hiatal hernia.
5. Post-bulbar stenotic area in the duodenum.
6. Blindness secondary to glaucoma, both eyes.
7. Organic brain syndrome.
8. Social deprivation.

She was constantly falling down and unable to care for herself. A nursing care plan done by a registered nurse on the day of admission included as problem #2:

PROBLEM: Episodes of unresponsiveness. History of falls.

GOAL: Will not injure self from fall, ongoing.

Month:	Department/Service:
	Overall Analysis

I. *Process Monitoring*

Conclusion:

Action:

Follow-up:

SOURCE: Courtesy of the University of South Alabama Medical Center, Mobile, Alabama.

Figure 21–7 • *University of South Alabama Medical Center Monthly Narrative Analysis of Process*

APPROACH: 1. Side rails up on bed.
2. Restrain PRN in chair.
3. Assist with ambulation.
4. Call bell within reach.

The formal plan was updated in writing every 3 months by policy.

Among the notes:

"This 93-year-old female is alert and oriented. Very friendly and enjoys attention. She attends large group activities with assistance. She attended the birthday party and also the Valentine party. Seems to enjoy parties and group singing. Plans: (1) visit, (2) assign volunteers to sit in once a week, (3) assist to large group activities."

Signed by Recreation Therapist

"1/15/90 3–11 T 97.4 P 88 R 18 BP 110/60. Ambulatory around room via walker. Call buzzer placed within reach. Explained to client how it is to be used and the reason she should cease climbing over side rails. States that she understands and would ring for assistance when needed. Diet and evening meds tolerated well. States that she is unable to see anything. Observation to continue."

Signed by an LPN

Subsequent notes record that Ms. Logan would not use call light and a nursing decision was made to create an environment that would be as safe as possible and allow Ms. Logan to be as independent as possible. The bed was positioned with one side rail up so she would exit and enter bed from the same side; furniture was placed to minimize falls; Ms. Logan was oriented to the room geography; her call bell was kept in reach and it was noted that this entailed the risk of a possible fall.

Records indicate that Ms. Logan enjoyed the nursing home environment, could perform most of the ADL herself, and was observed for falls and safety.

During a 22-month period, brief entries were made in chart daily by LPNs and RNs. Nurses' aides checked off ADLs each shift. A typical biweekly summary reads:

"September 25, 1990, Wt 118 lbs, BP range 110/70–130/60. This ambulatory client's condition appears stable. Was granted a 3-day pass with daughter on 8/13/90. Returned to facility in satisfactory condition. Appeared cheerful and stated that she really enjoyed herself. Sight is blind. Skin turgor good for age and diagnosis. Speech is clear. Tissues normal. Hears well. Is alert and oriented in spheres X III. Meals fed per self are usually taken well. ADLs are assisted with by staff. Enjoys attending planned activities about facility, especially those of a religious nature. Surroundings are kept hazard-free. Ambulates to toilet in room PRN. Will continue to observe and render care."

Signed by an LPN

During a period of 72 months, Ms. Logan fell twice. She was appropriately examined and treated both times. The second time she fell and fractured her right hip. She was treated successfully and was still living as of July 1990. The family sued the nursing home because nursing personnel "Negligently or wantonly failed to exercise due care in the care and treatment of the plaintiff in that she was allowed to fall from her bed onto the floor, or to some other hard object, and as a proximate consequence of said negligence or wantonness, she received the broken right hip, and she has suffered excruciating physical pain and mental anguish, and is still suffering and will continue for the remainder of her life to suffer from such pain and mental anguish."

3.1 As an expert nurse witness how would you defend the nursing staff?

3.2 What are the implications for quality assurance?

3.3 What are the implications for risk management?

4. Read one of the following articles and prepare an abstract of approximately one page, double spaced, that summarizes the key points made by the author.

G. Marker, "The Marker Model: A Hierarchy for Nursing Standards," *Journal of Nursing Quality Assurance,* Feb. 1987, 7–20.

Any recent article from the *Journal of Quality Assurance* or *QA Review,* or other recent articles on quality assurance in nursing journals.

NOTES

1. M. J. Zimmer, "A Model for Evaluating Nursing Care," in *Management for Nurses: A Multidisciplinary Approach,* M. S. Berger, D. Elkart, S. C. Firsich, S. B. Jordan, and S. Stone, eds. (St. Louis, MO: C. V. Mosby, 1980), 47–52.
2. L. F. Maciorowski, E. Larson, and A. Keane, "Quality Assurance: Evaluate Thyself," *Journal of Nursing Administration,* June 1985, 38–42.
3. L. Edmunds, "A Computer Assisted Quality Assurance Model," *Journal of Nursing Administration,* Mar. 1983, 36–43; A. DeLotto, "Examining Quality of Care Becomes Top Industry Priority," *Amherst Quarterly,* Winter 1988, 1–3.
4. B. J. Curtis and L. J. Simpson, "Auditing: A Method for Evaluating Quality of Care," *Journal of Nursing Administration,* Oct. 1985, 14–21; M. A. Wandelt and M. D. Phaneuf, "Tools for Evaluation," in *Management for Nurses,* op. cit., 229; H. S. Rowland and B. L. Rowland, *Nursing Administration Handbook,* 3d ed. (Rockville, MD: Aspen, 1992), 367–393.
5. Ibid.
6. Ibid.
7. Curtis and Simpson, op. cit.
8. Edmunds, op. cit.
9. H. S. Rowland and B. L. Rowland, eds., "Quality Assurance," *Hospital Legal Forms, Checklists, and Guidelines* (Rockville, MD: Aspen, 1988), 26:1–26:14.
10. S. R. Edwardson and D. I. Anderson, "Hospital Nurses' Valuation of Quality Assurance," *Journal of Nursing Administration,* July-Aug. 1983, 33–39.
11. Ibid.
12. B. H. Munro, "A Useful Model for Program Evaluation," *Journal of Nursing Administration,* Mar. 1983, 23–26.
13. Rowland and Rowland, *Nursing Administration Handbook,* op. cit.
14. Edmunds, op. cit.
15. D. C. Coddington and K. D. Moore, "Quality of Care as a Business Strategy," *Healthcare Forum Journal,* Mar.-Apr. 1987, 29–32.
16. Ibid.
17. R. Levy, "The Go-Go World of the Risk Manager," *Dun's Review,* Nov. 1967.
18. G. W. Poteet, "Risk Management and Nursing," *Nursing Clinics of North America,* Sept. 1983, 457–465.
19. Ibid.
20. A. P. Sielicki, "Current Philosophy of Risk Management," *Topics in Health Care Financing,* Spring 1983, 3.
21. Rowland and Rowland, eds., *Hospital Legal Forms, Checklists, and Guidelines,* op. cit., 28:1–28:58.
22. Sielicki, op. cit.
23. "QAs Pave the Way: The Quest for Quality," *Hospital Profiles,* Alabama Hospital Association, Dec. 1987/Jan. 1988, 1, 4–5.
24. Poteet, op. cit; Rowland and Rowland, op. cit; and K. H. Henry, ed., *Nursing Administration and Law Manual* (Rockville, MD: Aspen, 1985), 9:1–9:39.
25. Ibid.
26. Ibid.

FOR FURTHER REFERENCE

Allio, R., "Forecasting: The Myth of Control," interview with Donald Michal, *Planning Review,* May 1986, 6–11.

Blake, P., "Incident Investigation: A Complete Guide," *Nursing Management,* Nov. 1987, 36–41.

Breland, D., "Medical Care Crisis Feared in State," *Mobile Register,* Sept. 25, 1985, B1, B6.

Buros, O. K., *Mental Measurements Yearbooks* (Highland Park, NJ: Gryphon Press, 1938, 1940, 1949, 1953, 1959, 1965, 1972, 1978).

Chun, K. T., Cobb, S., and French, J. R. P., Jr., *Measures for Psychological Assessment: A Guide to 3,000 Original Sources and Their Applications* (Ann Arbor: Institute for Social Research, University of Michigan, 1975).

Deep, W. M., "Dilemma of a Malpractice Insurer's Appointed Defense Attorney," *PLN* (Insurance Corporation of America), Sept. 1985, 2–5.

Hermon, S. A., "QA at St. Joseph's—Every Nurse's Responsibility, Every Nurse's Obligation," *Nursing Directions* (St. Joseph's Hospital Centers), July 1987, 1–3.

Joint Commission on Accreditation of Healthcare Organizations, *Quality Review Bulletin* (875 North Michigan Avenue, 22nd Floor, Chicago, IL 60611).

Joseph, D., and Jones, S. K., "Incident Reporting: The Cornerstone of Risk Management," *Nursing Management,* Dec. 1984, 22–23.

Kinloch, K., "For Nurses Only: Should Nursing Administrators Use Incident Reports as a Risk Management Tool?," *Canadian Nurse,* Nov. 1982, 16–17.

Larson, E., "Combining Nursing Quality Assurance and Research Programs," *Journal of Nursing Administration,* Nov. 1983, 32–34.

"Malpractice Crisis Threatens Health of Medical Profession," *Alexian Way,* Summer 1985, 3–9.

Purgatorio-Howard, K., "Improving a Quality Assurance Program," *Nursing Management,* Apr. 1986, 38–40, 42.

"QAs Pave the Way: The Quest for Quality," *Hospital Profiles* (Alabama Hospital Association, Dec. 1987/Jan. 1988), 1, 4–5.

Renzulli, J. S., *A Guidebook for Evaluating Programs for the Gifted and Talented* (Ventura, CA: Office of the Ventura County Superintendent of Schools, 1975).

Renzulli, J. S., "Key Features: A Practical Model for Program Evaluation," *Curriculum Trends,* Feb. 1972, 1–6.

Schuman, J. E., Ostfeld, A. M., and Willard, H. N., "Discharge Planning in an Acute Hospital," *Archives of Physical Medicine and Rehabilitation*, July 1976, 343–347.

Smeltzer, C. H., Geltman, B., and Rajki, K., "Nursing Quality Assurance: A Process, Not a Tool," *Journal of Nursing Administration*, Jan. 1983, 5–9.

Spicer, J. G., and Lewis, G. M., "Using Theory to Promote Change," *Nursing Administration Quarterly*, Winter 1981, 53–57.

Ward, M. J., and Lindeman, C. E., eds., *Instruments for Measuring Nursing Practice and Other Health Care Variables*, 2 vols., DHEW Publication No. HRA78-53 (Hyattsville, MD: U.S. Dept. of Health, Education, and Welfare, 1979).

Wolff, G. M., "Systems Management: Evaluating Nursing Departments as a Whole," *Nursing Management*, Feb. 1986, 40–43.

Performance Appraisal

INTRODUCTION

Performance appraisal is a control process in which employees' performances are evaluated against standards. The literature on performance appraisal is voluminous, indicating its value to management. Considerable research has been done on various aspects of the performance appraisal process.

Neither employees nor managers like performance appraisal. Some employees view performance appraisal as being more valued by top management than by themselves and their supervisors. Some managers do not like to do performance appraisals because it makes them feel guilt: "Did I do justice by the employee?" As writers of performance appraisals, managers are concerned that they may "cast something in stone" that is inaccurate, may be criticized on written grammar and spelling, or say something illegal about the ratee or that may not be able to be substantiated.[1] Other managers are afraid of employees' reactions to ratings. Also, performance appraisal requires careful planning, information gathering, and an extensive formal interview, a time-consuming process. Managers usually perform activities of short duration, attend ad hoc meetings, perform nonroutine behavior, and focus on current information, all short-term activities in comparison with ongoing performance appraisal.[2] Furthermore, the process is usually not interactive, moves slowly, is passive, is isolated, and is not oriented toward people.[3]

Measurement of performance is imprecise. Often the focus is on the format, not the people. In some organizations the human resources department sends the rating forms to the departments shortly before the end of the fiscal year. They have to be completed immediately and are done with little or no training and preparation of either rater or ratee. The result is distrust by employees and dread by managers.

A survey of Fortune 1300 companies (1000 industrial and 300 nonindustrial) indicated that 29 percent of hourly workers are not evaluated by a formal appraisal system. Thirty-nine percent of respondents indicated that, where used, performance appraisal systems are "extremely effective" or "very effective." They are underappreciated.[4]

Performance appraisal systems require top management commitment. They can be tied to the planning cycle by relating them to personnel budgets or including them as a management plan.

PURPOSES OF PERFORMANCE APPRAISAL

Performance appraisal is a nurse manager's most valuable tool in controlling human resources and productivity. The performance appraisal process can be used effectively to govern employee behavior in order to produce goods and services in high volume and of high quality. Nurse managers can also use the performance appraisal process to govern corporate direction in selecting, training, guiding career planning, and rewarding of personnel. The Fortune 1300 survey indicated that 80 percent used appraisal systems to justify merit increases, provide feedback, and identify candidates for promotion, all considered short-range goals. They were linked to long-range goals of performance potential for succession planning and career planning, but could be much more useful in strategic planning. Fifty-eight percent used performance appraisal to identify strengths and weaknesses, while 39 percent used it for career planning. Eighty-nine percent used it for general guidelines for salary increases, while only 1 percent used it for forced distribution for bonuses. Forced distribution sets a limit on the number of high-level ratings.[5]

In addition to being used for promotions, termination, selections, and compensations, performance monitoring has been found to make employees effective. It is a managerial tool that can facilitate performance levels that achieve the company's mission and objectives.[6]

Appraisal systems are needed to meet legal requirements including those for standardized forms and procedures, clear and relevant job analysis, and trained raters. When they do not, disciplinary actions including termination do not stand up in court.[7]

Motivation

A goal of performance appraisal is to stimulate motivation of the employee to perform the tasks and accomplish the mission of the organization. Promotions, assignments, selection for education, and increased pay are among the goals of the employee that stimulate this motivation. If performance appraisal is to improve performance, the science of behavior technology should be used. This science has as its basis the premise that consequences will influence behavior. People will work more willingly if supervisors or managers exercise concern for their feelings and needs. A basic question here is, what rewards will the employee work for?

The Xerox Experience. Before 1983, Xerox had a traditional appraisal system tying merit pay increases to performance rating. Employees were dissatisfied with the lack of an equitable rating distribution. Ninety-five percent of employees were at the 3 or 4 level of a four-level rating system. Forced distribution was used to control the numbers of employees above or below a specific level. There were no preplanned objectives, the focus being on the summary rating. A task force was used to develop a performance feedback and development process with the following characteristics:

1. Objectives were set between manager and employee.
2. The evaluation was documented and approved by a second-level manager.
3. An appraisal review was held at the end of 6 months, with review and discussion of objectives and progress. The written report was signed by both.
4. A final review was held at 1 year.
5. The process emphasized performance feedback and improvements.
6. A merit increase discussion was held 1 to 2 months later.
7. There was agreement on personal goals related to communications, planning, time management, human relations, and professional goals (specialty and job).
8. There were financial and human resource management objectives.
9. Managers were trained in the process.

Regular surveys of the Xerox system indicated that 81 percent of employees understood their work group objectives better, 84 percent considered appraisal fair, 72 percent understood how merit pay was determined, 70 percent met personal and professional objectives, and 77 percent favored the system.[8]

Other Purposes of Performance Appraisal

An effective appraisal generates understanding and commitment, leading to productivity. Career development and performance appraisal support each other if they share objectives, recognition, concern, and communication. Usually nurse managers take charge of performance appraisal while employees take charge of career development. They can be brought together for mutual benefit.

Talent development can be a mutual goal and benefit of the two programs. Performance input supports future options and paths for future growth and development of employees.[9]

Performance appraisals can also be used to confirm hiring decisions. This is particularly true when new employees have a probationary period before becoming permanent. This is a crucial period as employees can be terminated without the extended termination process. Effective nurse managers will use this period to counsel and coach the employee to effective performance. The performance appraisal will document the process.

DEVELOPING AND USING STANDARDS FOR PERFORMANCE APPRAISAL

Performance Standards

Performance standards are derived from job analysis, job descriptions, and job evaluation and other documents detailing the qualitative and quantitative aspects of jobs. They are established by authority, which may be the agency in which they are used or a professional association such as the American Nurses' Association (ANA). They are measuring sticks for qualitative and quantitative evaluation of the individual's performance. They should be based on appropriate knowledge and practical enough to be attained. Like other documents, they must be kept up to date. Job or performance standards for the nurse manager may be developed using the ANA *Standards for Organized Nursing Services and Responsibilities of Nurse Administrators Across All Settings.*

Performance standards are written for a job and are used to measure the performance of the individual filling the job. Employees should know that these standards are being used and what they are. They may be asked to bring them to their supervisor for scheduled counseling. They may also be asked to list their accomplishments in relation to the standards. This makes performance counseling less of a threat and allows employees to recognize and discuss their accomplishments. They may be guided into recognition of those areas where their performance falls short and to voice goals for improvement in these areas. This method of using performance standards has been found to be effective.

The ANA Congress for Nursing Practice has developed and published standards of practice in several areas: nursing practice, community health nursing practice, geriatric nursing practice, maternal-child health nursing practice, psychiatric-mental health nursing practice, medical-surgical nursing practice, emergency room nursing practice, cardiovascular nursing practice, orthopedic nursing practice, operating room nursing practice, and others. The ANA *Standards of Clinical Nursing Practice* can be used in the development of performance standards.

Figure 22–1 is an example of performance standards for a clinical nurse.

Job analysis, job descriptions, and job evaluations are important sources of standards for performance evaluation.

Job Analysis

Edwards and Sproull list "objective performance dimensions, developed by management and employees" as a necessity for effective performance appraisal. These dimensions are developed from job analysis. "Performance criteria should be: (1) measurable through observation of behaviors of the job, (2) clearly defined, and (3) job-related." Nurse managers and nursing employees would agree on the meaning and priority of each measurement. These standards need not be quantifiable but must be keyed to observable behavior:[10]

Observable Behavior → Job Analysis
→ Job Standards

Basing performance appraisal on job analysis makes it more relevant and establishes content validity.[11] Job analysis systematically gathers information about a particular job. It "identifies, specifies, organizes, and displays the duties, tasks, and responsibilities actually performed by the incumbent in a given job."[12]

The job analysis will reveal overlaps among jobs so that they can be modified. It can be used to improve efficiency and proficiency by identifying skills certification, altering staffing levels, reassign-

Performance Standards

1. Type of work: Nursing care of patients.

   Major duty: Performs the primary functions of a professional nurse (50 percent of working hours).

   a. Obtains nursing histories on all newly admitted patients.
   b. Reviews nursing histories of all transfer patients.
   c. Uses nursing histories to make nursing diagnoses determining patients' needs and problems.

   Using this information:

   d. Initiates a nursing care plan for each patient.
   e. Lists goal(s) for each nursing need or problem.
   f. Writes nursing prescription or orders for each patient to meet each need or problem and goal.
   g. Applies the plan of care, giving evidence of knowledge of scientific and legal principles.
   h. Executes physicians' orders.

2. Type of work: Management of nursing personnel.

   Major duty: Plans nursing care of patients on a daily basis (14 percent of working hours).

   a. Rates each patient according to number and complexity of needs and goals.
   b. Knows abilities of each team member.
   c. Makes a daily assignment for each team member.
   d. Discusses assignment with each team member at the beginning of each shift.

      1. Listens to taped report with team members.
      2. Sees that team members review physicians' orders and nursing care plans.
      3. Answers questions arising from these activities.

   e. Confers with clinical nurse manager and unit clerk periodically to ascertain whether there are any new orders.
   f. Plans for a team conference at a specific time and place and tells team members.
   g. Incorporates division and unit philosophy and objectives into team activities.
   h. Assists with assignment of LPN and RN students, including them as active team members according to their backgrounds and learning needs.

3. Type of work: Management of nursing personnel.

   Major duty: Supervises team activities (10 percent of working hours).

   a. Makes frequent rounds to assist team members with their care of patients. At the same time, talks to and observes patients to determine:

      1. New needs or problems.
      2. Progress. Confirms these observations with patient if possible.

   b. Conducts 15- to 20-minute team conference using a specific agenda that has been made known to team members at previous day's conference.

      1. Involves all team members.
      2. Solicits comments on new problems or special problems of patients and updates selected nursing care plans as needed.
      3. Assigns roles for next day's team conference.

   c. Writes nursing progress notes and updates remaining nursing care plans.

      1. Assists technicians with writing notes as needed for training. Otherwise reads and countersigns their notes. Writes own notes.
      2. Updates those nursing care plans not done at team conference. Recognizes this is a professional nurse's responsibility.
      3. Reads notes of LPNs and RNs.

   d. Communicates nursing service and hospital policies to team members on a daily basis through referral to such information as daily bulletins, minutes of meetings, and changes in regulations.

4. Type of work: Management of equipment and supplies.

   Major duty: Identifies needs; plans and submits requests for new and replacement equipment and supplies to clinical nurse manager (1 percent of working hours).

   a. While working with team members, identifies malfunctioning equipment and supply shortages and reports same to clinical nurse manager and unit clerk on a daily basis.

Figure 22–1 • *Performance Standards—Clinical Nurse*

b. Submits requests for new equipment and supplies to clinical nurse manager on a quarterly basis.

5. Type of work: Training.

Major duty: Identifies training needs of team members and plans activities to meet needs (5 percent of working hours).

a. Identifies specific training needs of individual team members through daily observation of their performance and interviews.
b. Evaluates performance through use of performance standards. Makes these standards known to each team member and holds them responsible for meeting standards.
c. Plans counseling and guidance of each team member on an individual basis, and at least quarterly.
d. Plans and conducts unit in-service education programs at least monthly. Involves team members.
e. Recommends team members for seminars, short courses, college programs, and correspondence courses.
f. Thoroughly orients all new team members. Conducts skill inventory during initial interview and plans on-the-job training for those needed skills in which team member is not proficient.
g. Submits budget requests for training materials and programs to clinical nurse manager annually.
h. Makes reading assignments and allows time for team members to use library resources.

6. Type of work: Planning patient care.

Major duty: Coordinates nursing resources essential to meeting each patient's total needs and goals (5 percent of working hours).

a. Consults with patients' physicians daily.
b. Requests consultations of clinical nurse specialists. This may include clinical nurse specialists in pediatrics, mental health, adult health, radiology, public health, and rehabilitation.
c. Consults with other personnel as needed, including chaplain, social worker, recreation worker, occupational therapist, physical therapist, pharmacist, and inhalation therapist. Coordinates with

physicians and clinical nurse manager as needed.
d. Supports philosophy of having unit clerks assume nonnursing activities by assisting with their training as needed on a daily basis, to help them become proficient in their duties.
e. Aggressively pursues having unit clerks do administrative tasks and nursing team members perform the primary functions of nursing. The latter most commonly occurs at patients' bedsides.

7. Type of work: Teaching patients.

Major duty: Teaches patients to care for themselves after discharge from the hospital (5 percent of working hours).

a. Plans teaching as a major rehabilitation goal of each newly admitted patient. Includes it as part of nursing assessment and enters it on the nursing care plan.
b. Reviews and updates teaching plans daily.
c. Involves resource people in teaching program.
d. Refers cases to visiting nurse for follow-up.
e. Makes follow-up appointments for assessment of progress toward nursing goals with a clinical nurse.
f. Involves families in teaching as indicated.

8. Type of work: Evaluation of care process.

Major duty: Conducts audits of nursing care (3 percent of working hours).

a. Audits nursing records on a daily basis.
b. Performs bedside audit on a weekly basis.
c. Audits closed charts of discharged patients on a monthly basis.
d. Reviews patient questionnaires.
e. Discusses results of all audits with team members as a group and on an individual basis.

9. Type of work: Personnel administration.

Major duty: Rates performances of team members (2 percent of working hours).

a. Writes performance reports.
b. Discusses reports with individuals to learn their personal goals.

10. Type of work: Self-development.

Major duty: Pursues a program of continuing education activities (5 percent of working hours).

a. Sets own goals for self-development including a reading program and a set of

Figure 22–1 (*Continued*)

educational goals for short courses, conventions, workshops, college courses, and management courses.
  b. Participates in division and departmental in-service education programs.
  c. Participates in nursing service committee activities.
  d. Participates in research projects.
  e. Participates as a citizen in the community through involvement in professional

organizations and service projects.
  f. Assumes responsibility for knowledge of, progress in, and use of community resources such as:
   1. Health groups.
   2. Civic groups.
   3. General education groups.
   4. Nursing recruitment.
   5. Others.

Figure 22–1   (Continued)

ing staff, selecting new employees, altering management, establishing training objectives and standards, developing career ladders, and improving job satisfaction.[13]

A procedure for doing job analysis is as follows:

1. Name the job specifically, e.g., nurse manager, oncology.
2. Go to the work place, identify the target nurses working in the job family, and talk to them. Ask these questions:

   2.1 What are the characteristics of a good clinical nurse?
   2.2 What are the characteristics of a poor clinical nurse?
   2.3 How does a good clinical nurse differ from a poor clinical nurse?
   2.4 How does a good clinical nurse perform tasks better than others?
   2.5 Give examples of effective performance by a clinical nurse.
   2.6 Why is this clinical nurse effective?
   2.7 Give examples of ineffective performance by a clinical nurse.
   2.8 Why is this clinical nurse ineffective?
   2.9 Describe a clinical nurse who performs the job better than anyone else. Why?
   2.10 What job skills would you look for if you had to hire someone to do clinical nursing? Why?
   2.11 Describe the prior training or experience needed to effectively perform clinical nursing. Why is this so?

3. Have the job incumbents list all duties, tasks, and responsibilities (DTRs) that they perform. Do for a specific time period.
4. As manager, list all DTRs that the job incumbents perform. Do by observation for specific time period coinciding with incidents. These can be prepared one to each index card.
5. Compare the two lists and aim for consensus between job incumbents and manager.
6. State the duties, tasks, and responsibilities in specific, clear behavioral terms.
7. Determine the four to eight job task categories to be used such as: managerial, direct care, maintenance, and interpersonal.
8. Classify each DTR into the four to eight core job categories.
9. List the DTRs by priority. Use consensus. This will improve efficiency.
10. Evaluate DTRs for specificity indicating how and when they will be performed.
11. Review with the team, eliminating those with low priority. Rewrite items as needed, making each a unique job skill stated in understandable language.
12. Set standards of performance, including the percentage of time each is to be done.
13. List constraints: education, experience, physical, and emotional.
14. Write a summary of the unique facets of the job.
15. Prepare a job analysis questionnaire and administer it to all personnel with the same job title.[14] See Figure 22–2 for format.

Job analysis leads to a job description of the work expected by the institution, which can be used for performance appraisal.

Job Descriptions

The Job Description as a Contract.   A job description is a contract that should include the job's functions and obligations and tell the person to whom the worker is responsible. It is a written report out-

Title: Head Nurse

A. Check here if you ever do the task in your present job.	B. Relative Time Spent			C. Training Emphasis		
	Lo 1 2 3	Avg 4 5 6	Hi 7 8 9	Lo 1 2 3	Avg 4 5 6	Hi 7 8 9

___ 1. (List DTRs)

___ 2.

Figure 22–2 • Job Analysis Questionnaire

lining duties, responsibilities, and conditions of the work assignment. It is a description of a job and not of a person who happens to hold that job. "That many executives recognize the importance of obtaining good position descriptions is reflected in a survey made several years ago by the American Management Association. In this study, seventy firms reported a median fee of $20,000 paid to management consultants for preparation of their job descriptions. Most significantly, 95 percent of the respondents reported that the expenditure was 'definitely worthwhile.' In two instances the fee paid for this service approached $100,000."[15] Most formats include a job title, statements of basic functions, scope, duties, responsibilities, organizational relationships, limits of authority, and criteria for performance evaluation.

What Are Job Descriptions Used For? Job descriptions are used for many purposes:

1. To establish a rational basis for the salary structure, thus showing why one job pays more salary then another. For example, job descriptions should show why a clinical nurse manager earns less than a director of nursing.
2. To clarify relationships between jobs to avoid overlaps and gaps in responsibility.
3. To help employees analyze their duties so that they will have a better understanding of their jobs.
4. To help define the organizational structure and support or give evidence for its revision.
5. To reassign and fix functions and responsibilities in the entire agency.
6. To evaluate job performance.
7. To orient new employees to jobs.
8. To assist in hiring and placement of employees.

9. To establish lines of promotion within the department.
10. To identify potential training needs.
11. To critically review the existing nursing practices within the agency.
12. To maintain continuity of all operations in a changing work environment.
13. To improve the work flow.
14. To provide data as to proper channels of communication.
15. To develop job specifications.
16. To serve as a basis for planning staffing levels.

Introduction of a system using job descriptions requires planning and should be built into the operational or management plan for accomplishment of departmental objectives.

A format is needed for quality and thoroughness of job descriptions. Kennedy recommends the following parts:

1. Header: job title, name and location of incumbent, immediate superiors.
2. Principal purpose or summary; overall contribution of incumbent.
3. Principal responsibilities, including percent of time spent on each.
4. Job skills: knowledge, skills, and education.
5. Dimension or scope: quantifies such areas as the budget, size of reporting organizations, impact on bottom line.
6. Organization chart.
7. Problem-solving examples.
8. Environment.
9. Key contacts.
10. References guiding incumbent's actions.
11. Supervision given and received.[16]

Job descriptions can be written to comply with some legal, regulatory, and accrediting requirements. The following are examples:

1. Licensing laws of the state, rules of accrediting agencies, and of Medicare and Medicaid can be met through job descriptions.
2. They can be used for job rating and classification.
3. They can be used to determine whether jobs are exempt or nonexempt.
4. They can be used in recruitment, selection, evaluation, and retention.[17]

Figure 22–3 presents a job description for a bedside nurse in a U.S. hospital about 1887.

Figure 22–4 is a job description for a generalized clinical nurse in 1992.

Job Evaluation

Job evaluation is a process that measures exact amounts of base elements found in jobs. Laws require men and women to be paid equally for equal work requiring equal skill, knowledge, effort, and responsibility under similar working conditions. This is an important factor in the fight to achieve pay equity for women and hence for nurses.[18]

TRAINING

A lack of training is considered a management and organizational shortcoming in which managers allow employees to give unsatisfactory performance. Unsatisfactory performance allowed to exist indicates substandard management. Nurse managers should be educated to do effective performance appraisals that will maintain employees' productivity. Training will entail coverage of such subjects as motivational environment, appropriate job assignment, proper supervision, establishing job expectancies, appropriate job training, interpersonal relationships, interviewing, coaching, counseling, and performance appraisal methods.

Training raters makes performance appraisal work. The goal of such training is improved productivity. A 2-day training program can give nurse managers a conceptual understanding of performance appraisal as a management system for transmitting, reinforcing, and rewarding the behaviors desired by the organization. Raters need to know how performance appraisals will be used. Research indicates that raters have been found to vary ratings depending on their uses. Refresher

In its publication *Bright Corridor*, Cleveland's Lutheran Hospital published this job description for a bedside nurse in a U.S. hospital about 1887:

In addition to caring for your fifty patients, each bedside nurse will follow these regulations:

1. Daily sweep and mop the floors of your ward, dust the patient's furniture and window sills.

2. Maintain an even temperature in your ward by bringing in a scuttle of coal for the day's business.

3. Light is important to observe the patient's condition. Therefore, each day fill kerosene lamps, clean chimneys, and trim wicks. Wash the windows once a week.

4. The nurse's notes are important in aiding the physician's work. Make your pens carefully, you may whittle nibs to your individual tastes.

5. Each nurse on day duty will report every day at 7:00 A.M. and leave at 8:00 P.M., except on the Sabbath, on which day you will be off from 12:00 noon to 2:00 P.M.

6. Graduate nurses in good standing with the director of nursing will be given an evening off each week for courting purposes, or two a week if you go regularly to church.

7. Each nurse should lay aside from each pay day a goodly sum of her earnings for her benefits during her declining years, so that she will not become a burden. For example, if you earn $30 a month you should set aside $15.

8. Any nurse who smokes, uses liquor in any form, gets her hair done at a beauty shop, or frequents dance halls will give the director of nurses good reason to suspect her worth, intentions, and integrity.

9. The nurse who performs her labors, serves her patients and doctors faithfully and without fault for a period of 5 years will be given an increase by the hospital administration of $.05 a day, providing there are no hospital debts that are outstanding.

Figure 22–3 • 1887 Job Description

training is recommended after one year. Performance appraisal training can be conducted with other management development programs.[19]

FEEDBACK

Feedback has been discussed in the section on management by objectives (MBO) in Chapter 14, a

Title: Generalized Clinical Nurse (GCN)

General Description. The GCN is a professional nurse with academic preparation at the BSN level or above, who provides expert nursing care based on scientific principles; delivers direct patient care and serves as a consultant or technical adviser in the area of health professions; and serves as a role model in the leadership, management, and delivery of quality nursing care by integrating the role components of clinician, administrator, teacher, consultant, and researcher.

Qualifications:

I. Educational:
   A. Graduation from an accredited school of nursing.
   B. Bachelor of Science in Nursing degree required.

II. Personal and Professional:
   A. Current state professional nursing license.
   B. Knowledge of and experience in preventive care (screening and teaching).
   C. Demonstrated knowledge and competence in nursing, communication, and leadership skills.
   D. Ability to analyze situations, recognize problems, search for pertinent facts, and make appropriate decisions.
   E. Ability to coordinate orientation and continuing education of clinic staff using appropriate teaching strategies.
   F. Ability to apply principles of change, organizational theory, and decision making.
   G. Membership and participation in professional organizations desirable.
   H. Recognition of civic responsibilities of nursing.
   I. Ability to communicate effectively both in writing and verbally.
   J. Evidence of professional manner and conduct.
   K. Optimum physical and emotional health.

Organizational Relationships. The GCN is administratively responsible and accountable to the nurse administrator. The GCN is responsible for assessing, teaching, coordinating, providing appropriate care, and making referrals when necessary.

Activities:

A. Clinician
   1. Give direct patient care in selected patient situations and serve as a behavioral model for excellence in practice.
   2. Assist the nursing personnel in assessing individual patient needs and formulation of a plan of nursing care; write nursing orders, when appropriate, for implementation of nursing plan; and assist the nursing personnel in documenting the effectiveness of the individualized care.
   3. Set, evaluate, and reevaluate standards of nursing practice; communicate these standards to the nursing personnel; and change standards as necessary.
   4. Evaluate nursing care given to patients within the clinical area (assessing and teaching); when appropriate, make recommendations for improvement of that care.
   5. Function as a change agent; identify the barriers to more comprehensive health care delivery, modify behavior, and introduce new approaches to patient care.
   6. Collaborate with other health care providers and make appropriate referrals when necessary.

B. Teacher
   1. Provide an atmosphere conducive to learning.
   2. Teach appropriate prevention measures to clients.
   3. Direct the orientation of new staff and student nurses to ease their role transition and improve their skills, attitudes, and practices.
   4. Consider the needs of the adult learners (nursing personnel) as well as the clinicians' knowledge and expertise when planning continuing education to the clinical practice.
   5. Initiate or assist with the planning, presenting, and evaluating of continuing education programs for clinic staff.
   6. Guide and assist staff and nursing students as they assume the responsibility of patient teaching.

C. Administrator
   1. Function as a change agent and appraise leadership, communication, and change

Figure 22–4 • *Position Description*

processes in the organization and assist with direct strategies for change as necessary.

  2. Work collaboratively with hospital personnel and other healthcare providers in planning care and making referrals.

  3. Make recommendations relative to improving patient care and staff and student requirements to the appropriate administrative personnel.

  4. Support and interpret the clinic policies and procedures.

D. Self-Development

  1. Assume responsibility for identifying own educational needs and upgrade deficit areas through independent study, seminar attendance, or requesting staff development programs.

  2. Evaluate own nursing practice and instruction of others and the effect these have on the quality of patient care.

E. Consultant

  1. Conduct informal conferences with nursing personnel concerning patient care of specific health problems, the problem patient, or other pertinent problems

related to nursing as suggested by the staff.

  2. Assist personnel to develop awareness of community agencies/resources available in planning patient care.

  3. Serve as a resource person to patients and their families.

F. Researcher

  1. Determine research problems related to preventive care, nursing clinics, etc.

  2. Conduct research studies to upgrade independent nursing practice.

  3. Demonstrate knowledge of the current research applicable to the clinical area and apply this knowledge in nursing care when appropriate.

  4. Research clinical nursing problems through the development and testing of relevant theories, evaluation, and implementation of research findings for nursing practice.

  5. Promote interest in reading and reviewing of current publications dealing with the delivery of preventive care to ambulatory patients.

Figure 22–4 (*Continued*)

process used in performance appraisal, particularly among management personnel.

Feedback can be provided through coaching, counseling, and interviewing.

Coaching

The appraisal rater is a leader and a coach. Coaching for job performance is similar to coaching for athletic performance. As a coach the rater does continuous reinforcement of tasks done well and helps with other tasks. In addition the rater uses knowledge of adult education to train the employees to accomplish assigned work, does two-way communication, and has the necessary resources to do the job.

Coaching can include walking around to observe and listen for examples of work, good or bad. The rater coach praises the good and helps improve the bad with a joint action plan. Coaching makes performance evaluation useful.[20]

Coaching is year-long evaluation and discus-

sion of performance. It eliminates surprises. Progress discussions can be brief, regular, frank, open, factual, and include the employee's viewpoint. In the latter instance the rater does not try to achieve truth but to discuss perception. The coach also removes obstacles to satisfactory performance. If the consequences are not working to improve unsatisfactory performance, the coach changes them. The ultimate resort is to transfer or terminate the employee.[21]

Counseling

Counseling can be the most productive function of supervision. Counseling interviews are for the purpose of advising and assisting an individual to grow and develop self-direction, self-discipline, and individual responsibility. The counseling interview is a helping relationship involving direct interaction between the counselor (rater) and the counselee (ratee). In a counseling interview there is a personal face-to-face relationship. One person helps another recognize, accept, examine, and solve a certain problem.

Nursing managers can use the counseling interview to offer support and:

- Help workers get realistic pictures of themselves, their abilities, their potential, and their deficiencies.
- Explore courses of action.
- Explore sources of assistance.
- Accept incontestable limitations and learn to live with them, whether physical, emotional, or intellectual.
- Make choices and improve capabilities.

Interviewing

Interviewing is covered in Chapter 5. The problem-solving approach is also more effective than "tell and see" or "tell and listen" appraisal interviews. High ratee participation produces greater rater satisfaction. The problem-solving rater has a helpful and constructive attitude; does mutual goal setting with the ratee; focuses on solutions of problems; and acts with the knowledge that harsh criticism does not improve behaviors.[22]

PEER RATINGS

Research has shown that an individual's peers, the people a person works with from day to day, are a more reliable source for identifying the capacity for leadership than are the person's superiors. The armed services have found that peer nominations on leadership are significant predictors of future performance. Democratic procedures, having peers select the person to be promoted, would probably be threatening to many nurse managers. It has been found that peer selection differs little from selections of superiors. Occasionally peers see a member of their group as a leader when superiors do not. Peer rating is valid if the members of the group have sufficient interaction and they are reasonably stable over time. It is also valid if the position is important within the organization. Peer rating does help identify potential leaders who go unnoticed by superiors. Where several individuals are equally qualified for a position, peer ratings may single out the one with the highest informal leadership status.[23]

Peer rating is the professional model of appraisal used by physicians. It is gaining in interest and use among professional nurses. It is advocated as part of a system to make performance appraisals more objective, the theory being that multiple ratings will give a more objective appraisal. They can be obtained from multiple managers, projects leaders, peers, and even patients.[24]

SELF-RATINGS

Self-rating is another method of performance appraisal that is little used. In the Fortune 1300 study, 96 percent of appraisals were done by the immediate supervisors.[25] Problems with self-rating are the same as with supervisory rating, indicating the need for training of the self-rater as well as the supervisory rater.[26]

Employee-developed performance appraisals have been found to be tougher than those of supervisors. Employees are the subject matter experts and do wider coverage of their jobs. Proactive, they establish expectations beforehand. Appraisal interviews are done after self-evaluation. They are done with a common agenda and without surprises, so conversations are more productive. Objectives are under the employee's control. The job elements and performance indicators come from both employees and supervisors so they are legally defensible, broad in perspective, and elicit employee commitment.[27]

Self-evaluation can be developed by using small groups. Having a good job description facilitates development of good behavioral-expectation appraisal forms. They become customized for each position. The human resources department can provide a facilitator and other support. Some questions that will facilitate performance indicators are:

- Think of who has been most effective at this element or task. What behaviors and results can you cite to support your choice?
- Think of the behaviors or results that made you say to yourself, "It would be good if everyone did that."
- What are the "tricks of the trade" related to this task or element?
- Think about times when you do this well and other times when you are not as successful. What causes the difference?
- How is the average performer different from the excellent one?
- If you were training someone, what would you emphasize?[28]

Self-rating has been found to be threatening as the employee places himself or herself in view of others. It is a participative management approach that research supports. Employees who view the organization as being open are more favorable to participative performance appraisals.[29]

Employees can be trained to research their own performance and the work environment. They can make self-assessments against goals and expectations and analyze them. Employees can also be trained to influence management communication skills and to provide information and advice, express their needs, and learn the style of influence to use on the manager. Thus employees become proteges of proactive performers.[30]

PERFORMANCE EVALUATION PROBLEM AREAS

It is largely assumed that merit rating systems of performance evaluation help to develop subordinates and prepare to attest to their readiness for pay increases, promotions, selected assignments, or penalties. When such systems have been scrutinized, three main problem areas have been found:

1. Subordinates have not been motivated to want to change.
2. Even when people recognize a need for a change, they are unable to do so.
3. Subordinates become resentful and anxious when the merit system is implemented conscientiously.[31]

Contrast these two situations. The same job standards are applied in each case. In the first situation the subordinate is handed a completed rating form and is told to read and sign it. She does so but immediately appeals to the next highest level of supervision, saying that it is the lowest rating she has received in 15 years of work and she has never been counseled that the quality of her performance has been slipping. Even though the situation is resolved in favor of the subordinate, she is no longer satisfied to work for the supervisor and has to be transferred.

In another situation the job standards are discussed with the subordinate before they are used. The subordinate is asked to identify those performance factors and responsibilities that are really important to the success of the unit. She is asked to write out the goals of her job as she sees them. They are fully discussed between supervisor and subordinate. Progress is discussed on request of the subordinate and at stated intervals. As a result the subordinate is assisted in planning educational activities that she will accomplish in preparation for the career she desires.

Which situation meets the criterion of an effective performance appraisal?

There are many pitfalls and deficiencies in performance appraisal. Many managers defend it as a system for improving performance. As used, it probably has negative influences, since most people know their shortcomings better than a supervisor. Criticisms by people who have not been adequately trained to manage an appraisal system cause employees to be anxious and frustrated, to feel themselves failures, and, in some cases, to withdraw.

What are the weaknesses? The rater is influenced by the most recent period of performance, an influence that may be positive or negative. Without objective measurements and records, raters tend to focus on the few outstanding activities that are vivid in their minds. Personal feelings influence raters, causing positive or negative halo effects. In many instances the performance is appraised without clear job definitions, job descriptions, and job standards. The employee seldom knows the yardsticks by which performance is being measured. Raters are either lenient or tough, resulting in a great variance in value judgments. Attitudes about whether the employee deserves a pay increase influence the rater. Some managers believe that all employees are average, and they project their beliefs by rating all alike.[32]

Other rating errors include:

- Leniency/stringency error. Raters tend to assign extreme ratings of either poor or excellent.
- Similar-to-me error. Raters rate according to how they view themselves.
- Central tendency error. All ratings are at the middle of the scale.
- First impression error. Raters view all early behavior that may be good or bad and rate all subsequent behaviors similarly.

Other problems of performance appraisal include racial bias, focus on longevity, and complacency of managers. In their usual form they are intrinsically confrontational, emotional, judgmental, and complex. A survey of 360 managers in 190 corporations indicated that 69 percent viewed objectives as unclear; 40 percent saw some payoff but 29 percent saw minimal benefits; 45 percent were only partially involved in setting objectives for their own performance; 81 percent indicated regular progress reviews were not conducted; 52 percent said guidelines for collecting performance data were haphazard or nonexistent; a scant 19 percent viewed performance appraisal as properly planned; and only 37 percent viewed meetings as highly productive, while 30 percent saw no worthwhile results.[33]

Performance appraisals are extrinsically affected when format is improper due to lack of manager preparation, confusion about objectives, once-a-year activity; and over-reliance on forms. Also, there is the extrinsic area of inappropriate values and attitudes: avoidance of conflict to avoid unpleasantness; lack of respect in failing to take appraisal seriously; and, misuse of power causing the ratee to be beaten down, resentful, and uncommitted.[34]

EFFECTIVE MANAGEMENT OF PERFORMANCE APPRAISAL

How do we overcome these pitfalls or deficiencies? First, we must be aware of them. Second, we can learn the management-by-objectives approach and treat people as people. Employees will know by what yardsticks they will be measured. The appraisal will be a joint project. It will be a helpful situation for rater and ratee. Usually, if the situation is working right, ratees will push themselves.

A complex and lengthy evaluation form has not proved effective in rating personnel. Many managers have reduced their rating system to a limited checklist and a write-up that asks for strengths and weaknesses with specific examples to justify each. Many managers will agree to the following principles for a rating system:

1. It should be a simple and effective plan.
2. The procedures and uses of the plan should be understood and agreed on by line management.
3. Factors to be rated should be measurable and agreed on by managers and subordinates.
4. Raters should understand the purpose and nature of the performance review. They should be taught to use the system, observe, write notes including a critical incident file, organize notes and write evaluations that include examples of evidence, edit their reports, and conduct effective review interviews.
5. Raters should understand the meanings of the dimensions rated including their relative weights. Managers are reported to be able to

distinguish between only three levels of performance: poor, satisfactory, and outstanding.
6. Criticism should promote warmth and the building of self-esteem with both the rater and the ratee.
7. The process should be organized and used to manage people on a daily basis.
8. Praise or suggestions for improvement should be done at the time of the event.
9. Standards of performance should be set and modified at the time of the event.
10. Performance standards should be valid, reliable, and fair.
11. Managers should be rewarded for good performance evaluation skills.
12. Professionally accepted procedures should be used for job analysis, developing job-related observable performance criteria, and job classifications. This approach ensures fairness as processes are applied systematically and uniformly throughout the organization.
13. Use a fair employment posture committed to equal opportunity. A conscientious and equitable appraisal system reduces lawsuits and assures fairness and confidence.
14. Measure work output, not habits and traits such as loyalty *unless* they are described by observed behavior examples.
15. Use multiple ratings including those of ratees' subordinates.[35]

SUMMARY

Performance appraisal is a major component of the evaluating or controlling function of nursing management. It is disliked by both raters and ratees. If used appropriately and conscientiously the performance appraisal process will govern employee behavior to produce goods and services in high volume and of high quality.

Purposes or uses of performance evaluation are multiple. In nursing it is used to motivate employees to produce high-quality patient care. The results of performance appraisal are often used for promotion, selection, termination, and improving performance.

Performance appraisal is a part of the science of behavioral technology and should be viewed as part of that body of knowledge that relates to the management of human behavior. Nurse managers need this knowledge to manage the clinical nurse effectively and efficiently as a human resource.

When used for merit pay increases—a retrospective use—performance appraisal should be separated from that which looks to the future. Output-based pay plans have been more effective than time-based pay plans.

Performance appraisal should be done as a system with:

1. Clearly defined performance standards developed by rater and ratee.
2. Objective application of the performance standards—both rater and ratee measuring the latter's performance against the standards.
3. Planned interval feedback with agreed-on improvements when indicated.
4. A continuous cycle. Raters and ratees should trust each other.

Job analysis and job description are essential instruments of behavioral technology used in performance appraisal. They provide objectivity and discriminate among jobs.

Coaching, counseling, and interviewing are skills of an effective performance appraisal system. In addition to supervisor ratings, performance appraisal can include peer ratings, and self-ratings. Problems with performance appraisal systems include poor preparation of raters and ratees, problems of recency, positive and negative halo effects, lack of use of standards, leniency/stringency errors, similar-to-me errors, central tendency errors, and first impression errors.

A simple, well-planned performance appraisal system can be devised. It will be successful when understood by employees and will require considerable supervisory effort using nursing management theory.

EXPERIENTIAL EXERCISES

1. Read the following account of the development and use of performance standards and then answer the questions that follow.

Ms. Heller, RN, was director of nursing in a community hospital with a 180-bed capacity. She wrote job descriptions and performance standards for all the jobs in her department. When they were printed, she had her secretary send a copy of the appropriate job description and performance standard to each employee. Copies were placed in each policy book within the department. Also, she gave the remaining ones to the in-service education co-ordinator to give to each new employee during orientation. Many employees were resentful of the new standards and voiced complaints that they were not appropriate to their jobs and so would be impossible to meet. Ms. Heller did not publish or furnish instructions for their use.

Place a check in the blank beside each statement that supports Ms. Heller's actions as being effective.

____ 1.1 The performance standards were established by authority.

____ 1.2 They will be useful measuring sticks for qualitative and quantitative evaluation of individual performance.

____ 1.3 They are based on appropriate knowledge and are practical enough to be attained.

____ 1.4 Employees know what standards are being used to evaluate their performances.

____ 1.5 Standards are being used for counseling.

____ 1.6 Employees will use the standards for improving their performances.

____ 1.7 This method of using job descriptions and performance standards will increase productivity and make work more satisfying to employees.

2. Group Exercise

2.1 Form groups of five to eight persons.

2.2 Elect a leader to keep the project going to completion.

2.3 Elect a recorder to keep a record of activities.

2.4 Use the procedure for doing a job analysis described in the "Job Analysis" section in this chapter. To facilitate the process, each group member can interview one nurse.

2.5 Analyze and compile the answers to the eleven questions in step 2.

2.6 Collect data on duties, tasks, and responsibilities from these nurses. This can be done with ruled paper, pencils, and clipboards.

2.7 Complete steps 5 through 14.

2.8 Use the format of Figure 22–2 to prepare a job analysis questionnaire. Do it for a clinical nurse. Each item from Figure 22–1 could be a duty, task, or responsibility (DTR).

2.9 Write the job description for a clinical nurse using the completed job analysis.

3. Examine a job description for a clinical nurse in the institution in which you work as a student. Answer the following questions about it.

3.1 What is the job title?

3.2 How are the statements of basic functions described?

3.3 How is the scope of the job defined?

3.4 How are the duties listed?

3.5 How are the responsibilities defined?

3.6 How are the organizational relationships defined?

3.7 How are the limits of authority defined?

3.8 How could the criteria for performance evaluation be identified?

NOTES

1. S. Krantz, "Five Steps to Making Performance Appraisal Writing . . . ," *Supervisory Management*, Dec. 1983, 7–10.
2. R. Zemke, "Is Performance Appraisal a Paper Tiger?" *Training*, Dec. 1985, 24–32.
3. Krantz, op. cit.
4. C. J. Fombrun and R. L. Land, "Strategic Issues in Performance Appraisal: Theory and Practice," *Personnel*, Nov.-Dec. 1983, 23–31.
5. Ibid.
6. C. E. Schneier, A. Geis, and J. A. Wert, "Performance Appraisals: No Appointment Needed," *Personnel Journal*, Nov. 1987, 80–87.
7. Zemke, op. cit.
8. N. R. Deets and D. T. Tyler, "How Xerox Improved Its Performance Appraisals," *Personnel Journal*, Apr. 1986, 50–52.
9. B. Jacobson and B. L. Kaye, "Career Development and Performance Appraisal: It Takes Two to Tango," *Personnel*, Jan. 1986, 26–32.
10. M. R. Edwards and J. R. Sproull, "Safeguarding Your Employee Rating System," *Business*, Apr.-June 1985, 17–27.
11. S. Price and J. Graber, "Employee-Made Appraisals," *Management World*, Feb. 1986, 34–36.
12. D. Ignatavicius and J. Griffith, "Job Analysis: The Basis for Effective Appraisal," *Journal of Nursing Administration*, July-Aug. 1982, 37–41.
13. J. Markowitz, "Managing the Job Analysis Process," *Training and Development Journal*, Aug. 1987, 64–66.
14. Ignatavicius and Griffith, op. cit.; Markowitz, op. cit.; E. P. Prien, I. L. Goldstein, and W. H. Macey, "Multidomain Job Analysis: Procedures and Applications," *Training and Development Journal*, August, 1987, 68–72.
15. C. Berenson and H. O. Ruhnke, "Job Descriptions: Guidelines for Personnel Management," *Personnel Journal*, Jan. 1966, 14–19.
16. W. R. Kennedy, "Train Managers to Write Winning Job Descriptions," *Training and Development Journal*, Apr. 1987, 62–64.
17. H. S. Rowland and B. L. Rowland, eds., *Hospital Legal Forms, Checklists, and Guidelines* (Rockville, MD: Aspen, 1987), 23–28.
18. A. Waintroob, "Comparable Worth Issue: The Employer's Side," *Hospital Manager*, July-Aug. 1985, 6–7.
19. D. C. Martin and K. M. Bardol, "Training the Raters: A Key to Effective Performance Appraisal," *Public Personnel Management*, Summer 1986, 101–109.
20. Schneier, Geis, and Wert, op. cit.
21. V. D. Lachman, "Increasing Productivity through Performance Evaluation," *Journal of Nursing Administration*, Dec. 1984, 7–14.
22. Martin and Bardol, op. cit.
23. G. S. Booker and R. W. Miller, "A Closer Look at Peer Ratings," *Personnel*, Jan.-Feb. 1966, 42–47.
24. M. G. Friedman, "10 Steps to Objective Appraisals," *Personnel Journal*, June 1986, 66–71.
25. Fombrun and Land, op. cit.
26. Zemke, op. cit.
27. Price and Graber, op. cit.
28. Ibid.
29. M. P. Lovrich, "The Dangers of Participative Management: A Test of Unexamined Assumptions Concerning Employee Involvement," *Review of Public Personnel Administration*, Summer 1985, 9–25.
30. Jacobson and Kaye, op. cit.
31. W. M. Fox, "Evaluating and Developing Subordinates," *Notes & Quotes*, Apr. 1969, 4.
32. J. C. Coyant, "The Performance Appraisal: A Critique and an Alternative," *Business Horizons*, June 1973, 73–78.
33. R. E. Lofton, "Performance Appraisals: Why They Go Wrong and How to Do Them Right," *National Productivity Review*, Winter 1985, 54–63.
34. Ibid.
35. Krantz, op. cit.; Martin and Bardol, op. cit.; C. Logan, "Praise: The Powerhouse of Self-Esteem," *Nursing Management*, June 1985, 36, 38; Friedman, op. cit.; Schneier, Geis, and Wert, op. cit.; Edwards and Sproull, op. cit.; E. Y. Breeze, "The Performance Review," *Manage*, Feb. 1968, 6–11.

FOR FURTHER REFERENCE

American Hospital Association Council on Nursing and the American Organization of Nurse Executives, *Guidelines: Role and Functions of the Hospital Nurse Executive* (Chicago: American Hospital Association, 1985).

Balcazar, F., Hopkin, B. L., and Suarez, Y., "A Critical, Objective Review of Performance Feedback," *Journal of Organizational Behavior Management*, Fall 1985/Winter 1985–1986, 65–89.

Blai, B., "An Appraisal System That Yields Results," *Supervisory Management*, Nov. 1983, 39–42.

Brethower, D. M., and Rummler, G. A., "For Improved Work Performance: Accentuate the Positive," *Personnel*, Sept./Oct., 1966, 40–49.

Coaly, P. R., and Sackett, P. R., "Effects of Using High- Versus Low-Performing Job Incumbents as Sources of Job Analysis Information," *Journal of Applied Psychology*, Aug. 1987, 434–437.

Davis, D. S., Greig, A. E., Burkholder, J.,and Keating, T., "Evaluating Advanced Practice Nurses," *Nursing Management*, Mar. 1984, 44–47.

Fouracre, S., and Wright, A., "New Factors in Job Evaluation," *Personnel Management*, May 1986, 40–43.

Helton, B. R., "Will the Real Knowledge Worker Please Stand Up?," *Industrial Management*, Jan.-Feb. 1987, 26–29.

"How to Establish the Comparable Worth of a Job—Or One Way to Compare Apples and Oranges," *California Nurse*, Mar./Apr. 1982, 10–11.

Idaszak, J. R., and Drasgow, F., "A Revision of the Job Diagnostic Survey: Elimination of a Measurement Artifact," *Journal of Applied Psychology*, Feb. 1987, 69–74.

Kirkpatrick, D. L., "Performance Appraisal: When Two Jobs Are Too Many," *Training*, Mar. 1986, 65, 67–69.

Kopelman, R. E., "Job Redesign and Productivity: A Review of the Evidence," *National Productivity Review*, Summer 1985, 237–255.

Kopelman, R. E., "Linking Pay to Performance Is a Proven Management Tool," *Personnel Administrator*, Oct. 1983, 60–68.

Lawler, F. E., III, "What's Wrong with Point Factor Job Evaluation?," *Management Review*, Nov. 1986, 44–48.

Lee, M. A., "How to Use Job Analysis Technique," *Restaurant Management*, Apr. 1987, 84–85.

Levenstein, A., "Feedback Improves Performance," *Nursing Management*, Feb. 1984, 65–66.

Meyer, A. L., "A Framework for Assessing Performance Problems," *Journal of Nursing Administration*, May 1984, 40–43.

Murphy, K. R., Gannett, B. A., Herr, B. M., and Chen, J. A., "Effects of Subsequent Performance on Evaluation of Previous Performance," *Journal of Applied Psychology*, Aug. 1986, 427–431.

Pollock, T., "Are You Getting Better?," *Production*, Aug. 1985, 33.

Pollock, T., "The Fine Art of Speaking from a Desk," and "How Do You Look to Your Boss?" *Production*, July 1985, 27–29.

Ratcliffe, T. A., and Logsdon, D. J., "The Business Planning Process—A Behavioral Perspective," *Managerial Planning*, Mar./Apr. 1980, 32–38.

Reed, P. A., and Kroll, M. J., "A Two-Perspective Approach to Performance Appraisal," *Personnel*, Oct. 1985, 51–57.

Schnake, M. G., and Dumler, M. P., "Affective Response Bias in the Measurement of Perceived Task Characteristics," *Journal of Occupational Psychology*, June 1985, 159–166.

St. John, W. D., "Leveling with Employees," *Personnel Journal*, Aug. 1984, 52–57.

TNA's Professional Services Committee, "Nurses and the Comparable Worth Concept," *Texas Nursing*, Apr. 1985, 12–16.

Weingard, M., "Establishing Comparable Worth through Job Evaluation," *Nursing Outlook*, Mar./Apr. 1984, 110–113.

Answers

ANSWERS FOR CHAPTER 1

5.1 The group with which she is working has asked for 4 weeks' time to do its work.

5.2 She has asked for recommendations and has given a group a specific assignment related to changing the future work of professional nurses.

5.3 No changes have yet been made. Personnel are still performing their daily work.

6.1 She has asked a group of nurses to identify activities that are in need of change because these activities are low producers.

6.2 One of the suggestions involves different rates for care, the lowest rate being charged to patients when their families perform special care for them. The suggestion for primary care by RNs and elimination of evening and night supervisors may result in a saving because fewer high-salaried RNs will be needed. This saving may also provide for the next salary increases of all nursing personnel.

6.3 Maximum use will be made of intensive care areas. The result will be better use of all categories of nursing personnel. Clinic nurses will be involved in primary care. Patients will be motivated to participate in their care as will their families.

    6.4.1 Innovation

    6.4.2 Training

ANSWERS FOR CHAPTER 3

<u> f </u> 3.1 New programs could be developed to meet identified health care needs.

<u> g </u> 3.2, <u> a </u> 3.3, <u> e </u> 3.4, <u> d </u> 3.5,

<u> c </u> 3.6, <u> b </u> 3.7.

Some of these objectives are not as clearly stated as they could be; however, each was fully

developed in the operational plan for its accomplishment.

6.1 You should have crossed out "to make a profit." The division of nursing exists for the good of the people. It is good business to make a profit doing it.

6.2 You should have crossed out "Unlike" and "no impact on society." Like business and industry, the division of nursing has a social impact on society because it provides health care services. All of business and industry have an economic impact on society by employing people and by providing desired goods and services.

6.3 You should have crossed out "does not produce an impact." The division of nursing produces an impact on society because of the number of people employed there.

6.4 You should have crossed out "do not have." Used disposables such as syringes and needles, contaminated dressings, and other waste products and pollutants from the division of nursing have an impact on society.

6.5 You should have crossed out "business and industry" and "nursing services." People may view the division of nursing as more concerned with the quality of life than economic institutions of the business world.

6.6 You should have crossed out "make a profit for the stockholders and the business." It is the business of nurse managers to satisfy the needs of patients.

ANSWERS FOR CHAPTER 4

<u>   </u> 1.1, <u> √ </u> 1.2, <u>   </u> 1.3.

<u>PP</u> 2.1, <u>PP</u> 2.2, <u>PP</u> 2.3, <u>MS</u> 2.4,

<u>MS</u> 2.5, <u>MS</u> 2.6.

<u> + </u> 3.1, <u> − </u> 3.2.

ANSWERS FOR CHAPTER 6

- 1.1 Plan for every activity and for every penny that will be spent.
- 1.2 The budget is the financial plan for accomplishing objectives.
+ 1.3 The budget is financed through fringe benefits of health insurance, salaries to workers, gifts, and taxes.
- 1.4 Something could be done in this area if creative and collective thinking were applied to developing new ways of delivering health care services. Clients and families could be much more involved and nurses better used.
- 1.5 They need to be continually monitored and revised.

+ 1.6, + 1.7, + 1.8.

ANSWERS FOR CHAPTER 7

7. Variations of the following are acceptable as it is a thinking question, not aimed at neuronursing care.

Level of consciousness: Check for alertness/lethargy.

Nutrition: Enteral feeding pump, tube care, residual checking, tube placement.

Skin: Turn q2 hours, decub care, inspection of skin, TED hose application, air mattress.

Respiratory: Trach care and trach tie changing, emergency trach insertion, CPR, positioning of airway, suctioning.

Elimination: Condom cath care, bowel program, transfer to bed pan, perineal skin care.

Medication: Auscultation for tube placement, administration meds syringe method per tube and flushing.

8. One-on-one involvement with Mrs. O, M-I-L, and mother; written plan for all procedures.

9. Enteral: aspiration precautions, bloating, occlusion of tube, reinsertion of tube.
Trach care: maintaining airway, changing trach ties, occlusion, CPR, and Ambu bagging technique.

10. Department of Social Services/Human Resources for community follow-up; all counties in the United States have this service.

In-home support or respite service if available in the community. County mental health department for individual or group support. Some communities have head-injured support groups for families.

ANSWERS FOR CHAPTER 8

- 1.1 This situation is sometimes encountered but is not desirable.
- 1.2, + 1.3, + 1.4.
- 2.1, + 2.2, - 2.3, + 2.4,
- 2.5
+ 2.6 At least they will be less resentful and irritated.
- 3.1 Goals should be made known to all nursing personnel.
+ 3.2
- 3.3 They should be consistent.
+ 3.4, + 3.5, - 3.6.

State nurse practice act requirements are mandatory. JCAHO standards are obligatory only if accreditation by that agency is desired. Professional nursing standards are neither mandatory nor required for accreditation. They are standards that imply an ethical responsibility and a commitment to a profession. More and more they form the basis for state nurse practice acts and for JCAHO accreditation.

4. You should have crossed out:

4.1 a policy book.
4.2 all organizational policies.
4.3 for the nursing service only.
4.4 the director of nursing.

5. Yes, a policy exists even though it is not written. Some policies of management are transmitted or communicated through management actions. This is an area for a personnel policy particularly because a job probably depends on the outcome of the test. The test is good practice, but lack of a policy promotes grounds for a labor grievance.

___ *6.1,* __+__ *6.2,* ___ *6.3,* __+__ *6.4,*

___ *6.5,* __+__ *6.6.*

ANSWERS FOR CHAPTER 9

Because this chapter is on decision making, your group, individual, and instructor decisions will contribute to correct answers.

ANSWERS FOR CHAPTER 10

__b__ *1.1,* __d__ *1.2,* __a__ *1.3,* __c__ *1.4.*

___ *2.1* Many of the changes occurring in nursing relate to methods and procedures for operating machinery and equipment as well as to standards concerning organizational structure and work relationships of employees.

___ *2.2* Most nursing employees work in environments in which they learn to perceive change as a threat to achieving their personal goals.

__+__ *2.3,* __+__ *2.4,*

___ *2.5* People resist change because they do not know how it will affect them, and they have had previous bad experiences resulting from change.

__+__ *2.6,* __+__ *2.7.*

__f__ *3.1,* __a__ *3.2,* __g__ *3.3,* __b__ *3.4,* __e__ *3.5,*

__c__ *3.6,* __d__ *3.7.*

4. You should have crossed out:

4.1 1, 20.

4.2 loyalty to the organization for which they work.

4.3 being told how they will practice nursing.

4.4 holding fast to their authoritarian management practices.

4.5 Ritual and job security.

4.6 ignore the needs and goals of the worker while focusing on those of the organization.

5.1 None. Even when the public announcement was made, no indication was given of plans to retain, retrain, or reorganize the staff.

5.2 Authoritarianism was indicated by the director of nursing's telling clinical nurse managers that the administrator would make an announcement at an appropriate time and until then the staff should continue with its work. It was also indicated by the arbitrary newspaper announcement.

5.3 Apprehension was promoted during the time rumors were rampant. Top managers did not act to find out what was troubling and agitating employees. Communication was not even one way.

5.4 Distrust and lack of confidence resulted from the fact that top managers, including the director of nursing, failed to inform employees of their plans, failed to obtain employees' assistance and support, and failed to assure employees of future employment.

5.5 The lack of communication and the resulting rumors would indicate that top management did not recognize that managers and workers were interdependent or that they shared responsibility for the success of the organization.

5.6 She did not act, and as a result there were multiple groups gossiping at every opportunity. This kind of atmosphere promotes the formation of formally organized labor groups, professional and nonprofessional, and generates union activity.

5.7 There was no sharing of control and responsibility. A concerned staff could assist in resolving most or all of the problems and could be involved in planning that would end in a smooth transition to a new organization and mission.

5.8 Because there was no bargaining or problem-solving discussion, the chance for conflict was greatly increased.

5.9 The opposite was true. Consumers were informed of the changes that would affect them; employees were not.

5.10 Top management's philosophy and practice was clearly indicated by the fact that they did not take employees into their confidence; top management shared neither management decisions nor the making of those decisions. Their actions would promote disloyalty as well as a lack of credibility in employees' minds and set the stage for labor grievances.

ANSWERS FOR CHAPTER 11

1.1 The organizational structure was poor because the philosophy and objectives were weak. They were either poorly defined or a paper exercise. They certainly were not used to give direction to the nursing organization.

1.2 The Chair noted the organizational structure to be sure that lines of authority were unclear at top management and operating management levels. Nursing management was absent from outpatient services. Planning within the division was nonexistent. Little or no direction stemmed from the philosophy and objectives.

1.3 The Chair's next steps will be to itemize key activities, formulate a strategy, and list what the present, future, and actual business of the division should be.

____ − 2.1 Philosophy represents beliefs or values important to the quality of care aimed for in the objectives.

__+__ 2.2, __+__ 2.3, __−__ 2.4.

__c__ 3.1 Most hospital-acquired infections are related to poor hygiene and careless housekeeping activities.

__d__ 3.2, __b__ 3.3,

__a__ 3.4 The result should be more direct nursing care hours available to practice the primary functions of nursing.

4.1 Mr. Bishop insists that supervisors do performance counseling and recommend personnel actions.

4.2 He cuts off direct communication between department heads. They can be given guidelines as to what requires top management approval.

____ 5.1 A team is usually small.

__✔__ 5.2

____ 5.3 Members of a management team would usually come from different areas of an organization.

__✔__ 5.4, __✔__ 5.5.

ANSWERS FOR CHAPTER 12

6.1 A definitive agenda is drawn up but is never sent to the attendees.

6.2 The secretary and clerk-typist prepare the meeting room beforehand.

6.3 She always learns the subject matter.

6.4 The agenda items are not timed, and the meetings run to two hours although planned for one hour.

6.5 She does not referee and set the pace of the meetings but allows arguments to go on.

6.6 There are arguments; however, there is no evidence of lively participation being promoted by the Director of Nursing.

6.7 She listens to what they have to say.

6.8 There is none. Few matters are ever settled.

6.9 There is none. Achievement of the purposes is seldom evaluated.

ANSWERS FOR CHAPTER 13

__f__ 6.1, __c__ 6.2, __d__ 6.3, __a__ 6.4,

__b__ 6.5 __e__ 6.6.

These were the intended answers. If you selected others and are comfortable with your decision, let them stand.

9.1.1 Assets:
 a. A nursing history is taken.
 b. The patient's spouse is involved.
 c. Most of the technical aspects of nursing care are being done.

9.1.2 Defects:
 a. There is failure to carry through the nursing history to nursing diagnosis and prescription.
 b. Total patient care is lacking.
 c. One would question the effectiveness of the quality assurance program.
 d. Accountability is lacking.
 e. There is a lack of attention to outcomes, to evaluation of applied care.

9.2 Theories that could be applied related to the interlocking major concepts of responsibility, authority, autonomy, and accountability. Supervision appears to be absent. Training and supervision should focus on such concepts as job enrichment, personalization, total patient care, and others. Discuss a remedy with your group.

ANSWERS FOR CHAPTER 14

2. The answer is the student's or group's conclusion. An effective nurse manager will find out if any problem exists that can be resolved to retain Ms. Lynd. Otherwise, the head nurse will facilitate the transfer with good will.

✔ 4.1.1 Delegating. However, if you selected all four, you are also correct. Mr. Thompson is delegating and this delegating is being done to give him more time to manage his department and to train and motivate his clinical RN staff.

ANSWERS FOR CHAPTER 15

1. Using Stogdill's definition of leadership, the following points can be made:

   1.1.1 There is a group of people—a nursing staff.
   1.1.2 They do not appear to set or achieve goals. Mr. Kelly believes that physicians will do all the health teaching. Patient teaching should be a part of an individualized plan of nursing care.
   1.1.3 Mr. Kelly is not influencing the group toward setting and achieving goals for patient teaching.
   1.1.4 There are personnel with differing responsibilities: head nurse, clinical nurse manager, and nursing staff.

2. Ms. Castro influenced her nursing personnel, who understood her communication as to what the primary functions of nursing were. She provided them with resources for performing those functions by relieving them of nonnursing duties and focusing on mission, philosophy, and goals. The results indicated they believed the behavior asked of them was consistent with

their personal values and interests, and with the purpose and values of the organization.

 d 4.1, a 4.2, b 4.3, c 4.4.

5.1 Both used the job performance standards as a point of reference during the counseling session.

5.2 She discussed in detail the need for Ms. Walters to establish a counseling program for her people.

5.3 She complimented her on the progress she had made and on her enthusiasm and productivity.

5.4 Her complimentary remarks plus her interest and the tone of discussion would indicate to Ms. Walters that Ms. Walsh cared for her.

5.5 She gave her free rein to develop her personal plan for counseling subordinates.

5.6 Nothing in the narrative would indicate otherwise, and Ms. Walsh used her counseling of Ms. Walters to develop the concept of individual counseling for all employees.

5.7 Ms. Walters gained satisfaction from the counseling and recognized this. She learned it can be beneficial to personnel. Ms. Walsh learned through her success at counseling with Ms. Walters.

5.8 The entire narrative depicted confidence and optimism.

5.9 Ms. Walters appeared to have expressed her thoughts in detail with regard to both her accomplishments and her plans.

   6.1.1 A professional nurse of stature who can rally other nurses. This has occurred when an institution was in danger of financial collapse and when autonomy of nurse licensure was threatened by legislation giving control to other groups.
   6.1.2 Nurses of outstanding ability and character, both managers and practitioners. A public health nurse leader in a small town in Texas achieved expansion of health services through her appeals to community groups, including local government officials.
   6.1.3 Popular attitudes of enthusiasm or negation for health care services provided by nurses. This is occurring as consumers are demanding the kind of care delivery

services provided by nurse-midwives. States are passing laws making it easier for nurse-midwives to practice. (Your answers may be different from these examples.)

d 8.1, c 8.2, a 8.3, e 8.4,

b 8.5

____ 9.1 False. Perceptions of leaders by the constituents are relative to their power.

____ 9.2 False. A strong structural assignment gives less power to the leader.

✓ 9.3 True.

____ 9.4 False. People should all be made as independent as possible.

✓ 9.5 True.

____ 9.6 False. When the leader has great influence over group members, a task-oriented leadership style works best. When the leader has moderate influence over group members, a relationship-oriented style works best.

✓ 9.7 True.

____ 9.8 False. Coercive power leads to passive-aggressive behavior and decreases productivity.

✓ 9.9 True.

✓ 9.10 True.

ANSWERS FOR CHAPTER 16

a 1.1, c 1.2,

b 1.3 Although there may be some bias on the part of the clinical nurse manager, she should be consulted, and if modification of her position is in order, she should be allowed to correct the situation herself.

b (or c) 1.4 This could be settled by discussing with the nurse the times the girl friend could visit, such as during a coffee break or at meal time. The place of such

meetings should also be established.

c (or b) 1.5 Although no one may be entirely satisfied, all parties should be handled with dignity.

a 1.6 The answer is to restructure the organization to best use the nurse's time.

2.1 She had a hypothesis that she may have had enough RNs but that they were not performing primary nursing duties.

2.2 She employed a qualified nurse to perform a staffing study. This was comprehensive in its attempt to gather facts about quantity of care needed by patients, quality of care as perceived by patients, nurses, and physicians, and activities performed by nurses.

2.3 She started with a large generalization, but she planned to gather enough facts to expand into generalizations about the entire department, and this occurred. Actually her theories were proved, and the generalization expanded into theories about other departments. This generated a plan that would modify the entire inpatient service.

2.4 The study explored the literature on the subject as a basis for deciding how it would be accomplished. Instruments were designed to collect needed facts, which were analyzed, and conclusions were drawn.

2.5 The entire study was done using basic research rules. Instruments designed to collect data were based on modifications of tested instruments used in other studies.

2.6 She employed a qualified person to perform the study and supported her with volunteer RNs to assist with data collection.

2.7 She involved her nursing staff in the study and solicited and received their input into the final plan.

2.8 This was intended but it could not be done until it was prepared so that the hospital administrator would have a finished product to work with. Many of the facts can be applied to human uses by the director of nursing if the entire plan is disapproved by the hospital administrator.

2.9 Involvement of nursing personnel in the study

plus their consultation by the director of nursing served notice that change was intended and forthcoming. They will be ready to participate in application of the plan.

____ 3.1, ✔ 3.2.

4.1 Ms. Sanchez's preparation of an agenda and her open invitation to discuss the department's mission, philosophy, objectives, and operational plan encouraged communication by encouraging the clinical nurse managers to give opinions and make recommendations.

4.2 The clinical nurse managers were given an opportunity to study the agenda for a week and to bring suggestions for activities that would benefit themselves and the entire nursing staff. They took advantage of this opportunity to make many suggestions.

4.3 The entire meeting was conducted in an environment that encouraged expression by the clinical nurse managers. They produced in the area of policies related to job standards, rating, and promotion. They assisted Ms. Sanchez by developing a program for her to discuss the mission, philosophy, objectives, and operational plan.

4.4 The nurse manager group has set timetables to accomplish statements of mission, philosophy, objectives, and operational plans for each of their units. They will involve their staff, and they will make recommendations for changes in other policies.

4.5 The meeting has been conducted in an orderly manner due to the early publication of an agenda. It has been productive, and the freedoms encouraged by Ms. Sanchez will lead to involvement of all nursing personnel in the achievement of personal objectives as well as imaginative change in the entire department of nursing and how it delivers health care services to patients.

5.1 Ms. Rather.

5.2 She is learning how her employees want to feel and to use those tools that will enable them to achieve satisfaction of their feelings. They will feel accepted. Both clinical nurse managers are helping their personnel perform their jobs and are recognizing satisfactory performance. Ms. Rather probably attempts to figure out why her people react the way they do to their work situations. She will figure out which need is prepotent and strongest at the time.

7. Rumors stymie motivation by distracting people. This is a technique for rumor control.

ANSWERS FOR CHAPTER 17

1.1 The team members decided that all oncoming personnel would be listeners, and they outlined the contents of reports. They also decided against taping physicians' and nurses' orders. Standards for evaluation of reports are not mentioned but are important.

1.2 Team members decided to write objectives for the reports, and they decided that the main purpose of the reports was to give them needed information to do their day's work. Standards of evaluation are not mentioned, but a schedule should be set up for review of the process to determine periodically whether objectives are being met.

1.3 Team members decided on an outline of information to be included in the report.

1.4 The question was not answered. Notes would be made, however, on the items contained in the outline.

1.5 She was working in the area during the report, and critiques of recordings were decided on. This would indicate how the recorder made her voice work for her.

1.6 She could not, but in face-to-face communication, eye contact by the speaker helps keep the listener alert and interested.

_e_ 2.1, _a_ 2.2, _b_ 2.3, _c_ 2.4, _a_ 2.5 _d_ 2.6.

3.1 It describes the current problems and the nursing actions taken to resolve them—nursing diagnosis and prescription.

3.2 The nursing problems and solutions are relevant and have value and purpose. Past progress notes are not duplicated. Omission of the hospital day number may or may not be important. Progress reports should have been made by evening and night nurses. The director of nursing would gain knowledge of the unit workload through these progress reports and similar information on other patients.

ANSWERS FOR CHAPTER 18

1. Possible answers may include:

    Memorandums and letters
    Forms management
    Budget analysis
    Statistical analysis
    Patient classification
    Personnel scheduling
    Personnel staffing
    Order management
    Nursing care plans
    Patient care worksheets
    Medication admission records
    Researching publications
    Expenses management
    Materials management
    Address management
    Personal inventory management
    Electronic mail

    1.1 Memorandums and letters: Personal, departmental and organizational
    Forms management: Departmental and organizational
    Budget analysis: Personal and departmental
    Statistical analysis: Personal, departmental and organizational
    Patient classification: Departmental
    Personnel scheduling: Departmental
    Personnel staffing: Departmental
    Order management: Departmental and organizational
    Nursing care plans: Departmental
    Patient care worksheets: Departmental and organizational
    Medication admission records: Departmental and organizational
    Researching publications: Personal, departmental and organizational
    Expenses management: Personal, departmental and organizational
    Materials management: Departmental and organizational
    Name, address, and telephone management: Personal and departmental
    Personal inventory management: Personal
    Electronic mail: Personal, departmental and organizational

1.2 A microcomputer can be used to perform the following tasks:

- Memorandums and letters
- Forms management
- Budget analysis
- Statistical analysis
- Personnel scheduling
- Personnel staffing
- Medication administration records
- Researching publications
- Expenses management
- Address management
- Personal inventory management

A mainframe computer can be used to perform the following tasks:

- Budget analysis
- Statistical analysis
- Patient classification
- Order management
- Nursing care plans
- Patient care worksheets
- Materials management
- Electronic mail

2. Money spent on computers and information management is often dependent on the organization's philosophy. Some organizations centralize the computer budget, while others decentralize it. The philosophy of upper management is also a factor in how much money is spent. Some upper management personnel are big proponents of computerization, while others tend to believe computer costs outweigh benefits.

    2.1 A hospital's computer budget will vary from one organization to the next. Roughly speaking a computer budget may be from 2 to 10 percent of the total operating budget.

3. There may not be any specific laws requiring hospitals to use computerized information systems. Most regulations and guidelines that dictate the use of computerization relate to the assurance of quality patient care and accurate patient billing.

    3.1 Computerized patient billing is essential for managing today's complex and readily changing billing requirements. Electronic billing may increase the hospital's chances of capturing correct information, and may decrease the billing payment turn-around time by 50 percent.

3.2 Governmental agencies such as the Social Security Administration and the Joint Commission for the Accreditation of Healthcare Organizations may have regulations and guidelines that compel computerized information management.

4.1 Applications common to an entire organization may include:

- Master patient index inquiries
- Patient account inquiries
- Order management
- Materials management
- Census inquiries
- Budgeting
- Electronic mail

4.4 Departments that may have their own computer information systems include:

- Pharmacy
- Clinical laboratory
- Diagnostic radiology
- Medical records
- Nursing services

5. Microcomputers can manage the following functions:

- Pharmacy functions
- Clinical laboratory functions
- Diagnostic radiology functions
- Medical records abstracting
- Medical records tumor registry

6. Laser scanners can manage the following information:

- Medical records tracking
- Radiology film tracking
- Supply processing and patient charging
- Inventory management

7. Personal information applications that could be implemented on a microcomputer may include:

- Personal memoradums and letters
- Personal budgeting
- Personal addresses and telephone numbers
- Personal inventory

8. Applications for the use of a spreadsheet may include:

- Departmental budgeting
- Departmental statistics, such as in the emergency department. Triage numbers, deaths, OBs, and admits may all be included. See Figure 18–2.

- Insurance auditing, such as the verification of patient charges by department.

9. Examples may include:

- Top margin of 2.5″, left and right margins of 1″, single line spacing, Courier 10 cpi type style.
- Top margin of 1″, left and right margins of 1.5″, 1.5 line spacing, Helvetica Bold 12 and Times Roman Italic 12 type styles.
- Top margin of 1″, left and right margins of 1.75″, 1.75 line spacing, Letter Gothic Bold 12 and Prestige Elite 10 type styles.

Note the differences among Figures 18–8, 18–9, and 18–11.

10. An example may include the following data: Five lines with: your name, title, company name, street, city, state, and zip code.

11. For example, Display Write 4 and Wordperfect 5.1 both have spelling functions.

11.1 Both word processing programs have supplements for storing words that are not in the dictionary, and both provide the capability to create and use multiple supplements.

11.2 Various aspects of spelling functions are:

- Replacing an incorrectly spelled word with its correct spelling by choosing it from a list of words.
- Editing an incorrectly spelled word that is not found in the dictionary.
- Adding a new word to the dictionary.
- Skipping a new word without adding it to the dictionary.
- Counting the number of words spell checked.

12. The association of a set of items or characters as a single unit (e.g., words, lines, paragraphs, and pages).

12.1 The smallest block could be a single character. The largest block could be the whole document.

12.2 Block functions you can perform may include:

- Copy
- Move
- Delete
- Append

- Retrieve
- Upper/lower case translations

13. Searching tasks may include simply finding some text or actually finding it and replacing it with some different text.

14. Applications that may be kept manually and could be converted to a database management system include:
   - Personnel records
   - In-service education records
   - Departmental inventory
   - Travel expenses
   - Budget analysis

15. Computerized applications that could be used in patient care management include:
   - Patient care profile
   - Order management
   - Medication administration records
   - Discharge planning

16. Quality benefits a nurse may receive from use of a computer include:
   - Improved quality in the delivery of patient care
   - Improved quality of work life

17. The clinical nurse can use the computer to increase work effectiveness. Clinical data can be collected and input for analysis and the formulation of treatment plans. Quantitative decision analysis can be used to support clinical judgments. Automated consultation can help manage the preparation and delivery of drugs. Computers can be programmed to screen for interactions among multiple patient orders.

18. The possible components of a patient care profile could include:
   - Identification data
   - Patient history
   - Activities of daily living
   - Active orders and treatments
   - Nursing care plan and progress notes
   - Discharge planning
   18.1 Identification data should provide the patient's account and medical record numbers, DOB, race, sex, weight, height, medical service and physician, and diagnosis.

The patient history should review the patient's lifestyle, health awareness, and illness leading to the clinical visit.

Activities of daily living relate to the monitoring of vital signs, mobility, hygiene, fluids, nutrition, and sensory deficits.

Active orders and treatments would identify orders and treatments in progress.

The nursing care plan identifies and lists desired nursing goals and planned nursing interventions. Progress notes are objective and subjective observations made by the nurses.

Discharge planning identifies and lists nursing goals and interventions essential in preparing the patient for discharge.

18.2 Benefits of a Patient Care Profile may include:
   - Improved uniformity and accuracy of nursing documentation in medical records
   - A practical and efficient method of individualizing patient care
   - A source for nurse managers to use in assessing cost data
   - Improved accountability of nurses
   - Reduction of other forms and paperwork

19. Departments often determine what supply items are stocked and what their par levels are. Central supply then creates a department catalog, using the computer and the materials management system. Supplies are reviewed daily and requisitioned, via the computerized catalog, to maintain par levels. Miscellaneous supplies can be requisitioned by scanning the computerized inventory.

19.1 Patient-chargeable and departmental-chargeable items are requisitioned in the same manner. All items are charged to the department, and the department is responsible for recouping its own patient revenue.

19.2 Patient charges can be captured by placing service code numbers on patient charge documents. These documents are then sent to data processing for keypunch. Some departments do key their patient charges directly into the computer. An order management system is the best way to capture patient charges. Where the charge is generated is a byproduct of the order being generated and performed.

19.3 These records should be general revenue and statistics reports that are distributed to every department.

20. A number of nursing employees may work with computers and the organization's information environment. Certain nursing areas may have specialized computer systems such as infection control and staff development. The nurses in these areas must be capable of working with their systems.

20.1 Specialized nursing positions should also exist for working with the NMIS and the HIS. The HIS position would be held by the Nursing Coordinator. This person would be a liaison between HIS client personnel and HIS programming personnel.

ANSWERS FOR CHAPTER 19

− 1.1 The nurse manager should regard the employee who behaves defiantly as the cause of conflict.

+ 1.2 Yes, the cause is space.

− 1.3 It is an example of a defier who is a Competitive Bomber.

+ 1.4

___ 2.1 Planning, involvement of clinical nurses, and "voluntary" rotation will all prevent conflict.

✔ 2.2 The nurse manager should offer support by saying "How can I help you?" Telling the nurse to limit phone calls or keep her personal life separate from her professional life creates conflict. Find out what services the institution has, such as counseling, and what can be financially supported

through the employees' health service.

___ 2.3 Age and agility can be sources of conflict but not for these nurses.

✔ 2.4

ANSWERS FOR CHAPTER 22

✔ 1.1 The institution and the department of nursing constitute the authority.

? 1.2 Who knows? Employees did not participate in their development. They have no instructions for using them.

? 1.3 Again, who knows? They may not be relative to the jobs and performances required to meet the objectives of the department of nursing.

✔ 1.4, ___ 1.5, ___ 1.6,

___ 1.7 Probably most employees will consider them to be window dressing. They will take this attitude with them to other jobs.

3. Your answers will be peculiar to the actual job description. Possible answers are:

3.1 The title will be listed.
3.2 They may be stated in a "Job Summary."
3.3 They may be stated as an opening "subject" or in a full "Job Summary."
3.4 They may be listed as "Performance Requirements" or "Specific Duties."
3.5 They may be stated as "Performance Requirements" or "Responsibilities."
3.6 They may be stated as "Job Relationships."
3.7 They may be stated in "Job Summary," "Responsibilities," and/or "Job Relationships" sections.
3.8 The criteria for performance evaluation may be identified by the detail in which the "Specific Duties" are written. You may have stated examples in your answers.

Index

2
47